THE HISTORY OF ANESTHESIA

THIRD INTERNATIONAL SYMPOSIUM

PROCEEDINGS

ATLANTA, GEORGIA, 1992

CRAWFORD W. LONG
SESQUICENTENNIAL
MDCCCXLII – MCMXCII

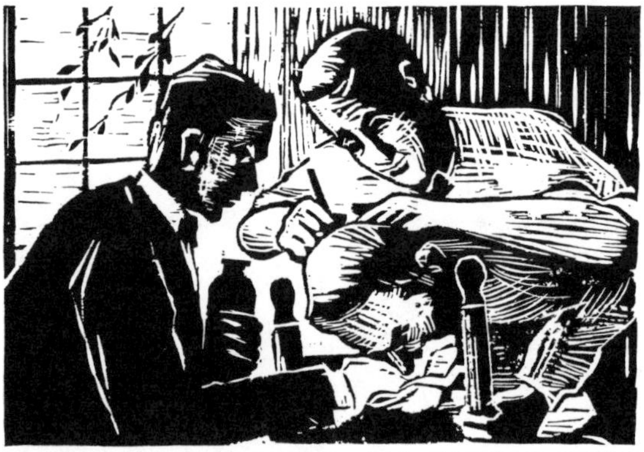

THIRD INTERNATIONAL SYMPOSIUM

THE HISTORY OF ANESTHESIA

ATLANTA, GEORGIA, U.S.A. – MARCH 27-31, 1992

Cover Illustration: CRAWFORD W. LONG, (1815–1878). This portrait hangs in the Crawford W. Long Hospital at Emory University, Atlanta, Georgia.

Photograph of portrait taken by Francis Long Taylor, daughter of Crawford W. Long.

THE HISTORY OF ANESTHESIA

THIRD INTERNATIONAL SYMPOSIUM

PROCEEDINGS
ATLANTA, GEORGIA
MARCH 27–31, 1992

B. RAYMOND FINK, Editor-In-Chief
LUCIEN E. MORRIS, Editor
C.R. STEPHEN, Editor

WOOD LIBRARY-MUSEUM OF ANESTHESIOLOGY

Hardbound Edition
Published by the
Wood Library-Museum of Anesthesiology
ISBN 0-9614932-5-9

Library of Congress Number 92-63246
ISBN 0-9614932-4-0

Printed in the United States of America

Published by:
WOOD LIBRARY-MUSEUM OF ANESTHESIOLOGY
520 North Northwest Highway
Park Ridge, Illinois
60068-2573

TABLE OF CONTENTS

TABLE OF TOPICS

Apparatus, Agents, and Techniques

Biography

Military

General

Foreword

Anniversaries are of the heart. The sesquicentennial of the prophetic exploit performed March 30, 1842 by Crawford Williamson Long (1815-1878) was fêted by the Third International Symposium on the History of Anaesthesia (TISHA). The opening day was devoted to Crawford Long: a plenary morning session on the man and his times, an afternoon visit to the Crawford W. Long Museum in Jefferson, and, the evening to a delightful original drama "Spit of the Devil" reenacting the historic event, specially written and produced through the initiative of John Steinhaus, chairman of the Organizing Committee. There was much wistfulness in Georgia as the symposium visited the site of that first-ever administration of anesthesia for a surgical operation. Had not Long in Jackson county been the unassuming rural forerunner to Boston City's Morton, Ericson to a latter-day Columbus? His reticence about his innovative exploits did not alter Long's priority as the world's first anesthetist, the world's first physician anesthetist. As it happens future jubilees will have added cause for celebration, for the British College of Anaesthetists received the coveted Royal Charter in London on October 4, 1992, a resplendent if distant outcome of the brilliant discovery in the United States which sheds adventitious radiance on Long.

But why did Crawford Long keep silent? Was he taking a leaf out of Humphry Davy's book? Long felt that his were minor operations, the sufferings he had prevented with the vapor of ether were still too small to merit public notice, an attitude reminiscent of Davy's toward "surgical operations in which no great effusion of blood takes place." The major operations of that time would surely be attended by much effusion of blood. All in all, Ogden Nash may inadvertently have summed it up quite well:

Take country people, they suffer stoically,
But city people prefer to live unheroically;
Therefore city dentistry is less painful,
Because city dentists find it more gainful.[1]

Many anniversaries do serve an educational goal. This one personifies a story that all practitioners of the specialty can identify with. Our daily errands of mercy are one with the aspirations of Long, Wells, and Morton, and we owe our ever-enlarging effectiveness to the endeavors of their successors, beginning with the Snows, the Pirogoffs, the Claude Bernards. The historical perspective deepens both our self-respect and the public's appreciation and confidence.

Garrison's Introduction to the History of Medicine starts the Modern Period with the nineteenth century. Examination reveals that the pace of science and technology accelerated enormously in the second half of that century, and one is tempted to speculate that the end of human helplessness in the face of pain must have greatly strengthened people's confidence in the power of the human mind to understand and control nature. If victory over pain was possible, all things became possible, although a recent special issue of Scientific American on Mind and Brain[2] admonishes that we will never fully understand the nature of consciousness or its suspension by anesthetics. More to the point, at the close of the Industrial Revolution, amid the mental ferment of the 1840s and the first blossoming of Animal Chemistry,[3] the Fullerian Professor of Physiology in the Royal Institution of Great Britain, William B. Carpenter, recapitulated the pre-anesthetic era view of the brain as follows:[4]

> In ordinary profound Sleep, which is a state of complete unconsciousness, it is evident that the Cerebral Hemispheres, and the Ganglia of Special Sense, are at rest; as the Cerebellum, also, may be considered to be: but the Medulla Oblongata and Spinal Cord must be in complete functional activity. The same is the case in profound Coma, resulting from the effusion of blood, or from narcotic poisons, but not affecting the power of breathing or swallowing.

Decidedly, the mindset of the period was fully prepared to embrace the coming discovery.[5] A sesquicentury later, although we interfere more scientifically with the elusive cerebral basis of consciousness, we feel more intensely than ever the responsibility involved in interrupting and restoring the operation of a human mind. Surely such an historical perspective is a necessary part of being a complete anesthesiologist.

TISHA throughout its many concurrent sessions of free papers, video-tapes, posters, exhibits, leavened with much pleasant international socializing, continually reminded us that we are bearers of one of western civilization's greatest single gifts to itself. The smorgasbord enjoyed in every room was delectable and will be vicariously savored even more intensely by readers of this volume.

The printed transactions of the first International Symposium on the History of Anaesthesia, held in Rotterdam in 1982 and organized by Joseph Rupreht and his fellow-scholars, M.J. van Lieburg, J.A. Lee, and W. Erdman, were arranged in five groups — Pioneers in Anaesthesia, Development of Technique, Regional Developments in Anaesthesia, The World Organization, and Humanism in Anaesthesia. The Proceedings of the Second International Symposium, held in London in 1987 and edited by R.S. Atkinson and T.B. Boulton, contained six sections — Special Presentations, Early Development of the Specialty, History of Anesthetic Agents, History of Anesthetic Apparatus, History of Resuscitation and Intensive Care, and Biography.

The ever-widening scope of anesthesiology and its history makes allocation of several TISHA papers to the above groups somewhat artificial. The subject is evolving too rapidly. The editors – C.R. Stephen and Lucien Morris for the Anesthesia History Association which organized the symposium and B. Raymond Fink for the Wood Library-Museum of Anesthesiology which is publishing these Proceedings – have – to expedite publication – accepted various tolerable departures from requested standards of style. The Table of Contents lists the papers in the alphabetical order of first authors and also in groups similar to the previous ones. The index includes key words from the titles as well as all of the authors.

B. RAYMOND FINK
Editor-in-chief

References

1. Nash O: The City. *in* The Ogden Nash Pocket Book. New York, Pocket Books Inc., p. 12, 1944.
2. Miller J: Essay. Scientific American 267:180 (Sept) 1992.
3. Liebig J: Animal Chemistry. New York. Wiley & Putnam, 356pp., 1842.
4. Carpenter WB: Principles of Human Physiology. Philadelphia. Lea & Febiger, p. 218, 1845.
5. Greene NM: A consideration of factors in the discovery of anesthesia and their effect on its development. Anesthesiology 35:515-522, 1971.

Acknowledgments

*The organizers wish
to thank the following
for important support:*

BAXTER HEALTHCARE
BOC HEALTHCARE
BURROUGHS WELLCOME
DU PONT PHARMACEUTICALS
JANSSEN PHARMACEUTICA
I C I PHARMACEUTICALS GROUP
ORGANON
MOSBY

THIRD INTERNATIONAL SYMPOSIUM ON THE HISTORY OF ANESTHESIA

Sponsored by

ANESTHESIA HISTORY ASSOCIATION

Co-sponsors

Georgia Society of Anesthesiologists
Greater Atlanta Society of Anesthesiologists
Departments of Anesthesiology
Emory University
Medical College of Georgia

Organizing Committee

John E. Steinhaus, Chairman
Betty, Bamforth, President
John Severinghaus, Vice President
Lucien Morris, Secretary-Treasurer
C.R. Stephens, Newsletter Editor
Selma Calmes, Publicity
Ray Fink, Publication
George Bause, Exhibits
Douglas Bacon

(Council Anesthesia History Association)

Norman Bergman, Chairman-Scientific Program
Leslie Rendell-Baker, Co-Chairman-Posters
Elizabeth Frost, Tech Exhibit
Jack Moyers, Co.Chairman-Financial Committee
Eli Brown, Co.Chairman-Financial Committee
Carl Smith, Chairman for Local Arrangements
Thomas Grisson, Business Manager
William Hammonds, President-Ga. Soc. Anes.
Ken Protas, President-G.A.S.A.
John Waller, Chairman, Department of Anesthesiology-Emory University
Robert Crumrine, Chairman-Department of Anesthesiology-Medical College of Georgia
Barbara Jones, Administrative Assistant

International Advisers

Prof. Miklon Tekeres–Hungary
Dr. Marion Kus–Poland
Dr. Barry Baker–New Zealand
Prof. J.L. Couper–South Africa
Dr. J.R. Maltby–Canada
Dr. A. Matsuki–Japan
Dr. J. Rupreht–The Netherlands
Prof. Ole Secher–Denmark
Dr. Torsten Gorhd–Sweden
Prof. Elena Damir–Russia
Dr. Thomas Boulton–England
Dr. Jonathan Wu–China
Prof. W. Rose–Germany
Dr. D.J. Wilkinson–England
Dr. Gwen Wilson–Australia
Dr. Carlos Parsloe–Brazil

THE FOUNDATION OF THE FACULTY OF ANAESTHETISTS OF THE ROYAL COLLEGE OF SURGEONS OF ENGLAND

AILEEN K. ADAMS
Cambridge, England, United Kingdom

The Royal Colleges occupy a unique position among the institutions concerned with standards of practice in the medical profession. They exist only in Great Britain and Ireland and in some countries previously under the influence of the British Empire. Their uniqueness derives from the fact that they were not bodies which were created to carry out the function of setting standards, rather they evolved from preexisting institutions that were formed as long ago as the Middle Ages. It is fascinating that the need for independent bodies to act as guardians of professional standards was recognised as long ago as the 12th and 13th centuries.

The Colleges are totally independent autonomous bodies, governed by their Fellows, receiving their income chiefly from their fellows' and members' subscriptions, but also backed up by the often large benefactions they receive because they are charities. They are answerable to no one except H M the Queen through the Privy Council, the body responsible for Royal charters. These are granted only to institutions that can show that their activities are directed solely for the common good, and not for the benefit of their fellows and members.

The functions of the Royal Colleges today include promotion of the highest possible standards of professional practice. They define these standards and uphold them in various ways, for example, by running educational activities themselves and by supervising the training programmes run by hospitals throughout the country. They conduct examinations, award diplomas, and grant specialist status to those who reach their standards. It should be stressed that the Colleges' right to do this is not absolute and has limited recognition in law, rather it is established by long tradition. The lack of legal rights, though, has not prevented them from exerting considerable influence both on doctors themselves and on those who provide medical services.

To see how this has arisen one needs to look at Europe in mediaeval times. As society emerged from its largely agrarian beginnings and started to form urban communities, so the need for some degree of specialisation emerged. Gradually there arose groups of different craftsmen, traders, learned professionals and others, who had a need to establish their credentials to protect the interests both of the group members themselves and society as a whole. In Britain, from about the 12th century onwards guilds of craftsmen were formed, many of which still exist today as the City Livery companies of London and other major cities. The function of the companies was to regulate practice, to define standards of training, and as far as possible to exclude from practice those who did not reach their standards. To some extent, therefore, they were elitist, keeping out the unqualified, but there is no doubt that they were proud of their skills and wished to maintain and improve them. Clearly, their aims were similar to those of our modern colleges. Additionally, they celebrated the feast days of their patron saints and made some provision for their more impoverished members.

Medicine was no exception in its need to control its practitioners. In earliest times medicine was practised largely by monks and priests, later it was taken over by lay physicians and apothecaries. Surgery, crude and primitive as it was, had humbler beginnings, being carried out by barbers who were often itinerants. The earliest surgical guild to be set up in Britain was the Company of Barbers incorporated in 1492. Little is known about this company, but as surgical skills developed so did the organisation of their practice, and in 1540 the Company of Barber-Surgeons was instituted and received its Royal Charter from King Henry VIII. The Barber-Surgeons required practitioners to have undergone a seven-year apprenticeship, and when they had passed their examination they then became freemen of the Company and eligible to be licensed to practice. The licensing at that time was in the hands of the Bishops, the Church thus retaining some of its influence. Inevitably, as surgery developed the interests of the barbers and the surgeons diverged, and after a series of disagreements they separated in 1745. The barbers retained their name and the Company of Barber-Surgeons still exists today as one of the London Livery companies, while a new body, the Company of Surgeons, was formed. This later became the Royal College of Surgeons, first of London, now of England (RCS). Thus, although the title of College was not given until 1800, the origins of the college are much earlier. Other bodies concerned with medicine arose even earlier, the Royal College of Physicians (RCP) dates from 1518, and the Society of Apothecaries from 1617. Both are still in existence.

In the past century, as specialisation has increased, many new medical Colleges have emerged, most of which in due course have received a Royal charter. These include the Obstetricians and Gynaecologists, the Psychiatrists, the Radiologists, and the Pathologists amongst others. Their functions are similar, and because they too are concerned solely with the promotion of high standards of patient care they have become respected and influential bodies. Government and others may not agree with advice from the Colleges, but they seldom ignore it, although one has to comment that, with the increasing commercialisation of medicine, this may not be so forever.

Anaesthesia has always been practised in Britain by medically-qualified doctors, as it still is, and amongst the earliest specialists were John Snow and Joseph Clover. By the end of the century there were sufficient anaesthetists to feel the need for an organisation devoted to the exchange of scientific knowledge. In 1893 the Society of Anaesthetists, the first anaesthetic society in the world, was formed in London by Dr Frederick Silk.[1] The Society flourished, and in 1908 it joined with other specialist societies to form the Royal Society of Medicine (RSM), still one of the foremost centres in the country for exchange of views on the art and science of medicine in all its aspects.

One of the few benefits of war is that they tend to produce rapid advances in surgical practice. The First World War showed the need for better anaesthesia, and one who took up this challenge was Sir Ivan (then Dr) Magill. As well as making numerous practical innovations, particularly in endotracheal intubation, Magill advocated that the way to raise the standard of anaesthesia was by better training, leading to a specialist diploma. The only institution which anaesthetists belonged to at the time was the RSM, and this did not allow for the conduct of examination, so Magill and others formed a new body, the Association of Anaesthetists of Great Britain and Ireland (AAGBI), one of whose objects was to set up a diploma. In fact it did not do so. Instead it approached the RCS because this College, in conjunction with the RCP, was experienced in conducting examinations for several diplomas, as well as for its own surgical Fellowship. The RC promptly accepted the need for a Diploma in Anaesthetics (DA), and the first examination was held in 1935. Later it co-opted an anaesthetist to its Council to assist in its deliberations. The DA fulfilled the needs of the specialty until after the Second World War. The decade of the 1940's had seen immense changes, not only in anaesthesia but in the whole of medical practice. Anaesthesia had been revolutionised by the introduction of curare in 1942, developments such as antibiotics and blood transfusion were changing surgery equally radically, while the preexisting system of providing medical services was increasingly unable to cope with these changes.

Until this time medical care had been provided in a two-tier service, private practice for the wealthy, and a free, or nearly free, system of hospital treatment given by specialists working without fee in the voluntary hospitals. There were few specialising in anaesthesia because there were few posts and these were poorly paid. There was little incentive to enter the field. Under the British system, surgeons were dependent on general practitioners for sending them private patients, so they in return asked these practitioners to give the anaesthetics, hence they received the fees. Consequently, the specialist anaesthetists could not supplement their meagre income from this source. The crucial factor for change was a political one, the determination of the newly-elected Labour government to bring in a National Health Service (NHS) freely available to all regardless of means. It soon became clear that anaesthesia was not going to be considered as one of the specialties within the NHS, and anaesthetists would still be doomed to inferior status and pay. Fortunately, the anaesthetists saw the dire consequences this would have on the development of the specialty and determined to aim for specialist recognition. Once again AAGBI approached the RCS to help them to set up an organisation that would demonstrate to the government that anaesthetists would achieve standards of training and practice similar to those of surgeons in the near future. The RCS responded by creating a suitable academic body, the Faculty of Anaesthetists, giving it authority to supervise and regulate training and to upgrade the DA to a standard similar to that of their surgical Fellowship. It was a great credit to all concerned that this was done so quickly, and in 1948, when the NHS came into being, anaesthesia was recognised as a full specialty, a major step forward in its professional advance.

Anaesthetists then had to show they were capable of achieving what they had promised, and fortunately, from among the few there were sufficient to form a high-calibre Board of Faculty under its first Dean, Dr Archibald Marston. This Board soon showed that anaesthetists were fully deserving of their new status. However, this was not enough, for standards of practice are dependent not only on the qualities of the leaders, but also on having sufficient numbers of skilled people available to treat patients throughout the country. Before the war these were very few, but the wartime Armed Services provided them. One of the important new developments in the Second World War was the formation of Field Surgical Teams consisting of surgeon, anaesthetist and supporting staff, to deal with casualties as near the front line as possible. The Army in particular had senior anaesthetists who not only set about the task of recruiting and training the large number required, but also of ensuring that they received appropriate recognition. These doctors became expert anaesthetists, often working under the most difficult circumstances in the field, and furthermore became enthusiastic for the specialty, and after demobilisation they were seeking employment as anaesthetists. It was the NHS with its large number of salaried hospital posts which provided this and gave the incentive to remain in the new specialty.

Thus, at least three factors came together in the immediate post-war period, the vast improvement in general anaesthesia due to the introduction of curare, the availability of large number of experienced anaesthetists from the Armed Services, and the academic framework provided by the new Faculty. All these came together and resulted in the enormous advances in research and practice which characterised the decades following the war, when far greater progress in anaesthesia was made in twenty or thirty years than in the whole of the hundred years following 1846.

The evolution of the Faculty within the RCS was marked by its steadily increasing autonomy, usually with the encouragement of the surgeons, though occasionally, it has to be said, they were obstructive. Its role remained similar to that of its parent body, but as would be expected of a new and advancing specialty, it has broken new ground and started new ventures. This evolution culminated in the establishment of the college of Anaesthetists in 1988, at first remaining within the RCS, but now an independent College which will soon move into its own premises, with the expectation of receiving the ultimate accolade of a Royal Charter.

References

1. Dinnick OP. The first anaesthetic society. Progress in Anaesthesiology. Excerpta Medica International Congress Series 200. 1968: 181-186.

Bibliography

Minutes of the Council of the Anaesthetic Section of the Royal Society of Medicine, Council of the Association of Anaesthetists of Great Britain and Ireland, Council of the Royal College of Surgeons of England, and of its Board and Faculty of Anaesthetists.

Cope, Z. The Royal College of Surgeons in England. A History. London: Anthony Blond. 1959.

JOSEPH THOMAS CLOVER
Some Aspects of his Personal and Professional Life

AILEEN K. ADAMS
Cambridge, England, United Kingdom

A portrait of Joseph Thomas Clover painted when he was about 18 years of age by his uncle is one of the less well-known but most attractive likenesses. It is housed in the College of Anaesthetists on long-term loan from the Clover family. When the Faculty of Anaesthetists was founded 44 years ago within the Royal College of Surgeons of England, they commemorated Clover by setting up a lecture in his name to be delivered biennially by a distinguished person associated with anaesthesia. To date twenty-six Clover lectures have been given. Much, therefore, has been written and spoken about him and his contributions to the art and science of anaesthesia are well-known. I shall therefore concentrate on some aspects of his life and times which have come from his unpublished papers and from the reminiscences of some members of his family.

Marston, the first Dean of the Faculty of Anaesthetists, in his inaugural Clover lecture in 1949[1] speculated that certain characteristics tended to run in families, and tried to show that Clover had inherited some scientific genes from his forebears. This is a little hard to sustain when we know so little about them, and the argument about whether heredity or environment is the more important is one in which I shall not engage today. We do, however, know that Joseph Thomas Clover was the second son born into a family of merchants in Aylsham, a market town in Norfolk. We know that his father was sufficiently well off to apprentice him at the age of 16 to Charles Gibson, a surgeon in Norwich, for a fee of £240, a sum equating today with between 11,000 and 12,000 dollars. From this beginning, Clover went on to qualify in medicine at University College Hospital in London, and ultimately to become one of the earliest specialist anaesthetists in Great Britain, following the example of John Snow. One can summarise his position in the history of anaesthesia by saying that, whilst his publications show him to be a lesser scientist than Snow, contemporary opinion suggests that he was a skilled clinician, careful and painstaking in his work, liked by his patients and appreciated by his surgeons. Detailed studies of the various pieces of apparatus he invented shows them to be original and ingenious in design, and fulfilling some but not all of the criteria we expect today. His vaporisers have stood the test of time, being in use either in their original or modified forms for at least 80 years. His ether inhaler was still listed, as late as the beginning of the Second World War, as part of the field equipment for anaesthetists in the Royal Air Force. Clover, therefore, can be regarded as a worthy successor to John Snow, making significant advances in both the art and science of anaesthesia.

Quite apart from these lasting contributions, Clover was certainly successful in his professional career. By modern standards his workload was small, about twelve anaesthetics per week, more than the eight averaged by Snow. But at this time surgical operations were rare occasions, the Glasgow Royal Infirmary being considered very advanced surgically in listing some 120 operations per year.[2] In addition, though, surgery on wealthier patients was often done either in the surgeons' rooms or in their own homes, for no one except the very impoverished would contemplate entering the poorly staffed unhygienic hospitals existing at the time. Clover was on the staff of University College and the Westminster and Dental Hospitals, but also included many private patients in his practice, even though this entailed extensive travelling around London by horse and carriage. This must have been exhausting for someone whose health was never good. However, he made time to design and evaluate new apparatus, to think about how to improve the safety of general anaesthesia, and to take part in lectures and discussions in learned societies. Among his many famous patients were members of the Royal Family, the Emperor Napoleon III, and Florence Nightingale, to name only a few.

We know sufficient of his family to assess whether, as Marston had asked earlier, they had acquired any of his personal qualities by heredity or environment, and also how well did he provide for them financially after his relatively early death. Clover liked to live well, though not extravagantly. When he became engaged to Mary Anne Hall, the daughter of a Cambridge don who became a canon of St Paul's Cathedral, he wrote to her "I like to see good house-keeping—as I like to see good painting and hear good music, in a word the best of everything is good enough for me—but I am not an epicure." The Clovers did live well in their home at 3 Cavendish Place. They had a good social life, numbering among their friends and acquaintances people from many walks of life, including Ruskin from the field of literature, Burne-Jones the artist, the Terrys from the theatrical world and Isambard Kingdom Brunel, the greatest engineer of his time. Clover's diaries and notebooks suggest that he could hold his own in this company, his drawings show considerable merit, and he used quotations showing he was well-versed in classical literature. His wife too was a good painter. A portrait she painted of Ellen Terry at the age of 15 was presented to the Old Vic Theatre Museum in Bristol by Clover's granddaughter Dorothea some years ago.

Clover married when he was 44, and died at the early age of 57 after several years of deteriorating health, leaving his widow with four children to bring up. The eldest was only nine years old, so there is not much family memory of their father, although Mary, the youngest, writing to Dr John Gillies when in her eighties, said that, although she was under six when her father died, she remembered him very vividly.

Clover was evidently careful with his money, keeping detailed records of his expenditures. After his death his will was proved in the sum of £27,932.14s.2d. This seems to have provided well for his widow, three sons and one daughter. All the sons went to a British "public" school, that is, a private independent one. No doubt the fees were as expensive then as they are now. All three repaid this expense by distinguishing themselves both as scholars and as sportsmen. Martin, the eldest, went to Shrewsbury School, was a good oarsman, stroking the school boat, and he played for their first football team. He went on to qualify in medicine, practicing as a doctor in Worcestershire, and he subsequently made the acquaintanceship of Professor Sir Robert Macintosh at Oxford. The second son, Harry, also was clever, he was an excellent cricketer, he won scholarships both to Winchester College and Cambridge University, took his degree and went into the Army, serving in the Boer War and winning a medal with three clasps. He then became a barrister, but it seems he was not suited for professional life, preferring to live on his private income and winning competitions at chess and bridge. Unfortunately, he drank heavily and was refused Army service in the First World War. It seems that he went downhill and died in 1923 at the age of 49 in Papworth Hospital, Cambridge, then a tuberculosis sanatorium. Alan, the youngest son, also went to Shrewsbury where he excelled at cricket and at cross-country running. He too went up to Cambridge and later was ordained an Anglican priest, continuing to play cricket and also writing poetry. Sadly, he became mentally unstable, and eventually died in a mental hospital. Thus, although Clover's three sons had much of their father's intellectual ability, only the eldest used it effectively, and even he was not exceptional.

It was their daughter, Mary, who inherited not only her father's academic abilities but also much of his pioneering spirit and immense capacity for work. She too went to Cambridge, graduating in mathematics from Girton College and remaining there for most of her long life, not as a scholar, but as an academic administrator of the greatest capability, being secretary of Girton College for 30 years. Many of the older dons remember her well, and I have heard many stories about her. Plainly, she was a lively character with enormous energy. Her obituary[3] sums her up well. "Working with Miss Clover was a lively experience. She throve on crises, and I sometimes suspected that she was postponing some urgent matter until the eleventh hour in order to have the excitement and challenge of a last-minute rush." When she started as secretary, the College had acquired a huge debt due to overspending on extending its buildings. She hurled herself with relish into the task of raising money, demanding, cajoling, threatening and persuading, and within a year had raised enough to clear the debt. During the First World War she became the administrator of a military hospital in Cambridge, liking to wear the Red Cross uniform because "it saved wasting time in the morning deciding what you were going to wear." She was one of the first women in Cambridge to own and drive a motor car, a yellow Morris she called "Phyllis," which she kept for very many years. Generations of staff and students had all sorts of adventures in Phyllis. Mary's paperwork shows her to have been meticulous, even obsessive. Perhaps these were qualities inherited from her father. Like many perfectionists, though, she was not easy to live with, and her family did not always appreciate her rather domineering efforts at organising their affairs. Nevertheless she always helped them out in crises, particularly looking after the families of Harry and Alan when they became ill. By the time she died in Cambridge in 1965 at 89 she had become something of a local legend.

Of Clover's eighteen direct descendents, only his eldest son Martin became a doctor, but one of his great-great-grandsons is now a second year medical student. One wonders whether he will be attracted to anaesthesia.

Historians of anaesthesia can be grateful to all four of Clover's children for enabling us to learn more about their father. Martin gave Sir Robert Macintosh all his father's notebooks and papers, together with some other memorabilia. The papers are now in the Woodward Biomedical Library of the University of British Columbia in Vancouver,[4] while several other items were presented by Sir Robert to the Faculty, now the College of Anaesthetists.

The second son, Harry, before his untimely death had married and fathered a son whose descendents include Anthony Clover, the present head of the family. He is particularly interested in his family history, and I am indebted to him for much of the information in this paper.

As for Alan, his daughter Dorothea is still alive and well, living in Bristol, and she too has donated mementoes of her grandfather to the Monica Britton Memorial Museum at Frenchay Hospital in Bristol, as well as telling me and others some of her memories.

Finally, Mary gave to Dr John Gillies in Edinburgh a photograph of her father now in the Anaesthetic Department of the Royal Infirmary, and she also gave to the Department at Addenbrooke's Hospital, Cambridge, some lecture notes in Clover's hand.

All therefore have added to our knowledge of their distinguished father, Joseph Thomas Clover, and have enabled us to build up a clearer picture both of Clover the anaesthetist and Clover the man.

Acknowledgments

I thank Anthony and Dorothea Clover for personal communications, Lady Ann Macintosh for access to Sir Robert Macintosh's papers, and Girton College, Cambridge, for access to Mary Clover's archive, and for their permission to quote.

References

1. Marston AD. The life and achievements of Joseph Thomas Clover. Annals of the Royal College of Surgeons of England 4: 267-280, 1949.
2. Sykes WS. Essays on the First Hundred Years of Anaesthesia. London: Churchill-Livingstone. 1960 1: 30.
3. Peace KM. Obituary. The Girton Review, Easter Term. 1965; 34-37.
4. Thomas KB. The Clover/Snow Collection. Anaesthesia 27: 436-449, 1972.

ANAESTHETIC LITERATURE OF 1892

C. N. ADAMS
Consultant Anaesthetist, Department of Anaesthesia
West Suffolk Hospital,
Suffolk, United Kingdom

In 1892 there were 44 States of the Union, the population of America was over seventy million, and that of Georgia was slightly under two million. It was a Presidential election year, with Benjamin Harrison, a Republican, being defeated by Grover Cleveland on November 8th. As in the previous election of 1888, there was no overall majority. The 51st Congress of 1890-91 under the Republicans had a prodigious legislative program and had been dubbed "The Billion Dollar Congress," and the newly elected speaker, Thomas B Reed of Maine, in 1892 called America "A Billion Dollar Country."[1]

It was a time of massive immigration into America, mostly by Europeans. In 1892, Ellis Island in New York was opened as the Federal Bureau of Immigration's receiving station. It could accommodate up to two ships and 7000 new arrivals per day.

To mark the 400th anniversary of Columbus' discovery of the New World, Chicago held a celebration in the form of the World Columbian Exposition. Here, the two most popular attractions were firstly the Ferris Wheel, a giant structure of 250 feet diameter with 36 boxes attached, and secondly an exotic dancer called "Little Egypt," who wore silk trousers and performed a "hoochee-coochee dance" of undulating movements.

A gasoline-powered motorcar, designed and built by the Duryea brothers, made its maiden run on September 22 in Springfield, Massachusetts. This is believed to be the first such run in America.

New Medical Inventions

Dr. John Philpots described his new stethoscope.[2] It consisted of two separate pieces of India-rubber tubing, each 2 feet 2 inches long with vulcanized earpieces at the upper ends. The lower ends were inserted into the chestpiece which measured seven-eighths of an inch. The whole instrument could be carried with ease in the waistcoat pocket or more conveniently in a pistol pocket made in the trousers. With the small chestpiece, it was now possible to ausculate the intercostal space and so detect mischief that an ordinary instrument would overlook and more importantly, there was no occasion to lean over the patient under examination, nor to inhale the patient's breath, "so frequently disagreeable."

It had been known for almost one hundred years that oxygen was a suitable antidote to asphyxia. This was originally described in Dr. Thomas Beddoes work, *"Considerations on the Medicinal Use and on the Production of Factitious Airs."* Although apparatus for the delivery of oxygen was available as early as 1817, its use had fallen into disrepute. In 1892, George Foy described his new apparatus for the inhalation of oxygen[3] and asked, "Is it too much hope that bottles of it to be kept in every operating theatre?" He commented that as a cardiac and respiratory stimulant there was no equal to oxygen, and that it appeared to play the part of a physiologic antidote to general anaesthetics.

"Anaesthetics, Their Use and Administration," by D.W. Buxton

In the preface to the second edition of his book, Dr. Buxton states that it was intended as a practical manual, rather than as a disputatious treatise. Appropriately, in the perspective of the current International Symposium, the first chapter of the book is devoted to a historical perspective on Anaesthetics.[4] Dr. Buxton started with the story from the Odyssey where Helen uses a sedative draught to "drown all sense of woe" and assuage the suffering of Menelaus. He described the use by the ancient Egyptians and Scythians of *Cannabis indica* which was burned and the fumes inhaled to alleviate pain. The Romans used powdered Memphis marble treated with vinegar to give a gas (carbonic dioxide) which was used to produce slight anaesthesia.

In the 16th and 17th centuries, patients were stupefied by compression of the cartoid arteries, so depriving the brain of blood. This practice may perhaps have been employed by the Assyrians in ancient times.

In 1784, James Moore, an English surgeon, suggested the compression of nerve trunks before incising the areas supplied by them. John Hunter actually used this method by compressing the sciatic and crural nerves before amputating a leg in St. George's Hospital.

Dr. Buxton attributed the start of modern anaesthesia to three men, Wells for nitrous oxide, Morton for ether, and Simpson for chloroform. The discovery of ether was initially credited to Djabar Yeber, an Arabian Chemist, and then in chapter IV to Valerius Cordus in 1540. This apparent contradiction is not further clarified.

In Chapter II, the preparation of a patient and choice of anaesthetic is described. Dr. Buxton bemoaned the fact that in 1892 the anaesthetist seldom had a choice over the timing of operation. He considered that a suitable hour was very important, as a weak patient should not be anaesthetised after a long fast, most particularly early in the morning. He pointed to the difference in effect of "anaesthetisation" when the patient is robust, and when he is an invalid.

Dr. Buxton advocated a light meal of soft and easily digested matters to be taken three hours before the surgeon should arrive. Examples included milk foods, strong beef tea, a light meal of fish, tea, coffee or cocoa. If the patient was weakly with feeble heart action, then a little good brandy or whisky was recommended. If the patient was very prostrate from vomiting, then iced brandy and soda should be given. In preparing the patient, reassurance with a few cheery words and if necessary, directions as to how the patient should take the anaesthetic would give him something about which to think.

In assessing the risks to the patient, the importance of pulmonary disease and renal disease were recognised and discussed. In both cases the A.C.E. mixture (8 parts ether to one part chloroform) was put forward as preferable to ether alone.

Children were felt to take chloroform and the A.C.E. mixture well, whilst ether was said to produce much bronchial trouble. After the age of six, a combination of nitrous oxide and ether was felt better, though children might strongly rebel against the face piece. We are reminded that deaths are by no means confined to adults.

The third chapter is devoted to nitrous oxide. In describing its physiologic action, Dr. Buxton stated that it appeared to suspend rather than extinguish vitality. He reported that, experimentally, plant seeds kept in nitrous oxide would not germinate but would remain uninjured indefinitely. He noted, however, that cold- and warm-blooded animals died when placed in pure nitrous oxide. Sir Humphrey Davy had shown that animals kept in a mixture of nitrous oxide and oxygen lived until the proportion of oxygen fell to 6 percent.

Nitrous oxide alone would produce anaesthesia which lasted only a minute, so for longer surgery the patient had to be allowed to almost resume consciousness before the gas was again applied. This process could be repeated. Dr. Buxton described his own apparatus for giving nitrous oxide alone. The apparatus was made by Mr. Blennerhassett of London. It comprised a silencer, the usual tripod, a steel bottle containing fifty gallons of nitrous oxide, a Cattlin's bag, a valve to admit air or nitrous oxide, and an ordinary Clover's face piece.

Dr. Buxton gave a description of each anaesthetic agent in turn. He commented methodically on chemical and physical properties, physiologic action, methods of administration, dangers and accidents, and after effects. Chloroform, ether and A.C.E. are included, as well as less commonly used anaesthetics such as amylene, ethidene chloride, and hydrobromic ether.

His method is well illustrated with the example of chloroform. The discovery of chloroform ($CHCl_3$) is attributed to Mr. Samuel Guthrie of Brimfield, Massachusetts, and independently Liebig, in 1831. Chemical and physical properties listed were a specific gravity of 1.497 at 62.5°F and vapour density 4.199 (Dumas), with an agreeable ethereal smell and a sweet taste. It was very volatile, but although mixing freely with air, pure chloroform vapour could only exist at 140°F. Physiologically, chloroform was said to be a solvent of blood corpuscles and a protoplasm poison. Prolonged inhalation was known to lead to fatty degeneration of the tissues, whilst inadvertent swallowing of a considerable quantity of chloroform would produce anaesthesia. In animals, inhalation soon caused dilatation of the ventricle, but withdrawal allowed the ventricle to return to normal size. A lethal dose of chloroform induced a fibrillary irritability of the heart. The action of chloroform on the nervous system was not known.

Dr. Buxton divided the stages of chloroform anaesthesia into five. The idea of five stages had been introduced by Snow in his book, *On the Inhalation of the Vapour of Ether in Surgical Operations,* of 1847[5] and would not alter until Guedel's description in 1920. Buxton started with stage one from the commencement of inhalation to impairment of consciousness; in stage two, mental powers are impaired though not suspended; in stage three, all voluntary movements are lost; in stage four, breathing is stertorous, the pupils dilated, and the muscles completely relaxed and flaccid; and stage five is the period of narcosis which "intervenes" before respiratory embarrassment and total cessation of breathing. We are told that, even after dyspnoea has passed into apnoea, the heart continues to beat for a brief while.

The means of chloroform administration discussed were Clover's chloroform apparatus, Snow's inhaler, Sansom's inhaler, Junker's inhaler, or an open method using a towel soaked in chloroform.

The list of complications after chloroform anaesthesia included vomiting, hysteria, jaundice, albuminuria, glycosuria, astigmatism, and even insanity!

In considering obstetric practice, Dr. Buxton thought chloroform preferable to ether. The A.C.E. mixture was also suitable. He asserted that chloroform should be withheld until the os uteri was fully dilated unless earlier pains were very severe. Rules guiding administration included a quiet room, avoiding distension of the bladder, deep anaesthesia if a meal had recently been taken because of the ensuing nausea. Statistical evidence suggested that maternal and perinatal mortality were no different from normal when chloroform was used.

Chapter XI is devoted to local anesthesia. Cocaine, the active principle from the leaves of *Erythroxylon coca,* was the sole local anaesthetic. It was first isolated by Gaedcke in 1855 (he called it erythroxyline) and then rediscovered by S.R. Percy of New York, who noted that it deadened the sensibility of the tongue. It is said to have come into use in the 1880s for producing local insensibility to pain. Methods of administration described were instillation into the eye, painting over mucous surfaces, and subcutaneous injections. Indications for usage were in ophthalmic surgery, operations about the larnyx and pharynx, on the urino-generative tract, in dental surgery, and for abscesses, boils and carbuncles. The physiological action of cocaine was to produce a marked depressing action upon the human heart. Other effects were severe headache, palpitation, tingling, formication, muscular weakness, cold sweats, extreme drowsiness and utter prostration. Nausea and vomiting sometimes occurred.

It is remarkable in the light of present day practice that the final chapter of the book is devoted to medico-legal aspects of the administration of anaesthetics. The chapter starts boldly, "The administration of an anaesthetic to a patient who is not a minor, against his will, constitutes an assault." Dr. Buxton recognised that subsequent struggling under narcosis was a different situation. In addressing prosecution for malpractice he noted that it rested with the anaesthetist to show the steps adopted were the best he could follow for the benefit of the patient. These included choosing the most suitable agent, administration with due skill and by an approved method, possession of all necessary facts with regard to the patient's bodily condition and making due allowance for these; and in the event of an accident the right and appropriate treatment with all promptitude.

So frequent were the charges of rape under anaesthesia that Dr. Buxton advised the greatest care and the presence of a third person. He stated that chloroform, ether, nitrous oxide, cocaine and other carbon compounds all possessed the property of exciting sexual emotions and in many cases produced erotic hallucinations.

Concerning the medico-legal aspects of death under anaesthesia, Dr. Buxton questioned, "who in the eye of the law is qualified to administer an anaesthetic?" He noted that butler, coachmen, dispensers and various unqualified persons were frequently permitted to give the anaesthetic. He felt that it was not the surgeon's responsibility, but that it could only be accomplished by one specially instructed and experienced in anaesthetics.

Finally he addressed the risks of self-indulgence in anaesthetics and the subsequent unfortunate addiction to chloroform, nitrous oxide and cocaine.

Deaths Under Anaesthesia

Though there was little to find in the American Journals of 1892, the *British Medical Journal* and the *Lancet* contained many reports of death associated with anaesthesia, and these articles provoked much discussion as to the cause, treatment and prevention of such accidents. At one inquest, the Coroner, Dr. Danford Thomas, estimated that the proportion of deaths under anaesthesia was one in every 4000 or 5000 cases.[6] A typical report[7] is that of a case which occurred at University College Hospital in London on Wednesday, March 9th. A young man of twenty-two who suffered from long-standing jaw mischief was anaesthetised with chloroform to facilitate the removal of some dead bone. No unusual symptoms occurred until the operation commenced and the gouge was applied to the carious bone. At this point respiration and the heart's action stopped. Though the operation was discontinued and attempts at resuscitation made, no pulse or heart's action could be detected.

In syncope or death under anaesthesia, the recommended courses of action were: massage over the heart[8]; inversion of the patient[9]; drawing the tongue forward, enemata of brandy, faradic current to the phrenic nerves, tracheotomy[10]; venesection of the external jugular vein, hot affusions to the chest followed by slapping with a cold wet towel, hypodermic injections with ether, inhalation of amyl[11]; flagellation[12]; or simply leaving the patient alone.[13]

In an attempt to relieve the monotony of the weekly publication of so many letters concerning death during "abnormal anaesthesia," Surgeon-Major Edward Lawrie of Hyderabad reported on three cases of "Normal chloroform anaesthesia."[14] The ages of the patients were 26 years, 32 years and 60 years, respectively, undergoing operations for acute abscess, aspiration of abscess of the liver, and excision of wen: all were completed uneventfully. In the same paper Lawrie also described a fatal accident during anaesthesia of an eighteen month old Hindu child for removal of calculus from the urethra. Anaesthesia appears to have taken only one minute to induce. In the twenty-minute procedure that followed, the infant's heart sounds were not heard and respiration became shallow and stertorous. Mouth-to-mouth resuscitation was applied without success. In this case, Lawrie commented on the inadequacy of note-taking as the student attending as note-taker was not accustomed to this process.

By drawing together scientific evidence from several sources, Dr Wilmot Buxton, in a paper in the *British Medical Journal,* attempted a physiological explanation of the question of death under anaesthesia.[9] He noted that, when asphyxia was not present, chloroform exerted an effect to weaken both the action of the heart and respiration. Furthermore, he ascribed this to a direct action of chloroform on the heart muscle. He believed that a fall in blood pressure placed the whole circulatory system at risk. He also questioned the effect that impurities in the chloroform might have on the patient.

Anaesthetics, a Necessary Part of the Curriculum?

In a paper read before the Thames Valley Branch of the British Medical Association,[15] Dr. J.F.W. Silk commented on the lack of teaching of anaesthetics in English medical schools. The instruction was limited to allusion during surgical lectures and then confined to the practical nature of administration. Thus, the knowledge imparted was of a functional rather than academic nature. In Scotland and Ireland the situation was worse as the prospectuses showed no aesthetic content whatsoever.

Dr. Silk felt that a systematic teaching of anaesthesia should be adopted by the medical schools. He gave as reasons the improvements in surgery, the increase in the number of anaesthetics, the importance of the subject, the improvements in methods of administration, the complicated nature of the process, and the attendant difficulties and dangers. In another letter to the *Lancet,*[16] Dr Silk also called for a separate section for anaesthetics at International Congresses. He supported this by stating that, in the recently published Report of the Berlin Congress of 1890, upwards of forty-five pages were devoted to anaesthetics.

Discussion

The *British Medical Journal* and the *Lancet* of 1892 contained many articles concerning death under anaesthesia. This subject was almost absent from the *J.A.M.A.* and *Boston Medical and Surgical Journal* in the same year. I found this omission surprising as chloroform would be banned only twenty years later by a Commission on Anaesthesia of the American Medical Association. Whilst Dr. Wilmot Buxton was contributing to an independent literature for anaesthesia, Dr. Silk was requesting that the subject be included in the training of medical students and that separate international meetings be held. Dr. Silk would in 1893 found the London Society of Anaesthetists, with Dr. Wilmot Buxton as treasurer. This society subsequently became the Section of Anaesthetics at the Royal Society of Medicine, London.

In devoting the first chapter of his book to a history of anaesthetics, the far-sighted Dr. Buxton demonstrated his interest in the history of anaesthesia.

We are continuing that process in this international meeting.

References

1. Brogan H. *Longman History of the United States of America.* 1st Ed. London: Longman Group Limited, 1985: p386
2. Philpots JR. A New Stethoscope, *Br Med J* i:562, 1892
3. Foy G. Apparatus for the inhalation of oxygen. *Br Med J* i:179-80, 1892
4. Buxton DW. *Anaesthetics; their uses and administration.* 2nd Ed. London: HK Lewis, 1892.
5. Snow J. *On the Inhalation of the Vapour of Ether in Surgical Operations.* London: John Churchill, 1847.
6. Anonymous. Deaths under chloroform. *Br Med J* i:134-5, 1892
7. Anonymous. Deaths under chloroform. *Lancet* i:709, 1892
8. Maas. The successful treatment of chloroform syncope by massage over the heart. *Boston Med Surg J* 126:590, 1892
9. Wilmot Buxton D. A discussion on the bearing of recent physiological and chemical research on the question of anaesthesia. *Br Med J* ii:933-9, 1892
10. Biddlecombe EH. Death under ether. *Lancet* i:412-3, 1892
11. Wood TJ. Death from chloroform. *Br Med J* i:711, 1892
12. Wilson AC. Syncope during the administration of ether. *Br Med J* i:443, 1892
13. Lawrie E. Death under chloroform. *Lancet* ii:115, 1892
14. Lawrie E. Cases of normal chloroform anaesthesia with a note of an accident from abnormal anaesthesia. *Br Med J* i:11-2, 1892
15. Silk JFW. Anaesthetics, a necessary part of the curriculum. *Lancet* i:1178-9, 1892
16. Silk, JFW. Anaesthetics at the international medical congress. *Lancet* ii:227-8, 1892

THE DELIVERY OF ANESTHESIA CARE DURING THE WAR OF THE REBELLION IN THE UNITED STATES OF AMERICA
Historical Episodes

MAURICE S. ALBIN
Professor of Anesthesiology and Neurological Surgery
The University of Texas Health Science Center at San Antonio
Department of Anesthesiology
San Antonio, Texas,
USA

While we reflect upon and celebrate the sesquicentennial of the first application of ether as an anesthetic agent by Crawford Williamson Long in 1842 (Fig. 1) it is important to remember that two decades later he too was caught in the conflict that was to rend the United States apart.

The outbreak of the Civil War caught both sides in this conflict totally unprepared to deal with the medical problems associated with the first "modern" war that employed high velocity missiles, ironclad ships, mobilization and movement of masses of troops using a railroad system and telegraphic communications. Unfortunately, the concept of aseptic surgery was not practiced and operative procedures were carried out with instruments, dressings and the hands of the surgeon that were not disinfected. Among Union troops it has been estimated that 65 percent of the deaths were due to disease, 15 percent died of wounds and 20 percent were killed in action.[1,2] The overall mortality due to specific types of wounds can be seen in Table I. In this essay we will touch on the use of anesthetics during this conflict, examine the contributions of individuals to the practice of anesthesia, discuss the development of narcotic addition during and after the Civil War and pay homage to our first military anesthetist.

Although ether had been used for surgical procedures since 1846 and chloroform since 1851 in the United States, there was a great deal of ignorance and overt hostility to their use when the Civil War started in 1861. This was in

TABLE I.
Overall Mortality According to Body Area

Spine	55.5%;	Chest	27.8%;	Abdomen	58.7%
Pelvis	29.7%;	Back	6.9%;	Head	28.9%
Face	5.8%;	Neck	15.0%;	Upper Extremity	6.5%
		Lower Extremity	13.8%		

TABLE II.
Number of Anesthetics According to Agent and Subsequent Mortality

- 80,000 Anesthetics Reported
- In 8,900 cases:

Chloroform	6,784	76.2%	37	0.54
Ether	1,305	14.7%	4	0.30
Mixture	811	9.1%	2	0.24

part due to the feeling by the American military surgeons during the Mexican American War in 1847 that ether was dangerous. Hammond notes that "In the Crimean War, it [chloroform] was used commonly and freely." He also states that ". . . MacLeod reports over 20,000 cases, with only a single fatality" during the Crimean War.[5] It has been calculated that at least 80,000 anesthetics were administered during the Civil War. The *Medical and Surgical History of the War of the Rebellion* (1883)[1] analyzed 8,900 cases of major surgery where anesthetics were used (Table II) with chloroform employed in 76.2 percent of the cases, ether in 14.7 percent and the mixture of the two in 9.1 percent. Chloroform was preferred because it had less bulk than ether, was easier to use because of its ability to produce a more rapid induction and due to it not being flammable. In spite of appalling operative conditions at the battlefield, the anesthetic mortality appeared to be relatively low. (Table II) Of the 37 deaths attributed to chloroform, six appeared to be due to an overdose and in one aspiration of vomitus occurred.[1] In the four deaths due to ether, an overdose occurred in one patient.

When the War of the Rebellion began in 1861, few of the Union Military Surgeons had more than a passing experience with the use of ether or chloroform. Nevertheless, the "Duties of the Operating Surgeon"[1] included:

"4. An operation being determined, he should have the patient properly placed upon the table and should judge of the practicality of administering anaesthetic and if their use is found necessary should superintend the administration.

5. The patient being etherized, the Surgeon proceeds with the operation that the case requires. . . ."[1]

Chisolm, Hammond and Long

In 1861, four months after the battle at Fort Sumter, the Confederate Surgeon Julian John Chisolm, published *A Manual of Military Surgery For the Use of Surgeons in the Confederate Army*[3] which went through three editions.[4] Chisolm was a strong believer in the use of chloroform, having great personal experience and being skillful in its application. Because the South had depended upon the North for most of its medical supplies, and since the North blockaded the southern ports, Chisolm realized the need to conserve the use of chloroform. With this in mind he developed a nasal inhaler (Fig. 2) in which chloroform was dropped on a metallic sieve, the body of the inhaler containing packed cotton-wool. Besides this nasal inhaler, Chisholm also designed a funnel vaporizer for chloroform. After the Civil War, he became the Dean of the School of Medicine of the University of Maryland and was among

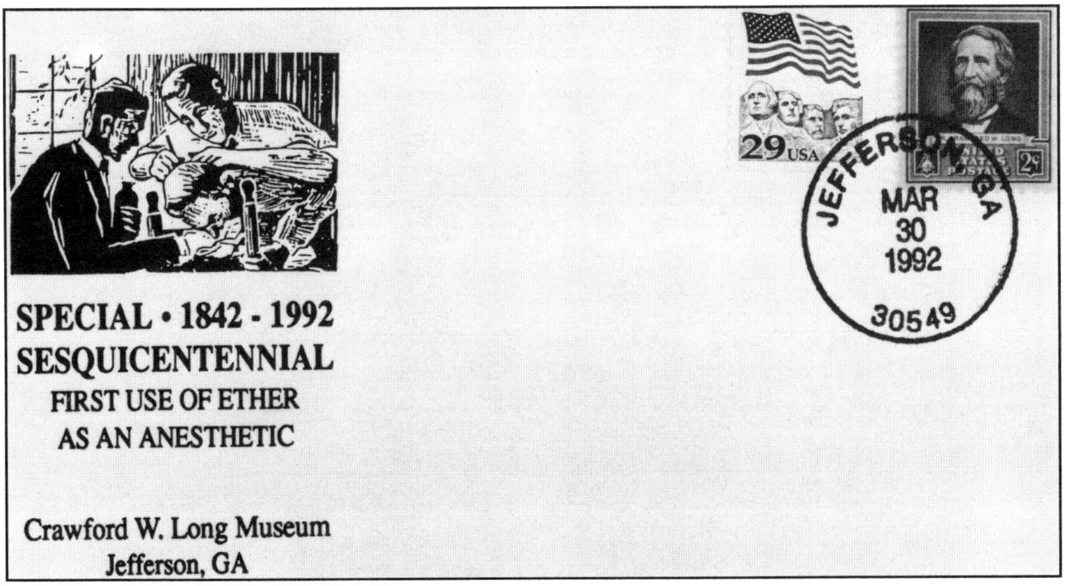

Fig. 1. First day cover celebrating the sesquicentennial of the first use of ether for a surgical procedure by Crawford Long in Jefferson, Georgia.

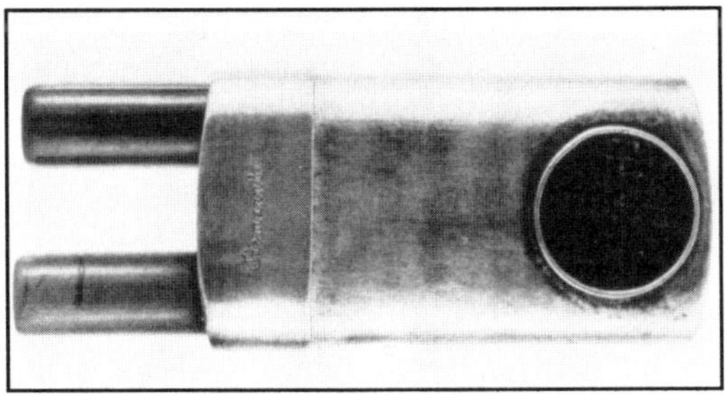

Fig. 2. The Chisolm inhaler. This device was used for the nasal inhalation of chloroform.

the first in the United States to use cocaine anesthesia for opthalmic surgery.[4]

William A. Hammond, M.D., had been Surgeon-General of the United States Army and responsible for initiating many of the reforms in the Union Army Medical Corps including the development of an ambulance corps, a general hospital system and setting up pavilion hospitals. In 1864 Dr. Hammond edited the *Military Medical and Surgical Essays*[5] which contained a chapter on "Pain and Anesthesia." In this section Hammond rebuts the concepts that pain is a stimulant against shock and expressed sensible and up-to-date criteria in the administration of anesthetics. He stated that "Anesthetics, when properly used are perfectly safe" and "—to exhibit anesthetic vapors too rapidly is to incur the danger of asphyxia." Concerned with the problem of vomiting and aspiration Hammond noted "—as he is much more likely to vomit when the stomach is full, he should not be allowed food for some hours previous to inhalation." Hammond appeared to be familiar with all the current anesthetic agents available when he said, "—I have carefully tested the power of other agents, such as nitrous oxide, to produce insensitivity to pain, but still consider none of them deserving of mention when compared with chloroform or ether."

On March 30, 1992, we celebrated the sesquicentennial of the first use of ether as an anesthetic for a surgical procedure when Crawford Williamson Long, M.D., living in Jefferson, Georgia, removed two tumors from the neck of James Venable.[6] (Fig. 3) Long did not serve in the Confederate Army during the Civil War and lived in Athens, Georgia during that period. In 1850, he spent a year in Atlanta and returned to Athens where he and his brother H.R.J. Long bought out two physicians and pharmacists and developed the largest wholesale and retail drug store in northeast Georgia. Of

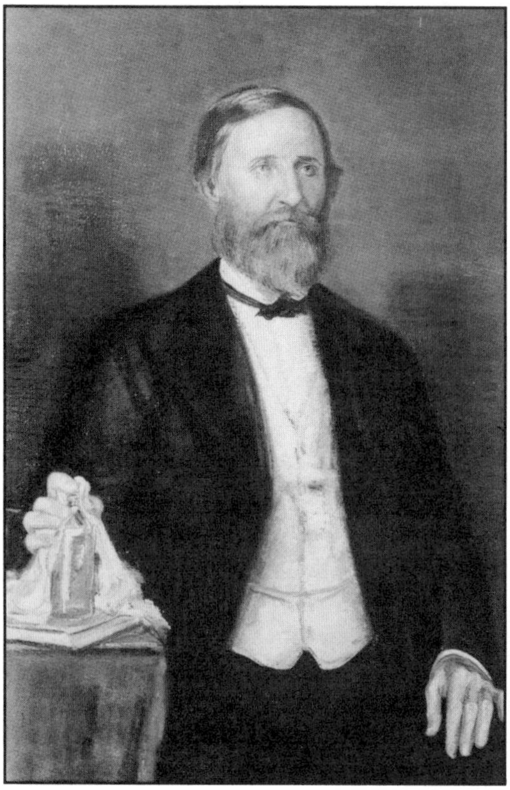

Fig. 3. Painting of Crawford W. Long

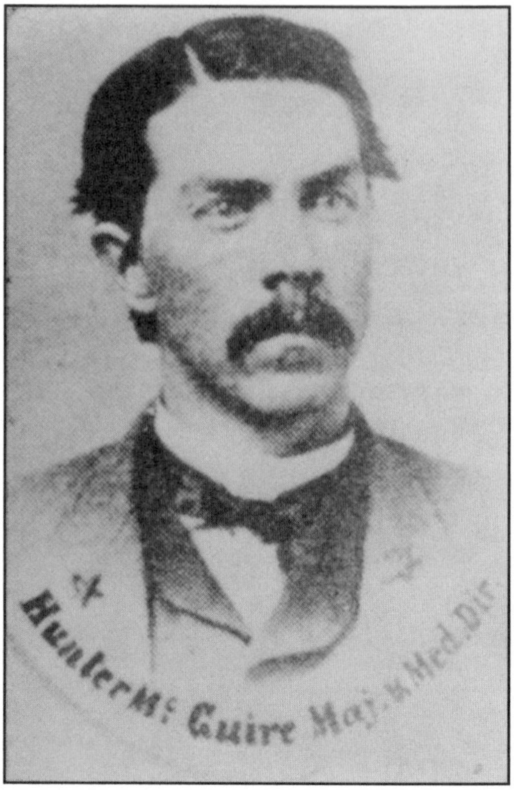

Fig. 4. Hunter Holmes McGuire, M.D.

interest is that just prior to the outbreak of the Civil War he purchased a large consignment of drugs from the North which reached Savannah, Georgia, soon after the fall of Fort Sumner. This shipment contained a large quantity of drugs, including ether, chloroform, carbolic acid and iodine and was confiscated by the Confederate Government for use by the military. Thus, his foresight in ordering ether and chloroform undoubtedly saved many Confederate soldiers from the dreaded experience of having surgery without anesthesia.

Hunter Holmes McGuire, M.D. and Thomas J. "Stonewall" Jackson

Hunter Holmes McGuire was the son of Dr. Hugh McGuire, who like Crawford W. Long, was a graduate of the University of Pennsylvania School of Medicine and a medical pioneer.[7,8] He was the first Virginian to perform a cataract operation and the first physician in the United States to operate on a patient with a club foot. McGuire *fils* studied medicine at Jefferson Medical College in Philadelphia and returned to Richmond, Virginia, prior to Christmas, 1859, completing his medical education, and becoming a member of the Faculty at Tulane University School of Medicine in New Orleans. Hunter Holmes McGuire became the Surgeon to Stonewall Jackson's Brigade and participated in his campaigns. (Fig. 4) McGuire was not only responsible for the medical care of the Brigade but also was the personal physician to Jackson. (Fig. 5) During the Shenandoah Valley campaign, Jackson's troops fought seven battles in a period of 48 days and marched 700 miles, defeating the Union armies containing as many as 70,000 troops with a Confederate Brigade containing not more than 15,000 soldiers. The medical problems faced by Dr. McGuire were certainly significant, often helped by large amounts of medical booty captured from the retreating Union armies. On Saturday, May 1, 1863, Jackson defeated the Federal troops west of Chancellorville and when returning from the front line at 8:00 P.M. was fired upon by his own troops. He was struck by three musket balls, one through the left arm that severed a major artery, one between the elbow and the wrist and the third entering the palm of the right arm. Jackson fell from his horse and when moved to a litter was subjected to artillery fire and fell from the stretcher when a bearer was killed. Jackson was then taken to a hospital at Wilderness Run near Fredericksburg and Hunter Holmes McGuire narrates that "at two o'clock Sunday morning Surgeons Block, Walls, and Coleman being present, I informed him that chloroform would be given him and his wounds examined. I told him that amputation would probably be required, and asked if it was found necessary, whether it should be done at once. He replied promptly, "yes, certainly; Doctor McGuire, do for me whatever you think best." Chloroform was then administered, and as he began to feel its effects, and its relief to the pain he was suffering, he exclaimed, "What an infinite blessing," and continued to repeat the word "blessing," until he became insensible. The round ball (such as is used for the smoothe bore Springfield musket) which had lodged under the skin upon the back of his right hand was extracted first. It had entered the palm, about the middle of the hand, and had fractured two of the bones. The left arm was then amputated, about two inches below the shoulder, very rapidly, and with slight loss of blood, the ordinary circular operation having been made. There were two wounds in this arm, the first and most serious was about three inches below the shoulder-joint, the ball dividing the main artery, and fracturing the bone. The second was several inches in length; a ball having entered the outside of the forearm, an inch below the elbow, came out upon the opposite side, just above the wrist. Throughout the whole of the operation, and until all the dressings were applied, he continued insensible." The surgical procedure went well and so did the convalescence, but unfortunately, Jackson developed pneumonia probably due to a contused lung caused by the fall from the litter. Jackson died on Sunday, May 10, 1863 saying "It is the Lord's Day; my wish is fulfilled. I have always desired to die on Sunday." After the war Hunter Holmes McGuire served as President and Professor of Surgery at the Medical College of Virginia in Richmond.

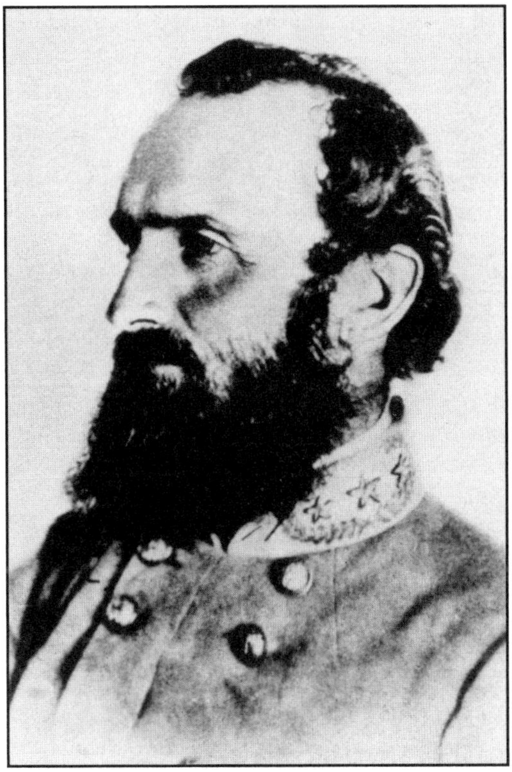

Fig. 5. Thomas J. "Stonewall" Jackson

"Opium Eaters" and "Morphinists": Analgesics and Chemical Dependence During the Civil War

In 1806, Serturner extracted morphine from opium and by 1853, the hollow needle (Alexander Wood) and hypodermic syringe (Charles Gabriel Pravaz) had been developed. Opium and opium products had been used extensively for analgesia beginning in the 1840's with resulting addiction of the so called "opium-eaters." Interestingly, it was thought that opium addiction could be treated by morphine injection. On the battlefield, morphine salts were often dusted into the surfaces of the wounds and also injected using the hypodermic syringe which became an integral part of the surgical kit of the Union surgeons near the end of the war.[9] By the conclusion of the war many soldiers became addicted to morphine. This problem was not helped by the fact that opiates were not controlled and easily available. Crothers, in 1902 said that "Many veterans of the Civil War became morphinists to relieve the pain and sufferings received in service, and the addiction is often concealed to prevent the possibility of imperiling their application for pension."[9] In fact, the addicted soldier was said to have "soldiers disease" or the "army disease." Opium supplies were not only imported but also grown and obtained in the West, South and New England states. In 1868, Horace Day wrote that[10] "The numbers of confirmed opium eaters in the United States is large, not less, judging from the testimony of druggists in all parts of the country as well as from other sources, than eighty to one hundred thousand. . . . The events of the last few years (Civil War) have unquestionably added greatly to their number. Maimed and shattered survivors from a hundred battlefields, diseased and disabled soldiers released from hostile prisons, anguished and hopeless wives and mothers, made so by the slaughter of those were dearest to them, temporary relief from their sufferings in opium."

Morton and the Battle of the Wilderness and Spotsylvania Courthouse

From May 5th to May 6th, 1864, a terrible battle took place pitting Grant (with 120,000 men) against Lee (with 66,000 men) in an area of Virginia called the Wilderness.[11] In this two day battle more than 17,600 Union and 7,500 Confederate troops were casualties. The war continued as Lee retreated to the Spotsylvania Courthouse. In these battles, the Dentist, William T.G. Morton from Boston who demonstrated the use of ether on October 16, 1846 at the Massachusetts General Hospital, spent many days administering ether and describes his experiences thusly:[12]

> Upon the arrival of a train of ambulances at a field hospital, the wounds are hastily examined, and those who can bear the journey are sent once to Fredericksburg. The nature of the operations to be performed on the others is then decided upon, and noted upon a bit of paper pinned to the pillow or roll of blanket under each patient's head. When this had been done, I prepared the patient for the knife, *producing perfect anaesthesia in the average time of three minutes.* [italics mine, MSA] and the operators followed, performing their operations with dexterous skill, while the dressers in their turn bound up the stumps.

In many ways Morton must be considered as the first Military Anesthetist since he dedicated himself solely to the practice of anesthesia on the battlefield. (Fig. 6) During this time he worked from dawn to dusk giving ether anesthesia and it has been estimated he gave his merciful anesthetic to more than 2,000 of the wounded, both Union and Confederate.

Morton was an unfortunate and depressed

Fig. 6. William T.G. Morton, D.D.S.

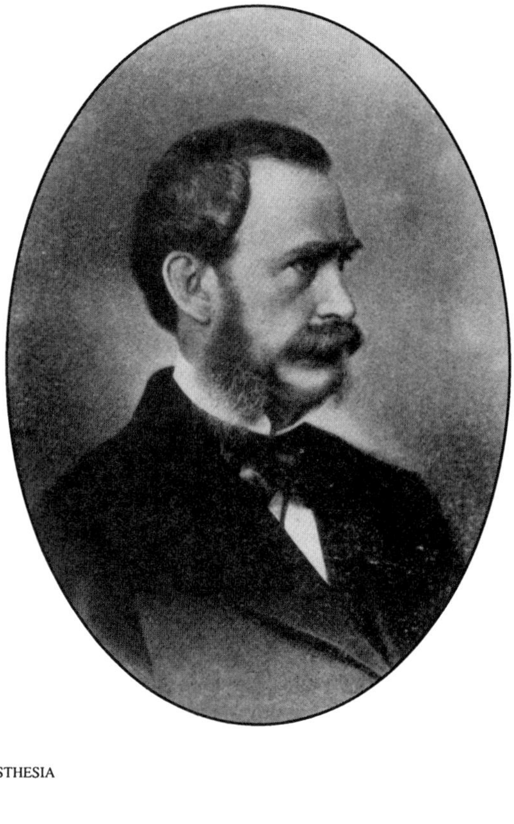

individual who felt he was robbed of the recognition due him as the true father of surgical anesthesia and he spoke of his work on the field of battle by declaring,

> For myself I am repaid for the anxiety and often wretchedness which I have experienced since I first discovered and introduced the anesthetic qualities of sulfuric ether, by the consciousness that I have been the instrument of averting pain from thousands and thousands of maimed and lacerated heroes, who have calmly rested in a state of anaesthesia while undergoing surgical operations, which would otherwise have given them intense torture. They are worth of a nation's gratitude — happy am I to have alleviated their sufferings.

References

1. The Medical and Surgical History of the War of the Rebellion. Part III. Volume II Surgical History. Second Edition, Joseph K. Barnes, George A. Otis, D.L. Huntington, Editors, Washington, Government Printing Office, 1883, 887-989.
2. Gillett MC: The Army Medical Department 1818-1865. Washington, D.C. U.S. Govt. Printing Office, 1987, pp. 371.
3. Chisolm JJ: A Manual of Military Surgery for the Use of Surgeons in the Confederate Army; with an appendix of the Rules and regulations of the Medical Department of the Confederate Army, Charleston, Evans and Cogswell, 1861, 1st Edition.
4. Worthington Jr. WC: Confederates, Chloroform, and Cataracts: Julian John Chisolm (1830-1903) Southern Medical Journal 79: 748-752, 1986.
5. Military Medical and Surgical Essays Prepared for the United States Sanitary Commission, William A. Hammond, Editor, Philadelphia, J.B. Lippincott, 1864, 385-399.
6. Taylor FL: Crawford W. Long and the Discovery of Ether Anesthesia. New York, Paul B. Hueber, 1928, pp. 237.
7. Schildt JR: Hunter Holmes McGuire; Doctor W. Grey. John W. Schildt, Chewsville, MD, 1986, pp. 135.
8. Hassler, WW: Dr. Hunter Holmes McGuire: Surgeon to Stonewall Jackson, the Confederacy and the Nation. Virginia Cavalcade 32: 52-61, 1982.
9. Quinones, MA: Drug abuse during the Civil War (1861-1865). Int J Addictions 10:1007-1020, 1975.
10. Day H. The opium habit, 1968. In: Terry C, Pellens M, the OPIUM PROBLEM, Montclair, N.J., Patterson-Smith, 1970.
11. Graham M, Skoch G: GREAT BATTLES OF THE CIVIL WAR, New York, Beekman House, 1980.
12. Morton WTC: The first use of ether as an anesthetic at the Battle of the Wilderness in the Civil War (an abstract from an unpublished paper by the late WTG Morton written after the Battle of the Wilderness in May, 1864, and furnished for publication by his son, Dr. Wm. J. Morton of New York City) JAMA, April 23, 1904, 1070-1075.

SOME ORIGINAL CONTRIBUTIONS OF LATIN AMERICANS TO EPIDURAL ANESTHESIA

J. ANTONIO ALDRETE
Director, Pain Management Center and Anesthesiology
Humana Hospital — Destin, Destin, Florida, USA

Most books, chapters and reviews concerning the history of anesthetia tend to limit their information to literature sources in the English language. Though the media in this language is abundant, most of the searches come from "indexed" journals and magazines.

Since the Current Index Medicus excludes many medical publications, many valuable and original contributions made by colleagues from other-language speaking countries remain ignored. This is a sad commentary on our specialty in an era of stimultaneous translation and communication. This presentation is made with the purpose of recognizing that there is a breakdown in communications, in the hope that in the future this will be corrected.

1926, Alberto Gutierrez (Bs. As. Argentina): Described the method of "The Hanging Drop" to identify the epidural space (ES). He also noted that the distance between the skin and the ligamentum flavum (LF) could range from, 2.5 to 12.5cm, but in 80 percent of patients was between 3.5 and 5.0cm.[1]

1939, Alberto Gutierrez (Ts. As. Argentina): founded the first Anesthesia Journal called *Revista Argentina De Anesthesia,* which is still published today.

1933, L.E. Ontaneda (Bs. As. Argentina): Measured pressures at different levels of the epidural space, using an aneroid manometer. He found pressures ranging from -3 to -9cm H20.[2]

1937. Murillo Graga (Sao Paolo, Brazil): Noticed quivering of the latissimus dorsi muscle after injections of local anesthetic into the epidural space as an early sign of the onset of an epidural block. He attributed it to the entry of the cold local anesthetic solution into the ES.[3]

1943, E. De Souza (Rio de Janeiro, Brazil): Attached an inflatable balloon connected to a stopcock. which deflated at the entry of the needle into the Epidural space. This is the first description of this device, preceding its description by Sir R. Macintosh by 8 years.[4]

1945, B. De Almedia (Sao-Paolo, Brazil): Proposed a rubber band attached to a syringe. It spontaneously advanced the plunger as the needle entered the epidural space.[5]

1947, in Cuba, M. Martinez Curbelo (La Havana, Cuba): Used a ureteral catheter in the epidural space, producing continuous placed epidural anesthesia; published in *Anesthesia and Analgesia* in 1949.[6]

1933, M. Martinez Curbelo (La Havana, Cuba): Described the supraclavicular brachial plexus block done with the patient sitting up.[7]

1949, Armando Fortuna (Santos, Brazil): Reported successful epidural blocks in pediatric surgical patients.[8]

1958, Juan Nesi (Bs. As. Argentina): Pointed out that a bubble in a fluid filled syringe does not compress when a needle penetrates the ligamentum flavum.[8]

1964, F. Bustos (Bs. As. Argentina): Described the "Sign of Foam" after injecting first air, then fluid; foam exits at the hub of a needle.[9]

1967, Jose Usubiaga, Lilia Usubiaga and Jaime Wikinski, (Bs. As. Argentina): Treated post-lumbar puncture headache with saline solutions.[10] Also, they conducted an extensive review of complications of epidural and spinal anesthesia.[11] Quantitated transfer of local anesthetics from epidural space to CSF.[12] The same team also studied the placental transfer[13] and action of local anesthetics on the neuromuscualar junction.[14]

1967, Ricardo Sanchez, L. Acuna, Y. Rocha (Mexico City): Noted that when advancing epidural catheters 20 cm, 48 percent went cephalad, 33 percent coiled, 12 percent kinked and 6 percent went out of the spine.[15]

1967, R.J. Plaza-Quijada (Caracas, Venezuala): Reported the sign of the foam coming out of a catheter in the epidural space.[16]

1969, M. Llerena (Mexico City): Using a male connector of an IV tubing, then made a loop, the soft tubing was filled with water, the liquid column disappeared, when the needle penetrated the epidural space.[17]

1969, To differentiate fluid coming out of an epidural needle, Andrade injected it intradermally. If it did not produce anesthesia, it was CSF.[8]

1971, C. Castános and A. Sagarnaga (La Paz, Bolivia): Auscultated, amplified and recorded a "click" produced as the needle penetrated the ligamentum flavum.[18]

1972, D. Andrade Marcano (Maracay, Venezuala): Showed changes of pressure in the epidural space, as produced by position changes, flexion and hyperextension of the spine.[19]

1975, Anibal Galindo (Bogota, Colombia): Showed the importance of spinal root diameter in relationship to onset of epidural anesthesia and concentration of local anesthetic.[20]

References

1. Gutierrez A: Valor de la aspiracion liquida en el espacio peridural en la anesthesia peridural. Rev Circ 12: 225-30, 1933.
2. Ontaneda LE: Tension del espacio epidural. Su importancia practica en la anestesia epidural metamerica. Rev Arg. Circ. 12:588-97. 1933.1
3. Meira, DG: Irigens e evolucao da anestesiologia brasileira, Grafica Editora Arte Moderno, Rio de Janeiro, 1981.
4. De Souza E: Puncao extraduaral Tecnica de un novo sinal. Rev. Bras. Circ. 12:120, 1943.
5. Andrade Marcano D: Bibliografia anestesica Venezolana. Actas del VIII Congreso Latinoamericano y II Venezolano de Anestesiologia, 2:393-413, 1966.
6. Martinez Curbelo M: Continuous peridural segmental anesthesia by means of a ureteral catheter. Anesth Analg, 28: 1-4, 1949.
7. M. Martinez Curbelo: Nueva tecnica de la anestesia del plexo braquial: Ventajas de esta anestesia regional en cliniqea ortopedica. Rev. Med. Cubana 1933.
8. Andrade Marcano, D: Anestesia peridural in Texto de Anesthesiologia Teorico-Practica, JA Aldrete (ed). Salvat Mexicana de Ediciones, S.A. de C.V. Mexico City: Vol I 1986, P 675-756.1.
9. Bustos F: El signo de la burbuja o de la espúma en la anestesia peridural. Rev Argent Anest 24:147-50, 1964.
10. Usubiaga JE, Usubiaga LE, Brea L: Effect of saline injections on epidural and subarachnoid space pressures and relation to post spinal anesthesia headache, Anesth Analg 46:293-6, 1967.

11. Usubiaga JE: Neurologic complications after epidural anesthesia. Anesthesiology Clinics, 1:1-123, 1977.
12. Usubiaga JE, Wikinski JA, Wikinski A, et al: Transfer of local anesthetics to the subarachnoid space and mechanisms of epidural block. Anesthesiology 25:752-9, 1964.
13. Usubiaga JE et al: Passage of procaine and paramino benzoic acid across the human placenta. Am J. Obstet Gynecol 100:918-21, 1968.
14. Usubiaga JE et al: Prevention of succinylcholine fasciculation by local anesthetic agents. Anesthesiology 26:3-6, 1965.
15. Sanchez R, Acuna L, Rocha F: An analysis of the radiological visualization of the catheters placed in the epidural space. Br J. Anaesth 39:485-9, 1967.
16. Plaza-Quijada RJ: Proposicion de un signo para identificar la colocacion correcta de un cateter en el espacio peridural. Rev. Venez Anest 2:57-62, 1967.
17. Llerena M: Un recurso mas para localizar el espacio extradural. Rev. Mex. Anest 18:353-4, 1969.
18. Castanoa C, Sagarnaga A: Sinal acustico para identificacao do espacio extradural. Rev. Bras. Anest. 21:886-9, 1971.
19. Andrade Marcano D, Gutierrez H, Espinal M: Registro y modernas interpretaciones de la presion negativa del espacio peridural. Mem Congreso Venezolano Anest. p. 148-54, 1972.
20. Galindo A, Hernandez J, Benavides O, et al: Quality of spinal extradural anesthesia: The influence of spinal nerve root diameter. Br J Anaesth, 47:41-7, 1975.

SOME ORIGINAL CONTRIBUTIONS OF LATIN AMERICANS TO ANESTHESIA BEFORE 1950

J. ANTONIO ALDRETE
Director, Pain Management
Center and Anesthesiology
Humana Hospital – Destin, Destin, Florida, USA

Writing about the history of anesthesia is an ongoing process. I do not know if we will ever know the whole set of facts. But the discovery process is what makes it interesting and tantalizing. That is why I have titled this presentation, "Some Original Contributions of Latin Americans to Anesthesia (before 1950)," because certainly we do not know now all the original contributions. Surely others will be found in the future and I hope to write about them.

For the record, as of 1986, the data concerning the first anesthetic administered in some of the Latin American countries are shown on Table I. In certain instances the details are scanty, but as more interest is aroused on the history of anesthesia in each country, more precise data will be reported.[1]

It also should be noted that the first anesthetic administered during a war was in the spring of 1847 during the Mexican-American War. Barton was sent by President Polk to Vera Cruz during the American occupation of this port. Barton taught US Army Surgeons, and probably some Mexican doctors also, how to give ether to wounded soldiers.[2]

In 1866, Pacifico Pereira (Bahia, Brazil) excised a sublingual osteoma of the mandible, using as anesthesia topically sprayed ether to produce localized freezing of the mucosa and underlying tissues.[3]

In 1882, A. Restrepo (Medellin, Colombia) proposed air insufflation through a tube with alternating compressions of ribs, sternum and epigastrium and mouth-to-mouth respiration.[4]

In 1891, Teodoro Castrillón (Bogota, Colombia) wrote a thesis on "Anesthesia in Altitude." He suggested that "Anesthetic vapors (Ether or Chloroform) must be given with air or oxygen since it is already decreased at this altitude" (8000 feet). He also described the electrical stimulation of the phrenic nerves in the neck on a patient who stopped breathing twice under chloroform anesthesia for an above-the-knee amputation.[5]

In 1899, Miguel Pereija, Miguel Couto and Antonio Leao (Rio de Janeiro, Brazil) anesthetized two Siamese xiphopags, Rosalina and Maria, so the surgeon, Alvaro Ramos, could separate them. They received chloroform.[6]

In 1900, Luis F. Bernal proposed in a case of cardiac arrest during anesthesia, to: a) stop the inhaled anesthetic; b) lower the head; c) restore respiration by tracheal insufflation of pleuric nerves 7 to 10 per minute; d) restore cardiac activity (open massage of the left ventricle); e) remove any secretions from the airway; f) inject stimulants (ether, caffeine, IV); and g) administer intravenously NaCL 0.7%.[4]

In 1903, the first anesthetic record from "The Casa de Misericordia" in Rio de Janeiro was written. The patient was Christina da Costa Rezende. She received general anesthesia, sulfuric ether. The duration was 1 hour, 13 minutes. The operation was not specified.[6]

In 1914, Luis Agote (Argentina) administered the first blood transfusion with sodium citrate in precise doses to Ramon Mosquera, who was the security guard from the Rawson Hospital.[7]

In 1927, Miguel Garcia Marin (Mexico City, Mexico) investigated the use of alcohol IV in cats, dogs, chickens, turkeys and monkeys; he arrived at a precise anesthetic dose. He administered it to 53 patients undergoing surgical procedures. He also pointed out the advantages of giving IV fluids during surgery.[8]

In 1927, Livet Araya and Luis Y. Pierron (Medellin, Colombia) applied electroanesthesia by inserting scalp electrodes, then passing what they called the "Araya" current. Manipulation and drainage of abscesses were done when unconsciousness was reached.[9]

In 1934, Juan Marin (Bogota, Colombia) proposed the routine use of precordial auscultation during anesthesia to "identify arrhythmias and cardiac arrest" in children and adult patients. This is the first recommendation of this monitoring practice.[10]

In 1934, Jose C. Delorme (Argentina) assembled an anesthetic machine with vaporizers for ether, chloroform and ethyl chloride, with tanks of oxygen and carbon dioxide, as well as a soda lime canister.[7]

In 1942, Oswaldo Vital (Rio de Janeiro, Brazil) extracted tubocurare from a plant of the strychnos variety. In 1945, he produced Dimethyl ether d-tubocurarine (Chondodendron platyphyllum) in 3:1000 solutions, marketed as "Kondocurare."[6]

Others usually receive credit for bringing back intravenous regional anesthesia after the earlier reports. Though published in an American journal in 1946, L.G. Herreros (Mexico City, Mexico), a military anesthesiologist, reported 104 cases of IV regional anesthesia with procaine and tetracaine; he is seldom recognized.[11] This report was followed in 1947 by Enzo Mourigan Canale (Montevideo, Uruguay), who published his experience in 55 cases of "Local Anesthesia by the intravenous route" with 0.5 procaine.12

In 1948, Blusque Castellano, Carlos Nesi and F. De Leonardis (Argentina) mastered the technique of intravenous procaine, thiopental and meperidine, which is still used today in Argentina.[13]

References

1. Aldrete JD: *Historia de la Anestesiologia.* In: Texto de Anestesiologia Teorico – Practica J.A. Aldrete. Editorial Salvat. Mexico City. 1986 p. 11-32.
2. Aldrete JA, Marron GA, Wright AJ; The first administration of anesthesia in military surgery. On occasion of the Mexican-American War. Anesthesiology 61:585-8, 1984.
3. Gaceta Medica de Bahia, 1866.
4. Alvarez T: Anotaciones para una historia de la Anestesia y Reanimacion in Colombia. University of Antioquia, Medellin. 1984.
5. Castrillón T: Contribución al estudio de la anestesia en las alturas. Contraindicación del cloroformo en la altiplanicie de Bogotá, 1891.
6. Meira DG: Origens e evoluçao da anestesiologia brasileira. Gráfica Editora Arte Moderno, Rio de Janeiro, 1981.
7. Venturini AH, y Fuentes OA: Historia de la Anestesiologia en la Republica Argentina. Rev. Arg. Anes., 37:139-54, 1979.
8. Garcia Marin M: Anestesia con alcohol intravenoso. Tesis Professional, Universidad Nacional Autonoma de Mexico, 1929.

9. Araya L, Pierron L: La Electroanesthesia con la corriente de Araya. Labor 5: 101-6, 1927.
10. Herrera Ponton J: Historia de la anestesia en Colombia. Rev. Col. Anes., 2:155-61, 1974.
11. Herreros LG: Regional Anesthesia by the intravenous route. Anesthesiology 7:558-60, 1946.
12. Pernin A., y Vega DE: Historia de la anestesia en el Uruguay, 1981.
13. Wikinski JA, Wikinski RL, Ceraso OL et al: General anesthesia with intravenous procaine. In Aldrete JA, y Stanley TH, (eds): Trends in intravenous anesthesia. Year Book Medical Publishers, Chicago, 1980. Pags. 189-215.

TABLE I.

DATA ON FIRST ANESTHETICS GIVEN IN LATIN AMERICA

Country, City	Date	Anesthetic	Patient	Operation	Anesthetist
Argentina, Buenos Aires	8/30/1847	Ether	30yr man	Corrected strabismus	Dr. Tuksbury
Brasil, Rio de Janiero	5/20/1847	Ether	–	Medical student	Dr. Roberto Haddock Lobo
Chile, Valparaiso	10/23/1848	Chloroform	90yr woman	Amputation arm	Dr. Fco. Javier Villanueva
Colombia, Bogota	1864	Chloroform	woman	Ovariectomy	
Cuba, La Habana	3/10/1847	Ether	–	–	Dr. Vicente Antonio de Castro
Ecuador	1888	Chloroform	–	–	–
Guatemala, Guatemala City	11/30/1847	Ether	–	–	Dr. Jose Luna
Mexico, Merida, Uc.	6/15/1847	Ether	man	Amputation arm	Dr. Jose Matilde Sansores
Salvador, San Salvador	1860	Chloroform	–	–	Dr. Emilio Alvarez
Uruguay, Montevideo	5/2/1847	Ether	injured soldier	Amputation arm in 4 minutes	Dr. Patricio Ramos
Venezuela, Maracaibo	1847	Ether	man	–	Dr. Blas Valbuena

ABOUT THE PARTICIPANTS IN THE HYDERABAD CHLOROFORM COMMISSIONS (1888–1889)

MOMIN ALI and ASRIT RAMACHARI
Hyderabad, Deccan, India

Within a few years of chloroform's introduction in 1847, and for decades afterwards, fears were expressed about the inherent safety of the agent, and these fears were usually coupled with conflicting opinions about how chloroform should be most safely given.

In 1888 and 1889 the chloroform controversy was given a powerful—if not vicious—twist from an unexpected quarter, namely Hyderabad. As a result, first one, and then a second scientific investigation was set up to enquire as the First and Second Hyderabad Chloroform Commissions. They are important in the history of anaesthesia, together being one of the factors which—for decades—perpetuated the myth of chloroform's innate safety. The Commissions were discussed in detail in the third volume of Sykes' Essays on the First Hundred Years of Anaesthesia.

Hyderabad is a city virtually in the middle of the Indian subcontinent. In the days of the British Raj, it was the capital of the independent Indian princely State of Hyderabad, which, for the last 20 years of the nineteenth century was ruled over by the Nizam, Mir Mehboob Ali Khan. Since it was an important but independent State, a British Minister (nowadays called an Ambassador) was accredited to Hyderabad, and he and his staff lived and worked there at the British Residency in Hyderabad city itself.

In 1885, Surgeon-Major Edward Lawrie, of the Indian Medical Service, was posted to Hyderabad as Surgeon at the British Residency. Within a short time, the Nizam (whose family and ministers Lawrie also looked after) had appointed him as Principal of the Indian Medical School in Hyderabad, and also Surgeon to the Afzal Gunj Hospital, which was the teaching hospital for its medical students. Lawrie was devoted to his patients, to his students, to his hospital and to the medical school in Hyderabad. He worked tirelessly on their behalfs until his retirement in 1902.

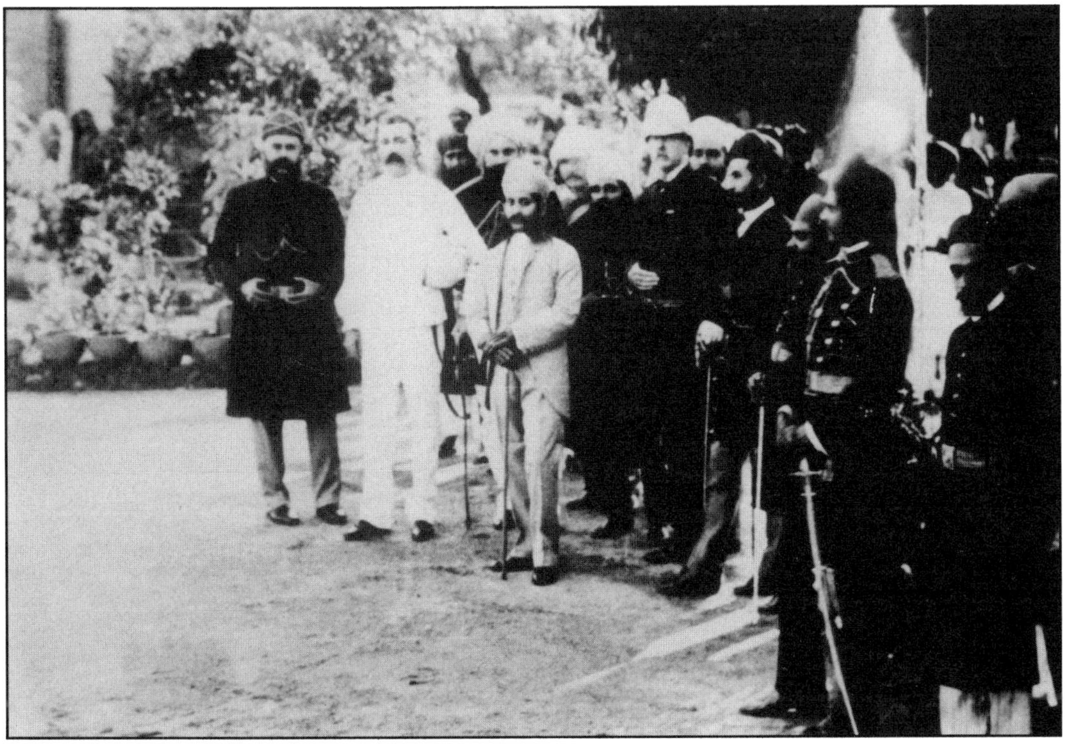

Fig. 1. The Nizam (the slightly-built figure with a cane almost in the center of the picture), the British Minister (in the pith helmet, and to the Nizam's left) and Edward Lawrie (in the white suit, and on the Nizam's right) at the Afzal Gunj Hospital in Hyderabad. They are awaiting the arrival of the Duke and Duchess of Connaught in January, 1889. Photographs such as this are to be found in the Indian National Archives in New Delhi, which is a rich and scarcely-tapped source of information about the Chloroform Commissions.

Throughout his professional life Edward Lawrie believed unswervingly in chloroform's absolute safety. He, and under his guidance, his Indian students and junior doctors, administered chloroform to thousands of patients at the Afzal Gunj Hospital. Using as an inhaler either a simple cloth or the locally-invented "Hyderabad Chloroform Cone," the mortality of chloroform given in Hyderabad (under Lawrie's autocratic direction) was negligible. Lawrie was stung by the doubts expressed in Britain about chloroform's safety, and concluded that his methods were far superior to those taught in England. He insisted that, if his method was followed, chloroform was perfectly safe. He strenuously denied that chloroform could ever cause sudden, primary cardiac standstill, and believed that any deaths which had occurred were due solely to overdose and respiratory depression.

In 1888, he persuaded the young and wealthy Nizam to pay for an animal investigation in Hyderabad, which Lawrie hoped would settle the argument once and for all. From the outset, Lawrie in his own mind equated this task with proving beyond doubt that his own view—that chloroform could do no harm—was correct.

This investigation, the First Hyderabad Chloroform Commission, was conducted by three of Lawrie's medical colleagues in Hyderabad. The President of the Commission was Patrick Hehir, a surgeon in the Indian Medical Service. He was assisted by Dr. Kelly and Dr. Chamarette. Dr. Hehir was a popular physician and author of a pamphlet on malaria and its treatment. His opinion on malaria was sought by Dr. Ronald Ross, concerning the likelihood of mosquitoes transmitting the disease. At the time of the two men's meeting (probably in India sometime between 1897 and

1898) Ross was working on malaria's spread at the British Cantonment of Secunderabad, which was adjacent to Hyderabad itself. Later, in 1902, Ross received the Nobel Prize for his work in discovering the cause of malaria. He was knighted (becoming Sir Ronald Ross) in 1911.

In 1888, the first Hyderabad Commission concluded that chloroform was entirely safe if given according to Lawrie's rules. Lawrie was reinforced in his opinion that the teaching methods of the London schools were defective, and argued that it was this that accounted for the higher chloroform mortality rate in England. Soon afterwards, Lawrie was presented with an irresistible opportunity to publicize his views more widely.

In January, 1889, the Duke and Duchess of Connaught (the Duke was one of Queen Victoria's sons) made an important and State Visit to Hyderabad. On several occasions photographs of various events were taken by the Nizam's royal photographer the renowned Rajadeen Dayal. Figure 1. shows the official reception group waiting to greet the Duke and Duchess at the Afzal Gunj Hospital. It shows, amongst others, the Nizam himself, Edward Lawrie and the British Minister.

Within a few minutes of this photograph's being taken, Edward Lawrie—in the presence of the Duke and Duchess of Connaught, at the Medical School's prizegiving—gave an address during which he once more inveighed against the London school's method of giving chloroform. It was an important occasion, and his remarks were reported in Britain by The Lancet, whose editor, nevertheless, remained unimpressed by the report and by the relative obscurity of the First Chloroform Commissioners, by whose work Lawrie set such store. Lawrie reacted by asking the Nizam to pay for an enlarged, second Commission whose members were to include an independent, eminent medical researcher to be nominated by The Lancet itself. Accordingly, the Second Hyderabad Chloroform Commission was constituted.

The members of the first commission joined in, but to add weight Lawrie himself and another of his senior colleagues in the Indian Medical Service—Surgeon Major Gerald Bomford—were also included, as was Dr. Rustomji (a Hakeem or locally trained doctor) who was the Indian Director of the Nizam's Medical Service. They were joined by Dr. Thomas Lauder Brunton.

Lauder Brunton had been chosen by The Lancet to be its independent expert, and he travelled to India (at the Nizam's expense) to join the Second Commission in its work. Brunton was an eminent physician, physiologist and pharmacologist. He was an authority on the action of drugs on the heart, and had written the then standard textbook on Therapeutics and Materia Medica. It was Brunton who had introduced amyl nitrite in the treatment of angina pectoris. Before he received The Lancet's invitation, Brunton had stated that, in his opinion, chloroform was dangerous, and that it could act directly to stop the heart.

In Hyderabad, Brunton was lavishly entertained by the Nizam's courtiers. Official receptions were given for Brunton by, amongst others, the Nizam's Prime Minister (Sir Asmanjah Bahadur) and the Revenue Minister (the Nawab Mohsin Ul Mulk). The receptions reflect the importance attached to the Second Hyderabad Chloroform Commission by the Nizam and his Ministers. The Commission was seen as a way of enhancing the medical reputation of Hyderabad.

The experimental work of the Second Hyderabad Chloroform Commission (which was led by Lawrie as its President) convinced Brunton that his previous opinion had been wrong. This was surprising, and probably owed much to Lawrie's forceful (if not bigoted) views on the subject. Nonetheless, Brunton readily agreed with the Second Commission's emphatic conclusion that chloroform was not directly injurious to the heart, and that it killed only by its effect on respiration. A complete *volte-face*.

Figure 2. shows the members of the Second Commission, together with others in Hyderabad who assisted the Commission's work. Standing between Edward Lawrie and Lauder Brunton is a lady dressed in a saree—Dr. Roopa Bai

Furdoonji. She was singled out for special mention by Lawrie in the final Report of the Hyderabad Chloroform Commissions and their work.

Lawrie encouraged Indian women to become doctors, and after they had qualified in Hyderabad arranged for some of them to receive further training in Edinburgh (the medical school from which he himself had qualified). Dr. Furdoonji later received part of her training in Edinburgh, and worked as a fulltime anesthetist at the British Residency hospital in Hyderabad. Possibly, she was the first lady physician anesthetist in the world. Dr. Furdoonji's dates of birth and death are unknown, and she was not married. However, a relative—Mr. Harmus Kausji—a historian who had worked at the Nizam's palace, and who died a few months ago at the age of 90, kept three of her original certificates. One, dating from the time of the Chloroform Commissions, is signed by Edward Lawrie as Principal of the Medical School and marks Dr. Furdoonji's attainments in Medicine. Another records her taking part in the Pathology course in Hyderabad, and a third (from the University of Edinburgh, in 1910) refers to her having passed the University's first professional examination in Chemistry.

A version of the Reports of the First and Second Hyderabad Chloroform Commissions was published in Hyderabad and, again at the Nizam's expense, copies were sent to leading medical centers and libraries throughout the world. Sir Asmanjah Bahadur (the Nizam's Prime Minister) took a keen interest in the proceedings of the Second Hyderabad Chloroform Commission. To add to their prestige, he wrote the Foreword to the Reports when they were published, in this form, in 1890.

The Nizam was a most generous benefactor of anesthesia and subscribed unstintingly to a noble cause—the underwriting of medical research into the very real and life-threatening problems associated with chloroform's use. That the Hyderabad Chloroform Commissions (for which he had made such handsome provision) failed to produce the correct answer was due to factors over which even the seemingly omnipotent Nizam held no sway. Nonetheless, the Nizam's good intentions, and the results to which they led, are an important part of the history of anesthesia.

Fig. 2. Edward Lawrie (seated, in the center) and Thomas Lauder Brunton (the bearded figure seated on Lawrie's left), together with others who assisted the work of the Second Hyderabad Chloroform Commission. Standing between Lawire and Brunton is Dr. Roopa Bai Furdoonji (see text).

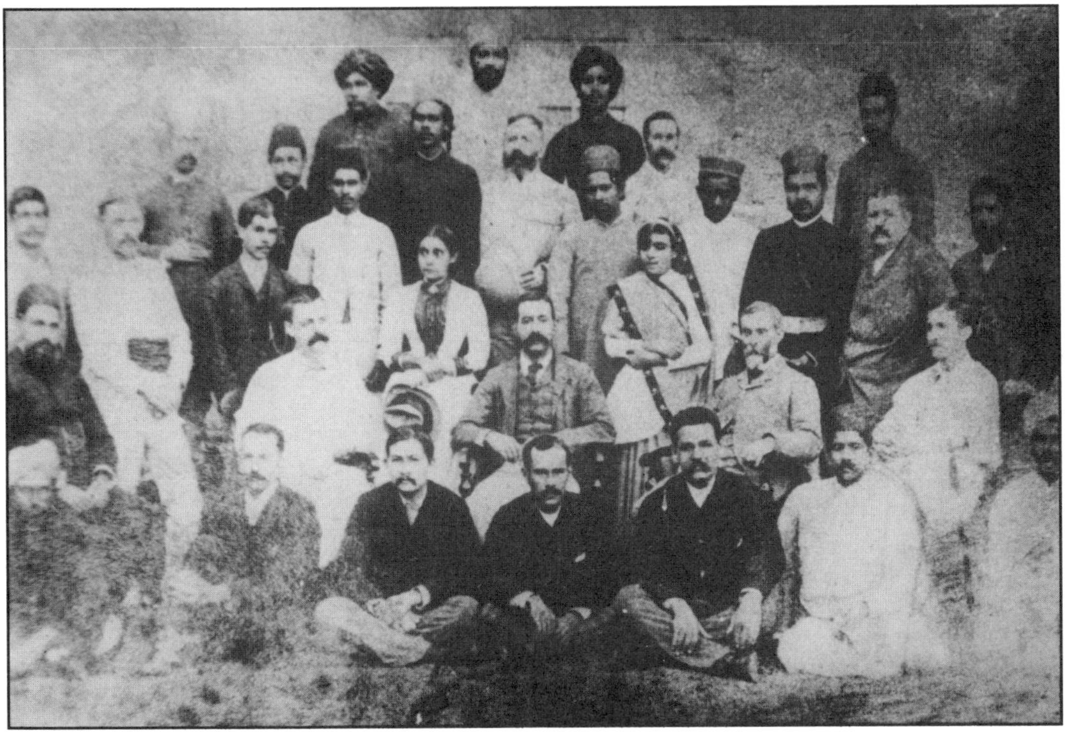

THE MERITS OF SAMUEL JAMES MELTZER AND JOHN AUER
For the Development of Apneic Oxygenation

K. AYISI and M. GOERIG***
Department of Anaesthesiology and Department of Cardiovascular Surgery***
University Hospital Hamburg, Germany

At the turn of this century, many surgeons became interested in thoracic surgery after anesthetic procedures had been improved and many hindrances no longer seemed unsurmountable. However, the overwhelming problem of pneumothorax remained unsolved.[1] Generally, it was an unwritten rule among surgeons to strictly avoid opening the chest cavity — *a noli me tangere* — was the order of the day.[2]

It was therefore not surprising that research was intensified throughout the world to find a solution. Indisputably before 1900, there were indices as to how the pneumothorax problem could be solved. Certain personalities are specifically to be remembered in this connection, such as the French research workers Eugène Louis Doyen (1859-1916), Théodore Tuffier (1857-1929), or the American surgeon Rudolph Matas (1860-1957).[1,3,4,5] The latter strongly recommended the use of the Fell-O'Dwyer (1849-1918) (1841-1891) apparatus.[6,7,8] Although their contributions were important, they did not gain general acceptance and were nearly forgotten.[9]

In Germany, the resident surgeon Ferdinand Sauerbruch (1875-1951), from the Surgical Department of the University in Breslau, which was then conducted by the outstanding Johannes von Miculicz-Radecki (1850-1905), developed the low-pressure-chamber resulting from a series of animal experiments.[10,11] This procedure became widely accepted and widespread. Ludolph Brauer (1865-1951), an internist of the University of Heidelberg at that time, developed and advocated his alternative, the so-called high-pressure technique, which appeared at the same time as Sauerbruch called attention to his procedure.[12] Sauerbruch, presenting brilliantly at congresses, vehemently rejected Brauer's method as "unphysiological".[3,10] Both techniques, however ,were feasible with expensive and complicated apparatus; but employing these in a general practice was unthinkable.[5]

The strong influence of Sauerbruch in Europe forestalled the technique of "high pressure" for many years.[10] Similarly, the technique of intubation narcosis, vehemently

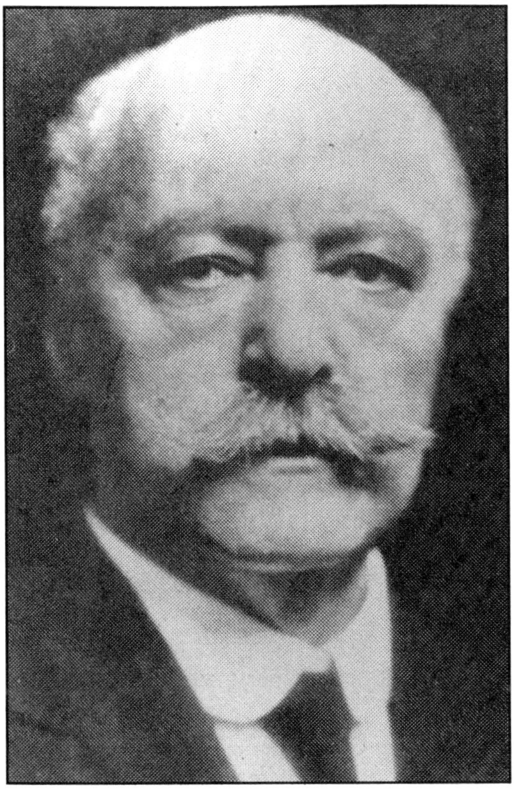

Fig. 1. Samuel James Meltzer (1851-1922)[55]

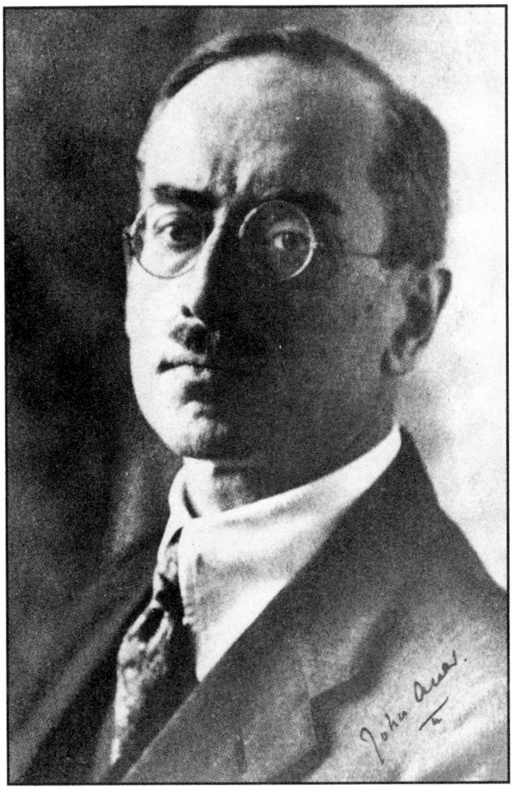

Fig. 2. John Auer (1875-1948)[23]

promoted by his German colleague, Franz Kuhn (1866-1929), met with Sauerbruch's rejection.[13,14,15,16,16]

At the time that the advantages and disadvantages of high pressure and low pressure chambers were being wrestled with at surgical congresses in Germany, two American physiologists, Samuel James Meltzer and John Auer, reported on the so-called "intratracheal insufflation technique" as a solution for the pneumothorax problem (Fig. 1, Fig. 2).[17] Both were then working at the Rockefeller Institute in New York.[18,19] Both had made detailed physiologic studies of an old procedure used for hundreds of years in animal experiments.

Biography: Samuel James Meltzer

Son of an orthodox Jew, Samuel James Meltzer was born March 22, 1851, in Trape near Kornos in Russia.[20,21,22] After completing high school in the German city of Königsberg, he started to study chemistry and then returned home, quite dissatisfied with his situation. He decided to study philosophy at the University of Berlin. For financial reasons, he gave up this plan and started medicine since this provided a more secure life. Under the lectureship of the leading physiologist at that time, Professor Hugo Kronecker, he presented his thesis in 1882. Meltzer then returned to Russia and worked for a short while as general practitioner before he decided to become a naval ship doctor on a transatlantic liner. In 1883, he settled in Harlem, New York, and worked once more as a general practitioner. On a part-time basis and bearing his own expenses, he carried out research in nearby hospitals, such as the Harlem Hospital, the Columbia Medical School and the Bellevue Hospital.

It is worth mentioning that, during the same period, the reputable pediatrician Joseph O'Dwyer was engaged with his first intubations in children at the Bellevue Hospital. Probably due to this, Meltzer became interested in this new medical field; he was looking for an alternative technique to the intubation procedure.[9] These important circumstances have never been discussed and pointed out before.

Later, Meltzer was invited by the Rockefeller Institute to take part in research in the Department of Physiology. From then until his retirement in 1919, he mainly was interested in circulation physiology and published more than 300 articles. Well-known and respected in many countries, and through his international contacts, he became the "Ambassador" of his institute.[2] Meltzer was named "one of the remarkable figures in American medicine, a brilliant investigator, a keen clinician, a scholar, author and organizer."[20] He indefatigably communicated his philosophy of life to his colleagues; the philosophy of "understand the fundamental to develop the practical."[21]

He won many awards and prizes, the highest of which should have been the Nobel prize, for which his former teacher Kronecker wanted to recommend him, but Meltzer refused. Meltzer died on November 7, 1920, a researcher who always said of himself, "Life means only the center of scientific activity."[21]

Biography: John Auer

John Auer was born March 30, 1875, in Rochester, N.Y.[23] He graduated in 1902 after medical training at the Universities of Michigan and Johns Hopkins. After a short period as house officer at Johns Hopkins, he began a research career at the Physiological Institute of the Rockefeller Foundation. Interrupted by short research terms at Harvard, he continued his research activities at the Rockefeller Institute. In 1922, he was appointed chief of the Pharmacological Institute at the St. Louis University School of Medicine. He retained this position until his death in 1948. Auer published more than 150 scientific papers related to problems concerning the heart, kidney, liver, gallbladder, digestive systems and respiratory organs. He also dealt with the phenomena of allergic related diseases and published a number of research papers in pharmacology, especially the muscle relaxant effects of magnesium. No less than his father-in-law, Meltzer, Auer received numerous awards and prizes.

A few weeks before his death, he became an honorary member of the St. Louis Society of Anesthesiologists "for his pioneering work in the field of anesthesiology." His "continued interest has proved a source of stimulation to the younger members in this field and has contributed greatly to this branch of medical science."[23]

The contributions of both Meltzer and Auer to the solutions of anesthesiologic related problems could not better be described. The following shows the concept of their intratracheal insufflation technique, and the relevance of the method, related to the background in those days, as compared to today's techniques.

The Meltzer-Auer Intratracheal Insufflation Technique

The method of intratracheal insufflation was already known to surgeons before Auer and Meltzer presented their detailed description.[1,3] It is cumbersome to argue about the first authors since the technique had been in used in animal experiments for hundreds of years. Both were performing animal experiments to study the mechanism of respiration in the presence of a double pneumothorax.[1,21] For its treatment they used the technique of Brauer using positive pressure.[17] They noticed that, "under certain conditions respiration can be carried on by rhythmical respiratory movements.[17] They were convinced of its effectiveness, as they had used curare to abolish any respiratory activity and, in spite of this, the animals survived. Primarily, both made a longitudinal slit in the trachea of the animal and then introduced a glass tube down to the tracheal bifurcation. Air "enters the trachea and reaches the bifurcation from which it returns through the space between the wall and tube." They continued to explain that it is "essential that the tube should fill out two-thirds of the lumen of the trachea, that the slit in the trachea be not too short and the pressure of the air . . . should amount to about 15 to 20 millime-

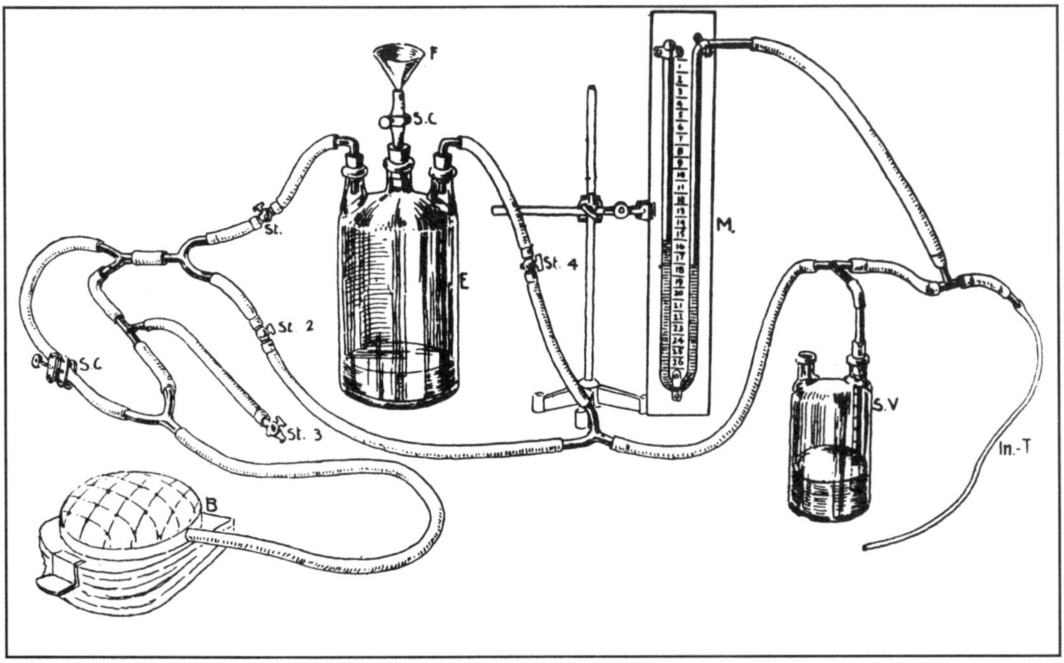

Fig. 3. Meltzer-Auer device for artificial respiration[45]

ters of mercury. Between the trachea and the pressure bottle, they interpolated a manometer, an ether bottle and a bottle with Ringer's solution to keep the mucous membrane of the trachea moist. When the air is thus circulating through the trachea the diaphragm descends, the thorax becomes moderately distended and the respiration mostly becomes very slow. . . . If the above described arrangement is carried out properly, the lungs retain their pink colour and the heart continues to beat regularly and efficiently for many hours (Fig. 3).[17] It is worth mentioning that both did not expressly hint that the insufflation of the air had to be interrupted every minute, thus allowing the lungs to collapse and to ensure an adequate removal of carbon dioxide.

Priority Discussions

The German surgeon, Franz Kuhn, reclaimed the priority of the insufflation technique, suggesting a similar technique, in which another smaller catheter should be inserted within the already positioned tracheal tube (Fig. 4a, 4b).[16,24,25] Especially for treatment of acute airway obstruction in emergency situations, Kuhn also saw many indications for the system, as optimal oxygenation, as well as an effective removal of carbon-dioxide, became possible.[25] Meltzer and Kuhn discussed their techniques in several articles, and it was Meltzer who questioned the efficacy of Kuhn's device.[26,27] Retrospectively, Meltzer's doubts were wrong.

First Clinical Realizations

It seems that the French surgeons, Lucien Barthélemy (1881-1949) and Marcel Dufour in Nancy, were the first to apply the intratracheal insufflation technique in humans in 1907. After digital intubation of the trachea with a thin catheter, chloroform was blown out of a Vernon-Harcourt Inhalator into the lungs.[28]

In 1909, new publications of successful insufflation anesthesia were published by the American neuro- and thoracic surgeon, Charles Elsberg (1871-1948), who had briefly worked at the surgical Department in Breslau under Johannes von Miculicz (1850-1905).[29,30,31,32] After detailed animal experiments in close association with Meltzer and Auer, Elsberg

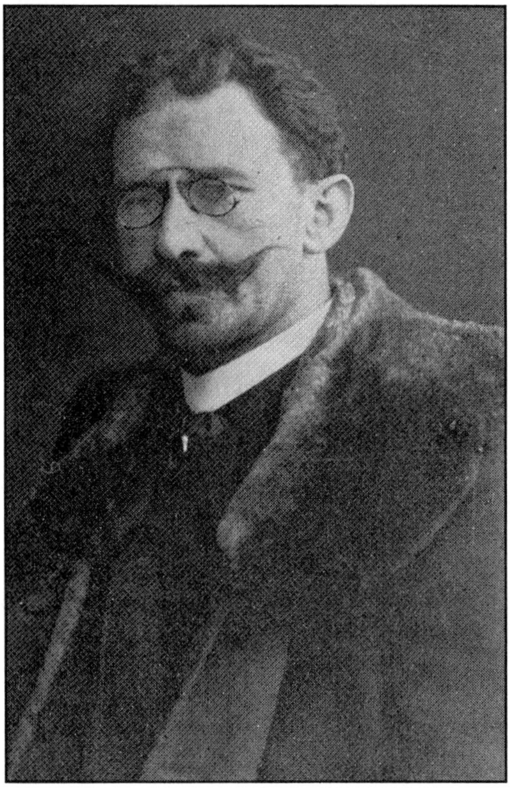

Fig. 4a. Franz Kuhn (1866-1929)[56]

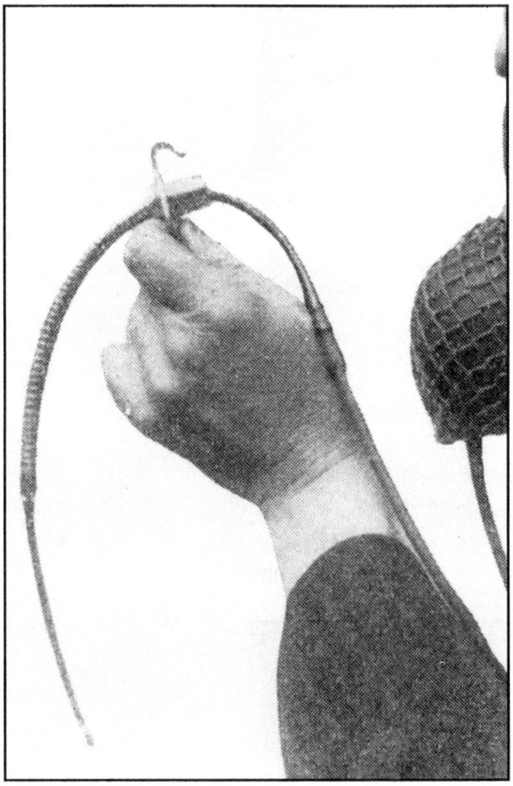

Fig. 4b. Scheme of Franz Kuhn's device[24]

applied the insufflation technique in a female patient with myasthenia gravis and he was able to insufflate her for hours before she died.[31,32] Motivated by this instance, he carried out intrathoracic surgery, exclusively using the insufflation method. A special insufflation apparatus was used to maintain a constant pressure with a maximum of 30 mm mercury, especially at the end of the operation, to close the pleural leaves.[32] In later years, many authors reported on the advantages of this method in pulmonary surgery.[33] Interestingly enough, the method was successfully used at that time to close a lung fistula, a technique not unusual today.[33] Repeatedly, reports were published on the low incidence of postoperative pulmonary infections when the insufflation technique had been used. Other authors saw a lower incidence of shock intraoperatively when using the method.[33] From today's point of view, this is difficult to understand. Probably, the main reason for these observed beneficial phenomena was the strict control of patients perioperatively, so that any acute obstruction of the respiratory tract could immediately be detected. Many other authors reported on the successful application of the technique in surgery.[34-41]

The German surgeon, Max Tiegel (1877-1952), even appealed for a wider scope of indications, to include cases of head injuries and in any airway obstruction through aspiration or membranes as in diphtheria.[42] By inserting the catheter deep enough, according to his observation, one could easily remove the obstructing foreign bodies. Tiegel went further and recommended the method in patients with tracheal stenosis caused by struma.[42]

Naturally, there were voices warning against the insufflation technique, especially of the dangers of traumatic injuries to the larynx and trachea.[16] Rupture of the lung, with the development of associated emphysema,

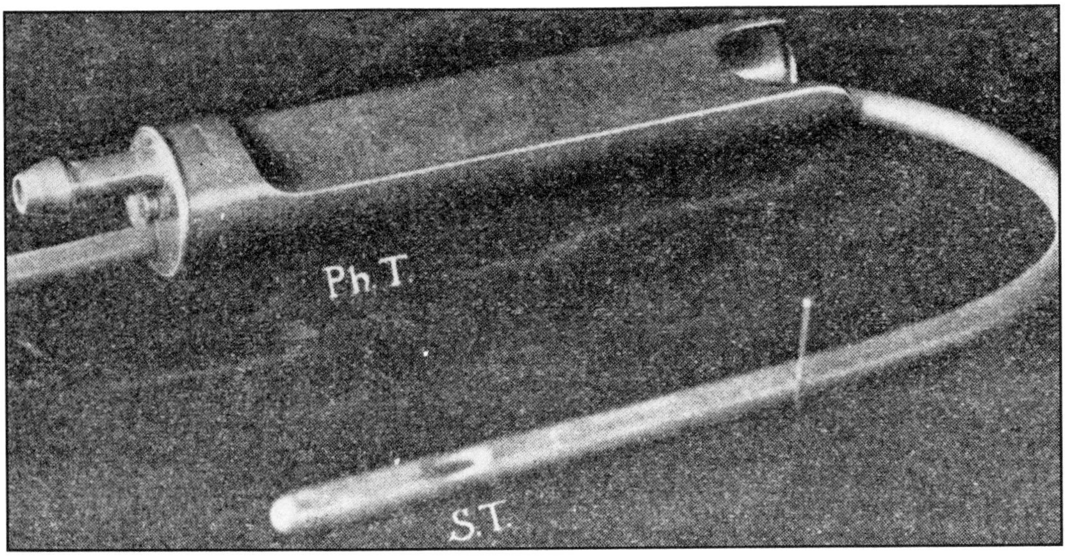

Fig. 5a. Meltzer's pharyngeal tube[46]

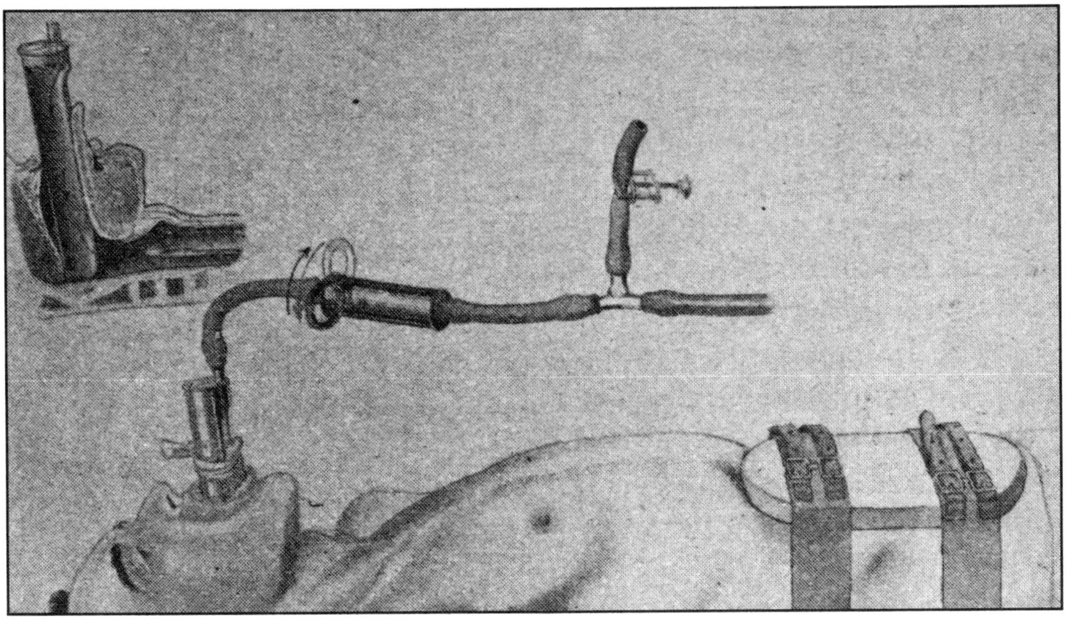

Fig. 5b Meltzer's pharyngeal tube *in situ*[46]

prompted others to appeal for cautious intubation, a fact which reflects on the lack of experience in those days with the atraumatic insertion of catheters into the trachea.[43] Usually ENT specialists did the intubations.[44] Meltzer recognized these mishaps and thought of a new technique, that of pharyngeal insufflation (Fig. 5a, 5b).[45,46]

Shortly after the detailed description of the intratracheal insufflation method was published, several types of apparatus were developed for its purpose (Fig. 6a, 6b).[47-52] In spite of the great difficulties involved with the positioning of the endotracheal catheter, the technique became widespread in a short period. In Europe, the method was received with skepticism, which

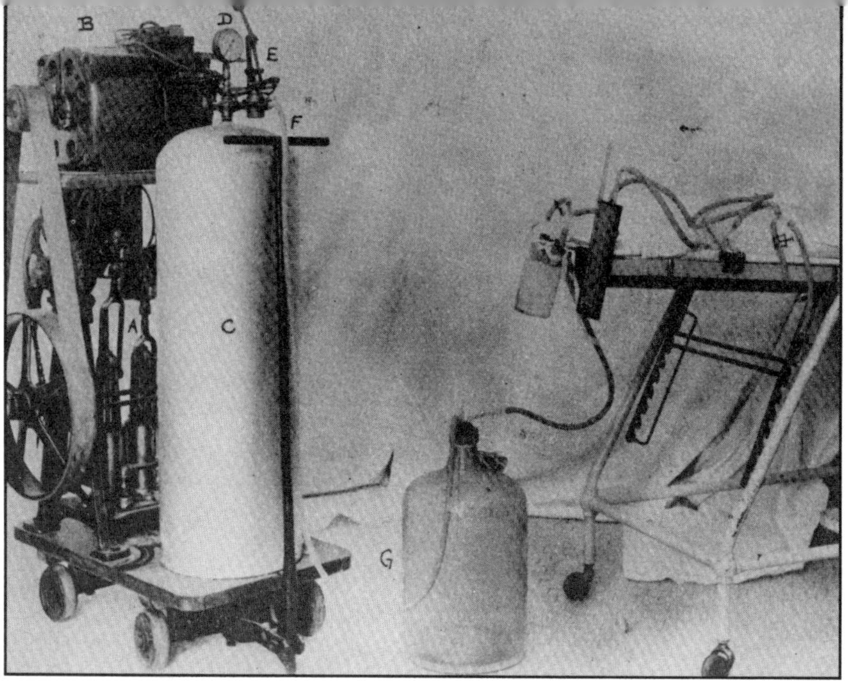

Fig. 6a. Elsberg's apparatus[31]

certainly was the result of the wrestling between the Sauerbruch and Brauer.[33] In the German literature, the technique was seldom mentioned and rarely applied, though thousands of surgical procedures were being carried out with it in the U.S. This reserved appraisal was intensified when the German surgeon, Carl Hirschmann, published his results of a study in which he had compared the effectiveness of the Meltzer-Auer insufflation method with other anesthesia techniques, from the point of blood-gas analysis.[53] He was able to demonstrate that the method of the American physiologists was ineffective for the removal of carbon dioxide when the patient had no spontaneous respiration. He was convinced that, especially for longer operations, the suggested interruptions of the insufflation were absolutely ineffective for the ventilation, resulting in a remarkable increase of carbon dioxide. Altogether, he saw many problems with the intratracheal insufflation technique and pleaded for the conventional anesthesia methods.

It should be noted that the insufflation technique is nowadays often used in combination with modern apparatus. The injector technique, firstly described by Sanders in 1967, is a modern derivation of the method described by Meltzer and Auer.[54]

The Meltzer-Auer insufflation technique had become an integral part of the

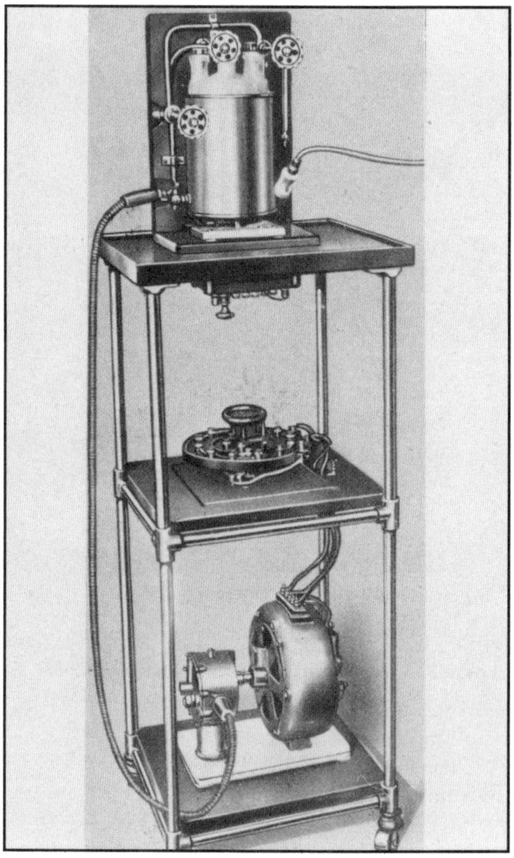

Fig. 6b. Robinson's device[50]

anesthesiologic "armamentarium anesthesiae" and that is why it is still successfully used.

References

1. Rendell-Baker L: History of thoracic surgery. In: Mushin WW; Rendell-Baker L, eds. The Principles of Thoracic Anaesthesia Past and Present. Oxford: Blackwell Scientific Publications, 1953.
2. Neugebauer J: Weltruhm deutscher Chirurgie – Johann von Miculicz. Haug Verlag, Ulm/Donau 1964.
3. Kieser F: Die Persönlichkeit und das Wirken Franz Kuhns. (Unter besonderer Berücksichtigung seiner Arbeiten zur Entwicklung der Intubationsnarkose.) med. Dissertion, University Düsseldorf 1964.
4. Fell GE: The Value of Forced Artificial Respiration (Fell-Method) in Life in Chloroform, Ether and Nitrous Oxide Narcosis. Together with an Account of a Remarkable Case, in which it was used for Three Days and Nights upon a Physician, Resulting in Saving his Life. Med Record, Philadelphia, Pa, May 30; 760, 1899.
5. Goerig M, Filos K, Ayisi K: George Edward Fell and the development of respiratory machines. In: The History of Anaesthesia. (1989) Ed. R.S. Atkinson and Th. B. Boulton: International Congress and Symposium Series Number 134 – The Parthenon Publishing Group, Carnforth, UK and New Jersey, USA 386.
6. Wiedemann K, Fleischer E: Zur Geschichte der Anästhesie in der Thoraxchirurgie. Pneumothoraxproblem, Intubation, Einlungenventilation. Anästh. Intensivmed. Notfallmed. Schmerztherapie 1:3, 1992.
7. Matas R: Intralaryngeal insufflation for the relief of acute surgical pneumothorax. Its history and methods with a description of latest devices for this purpose. JAMA 2:1468, 1900.
8. Ochsner A: In Memoriam: Rudolph Matas (1860-1957). J Thorac Surg 36:621, 1958.
9. Goerig M, Filos K, Renz D: Joseph O'Dwyer – Ein Wegbereiter der endotrachealen Intubation und Druckbeatmung. Anästh Intensivmed Notfallmed 5:244, 1988.
10. Nissen R: Erlebtes aus der Thoraxchirurgie. Thieme Verlag, Stuttgart 1955.
11. Sauerbruch F: Zur Pathologie des offenen Pneumothorax und die Grundlage meines Verfahrens zu seiner Ausschaltung. Mitt Grenzgeb Med Chir XIII: 399, 1904.
12. Brauer L, Petersen W: Über eine wesentliche Vereinfachung der künstlichen Atmung nach Sauerbruch. Hoppe Seyler's Zschr 41:299, 1904.
13. Kuhn Fr: Die Überdrucknarkose mittels peroraler Intubation. Zbl f Chir 42:1177, 1904.
14. Kuhn Fr: Lungenüberdruck mittels peroraler Intubation und kontinuierlicher Luftpuffung in dem Intubationsrohr. Zbl f Chir 26:788, 1908.
15. Sweeny B: Franz Kuhn. Anaesthesia 40:1000, 1985.
16. Goerig M: Franz Kuhn (1866-1929) zum 125. Geburtstag. Anästh Intensivmed Notfallmed Schmerztherapie 8:416, 1991.
17. Meltzer S, Auer J: Continuous Respiration without Respiratory Movements. J Exp Med 11:622, 1909.
18. Galishoff S, SA Meltzer, In: Dictionary of American Medical Biography. Vol II, ed. Martin Kaufman, Stuart Galishoff, Todd L. Savitt, Greenwood Press, Westport, Connecticut, London, England.
19. Galishoff S, John Auer, In: Dictionary of American Medical Biography. Vol II, ed. Martin Kaufman, Stuart Galishoff, Todd L. Savitt, Greenwood Press, Westport, Connecticut, London, England.
20. Kagan SA: Samuel James Meltzer (1851-1920). Med Rec 150:243, 1939.
21. Meltzer A: Dr. Samuel James Meltzer: Physiologist of the Rockefeller Institute. In: American Jewish Archives. Vol XLII, Spring/Summer 1990, NO. 1 Ed. J.R. Marcus. Hebrew Union College-Jewish Institute of Religion.
22. Meltzer A: Dr. Samuel James Meltzer and intratracheal anesthesia. J Clin Anesth 2:54, 1900.
23. Roth GB: John Auer 1875-1948. J Pharmacol Exper Therap 95:285, 1949.
24. Kuhn Fr: Lungenüberdruck mittels peroraler Intubation und kontinuierlicher Luftpuffung in dem Intubationsrohr. Zbl f Chir 26:788, 1908.
25. Kuhn Fr: Meltzer's Verfahren und die perorale Intubation. Zbl f Chir 3:73, 1912.
26. Kuhn Fr: Meltzer's Insufflation und meine perorale Intubation. Bln klin Wochenschr 38:1769, 1910.
27. Meltzer SJ: Erwiderung zu vorstehenden Bemerkungen des Herrn Kuhn. Bln klin Wochenschr 38:1770, 1910.
28. Barthélemy RL, Dufour M: L'Anesthésie dans la chirurgie de la face. Presse méd 15:474, 1907.
29. Alexander E: Charles Albert Elsberg, M.D. (1871-1948): Father of Spinal Surgery. Neurosurgery 20: 5:811, 1987.

30.
31. Elsberg CA: Zur Narkose beim Menschen mittelst der kontinuierlichen intratrachealen Insufflation von Meltzer. Bln klin Wochenschr 21:957, 1910.
32. Elsberg CA: Erfahrungen in der Thorax-Chirurgie mit der intratrachealen Insufflation von Luft und Aether. (Meltzer-Auer), mit Bemerkungen über den Werth dieser Methode für die allgemeine Chirurgie. Langenbeck's Arch f klin Chir XCVI:57, 1911.
33. Haberland HFO: Die Auer-Meltzer'sche intratracheale Insufflation. Ergeb Chir U Orthopäd 20:443, 1918.
34. Carrel A: Experimentelle intrathorakale Chirurgie mittels der Methode von Meltzer und Auer. Bln klin Wochenschr 47:565, 1910.
35. Fraenkel A, Körte W: Der gegenwärtige Stand der Lungenchirurgie. Bln klin Wochenschr 7:289, 1912.
36. Gelinskiy: Künstliche Atmung bei intrathorakalen Eingriffen. Bln klin Wochenschr 45:2093, 1913.
37. Lilienthal H, Elsberg CA: Erfahrungen am Menschen mit der Methode der intratrachealen Insufflation (Meltzer). Bln klin Wochenschr 21:958, 1910.
38. Lilienthal H, Elsberg CA: Erfahrungen am Menschen mit der Methode der intratrachealen Insufflation (Meltzer). Bln klin Wochenschr 21:958, 1910.
39. Nordmann O: Experimentelle Studien über die Thymusdrüse nebst Bemerkungen zu der Meltzer'schen intratrachealen Insufflation. Arch klin Chir 92:946, 1910.
40. Unger E: Zur Insufflationsnarkose (Meltzer) biem Menschen. Bln klin Wochenschr 2:1748, 1910.
41. Unger E, Bettmann M: Experimente zur Bekämpfung der Athemlähmung bei Gehirnoperationen mittels Meltzer's Insufflation. Arch f klin Chir 99:118, 1912.
42. Tiegel M: Der Wert der trachealen Insufflation für die Nachbehandlung Tracheotomierter. Zbl f Chir 40:1364, 1911.
43. Luke H: A case of extensive subcutaneous emphysema following intratracheal anesthesia, with recovery. Surg Gynecol Obstet 16:204, 1913.
44. Rendell-Baker L: Historical Background to Automatic Ventilation. In Mushin, W. W., Rendell-Baker, L., Thompson, P.W., Mapleson, W.W. Automatic Ventilation of the Lungs. Blackwell Scientific Publications, Oxford.
45. Meltzer SJ: Der gegenwärtige Stand der intratrachealen Insufflation. Bln klin Wochenschr 15:677, 1914.
46. Meltzer SJ: Pharyngeale Insufflation, ein einfacher Apparat für künstliche Atmung am Menschen; nebst Bemerkungen über andere Methoden der künstlichen Atmung. Bln klin Wochenschr 17:425, 1915.
47. Meltzer SJ: Simple devices for effective artificial respiration in emergencies, JAMA 60:1407, 1910.
48. Meltzer SJ: The value of continuous intratracheal insufflation of Air (Meltzer) in thoracic surgery, with description of an apparatus. Med Rec 77:493, 1910.
49. Fischer H; The continuous intratracheal insufflation (Meltzer-Auer) in intrathoracic operations in the human subject with description of an apparatus. Surg Gynecol Obstet 13:566,1911.
50. Robinson S: An apparatus for thoracic surgery under intratracheal insufflation or positive pressure; also for ether-anesthesia by mask, intrapharyngeal, intratracheal, and intrabuccal methods. Surg Gynecol Obstet 14:462, 1912.
51. Nordmann O: Thoraxwandresektion mit Melzerscher Insufflation. Dtsch med Wochenschr 8:360, 1913.
52. Cohen I, Cotton FJ, Boothby WM: Anesthesia by intratracheal insufflation. Surg Gynecol Obstet 13:572, 1913.
53. Hirschmann C: Der Charakter de Auer-Meltzer'schen intratrachealen Insufflationsnarkose nach blutgasanalytischen Untersuchungen. Bruns Beitr klin Chir 137:248, 1926.
54. Heijman K, Heijman L, Jonson A et al: High frequency positive pressure ventilation during anesthesia and routine surgery in man. Acta Anaesth Scand 16:176, 1972.

ONE HUNDRED THIRTY-FOUR YEARS OF EVOLUTION
The Buffalo General Hospital Anesthesia Experience

DOUGLAS R. BACON and RICHARD N. TERRY***
**Clinical Professor Emeritus SUNY at Buffalo*
***Assistant Professor of Anesthesiology SUNY at Buffalo, N.Y., USA*

In the corner of High and Elm Streets in Buffalo, New York the Buffalo General Hospital has stood since its dedication by former President Millard Fillmore on 24 June 1858. Buffalo's rail and water connections made the city a gateway on the Westward migration; merchants within the city were prosperous. Philanthropically, these canal trade businessmen as a reaction to the cholera epidemic of 1852[1] conceived and built the hospital from private contributions for the care of the indigent. A site was chosen near the then city limits, in the country air overlooking the harbor and the Western terminus of the Erie barge Canal. The new hospital (Fig. 1) was quickly integrated into the ten year old medical school. By 1869, the *Medical School Bulletin* would advertise that the "Buffalo General Hospital, which is but a few minutes walk from the college, will be open for clinical instruction."[2]

The Buffalo General has never known surgery without anesthesia. Yet, a study for anesthetics and anesthesia personnel serves as a microcosm of how anesthesia has evolved within teaching hospital in the United States. Influences are traced, from interns to nurses, to anesthesiologists, heard over the din of the surgeons' bellow for more "professional" anesthesia. Broadly, anesthesia at Buffalo General can be broken into four eras, by practitioners: interns, junior surgeons, nurses, anesthesiologists (Fig. 2). Along with these evolutionary personnel changes, the surgical case load has increased dramatically; from 19 cases a year in 1860 to over 20,000 in 1990 (Fig. 3).

Beginning with the first physician specialists, there have been five chairmen of a Department of Anesthesia: John Henry Evans, Paul W. Searles, Clarence J. Durshordwe, Richard N. Terry and Marcos M. Viguera. Parallelling the professionalization of anesthesia, case complexity has increased from simple incision and drainage of abscesses to heart transplantation. One hundred thirty-four years have witnessed enormous changes in anesthesia, and consequently immense transformations in the practice of surgery.

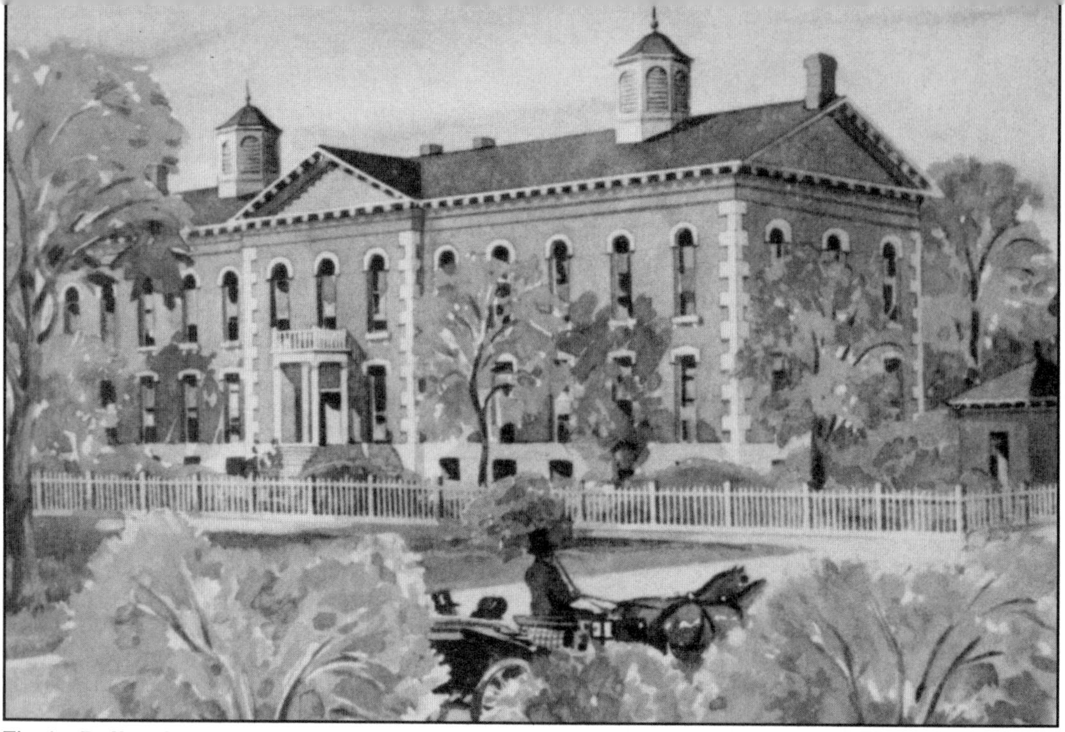

Fig. 1. Buffalo General Hospital *circa* 1865.

The Intern Era

The giving of anesthetics was often relegated to the least experienced physician practitioner. "Putting the patient to sleep" was considered far too simple a task to warrant the attention of an attending physician.[3] Although his first priority was riding the hospital's ambulance, the intern was given the responsibility of anesthetizing patients for surgery. Often poorly trained, for it would not be until 1913 that the Medical School in Buffalo would appoint faculty to address the issue of teaching anesthesia in the curriculum,[4] interns often could not create within the patient conditions conducive to prolonged surgery.

Addressing the problem of poor anesthetic care, the Buffalo General Hospital decided that the combination of overwork and lack of exercise affected the interns ability to properly anesthetize patients. A tennis court was built on hospital grounds with the objective of providing both exercise and a release from the pressures of internship. While surgeons' complaints concerning anesthesia did not diminish,[5] the patients objected to the noise created.

While to the operator and patient the anesthetic was of prime importance, surgical cases were not a large part of the hospital's activity. In 1860, the first year that surgical

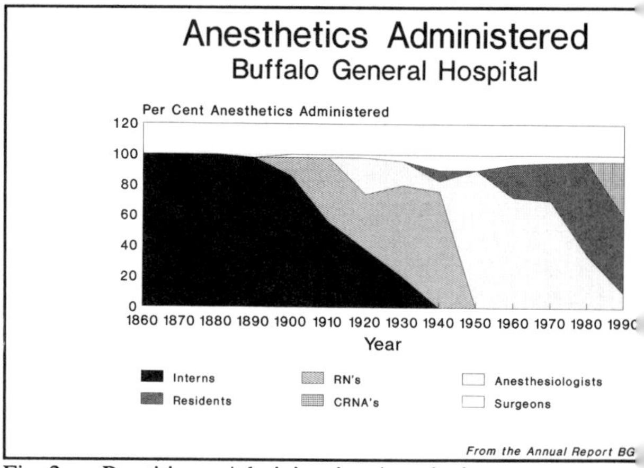

Fig. 2. Practitioner Administering Anesthetic, Buffalo General Hospital.

Fig. 3. Number of Anesthetics Buffalo General Hospital.

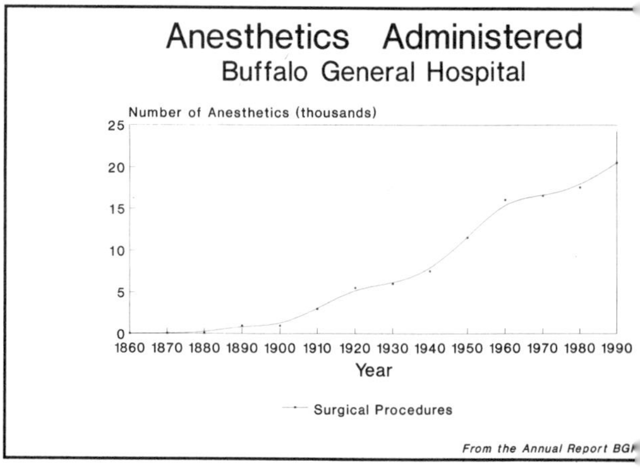

operations are recorded, 19 cases were performed. Twenty years later, in 1880, the case load had increased to 62 operations per year, an insufficient number for interns to achieve proficiency in the administration of ether. In 1883, there were 176 operations. The following year, 1884, which heralded the arrival of the renowned surgeon from Rush Medical Center in Chicago, Dr. Roswell Park, the case load rocketed to 217 operations.[6]

The Era of the Surgeon

The arrival of Roswell Park to the Buffalo General Hospital (BGH) in 1884 is pivotal to the anesthesia story. Trained at Rush Medical Center in Chicago, Park was devoted not only to surgery, but to improving the anesthetic care at the hospital, as well as scientific investigation within the specialty. Park's influence was immediately felt. He believed that young surgeons could learn at the head of the table, and consequently he set his junior staff to coach the interns giving anesthetics. Now, for the first time, there was someone senior in experience to help guide interns through the administration of an anesthetic.[7]

Secondly, with his appointment as Chairman of the Department of Surgery at the University of Buffalo School of Medicine, he began teaching medical students anesthetic techniques. Park often administered spinal anesthetics on his own patients.[8] Additionally, he published a monograph, the "Introduction of ether as an Anesthetic Agent," in 1896.[9]

Thirdly, Dr. Park increased the surgical case load at the hospital. Within three years of his arrival Buffalo General, for the first time, averaged one anesthetic per day. Eleven years after his Buffalo arrival, by 1895, an average of two surgical cases were done each day. Given his insistence on supervision, interns now had instruction in anesthetic technique. However, Park's extended surgical schedule also began to overwhelm the housestaff. By 1900, restless surgeons began to look to nurses to give their anesthetics, at the suggestion of Cleveland's Dr. George Crile when he was visiting Dr. Park.[10]

Enter the Nurse

The introduction of nurse anesthesia occurred concomitantly with both the advent of physician anesthesiologists, and the increased surgical volume. Not only did the number of surgical cases increase, but also the number of surgeons. Anesthesia demand exceeded the housestaff availability; its members could not cover their other responsibilities and give all the anesthetics. By the turn of the century, nurses were giving approximately 15 percent of the surgical anesthetics.[11]

Between 1900 and 1950, nurses were responsible for approximately 60 to 70 percent of all the anesthetics given. Indeed, these self-trained nurses were among the pioneers of their field. The nurses were called to give anesthetics for the surgeons' private patients, (house cases were the interns responsibility) and were responsible only to them. They billed independently, however.[12] By the late 1930s, these nurses were in the forefront of their professional society. In 1943, the American Association of Nurse anesthetists met at the Statler Hotel in Buffalo. Miss Dobbie, longtime nurse anaesthetist at BGH was one of the hosts.[13]

By 1950, anesthesiologists returning from military service began to assume a larger role giving anesthetics. These physicians established a residency training program, and, with the advent of group practice for anesthesiologists, nurses were gradually phased out by attrition. It was the opinion of the anesthesiologists that every patient deserved the services of a residency-trained anesthesiologist. Surgeons shared this view, for their cases had to be scheduled around the chronically understaffed anesthesia department. However, in 1980, the Buffalo General merged with the financially troubled Buffalo Deaconess Hospital, and the two anesthesia departments likewise combined. The long established CRNAs of the Deaconess group were welcomed at the Buffalo General as part of the merger agreement, and since have been responsible, under anesthesiologists supervision, for approximately forty percent of

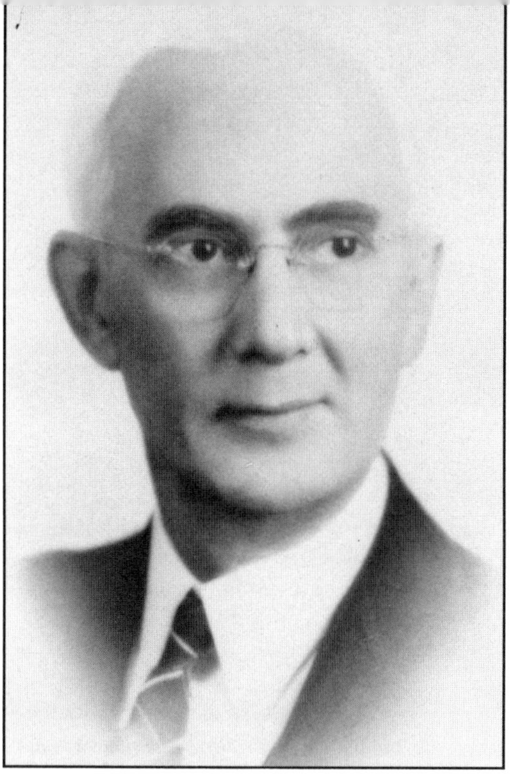

Fig. 4. John Henry Evans, M.D. (Photograph courtesy of the Buffalo General Hospital).

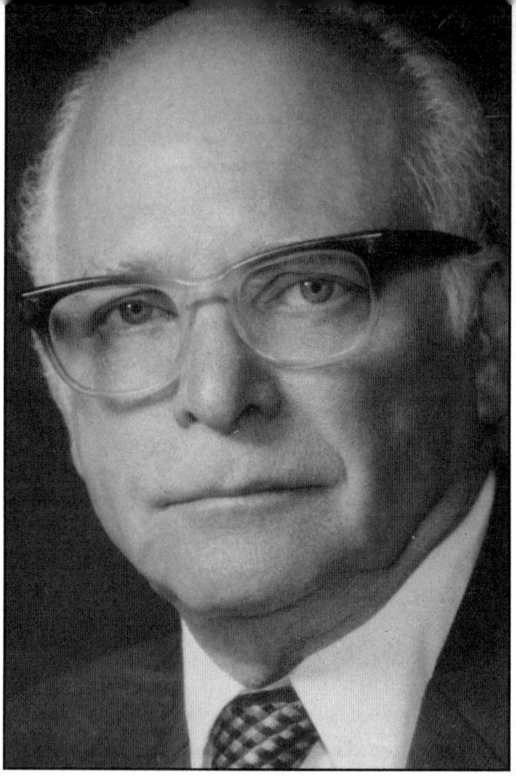

Fig. 5. Paul W. Searles, M.D. (Photograph courtesy of the Searles family).

the anesthetics given at the hospital, since the increased surgical load could not be sustained without the CRNAs' efforts.[14]

The Coming of the Anesthesiologist

Shortly before his death, Roswell Park arranged for the first physician specialists in anesthesia to begin practice at the Buffalo General Hospital. Grace Elmendorf and John Henry Evans (Fig. 4) began work in 1913. Additionally, Dr. Park arranged for Dr. Evans to become the first paid faculty member at the University of Buffalo School of Medicine. Slowly, under Dr. Evans guidance, the Department of Anesthesia emerged. By 1937, a residency training program was established, directed by Dr. Evans and his partner, Dr. Durshordwe.15

In 1937, Dr. Evans was replaced as Chairman by a Mayo Clinic residency trained physician, Paul W. Searles (Fig. 5). This heralded a major shift in philosophy, from self-trained to physicians with formal graduate training in anesthesia. Searles brought the astonishing new intravenous anesthetic thiopental with him from the Mayo Clinic. He soon inaugurated blood banking to the Buffalo General. Searles continued the strong link with the medical school, playing the dual role of University Chairman and Department head at the Buffalo General.

Before Searles had the chance to imprint his style upon the Hospital he entered military service. The hospital relied upon Dr. Evans in Searles' absence. When the war was over, Searles headed to another local hospital, taking the chair of the University Department with him.[16] Dr. Durshordwe (Fig. 6) assumed the leadership of matters anesthetic at the General. The residency swelled with the return of physicians from service, and many of the Armed Forces anesthesiologists completed their training at Buffalo General.

The 1950's witnessed a most startling revolution in anesthetic management. Succinylcholine, the new profound muscle relaxant, for the first time enabled routine endotracheal intubation of patients and also introduced the need for mechanical ventilation. The development of profound muscle relaxation and mechanical ventilation extended the range of surgical candidates both chronologically and anatomically. Those patients too old or infirm to have surgery before soon began to make their

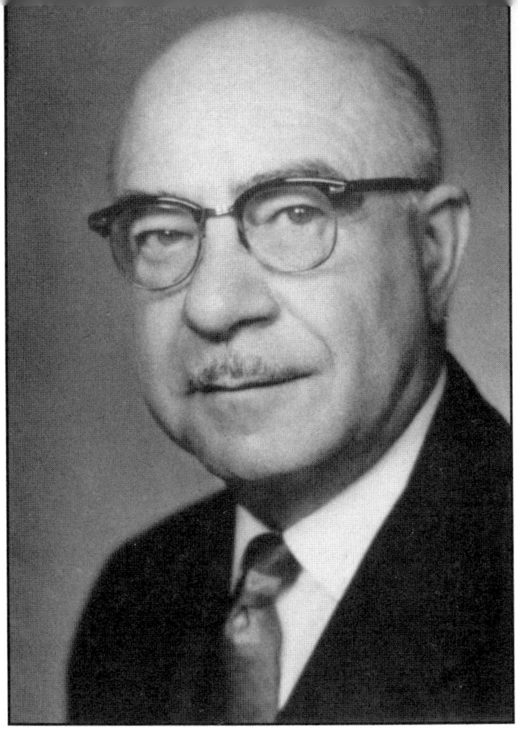

Fig. 6. Clarence Durshordwe, M.D. (Photograph courtesy of the Buffalo General Hospital).

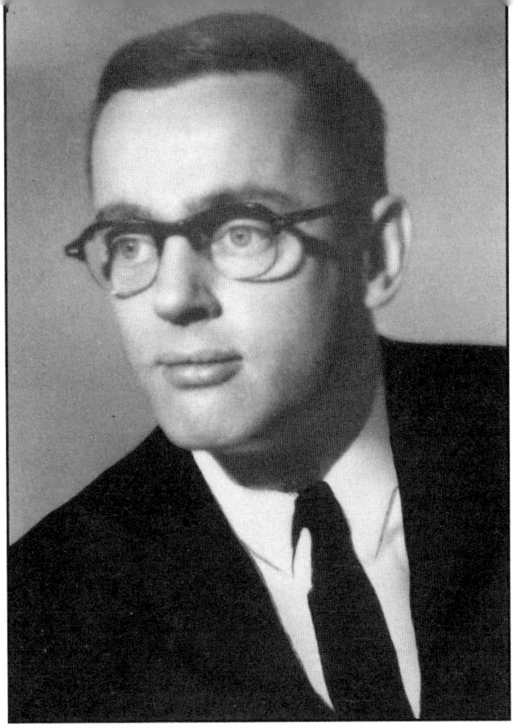

Fig. 7. Richard N. Terry, M.D. (Photograph courtesy of the Buffalo General Hospital).

way into the operating room.

In the early fifties three other profound changes occurred at the Buffalo General. First, Dr. Durshordwe stepped down as chief, and Dr. Richard Terry (Fig. 7) assumed the mantel of command. He began restructuring the department, and created the first organized residency program. Secondly, the volume of surgical cases, ever increasing pushed the anesthesiologists to change their mode of practice. No longer tethered to one surgeon, they formed a group, Buffalo Anesthesia Associates, to provide adequate day and night coverage to both BGH and Buffalo Children's Hospital.

Finally, in 1956, halothane, a revolutionary new inhalation agent was introduced into clinical practice and effectively ended the "tyranny" of the explosion hazard. Additionally, this agent provided a pleasant, smooth induction free from coughing, retching and vomiting combined with a reduced incidence of postoperative nausea and vomiting. Replacing explosive anesthetic agents, halothane permitted the employment of electrical apparatus safely in the operating room, and EKG monitoring slowly became standard. Surgeons were free to use electrocautery with abandon.

Yet, as the story of many innovations ends, the misfortune of halothane hepatitis struck the Buffalo General. An important member of the community was anesthetized for breast surgery. With no known medical or chemical problems, she died on the fourth postoperative day in overt liver failure. During a discussion of the case, a physician attributed the death to the agent, citing similarities to chloroform — both halogenated agents presumably metabolized in the liver. A second case shortly after the first caused the agent to be banned from the operating suite, despite the lack of a plausible explanation for the liver failure. Three agents were used to replace halothane with no increase in electrical hazards — nitrous oxide, meperidine and curare. This "new" method was soon also condemned for there was a substantial number of patients who recalled parts of their operations despite what appeared to be adequate anesthesia.

The 1960's were a period of growth for both the anesthesiologists (Fig. 8) at the Buffalo General and the hospital itself. Clinical practice demanded anesthesiologists at various locations, and even with imaginative scheduling and compromise the department barely managed to cover all but the obstetric suite consistently. Obstetric residents, supervised by the

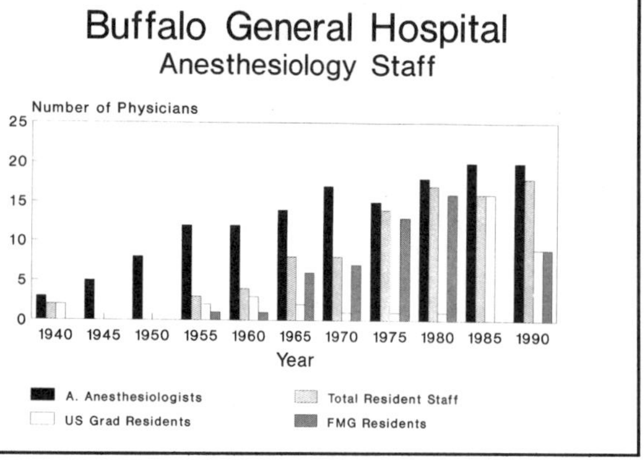

Fig. 8. Buffalo General Hospital Anesthesiology Staff.

Anesthesiology staff, provided a temporary solution, although much to the anxiety of the Medical Board of Trustees. During their unpaid laboratory rotation, supplemental income could be earned by the residents for providing anesthesia for the obstetrical patients. Proficiency gained during this period proved helpful to the young obstetrician on completion of his training, as several local hospitals could not provide obstetric anesthesia services. Junior attending obstetricians entering practice gave anesthetics to support themselves, often with heart in hand.[17]

The 1960s also witnessed the rise of the political influence of the Buffalo General anesthesiologists. Richard Ament became the third Buffalo anesthesiologist to be elected President of the New York State Society of Anesthesiologists, the second largest group of physician practitioners in the country. He followed the tradition of his partner, Richard Terry, who was president in 1954, and Paul Searles, who held the office in 1948.

Ament's election in 1967 heralded his arrival on the national political scene in anesthesia. Dr. Ament would continue his involvement in politics eventually becoming president of the American Society of Anesthesiologists in 1977.

During the 1970's BGH emerged as a tertiary care facility. Specialty care units, begun in the late 50's and early 60's blossomed into large divisions. The demand for anesthesia services in ancillary locations, such as urology, ophthalmology and oral surgery clinics, as well as in the X-ray Department created scheduling difficulties for a group committed to covering two hospitals leading to separation of the Buffalo General and Children's Hospital anesthesia groups. The residency training however remained united between the hospitals. The ultimate solution to the unresolved obstetric anesthesia coverage finally came when the State of New York closed the BGH's obstetric unit, ending the most vexing manpower problem for the anesthesiologists.

The 1980s were a decade of challenge for the hospital. In 1980, Dr. Terry retired as chairman after almost thirty years of service, continuing as a staff anesthesiologist while Dr. Viguera assumed the mantel of command. The year 1986 saw the unification of Buffalo General with the Buffalo Deaconess Hospital, involuntarily returning nurse anesthesia after an interval of thirty years. The nurses this time had formal training and licensure manifested in the CRNA title. Secondly, the anesthesia care team concept had been adopted, with each practitioner contributing a distinct function in anesthetic management.

Residency training at Buffalo General dramatically changed at the time as well. Traditionally the seat of the University's training program, the medical school's chair left with Searles and was soon located at another Buffalo hospital. In 1984 three of the four residencies in Buffalo were united under the auspices of the University. While the chair remained at the Erie County Medical Center, the Educational Program Director and his assistants were placed at the Buffalo General. BGH continued as one of the cornerstones of the program; today over half the anesthesia residents in Buffalo are, at any one time, at the Buffalo General.

The year 1985 saw the reintroduction of a multidisciplinary pain center, which had originally closed in the 1960's when the anesthesiologists deemed their mostly nerve block therapy to be ineffectual. With several thousand visits per year, the clinic remains a busy center within the hospital. Additionally, the pain team has taken an active role in the management of acute, iatrogenic surgical pain. The pain service has been an integral part of the residency training in Buffalo, and among the first fellowships established for training beyond the scope of residency.

The 1990s have further added to the challenges of the Anesthesia Department. Cardiac transplantation became a reality in 1989 at which time the Buffalo General was designated one of the state's two cardiac transplantation centers by the New York State Health Department. The anesthesia department is also expanding into the critical care units, with an attending anesthesiologist taking responsibility for the care rendered in the Cardiothoracic unit. While anesthesia residents have traditionally rotated through the intensive care unit, the department is now taking a more active role.

Conclusions

The Buffalo General Hospital story illustrates many of the salient features of the History of Anesthesiology in the United States. This story is unique in that the 134 year history is recorded in continuity. While the local flavors and personalities engender the special nature of this story, this history also is universal. The evolution of anesthesia at the Buffalo General Hospital has been repeated countless times in other locations, perhaps with different dates, but the cycles are similar.

Additionally, the Buffalo General Hospital anesthesia story as recounted here places emphasis on the last forty-five years of the story. It is perhaps because of the predominance of physicians during this time, such as were at the Buffalo General, which helped convince the world, one hospital at a time, one anesthetic at a time, of the value of physician anesthesia. The anesthesiologists' desire to innovate and attempt new techniques and develop new apparatus cannot be underestimated.

Finally, the Buffalo General story also demonstrates the need for political action. For without men like Searles, Terry and Ament, there would be no state and national organizations to help meet the needs of today's anesthesiologists. And, without political savvy within the hospital confines, pain teams could not function, and anesthesia would never have left the operating room. Foreign, political discernment, and technical excellence have combined to reward the Buffalo General and anesthesia with a rich colorful history.

References

1. *The Buffalo Medical Journal. passim*
2. Sesquicentennial Centennial Issue, *Bulletin of the Medical Society of Erie County,* p. 58.
3. Park R: Remarks upon the History and introduction of anesthesia in surgery. *Buffalo Medical Journal,* November 1896.
4. See Bacon DR, Yearly CK: Among the first: the career of John Henry Evans, M.D. *Anesth Analg* 72:684-92, 1991.
5. Minutes of Quarterly Meeting, Medical Staff, Buffalo General Hospital, September 1910.
6. *Annual Reports of the Buffalo General Hospital.* (1860-1992) Buffalo General Hospital Archives.
7. Minutes of the Medical Staff Meetings, Buffalo General Hospital, April 1908, p. 43.
8. Parmenter FJ: A brief analysis of 166 cases of sacral and 26 cases of spinal anesthetics in Urologic operations. *Buffalo General Hospital Bull.* 3:22-26, 1925.
9. Park R: Remarks upon the History and introduction of anesthesia in surgery. *Buffalo Med.,* November 1896.
10. Personal Communication, Machemer W. Chief of Surgery Buffalo General Hospital.
11. From the Operating Room Report in *Annual Report of the Buffalo General Hospital* (1860-1990), Buffalo General Hospital Archives.
12. Bill from Nurse Anesthetist Miss Dobbie to Charles Eschner for anesthetic February 19, 1927.
13. Annual Report for 1943. *American Association of Nurse Anesthetists.* Wood Library-Museum Collection, Park Ridge, Illinois.
14. Buffalo General Hospital, *Surgery Log Book,* 1937-38.
15. Bacon DR, Yearley CK: Among the first: the career of John Henry Evans, M.D. *Anesth Analg* 72:684-92, 1991.
16. Paul Searles, M.D. was the University of Buffalo Department of Anesthesiology Chairman until he left Buffalo in the late 1940s. E. Dean Babbage, M.D. was then chosen his successor to the University Chairmanship. From the time when Searles left the Buffalo General Hospital until July of 1992, the University Department Chairman of Anesthesiology and the Buffalo General Hospital Department Chairman have been two separate individuals.
17. Personal communication Ronald Batt, M.D.

THE PAPERS OF HELEN LAMB
Insights into Relationships Between Pioneering Nurses and Physicians and Anesthesia

MARIANNE BANKERT
Chicago, Illinois, USA

It is a happy coincidence that this symposium on the history of anesthesia is taking place in the month of March. This is because in this country March is Women's History month, and women have contributed much to anesthesia. At this conference, for example, are two extraordinary women who are distinguished pioneers in their respective countries: Dr. Gertie F. Marx of the United States and Dr. Doreen Vermeulen-Cranch of The Netherlands. On this occasion they merit a special salute.

Helen Lamb was another extraordinary woman in the field. As anesthetist for the eminent surgeon Evarts Graham (considered the father of modern chest surgery and the founder of the American Board of Surgery), she performed the anesthetic for the world's first successful pneumonectomy in 1933.

Her papers came to the American Association of Nurse Anesthetists after her death in 1979. The collection (which arrived in two cartons and was not inventoried until 1990) is remarkable in that it covers her entire career in anesthesia: from 1928, when she began her anesthesia studies with Agatha Hodgins, to 1976, when she received the AANA's "Agatha Hodgins Award for Outstanding Accomplishment." The papers not only illuminate her career, but serve as a microcosm of the experiences of pioneering nurse anesthetists.

By way of background, it is helpful to recall briefly how nurses came into the field of anesthesia in the United States, and to describe the professional climate that existed when Lamb practiced.

On October 16, 1846, one of the greatest moments in the history of medicine occurred. In the operating theater of the Massachusetts General Hospital, dentist William T. G. Morton successfully demonstrated surgical anesthesia. The great irony is that this gift to suffering humanity was plagued with controversy from the very beginning. There immediately arose a bitter — even deadly — struggle over credit for the anesthesia discovery: Morton, Horace Wells, Charles T. Jackson — all were involved in making that moment happen. There is also, of course, Crawford W. Long of Georgia, who used ether in his medical practice as early as 1842, but who said nothing until after the 1846 event in Boston. This is a subject that still stirs passion and debate among partisans of the various claimants.

Later in the century, as surgery developed and the need for professional anesthetists became clear, there arose another controversy — equally long-lived and often bitter: Who should administer anesthetics? Anesthesia, by that time, *was* recognized as serious business, but one that lacked medical status. It was the surgeon who captained the ship — and collected the large fees. There was no financial incentive for a person holding a medical license to assume the work. However, surgeons, in order to advance their specialty, needed reliable, professional anesthetists.

One American response to the challenge faced by medicine as a result of the anesthesia breakthrough was found in nurses. Thus, the first professional nursing specialty was called into being. And, in its origins, this decision *was* economic- and gender-based. It would be decades before the terms "physician" and "nurse" were not synonymous with "male" and "female" respectively.

Apart from the few physicians who had a genuine intellectual interest in anesthesia, it would take years for the economics of anesthesia to make it a viable area of practice for their colleagues. As this change took place, it was necessary for physician-anesthetists to establish their claim to a field of practice they had earlier rejected. To achieve this end, the accomplishments of outstanding nurse anesthetists had to be denied or denigrated or ignored.

But the quality of work of these nurses had made them the anesthetists of choice for many of the most brilliant surgeons. For example, visitors who came to the Mayo Clinic to learn surgical techniques from its renowned surgeons also saw the "peerless" administration of anesthesia by Alice Magaw and her nurse anesthetist colleagues. Thus, when Dr. George Washington Crile of Lakeside Hospital, Cleveland, wanted to develop nitrous oxide as an anesthetic agent, he imitated the Mayo example and chose a nurse to be his anesthetist. He selected Agatha Cobourg Hodgins. Hodgins, who came to establish the International Association of Nurse Anesthetists (later known as the American Association of Nurse Anesthetists), also had a commitment to education. With Crile, she founded a school of anesthesia at Lakeside in 1916. Its first graduating class consisted of six physicians, two dentists, and eleven nurses.

A leading force in the anti-nurse anesthetist activity was Dr. Ralph M. Waters. In 1927 he joined the faculty of the new medical school of the University of Wisconsin at Madison, and established the first medical residency in anesthesia. He has come to be known, therefore, as the "Father of Academic Anesthesia." Waters was not only anti-nurse anesthetist, he was anti-woman physician. In her impressive study, *American Medicine and the Public Interest* (New Haven: Yale University Press, 1971), historian Rosemary Stevens observed that pioneering male physicians in anesthesia had a special obstacle: seeking to gain status for anesthesia as a medical specialty, they had to "contend with the female image" of the field. For not only had nurses been drawn into the new and undervalued work, but, as anesthesiologist-historian Selma Calmes has detailed, so had female physicians.

It is a commonplace in the literature of sociology that work associated with women is less valued than that associated with men. It is not surprising, then, to find an antipathy to women in the comments of pioneering physician anesthetists. Calmes has noted for example, that Arthur R. Guedel wrote to Waters in 1931, "However I do not believe in women doctors." Waters responded, "You have nothing on me in your attitude towards that." And, later, Guedel once again, "I still feel as usual about women anesthetists."

To gain recognition for anesthesia as a

"science," the female image had to be eradicated. (Still later, this dynamic worked in reverse for female nurse anesthetists when male nurses began entering the field. The female nurses knew that the male presence would increase status and economic opportunities for all nurse anesthetists. This is one reason why, contrary to Calmes's assumption, there is no evidence that gender conflict has shaped the nursing group.)

This was the professional climate when Helen Lamb entered the field.[1]

She was the daughter of an Iowa country doctor of modest means. She recalled that, "It was never considered that I would do anything else besides enter nurse's training. From the time I was seven or eight years old, I went with my father on Saturday obstetrical calls — in a horse-drawn sleigh or carriage. I regarded it as a real privilege to clean my dad's office. He paid me fifty cents a Saturday, and I saved my money to buy a pair of silk stockings." (Interestingly, Lamb's brother, Charles, became a surgeon.)

After graduating from Christian Church Hospital School of Nursing, Kansas City, Missouri, Lamb borrowed money for tuition to enroll in a surgical nursing course at Barnes Hospital in St. Louis. At that time, a staff anesthetist trained both interns and nurses in anesthesia because, she noted, "many of the staff surgeons wanted their own anesthetists, and in most instances, they were nurse anesthetists." The noted plastic surgeon Dr. Blair invited Lamb to become his anesthetist; he said that his nurse would train her. But Lamb, being interested, instead looked for a school where she could study anesthesia. She learned of Hodgins's Lakeside School, and there began her studies in 1928.

During her stay in Lakeside, she realized that Barnes Hospital would "be an excellent place to come back to. . . . there were possibilities there."

Upon graduation, she did return to Barnes, and began a career of achievement in anesthesia research, practice, education, and professional organization. She founded the Barnes School of Anesthesia in 1929, and served as its director until her retirement in 1951. In 1931 she was one of the founding members of what came to be named the American Association of Nurse Anesthetists. She was chairman of the AANA Education Committee from 1932 through 1939, and was a major force in establishing the curriculum and minimum standards for schools of nurse anesthesia. Throughout her career at Barnes, she was anesthetist for Evarts Graham, and in that capacity performed the anesthetic for the world's first successful pneumonectomy in 1933. For more than twenty years, she collaborated with chemist Richard von Foregger in the development of anesthesia equipment. She served as president of the AANA from 1940-1942.

Lamb continued her professional development in part by visiting various surgeries, observing procedures and discussing cases. These were not always pleasant experiences.

In August, 1937, she visited the Madison Wisconsin General Hospital and observed an anesthetic procedure by Dr. Ralph Waters. In her notes from that visit, after describing the clinical data, she adds: "Waters was not cooperative, brought out a letter which explained why he did not want nurse anesthetists, would not discuss or answer questions asked on anesthesia. Was very evasive and vague."

On a visit to California in 1939, Lamb attempted to visit Dr. Arthur E. Guedel at his hospital. The visit did not take place. Guedel's letter to Lamb, dated July 25, 1939, explained,

> I am sincerely sorry that you did not call me up last Friday. I had the afternoon laid out for a good chat in my back yard. I am sorry that I was busy when you called Thursday. Now I feel that you feel that I was trying to sidestep you and you were either indignant or hurt.
>
> Believe me, although there is much feeling out here against the nurse anesthetist, and I am necessarily cautious because I am watched, I have the most wholesome respect for your work. I feel that the work of most medical anesthetists is inferior to yours. And, although I could not publicly have you as a visitor at the hospital, I would

> have enjoyed meeting you and talking with you. And it is true that I do not have any visitors M.D. or otherwise in my surgery.

On August 17, however, Foregger wrote to Lamb, and sent along excerpts from a Guedel letter to him dated July 24, 1939, with this account of the non-meeting: "Now for Helen Lamb. I respect her. She is the best nurse anesthetist in the world and better by far than many M.D. anesthetists. She called me up. I told her frankly that I could not entertain her at my hospital because I cannot entertain any anesthetists medical or otherwise. Of course the really good medical anesthetists who are ready for *advanced work* I permit to visit. But no others. I advised her to go to the County Hospital and call herself Dr. Lamb. I was nice to her. I asked her to call me on Thursday stating that I would like to meet her in my back yard. She called me and it happened that on that afternoon I had an emergency case and could not see her. I explained that to her but I feel that she, in her sensitive doubt, did not believe me. I asked her to call the next afternoon and waited at home all afternoon for her to call. She did not call and I have not heard from her since. I am going to write her a nice letter and present her with an autographed copy of my book. I respect her and don't want to be misunderstood. I am for ability regardless of degree or training. I hope that she remains friendly to you and to me."

Interestingly, while Foregger acknowledged to Lamb that passing along a letter not intended for her eyes was "a conventional breach," he did so with no apparent sense that Guedel's words added to the insult — nor even that there had been an insult. Foregger simply commented to Lamb: "Guedel was worried to have hurt your feelings, afraid you misconstrued. I know him well and know that he means whatever he says, and that he had no intention to avoid you."

As mentioned, for more than twenty years Lamb collaborated with Foregger in the development of anesthesia equipment. When the physician-anesthetist journal *Anesthesiology* was launched in 1940, Foregger planned his first advertisement in its pages. He chose to feature her design, but did not follow the custom of naming the person responsible for the work — for "reasons that need no explanation," he wrote to her in a letter of December 2, 1940.

In a subsequent letter to Lamb on December 6, he expressed his relief that the ad was "at last" on its way to the printer, and mused, "I wonder how disappointed you will be when you see it."

Lamb's informal response to Foregger dated December 5, 1940, makes clear that she understood his marketing decision: "There can certainly be no antagonism raised to *your* specification or design — whereas there might (would) be to *specification by* or *design for* some department with which some readers would be out of sympathy."

Foregger had written to Lamb that he wanted "to have an impressive ad for the first time in *Anesthesiology,* and of course, as you know without the least semblance to bill-boarding." The three-page ad is, in fact, very subtle. Page one (opposite the inside-cover masthead with the editorial board a who's who of pioneering physician anesthetists, including both Guedel and Waters) is a war-time appeal to patriotism ("The Spirit of Defense"). Pages two and three juxtapose "Progress in 1924" with that of "1940." The 1924 design is credited: "Designed upon specification of Dr. Ralph M. Waters, Madison, Wisconsin." The Lamb "1940" design is described: "Used with eminent satisfaction for more than a year in the thoracic surgery clinic of Dr. Evarts A. Graham at Barnes Hospital, St. Louis. (Quoted with permission.)"

Ironically, then, this equipment, presented to physician anesthetists in their new journal as the latest in scientific precision (as evidence of "the convincing gains of the last two decades") was designed by a female nurse anesthetist — at the time also president of the American Association of Nurse Anesthetists. But she received no credit " "for reasons that need no explanation."

References

1. Two excellent studies on women in the health care professions are Mary Roth Walsh, *Doctors Wanted, No Women Need Apply: Sexual Barriers in the Medical Profession, 1835-1975* (New Haven and London: Yale University Press, 1977) and Barbara Ehrenreich and Deirdre English, *Witches, Midwives, and Nurses, A History of Women Healers* (New York: The Feminist Press, 1973).

MEDICINAL USES OF SULFURIC ETHER BEFORE CRAWFORD LONG

NORMAN A. BERGMAN
Portland, Oregon, USA

In reviewing much of the written existing anesthesia history, it is easy to obtain the impression that diethyl ether was an obscure substance and a curiosity before those who received credit for "discovering" anesthesia used it for pain relief associated with operative procedures during the 1840's. This is certainly not true. Ether was actually a familiar substance which enjoyed wide medicinal use and had accumulated quite an extensive literature. This presentation will briefly recount some of the knowledge concerning either before it sprang into prominence as an anesthetic agent.

Diethyl ether (also called sulfuric ether because it was made from sulfuric [vitriolic] acid and alcohol) was first described by Ramon Lull, a Spanish mystic and philosopher, in the thirteenth century. Another worker associated with the early history of ether was Valerius Cordus. In his book, "De Artificiosis Extractionibus," which appeared in 1561 and 1571, he first gave instructions for preparing sulfuric acid (sour vitriol) and described some therapeutic applications of this substance. "Sweet oil of vitriol" (ether) could then be prepared from sour oil of vitriol and "strong very biting thrice purified wine." He explained how to separate the sweet oil of vitriol. The yield of ether from this reaction was small and the substance tended to evaporate easily. Cordus was not the first to synthesize ether, but he was the first to explain the method. He also described some of the physiologic responses to ether, such as mucus production. In addition, he proposed some therapeutic uses for ether, which included all situations in which sulfur was applied according to then current medical practice. Additional uses were in all body putrefactions, including plague, extraction of pus and mucus from the lung in pleurisy, and other applications. Ether could be taken internally: 2-3 drops in wine.[1]

Paracelsus (ca 1493-1541) knew of the narcotic and sedative properties of ether-like preparations that he obtained from the interaction of alcohol and sulfur, or alternatively, from

Valerius Cordus during a visit to Nuremberg or Leipzig.[2] Many extraneous products could be obtained during preparation of ether.[3] One such mixture was Hoffman's anodyne, which had rectified spirits (alcohol or brandy of some type), ethereal oil (ethyl hydrogen sulfate?) and ether. Paracelsus provided an unmistakable description of ether and considered several general medicinal uses for the substance. He identified ether as anodyne and stupefacient. An important connection of Paracelsus with anesthesia was his administration of ether to chickens, with an ensuing temporary state of stupefaction in them. He probably selected these animals to study because of the well known narcotic effect of hyoscyamus (henbane) upon them (an effect also called "mort aux poules").[4] He appeared to be familiar with administration of substances by inhalation, but gave the ethereal substance to his chickens orally. There is some question as to the nature of the substance given to the chickens since a modern investigator established experimentally that fasting chickens would not eat feed to which ether had been added, but would eat when it contained something like Hoffman's Anodyne. Nevertheless, Paracelsus is often acknowledged to be the first to describe the soporific properties of sulfuric ether.[5]

"Aether" was named in 1730 by Frobenius and some of its properties were described. He indicated that Sir Isaac Newton had been interested in this fluid.[6]

By the eighteenth century ether was extensively prescribed by a number of practitioners.

Michael Morris, in 1758, discussed medicinal uses of ether, which included local application in headache, toothache, earache and rheumatic pains in the neck, and internal administration in whooping cough, hysteria, syncope and lethargy.[7]

In 1761 Matthew Turner, a surgeon of Liverpool, published "An Account of the Extraordinary Medicinal Fluid Called Aether." He stated that he had used this substance for a considerable length of time in his practice. Previous writers on ether familiar to Turner had included Robert Boyle, Isaac Newton and Frobenius. The substance was prepared by the action of vitriolic acid (sulfuric acid), on vinous spirits (primarily alcohol). It was extremely flammable, being capable of igniting at the approach of a candle or of an electrified body. It was light and very volatile, a powerful solvent and extremely cold when dropped on the hand.

Clinical applications recommended by Turner were many. Ether was most useful in fits of all forms and in other nervous diseases. It was also recommended in a wide variety of arthritic, rheumatic, digestive and other types of disease. For any of these complaints, one teaspoon of ether could be taken internally once or twice daily. It could also be applied to the affected part or placed on a rag and inserted into the nostrils for inhalation. For deafness, ether could be instilled into the ear. Instructions for detecting "good" ether in terms of color, volatility and miscibility with water were presented. He was willing to sell ether for two shillings the ounce. It is of interest that dizziness or giddiness associated with ether inhalation is never mentioned by Turner. Virtually all other pneumatic physicians who employed inhalations of ether described these sensations.[8]

William Lewis, in 1761, mentioned "dulcified spirit of vitriolic acid" (ether) in his "Materia Medica." He believed that it was a curiosity and that not too much was known about its medicinal properties. Among the several therapeutic indications suggested for the substance were as a tonic, a cordial, and an anodyne. In addition, it could be rubbed on the temples to relieve headache. The dose for internal use was 3-12 drops in water.[9]

John Rotheram, writing in 1797, suggested that ether could be used as a solvent and also to promote perspiration and urinary secretion, ease pain and produce sleep. The dose was 80-90 drops in any convenient fluid.[10] William Withering also advocated ether inhalation in various types of pulmonary disease.[11] A distinguished chemist who undertook researches on ether was Antoine Lavoisier. He proposed several medicinal uses for the substance.[12] Another physician who is known to have prescribed ether early in the 19th century was Dr. Woolcombe of Plymouth. His experiences with ether were chronicled by Sir Thomas Watson.[13]

Ether was commonly prescribed as a "diffusible stimulus" within the context of the system of medicine of John Brown, that remarkable method of medical practice so popular among 18th and early 19th century physicians. Brown considered "diffusible stimuli" for use in "asthenic diseases."[14] The weakest degree of diffusible stimuli included white and red wines. Of the next order of magnitude on the stimulus scale were musk, volatile alkali and camphor, which had been incompletely tried. Next came ether, and strongest of all was opium. Other authors also believed that ether and opium had similar types of actions.

Dr. Robert John Thornton described Dr. Townsend's method for inhaling the vapor of sulfuric ether in certain respiratory diseases.[15] Thornton demonstrated the inflammability and explosiveness of ether. When one drop of ether was placed in one ounce of vital air (oxygen) in a vial and ignited with a glowing match, a violent explosion occurred.

Thornton indicated that Dr. Richard Pearson was treating a chest complaint with sulfuric ether inhalations. The patient reported a sensation of giddiness after each inhalation.

In the late 1820's, William Wright, aurist (ear specialist) to Queen Charlotte (wife of George III), wrote extensively on ether and nitrous oxide in the treatment of deafness and diseases of the ear. He commented on sedative properties of the vapor of sulfuric ether.[16]

The narcotic properties of ether and the reversibility of this action were clearly demonstrated during a lecture presented by Benjamin Collins Brodie (1783-1862) on Feb. 5, 1821, at the Royal College of Surgeons of England. He placed a guinea pig under a bell jar into which he introduced ether vapor. After about twelve minutes the guinea pig appeared motionless and dead. The animal was revived by removing it from the vapor and by application of artificial respiration. Brodie attributed these effects to specific actions of either—not to suffocation.[17]

The properties of ether were well known in New England in the first half of the nineteenth century. Eli Ives (1779-1861), professor of materia medica at Yale University, lectured on some general medicinal properties of ether before 1846. Ives characterized ether as the most diffusible stimulus known and states that its use was not followed by indirect debility. The cooling action of ether when applied to the skin was noted. It was useful when poured on the scrotum for strangulated hernia, and on the head for head pain. Inhalation of ether vapor was also valuable in the last stages of consumption. Ives appeared to have no idea about the central nervous system effects of ether.[18]

Dr. John Collins Warren Jr. indicated that Dr. J.C. Warren Sr., one of the physicians involved in William T.G. Morton's ether demonstration in 1846, had previously used ether in Boston to relieve the distress attending the last stage of pulmonary consumption. He mentioned a letter indicating that it had been so used, and that its effect in producing unconsciousness had been noted at the Massachusetts General Hospital in 1836.[19]

Dr. John Collins Warren Sr. is quoted as having commented on the soporific properties of ether in 1848: "its general properties have been known for more than a century, and the effects of its inhalation in producing exhilaration and insensibility has been understood for many years, . . ."[21]

Properties of ether, including its ability to stupefy, were well described in certain textbooks of materia medica in the first half of the 19th century. Examples were those by Townsend (1801) and Pereira (1842).

Discussion of the recreational use and abuse of volatile narcotic drugs is beyond the scope of this presentation. It should be noted, however, that nitrous oxide was the first such drug to be used in this manner. Michael Faraday, in 1818, published a brief communication announcing that the effects of ether on consciousness and mentation were similar to those of nitrous oxide. Since ether was much more readily obtainable than the gas, there was little impediment to the widening use of ether in "frolics" and entertainments.[20]

Thus, Crawford Long's anesthetic administered at Jefferson, Georgia, USA, in 1842 did not involve an obscure or exotic agent. The ether that he employed was one of the most familiar and widely used substances in the 19th century pharmacopoeia, and its actions on mentation and consciousness appear to have been well known.

References

1. Tallmage GK: The Third Part of the De Extractione of Valerius Cordus. Isis 7:394-411, 1925.
2. Leake CD: Valerius Cordus and the Discovery of Ether. Isis 7:14-24, 1925.
3. Robinson T: On the nature of Sweet Oil of Vitriol. J Hist Med 14:231-3, 1959.
4. Pagel W: Biographical Sketch of Paracelsus. In "Dictionary of Scientific Biography" N.Y. Charles Scribner's Sons. 1973.
5. Gravenstein J S: Paracelsus and His Contributions to Anesthesia. Anesthesiology 26:805-11, 1965.
6. Frobenius. An account of a Spiritus Vini Aethereus, together with several experiments tried therewith. Philosoph Trans 36:283-9, 1730.
7. Morris M: A letter from Michael Morris M.D. to the Medical Society describing the process for making Aether, with some observations on its medical use. Article XII, read Dec 18, 1758. Medical Observation and Inquiries by a Society of Physicians in London. 2:176-86, 1764. London, William Johnson, 1764.
8. Turner M: (Surgeon in Liverpool). An Account of the Extraordinary Medicinal Fluid Called Aether. City?. John Sadler. 1761.
9. Lewis W: An Experimental History of the Materia Medica etc. London. H. Baldwin. 1761.
10. Rotheram J: The Edinburgh New Dispensatory being an improvement of the New Dispensatory of Dr. Lewis. Ed. V. Edinburgh. William Creech. 1797.
11. Withering W: Description of a glass inhaler for pneumatic inhalation. Ann Med 3:447-51, 1798.
12. Fulton J F, Duveen DI, Klickstein HS: Antoine Laurent Lavoisier's "Réflexions sur les Effets de l'Ether Vitrilique et de l'Ether Nitreux dans l'Economie Animale." J Hist Med 8:318-23, 1953.
13. Watson T: Lectures on the Principles and Practice of Physic. London. Longmans Green and Co. 1871.
14. Brown J: The Elements of Medicine. Translated by Thomas Beddoes. Philadelphia. Thomas Dobson. 1806. p. 191.
15. Thornton RJ: Dr. Cullen's Practice of Physic etc. with notes explanatory and practical etc. . . . added the discoveries made in physic since the time of Dr. Cullen by. . . Trotter-Beddoes-Darwin - Thornton. London. E Cox and Son. 1816. p. 401.
16. Wright W: On the Varieties of Deafness and Diseases of the Ear, with Proposed Methods of Relieving Them. London. Hurst, Chance and Co. 1829.
17. Brodie BC: Effects of Ether on a Guinea Pig. (Handwritten manuscript of lecture notes illustrating effects of ether vapour inhalation on a GP.) London. Royal College of Surgeons. 1821.
18. Greene NM: Eli Ives and the Medical Use of Ether Prior to 1846. J Hist Med Allied Sci 15:297-9, 1960.
19. Warren J C: The Influence of Anaesthesia on the Surgery of the Nineteenth Century. (An Address delivered by the President of and to the American Surgical Association.) Boston. Privately Printed. 1906.
20. Warren JC: Etherization; with Surgical Remarks. Boston. William Ticknor. 1848.
21. Anon. (Faraday) v. Effects of Inhaling the Vapour of Sulphuric Ether. J. Science and Arts 4:158, 1818.

THE FIRST USE OF "INTOCOSTRIN" IN ANESTHESIA

RICHARD BODMAN
Dalhousie Society for the History of Medicine, Halifax, Nova Scotia, Canada

For three centuries after the discovery of the "New World" the weird and mysterious drug, curare, intrigued physiologists and physicians. The accounts of experiments by Waterton, Claude Bernard, Sir Henry Dale and the chemical analysis of the drug by Harold King in 1935 are well known. The explorer Richard Gill supplied the pharmaceutical company—ER Squibb—with raw materials from the Amazon basin, which enabled them to make a preparation described as "Intocostrin—an unauthenticated extract of curare." Lewis Wright, medical representative for the company, deserves the credit for promoting the use of this drug. He supplied it to A.R. McIntyre, a pharmacologist in Omaha, Nebraska, who encouraged A.E. Bennett, a psychiatrist, to use the drug to control the convulsions produced by the shock therapy with which he was treating schizophrenics. Prior to the use of curare Bennett had reported that 43-51 percent of his patients suffered compression fractures of the spine. This was eliminated by using small doses of curare to modify the convulsions; thus was demonstrated the first authentic and successful therapeutic use of curare in man. A film was made of this procedure and was shown at the meeting of the American Medical Association in New York in 1940.

Lewis Wright tried to persuade his anesthetic colleagues to use "Intocostrin." The response was cautious or incredulous. Harold Griffith had seen Bennett's film in New York and laughingly dismissed the idea of using it when his friend Lewis Wright approached him. However, back in Montreal he reviewed Bennett's papers and the film. "Well, I thought to myself, the worst it can do is to paralyse the patient's respiration and that is not a very serious concern for anesthetists, we control respiration every day in the operating room." Harold Griffith had a long experience of cyclopropane; since the first demonstration of its use by Ralph Waters in 1933, he had by 1941 used it in over 7000 anesthetics. He was familiar with the respiratory depressing effect of cyclopropane, but he always used an endotracheal tube and was used to ventilating the lungs

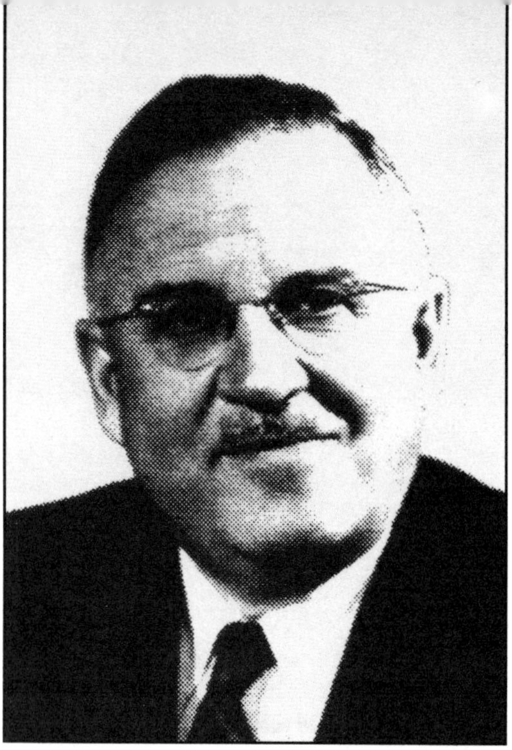

Fig. 1. Harold R. Griffith, M.D.

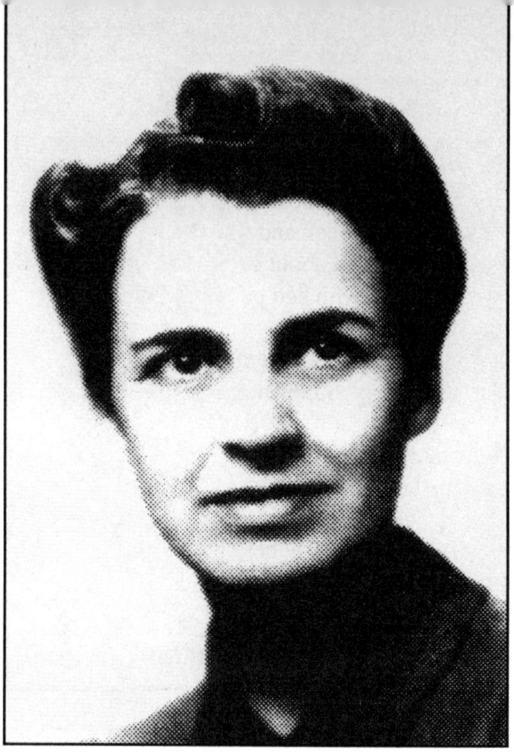

Fig. 2. G. Enid Johnson, M.D.

THE USE OF CURARE IN GENERAL ANESTHESIA
Montreal, Canada
Anesthesiology, Vol. 3, No. 4, pp 418–420, July, 1942.

by squeezing the breathing bag, a procedure he had perfected for upper abdominal surgery. He asked Lewis Wright for samples of "Intocostrin."

On a fateful day—23 January 1942—Harold Griffith selected for the experiment Mr B. Townsend, a muscular young man of 20 years, weighing 150 pounds, scheduled for appendectomy. He was premedicated with "Seconal" grains iii by mouth and 1/6 grain morphine with 1/150 grain atropine by injection at 9:15 a.m. An intravenous line was set up and the anesthetic administered by Dr Griffith's resident, Enid Johnson, commencing at 10:05 a.m. and using cyclopropane and oxygen. She intubated the patient—"we always intubated our patients"—and the surgeon commenced at 10.17. After 1 1/2 minutes Griffith injected 3.5 cc "Intocostrin" into the i-v line. There was no appreciable effect on the pulse or respiration, an after five minutes another 1.5 cc was given. In less than two minutes the abdominal muscles were quite relaxed and continued so for 20 minutes, "during which time the cyclopropane was lightened. . . there was no demonstrable change in pulse, blood pressure or respiration." The operation finished at 11.15 a.m. The surgeon, George Novinger, Harold Griffith and Enid Johnson were frankly amazed at the effect produced in so short a time. The procedure, which could have been quite difficult in this muscular young man with cyclopropane alone, was really made easy.

Harold Griffith and Enid Johnson were so impressed that, after completing a small series of 25 cases, they submitted a paper for publication to the journal "Anesthesiology," concluding "Intocostrin" would be ". . .of great value, and will give us a means of providing the surgeon rapidly with excellent muscular relaxation at critical times during certain operations."

Enid Johnson described their method. "We would intubate with cyclopropane in the anesthetic room, bring the patient into the operating room and when the surgeon was ready give the curare. Sometimes we would wait for the surgeon to make the incision and then give the curare if there was not enough relaxation. We did not give it to every patient."

The following Christmas, Harold Griffith

sent Enid Johnson a card, remarking "I was in New York last week and found all the anesthetists quite excited about curare—and some red faces on those who had passed it up before we started to use it!"

In 1943, Stuart Cullen, Professor of Anesthesiology at the University of Iowa, reported the use of "Intocostrin" in 500 cases, confirming Harold Griffith's findings. By this time the latter commented "I am beginning to believe now that curare may replace spinal anesthesia. So I really believe that curare is going to mean a very great change in our anesthetic methods." By June 1945, Sidney Newcomer, a Director of E R Squibb company, wrote ". . .the use of "Intocostrin" in anesthesia is mounting rapidly and we believe that it is well over 10,000 doses a month. . . we are preparing a book in which we shall give excerpts from all of the recent articles on curare. There are over one hundred of them. The interest in curare has increased so far beyond our expectations it is difficult for us to put it into vials fast enough to keep up."

In 1945, Harold Griffith, who was now a Wing Commander and Consultant in Anaesthesia to the Royal Canadian Air Force, asked the E R Squibb company to send samples of "Intocostrin" to Robert Macintosh, his opposite number in the Royal Air Force in Britain. In return Macintosh asked Griffith to submit a paper to the Lancet. This paper was published in July 1945; in it Griffith remarked ". . .we have used it more than 500 times. . . curare should not be made the excuse for a poor anaesthetic sloppily administered. . ."

Observations have been made belittling Harold Griffith; he has been described as an obscure family physician, implying he was an amateur in the anesthetic world. In fact he was a well respected member of the anesthetic community at the time; he was one of the earliest members invited by Ralph Waters to join the prestigious "Anesthetists' Travel Club." He had been President of the Twelfth Annual Congress of the International Anesthesia Research Society an the Associated Anesthetists of the United States and Canada at their meeting in Chicago in 1933. He probably had more experience of cyclopropane, intubation and controlling respiration than any other anesthetist, at a time when these procedures were quite rare. He readily acknowledged the important part played by the pharmaceutical firm of E R Squibb company in producing a usable preparation of curare and of the encouragement he received from his friend Lewis Wright. If we accept Sir William Osler's dictum, "In science the credit goes to the man who convinces the world, not to the man to whom the idea first occurs," there can be no doubt that Harold Griffith fully deserves the credit for introducing curare to surgical anesthesia. David Little, Associate Editor of the Survey of Anesthesiology in 1957, wrote, "The introduction of curare by Harold Griffith represented a milestone of progress in anesthesia without equal since the classic demonstration of ether a century before. The drug revolutionized the practice of anesthesia by permitting utter muscular relaxation without the necessity of resorting to deep and dangerous levels of anesthesia." Cecil Gray, Professor of Anaesthesia at Liverpool, England, described it as a "flash of inspired genius."

ASSOCIATED ANESTHETISTS OF THE UNITED STATES AND CANADA
(1925–1941)

RICHARD BODMAN
Dalhousie Society for the History of Medicine, Halifax, Nova Scotia, Canada

The Associated Anesthetists of the United States and Canada was a precursor, but not the parent, of the American Society of Anesthesiologists and the Canadian Anesthetists' Society. It owed its formation to the enthusiasm of Frank McMechan. This remarkable man graduated from the Medical School of Cincinnati in 1903 and at once began to specialize in anesthesia: "I found the profession rather amazed that a young doctor could fool away his time at anything so inconsequential as putting patients to sleep, but it was not long before some of the surgeons were completely won over." He developed a successful practice in Cincinnati, but was struck with ankylosing spondylitis and had to give up his practice in 1911. However, he had by this time made himself familiar with developments worldwide and with those interested in promoting research in anesthesia. He decided to devote himself to organizing anesthetic societies and editing a journal.

Together with James Gwathmey, author of the first American textbook of anesthesia, William Bainbridge, noted New York surgeon, and Yandell Henderson, respiratory physiologist of Yale University, application was made to the American Medical Association in 1911 to form a Section of Anesthesia. This was refused; anesthesia was not regarded as of sufficient importance to merit recognition. As a result, an independent American Association of Anesthetists was formed and held its first meeting in June, 1912, with Gwathmey as President and McMechan as Secretary.

Realizing the importance of communication to a growing specialty, McMechan, with the enthusiastic help of Dr Joseph MacDonald, editor of the American Journal of Surgery, started a quarterly supplement in October, 1914, titled the American Journal of Anesthesia and Analgesia.

McMechan was an indefatigable organizer; he established the Inter-State Society of Anesthetists (1915) comprising Ohio, Indiana and Kentucky, the three States adjacent to Cincinnati; this became the Mid-Western Association in 1924. In the east, the Long Island Society, which had become the New York Society of Anesthetists in 1911, formed part of the Eastern Society. The Southern Association of Anesthetists (1922) represented the Southern States, and the Pacific Coast Society (1922) the west. The Canadians formed the Canadian Society of Anaesthetists in 1920, although it only lasted until 1928 when it was absorbed as a Section of the Canadian Medical Association. There were many other local societies of anesthetists, often supported by members of the dental profession.

Not content with organizing regional societies, McMechan realized the importance of research; in this he was encouraged by commercial interests. At this time nitrous oxide was becoming available in cylinders and manufacturers were interested in producing apparatus for delivering nitrous oxide/oxygen mixtures for normal and operative obstetrics.

Endotracheal insufflation, pioneered by Charles Elsberg, a New York surgeon, required safe electric motors to pump ether into the lungs. The importance of suction to maintain clear airways became evident. A group of manufacturers met with McMechan in Cleveland, Ohio, in 1919, as a result of which the National Anesthesia Research Society was formed with McMechan as chairman, members being representatives of manufacturing industries, professional anesthetists and dentists and scientists. McKesson was a prominent member of this group as a practicing anesthetist and manufacturer of apparatus. Finally, the Society instituted Annual Congresses, the first of which was held in 1922, and commenced the publication of an independent journal—"Current Researches in Anesthesia and Analgesia." The success of these projects attracted many interested medical men, not only in the U.S. and Canada, but members were welcomed from Britain, the Commonwealth countries and Europe. The name was then changed to the International Anesthesia Research Society (I.A.R.S.) and overseas members were appointed to the Board. The membership included all those interested in promoting research in anesthesia—scientists, manufacturers, surgeons, dentists, as well as practising anesthetists. Membership in the American Association of Anesthetists was for medical practitioners whose principal interest was the practice of anesthesia, amongst them being a number of prominent Canadians. It was decided in 1925 to rename the society the Associated Anesthetists of the United States and Canada. This society was invited to take part in the annual meeting of the British Medical Association in Nottingham, England, in 1926. This implied recognition of the specialty of anesthesia by both the Canadian and the British medical professions.

The next fifteen years saw a continuing struggle to have anesthesia recognized as a legitimate specialty by the American Medical Association. McMechan continued to promote the I.A.R.S., the annual congresses, the journal, and the Associated Anesthetists of the United States and Canada, but he was leery of the American Medical Association because they would not recognize the specialty and they tolerated technician and nurse anesthetists.

Meanwhile, in the 1930's State Medical Boards were becoming more critical of medical practice, and it became clear that formal recognition of the status of anesthetists was necessary to negotiate fees and salaries in State hospitals. By 1936 the New York Society of Anesthetists had canvassed members throughout the U.S. and changes its name to the American Society of Anesthetists, incorporated in the State of New York. They were not in a position to negotiate as a national society.

Board certification in the specialties was the responsibility of the Council on Medical Education and Licensure of the American Medical Association, which at first refused recognition of anesthesia. In Canada the specialty was recognized by the Canadian Medical Association, but the Royal College of Physicians and Surgeons had yet to inaugurate certifying examinations in anesthesia. In Britain the Royal Colleges introduced a Diploma in Anaesthetics in 1935.

In the United States there were now two groups promoting the professional practice of anesthesia—the Associate Anesthetists and the American Society of Anesthetists. They were not mutually exclusive; in fact it was said that 80 percent of established anesthetists belonged to both—perhaps they were hedging their bets, but clearly a specialist would want to subscribe to the journal—Current Researches in Anesthesia and Analgesia— and attend the annual congresses; at the same time it would have been wise to join the American Society of Anesthetists, which was hoping to be recognized by the American Medical Association.

The two groups were both dedicated to the promotion of anesthesia, but their philosophies were somewhat different. The I.A.R.S. was ostensibly preoccupied with research and the development of the specialty, while the Associated Anesthetists represented the political wing of the group; both were internationally oriented and under McMechan's guidance fiercely independent.

On the other hand, the American Society of Anesthetists was deliberately formed as a national society in order to gain recognition by the American Medical Association, the state legislatures, which were increasingly involved in providing medical services, and the armed forces in case war should break out.

Both parties had set up Fellowships. McMechan's group established an International College of Anesthetists, with the designation F.I.C.A. The American Society of Anesthetists granted Fellowships, which were later attributed to the American College of Anesthetists—F.A.C.A. Both fellowships were at first awarded in consideration of experience and peer recommendation.

The possibility of affiliating the American Society of Anesthetists and the Associated Anesthetists of the United States and Canada was discussed. But events were running ahead of negotiations. In June of 1939 Frank McMechan died, sincerely mourned by all the anesthetic world. In September of that year Canada declared war and proceeded to call up to the Forces all able-bodied anesthetists, and initiated a training scheme to recruit more. By the time the United States was drawn into the war in 1941, the American Medical Association realized that the time had come to recognize the specialty; a Section of Anesthesia was established with John Lundy as secretary, and an independent Board of Anesthesiology was set up. In 1942 the U.S. Army and Navy also recognized anesthesiology as a legitimate specialty.

The possibility of the American Society of Anesthetists adopting "Current Researches" had been mooted, but was not pursued; instead the Society produced the first number of its own journal—"Anesthesiology"—in 1940. Finally, the society changed it name to the American Society of Anesthesiologists, Inc. (A.S.A.) in 1945.

McMechan's mantle fell on Harold Griffith. He traveled from Montreal as many as four times a year to Cleveland, Ohio, in support of McMechan's wife, Laurette, who continued to manage "Current Researches." In 1941 the Associated Anesthetists of the United States and Canada was formally absorbed into the I.A.R.S. The Canadian Anaesthetists' Society was formed in 1943 with Harold Griffith as president.

Anesthetists of Canada and the U.S. remained on cordial terms; half a dozen Canadians sat the first examination for the American Board in Anesthesiology. In 1941 the A.S.A. held its annual meeting in Montreal and elected the Canadian Wesley Bourne as President, the only non-American ever to hold that position.

The Associated Anesthetists of the United States and Canada had outlived its function, but its international, indeed ecumenical, reputation lived on in the I.A.R.S. Under Harold Griffith's guidance, the Society contributed enthusiasm and substantial financial assistance to the ultimate goal of founding a World Federation of Societies of Anesthesiologists.

I am indebted to the American Society of Anesthesiologists Inc. for granting me a fellowship to study at their Wood Library-Museum of Anesthesiology in Chicago.

FORMATION OF PRINCIPAL SOCIETIES IN THE UNITED KINGDOM CANADA AND THE U.S.A.

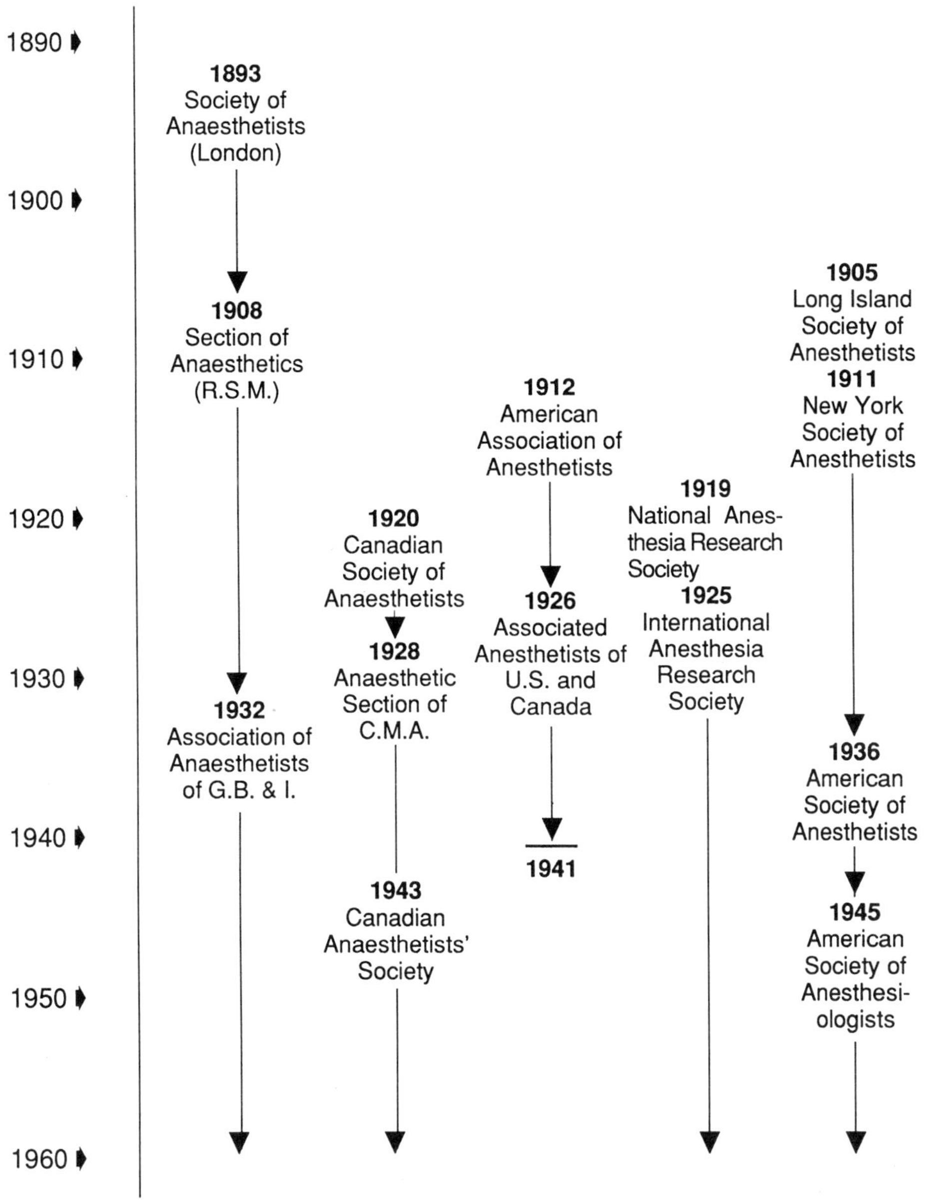

THE EARLY HISTORY OF BLOOD TRANSFUSION

THOMAS B. BOULTON
Association of Anaesthetists of Great Britain and Ireland, London, England, United Kingdom

The life of the creature is in the blood.
Leviticus 17, xi.

The transfusion of human donor blood to human patients is a vital procedure with which all modern physician anaesthetists are intimately concerned. The first human to human intravenous transfusion was reported on the twenty-second of December 1818 to the Medico-Chirurgical Society of London by James Blundell, lecturer in physiology and obstetrics to Guy's and St. Thomas' Hospitals in London.[1-7]

Blood has been recognized as of vital importance since the dawn of history. The ancients considered it to be the seat of the soul and believed that it carried within the mental and physical qualities of the donor. Egyptian princes bathed in blood to rejuvenate their mental and physical powers, and the Romans drank the blood of gladiators killed in the Arena. There was also an attempt to resuscitate the decrepit Pope Innocent VIII in the late 15th century with an oral draught of blood obtained from exsanguinated youths. There were vague suggestions of the possibility of injecting donor arterial blood into patients for therapeutic rejuvenation in the early 17th century, but there is no record of any practical attempt at transfusion.[3-7]

The experimental and practical application of animal-to-animal and animal-to-human intravenous transfusion had of necessity to await William Harvey's description of the circulation of the blood in 1616 and the careful experiments of the intravenous injection into veins in 1656 by the great scientist and architect Christopher Wren in Oxford, who devised practical equipment composed of goose quills and a dog's bladder.[3-7]

It was undoubtedly Wren's experiments which stimulated other members of the Royal Society of London, which had been formed in 1660, to experiment with blood transfusion. His contemporary Thomas Sprat tells us that Wren "was the first author of the noble anatomical experiments of injecting liquors into the veins of animals" and that "hence arose many new experiments, chiefly that of transfusing blood . . . that will probably end in extraordinary success."[8]

Richard Lower, a friend of Wren's and a fellow of the Royal Society, carried out the first experimental direct animal-to-animal blood transfusion in 1666. He overcame the problem of extracorporeal thrombosis which he encountered initially, by rapid direct transfusion through a short cannula from the carotid artery of a donor dog to the jugular vein of an exsanguinated recipient dog; the latter was consequently resuscitated.[3-7,9,10]

Priority for the first attempt at therapeutic blood transfusion must go to Jean Baptiste Denis of Paris.[3-8,11,12] Denis, having learnt about Lower's successful experiments, endeavoured to treat a seventeen year old youth with a fever by the transfusion of about 250 ml of blood from the carotid artery of a sheep on 15 June 1667. There was no obvious adverse reaction. Denis carried out several further transfusions to humans using both sheep and calf blood in 1667, but, not unnaturally, later patients suffered transfusion reactions with gross haematuria and two of them died. Denis was tried for murder and, although he was aquitted, the Faculty of Medicine in Paris condemned the procedure, and later an act of the French Chamber of Deputies prohibited further experimental blood transfusions in France.[3-8,10-14]

Lower demonstrated animal-to-man transfusion to the Royal Society in London, with the aid of Edumnd King, in 1667 in an attempt to transfer the docile nature of a lamb to Arthur Coga, a "mild melancholy insane man," by direct transfusion of blood from the carotid artery of the animal. The procedure was uneventful, although the mental condition of the patient was not improved. It is significant that neither Lower, despite his dog experiments, nor Denis appreciated that blood transfusion was a procedure indicated for acute loss of blood. They, like the ancients before them, regarded it as a fluid which could be used to transfer the physical or mental attributes of the donating animal to the patient. Animal to man transfusions were also carried out about this time in Germany and Holland.[3-8,14]

Little progress was made in the development of blood transfusion to man for 150 years after the debacle of the Denis transfusions, but authors of textbooks in the eighteenth century often included theoretical descriptions and fanciful pictures of the procedure.

The contribution of James Blundell

James Blundell (1790-1877) received his medical training in London and Edinburgh, as was not unusual in those days. He was well connected and had a considerable private income as well as a lucrative practice. He was the nephew of Dr. John Haighton, an eminent physiological investigator and vivisectionist, who had been a pupil of the great John Hunter. James Blundell succeeded his uncle as Lecturer in Physiology and Obstetrics at Guy's Hospital. He was 28 and had been in obstetric practice in London for about 4 years when he turned his attention to the question of blood transfusion; his interest being prompted by the many deaths which followed post-partum haemorrhage in those days.[15]

Blundell conducted a series of carefully planned animal experiments with dogs. This investigation constituted the first systematic study of blood transfusion. He first used the traditional direct method by connecting the artery of the donor dog to the recipient vein, but soon moved on to employ a cannula and graduated brass syringe. He was thus the first to be able to measure the quantity of blood transfused. He avoided coagulation by losing no time in transferring the donor blood to the recipient animal.[1,2,15-17]

The results of these animal experiments established the principles on which his subsequent clinical practice was based. He rejected the idea of the transfusion of animal blood to man, he established that venous blood had resuscitative powers equal to arterial blood and that relatively small volumes of blood compared with the loss which the recipient had suffered could tip the balance in favour of recovery. He appreciated that exclusion of air was important, but he established that small quantities of air injected into the circulation were not as lethal as had previously been believed.[1,2,15-17]

Blundell's first human to human transfusions were undertaken using the simple syringe technique, but he went on first to design a valved "Impellor" in an effort to reduce the danger of coagulation by ensuring that the blood was outside the body for the least possible time. Donor blood was shed into a conical receptacle surrounded by warm water which was thought to further retard coagulation, and immediately pumped into the patient using the syringe which was an intrinsic of the device.

The apparatus was equipped with a large screw so that it could be mounted on a chair.[2-7,15-17] Lastly, in 1828 he designed the "gravitator." The donor bled directly from a venesection into a receptacle and the blood flowed directly into the recipient under gravity, much as is the case with modern intravenous apparatus, except that there was no intervening drip chamber (see below).

Blundell's primary indication for transfusion was massive haemorrhage, but he did not entirely abandon the concept that blood had intrinsic life-giving properties. He regarded transfusion as a procedure of last resort. He recorded 10 transfusions in the period 1818 to 1828. One case of post-partum haemorrhage and one other patient were almost certainly already dead. Five of the remaining six patients which he transfused for haemorrhage survived. The other two transfusions were for puerperal fever and inanition; both survived the procedure but died from their primary diseases some hours later.[2,5,16-18]

Blundell does not seem to have encountered any transfusion reactions, but both the volumes transfused (120 to 480 ml) and the number of transfusions were numerically small. It is possible to calculate that, with a Western European population, the statistical chances of a major ABO incompatibility occurring is only 36 percent with uncrossmatched blood.[15]

Blood transfusion in the second half of the nineteenth century

Blundell was undoubtedly the father of modern transfusion; as Roussel wrote in 1877, "since the labours of Blundell transfusion has never been lost sight of in England and other countries."[19] His publications and already well established reputation as a scientist, surgeon and obstetrician brought gradual recognition of the value of transfusion as a treatment of last resort in continental Europe, the British Isles and the United States.[1,17]

A number of new devices were designed with a view to avoiding coagulation, the principal cause of technical difficulty, by rapid transference from donor to recipient.[3-7,20-25] Higginson of Liverpool used a version of his well known rubber syringe with ball valves to transfer venous blood from a warmed funnel in 1857.[20] Waller, Blundell's London contemporary, employed a syringe and three-way tap in 1859,[21] and two transfusions using a simple syringe were carried out during the War between the States in the eighteen sixties.[22] Roussel of Brussels described a rather elaborate instrument in 1867.[23] It applied suction over a donor vein to withdraw blood into a receptacle and then employed an indiarubber bulb pump to pump it into the recipient vein. This device is said to have been used in the field in the Franco-German War of 1870.[4] Avelin, another London obstetrician, devised a much simpler pumping device for vein-to-vein transfusion; it was successfully used to resuscitate a lady suffering from an inverted uterus due to post-partum haemorrhage by transferring 240 ml of blood from her gallant coachman.[24] Franz Gesellius of Leipzig was an advocate of warming blood to avoid clotting and surrounded his device with a hot water bottle.[25]

It is unfortunate that, despite the experiences of Denis and the careful scientific investigations of Blundell, animal-to-man transfusions continued to be employed up to the early eighteen seventies, particularly by German workers.[25,26] The published work of both Ponfick[27] and of Landois[28] finally ended this regrettable procedure.

Landois reviewed the total recorded world experience of 478 authenticated transfusions to man in 1875; 129 of these were of blood from animals (including the transfusions by Denis and Lower) and 347 of human blood.[28] Forty-three percent of the human-to-human transfusions survived and the patients were deemed to have improved, 52 percent were not improved or died later, the result in 15 patients (4.3 percent) was unknown, but only two (0.6 percent) were known to have died during the transfusion.

It must be remembered in considering the results that, on the one hand most of these transfusions were administered to patients *in extremis,* and on the other that often only very small quantities of blood were administered because of the practical difficulty of coagulation in the apparatus. This latter factor probably saved many lives!

Transfusion continued to be regarded as a procedure of last resort.[29] Isolated reports of success, particularly for the treatment of obstetric haemorrhage, continued[4] (for example Halsted (1852-1922) of Johns Hopkins transfused his sister with his own blood for post-partum haemorrhage in 1881),[30] but the full potential of blood transfusion could not be realised until the triple complications of coagulation, incompatibility and possible infection could be conquered. The possibility of infection, of which there is admittedly remarkably little evidence in early reports, was to be solved by the development of aseptic surgical technics in the last two decades of the nineteenth century; coincidentally, however, this of course brought with it more heroic surgery and a greater need for blood transfusion despite contemporary interest in saline infusions for the replacement of blood loss.[7]

The revival of direct artery to vein transfusion

George Washington Crile (1864-1943) of the Cleveland Clinic revived the procedure of direct artery-to-vein transfusion using the new aseptic technics early in the twentieth century from 1903 onwards.[31,32] Crile's secret was to use a specially designed short cannula which permitted continuity of the vascular intima. A number of American surgeons followed Crile's lead. The method of dealing with incompatibility was very crude. It was simply to apply what was described as the "biological test"; the transfusion was started and allowed to continue unless severe symptoms of incompatibility occurred. It is not surprising that there were fatalities!

Crile's indications for transfusion are interesting. His use of it for haemorrhagic shock, burns, anemia, leukemia, septicemia and even carbon monoxide poisoning are logical in the light of modern knowledge, but his trials of the procedure for sarcoma carcinoma, exophthalmic goitre, tuberculosis, eclampsia and pellagra show that the concept that blood contained some vital factor besides cells and hemoglobin was not yet completely abandoned in the early twentieth century.

Blood grouping

It is well known that Landsteiner (1868-1943)[33] described three of the major ABO groups in 1901 and that Cartello and Sturli[34] discovered the fourth group in 1902, but the practical application of grouping to clinical transfusion awaited the work of Jansky in Prague in 1907,[35] and, more importantly from the point of view of Great Britain and the United States, the independent publication by Moss[36] of Johns Hopkins in 1910. The Roman numbers which Jansky and Moss both initially allocated to designate the four groups were reversed so far as the O (universal donor) and AB (universal recipient) groups were concerned. This was obviously a very dangerous situation. Landsteiner, by then working in New York and sponsored by the American Association of Immunologists, suggested the ABO classification which was universally adopted in 1927.[13,37] It is incredible but true that Oehlecher of Hamburg was still describing a modified version of the biological test (the initial injection of 20 ml of blood at 2 minute intervals) in 1933.[38] The biological test was, of course, useless if the patient was moribund or anaesthetised.

Physical methods of avoiding coagulation

It was originally mistakenly believed that keeping blood warm would retard coagulation.[18,25] It is now known that there are good reasons for warming blood during transfusion, but preventing clotting is not one of them. The only recourse in the early days was therefore the rapid transference of blood from the donor to the recipient. Hewson,[39] an associate of the great surgeon John Hunter, working the in second half of the eighteenth century, showed that blood remains fluid so long as it is in contact with the vascular intima, and this fact was exploited by Crile in his direct transfusions.

Defibrination by beating the blood in a similar manner to beating an egg with a whisk was practised by some transfusionists from the very early days, but with only moderate success.[2-7,13] Reactions were frequent, possibly because greater quantities of incompatible blood were administered to the patient simply because it remained fluid, but, despite Blundell's early investigations,[18] the injection of small air bubbles produced in the process of defibrination were blamed for many of the reactions which occurred.[40] Moss[41] described a sophisticated method of defibrination by agitating with glass beads in 1914, and with his knowledge of blood grouping he was thus able to administer cross-matched blood without the danger of coagulation.

Another approach to avoiding coagulation was the use of a flask coated internally with paraffin wax, as described by Kimpton and Brown in 1914.[42] The glass cannula which formed an intrinsic part of the flask was first used to bleed the donor and then immediately transferred to the recipient's vein.

Chemical anticoagulants

The ultimate solution to the coagulation problem was, however, chemical by the removal of ionised calcium by citrate. This clinical breakthrough was achieved by Albert Hustin (1882-1967) of Brussels, who first used citrated blood for human transfusion in March 1914.[43,44] Hustin's contribution was the culmination of a very long story. Hunter's associate, William Hewson, had noted that neutral salts could prevent the coagulation of blood 140 years earlier in 1774,[39] nearly half a century before Blundell's first transfusion! John Braxton Hicks, like Blundell an obstetrician from Guy's Hospital, London, had used sodium phosphate empirically in 1868 to prevent clotting in three cases of post-partum haemorrhage.[45] It is true that all three patients died; however, they were *in extremis* and one of them lived for five days. There is nothing in the original paper to suggest that their deaths were due to the infusion of the inorganic phosphate, as has sometimes been suggested.[7,45,46] Two Swiss workers, Arthus and Pages, used sodium citrate in animal work in 1890,[47] and from then on the technic was well known to laboratory workers, but it was not applied to clinical medicine by Hustin for another twenty years. A comparison can be made with the long interval between the introduction of curare to animal experimentation and its use in clinical practice.[48]

Blood transfusion in the Great War 1914-1918

Providence had thus decreed that the two great problems which held back the development of human transfusion, major ABO incompatibility and extra corporeal clotting, were both solved on the eve of the Great War of 1914-1918.

Crile was in Paris for three months early in 1915 at the head of a civilian team from Lakeside Hospital in Ohio dealing with British Military casualties. He practised blood transfusion by the direct cannula method at that time and demonstrated his anesthetic technic of anoci-association to British Medical Officers, including the famous surgeon Colonel (later Lord) Moynihan.[29,49]

Crile returned to France in 1917 as a Consultant Surgeon in the United States Army. His No. 4 Base Hospital, which was once again formed from the staff of the Lakeside Hospital in Ohio, was the first US army unit of any kind, combatant or non-combatant, to reach France. It was initially attached to the British No. 9

General Hospital at Rouen. Crile was surprised to find that transfusion was not being used by the Medical Services of the British and French armies.[29]

A British physiologist, Captain Geoffrey Marshall (1887-1982), later well known as the leading chest physician Sir Geoffrey Marshall, was at that time investigating the large number of deaths during and after surgery in the British Military Hospitals in France.[50-53] The sort of problems which were being encountered were described in Marshall's classic paper in the *British Medical Journal* in 1917;[50] for example, there was the profound and sometimes fatal fall in blood pressure which occurred during surgery under spinal anesthesia in the hypovolemic patient due to abolition of sympathetic control of the vascular system; similarly, catastrophic hypotension often occurred in the postoperative period following deep ether anesthesia when the sympatheticomimetic effect of etherisation on cardiac output was withdrawn.[46,47]

Crile introduced blood transfusion using the new technics of cross-matching and citration both in the General Hospitals and in Casualty Clearing Stations. The British Medical Services adopted Crile's technics with alacrity. Marshall and others record that the improvement in the survival rate of the wounded men was dramatic.[29,53-56]

Captain Geoffrey Keynes (1887-1982), a young British surgeon, learned the technic of using citrated blood from another United States medical unit composed of doctors from Harvard, and applied his new knowledge with considerable success.[6,55]

Rous and Turner[57] of New York demonstrated in 1916 that the addition of glucose to the citrate solution extended the period for which blood could be stored outside the body. Captain Oswold Robertson, a Canadian, working with the United States Base Hospital in France, used this knowledge to organise the first bank of stored blood in 1918. Some of the blood was used after being stored for 28 days, but usually it was stored for 10 to 14 days.[6,7,58]

Keynes modified the flask designed by Robertson and added the familiar drip-chamber which had originally been designed by Laurie for subcutaneous saline infusions in 1909.[3,59] Keynes was a leading advocate of citrated blood transfusion in the United Kingdom after the Great War. He ultimately became Sir Geoffrey Keynes, one of the foremost British surgeons of his generation.[60] The Keynes' flask was standard equipment in British Hospitals in the nineteen twenties and thirties until it was replaced by gravitational systems such as that described by Marriott and Kekwick in 1935.[61] This technic bears a marked resemblance to Blundell's original gravitator with, of course, the addition of the drip-chamber.

Summary

Nineteen eighteen, one hundred years after Blundell undertook the first human to human blood transfusion in 1818, can be regarded as the year in which the early history of the procedure ended. The twin problems of coagulation and incompatibility, which had hindered development in the nineteenth century, had been solved by then and, in addition, a technic for banking blood for future use had been introduced. Sad to say, however, the lessons learned in war are often forgotten in peacetime. It was not until the Spanish Civil War (1935-1939) and the Second World War (1939-1945) that the technics of citration and refrigeration on a large scale were fully accepted and exploited.[6,7,62]

References

1. Blundell J: Experiments on the transfusion of blood by the syringe. *Medico-Chirurgical Transactions* 9: 56, 1818.
2. Jones HW, Mackmull G: The influence of James Blundell on the development of blood transfusion. *Annals of Medical History* 10: 242-8, 1928.
3. Keynes G: *Blood Transfusion.* London: Frowde and Hodder and Stoughton, 1922.
4. Kilduff RA, DeBakey M: *The Blood Bank and the Technique and Therapeutics of Transfusion.* St. Louis: Mosby, 1942.
5. Keynes G: The history of blood transfusion. *British Journal of Surgery* 31: 38-45, 1943-1944.

6. Keynes G. ed: *Blood Transfusion.* Bristol: Wright, 1949.
7. Hutchin MD: History of blood transfusion. *Surgery* 64: 685-700, 1968.
8. Sprat T: *History of the Royal Society*. London: 1667: 371.
9. Lower R: *Tractatus De Corde item De Motu & Colore Sanguinis et Chyli in eum Transitu.* London: Redmayne, 1669.
10. Hoff EC: The life and times of Richard Lower, physiologist and physician. *Bulletin of the Institute of History of Medicine*. Johns Hopkins University 4: 517-35, 1936.
11. Denis J: A letter concerning a new way of curing sundry diseases by transfusion of blood. *Philosophical Transactions,* 2: 489, 1667.
12. Keynes G: Tercentary of blood transfusion. *British Medical Journal* 4: 410-1, 1967.
13. Maluf NSR: History of blood transfusion. *Journal of the History of Medicine and Allied Sciences* 9: 59-107, 1954.
14. Hoff HE, Guillemin R: The first experiments on transfusion in France. *Journal of the History of Medicine and Allied Sciences,* 18: 103-24, 1963.
15. Boulton TB: Classical File. James Blundell MD, FRCP and the introduction of the transfusion of human blood to man. *Survey of Anesthesiology* 30: 100-6, 1986.
16. Blundell J: *Researches physiological and pathological; instituted principally with a view to the improvement of medical and surgical practice*. London: Cox, 1824.
17. Blundell J: Observations on the transfusion of blood, with a description of his gravitator. *Lancet* 2: 321-4, 1828-1829.
18. Blundell J; Successful case of transfusion. *Lancet* 1: 431-2, 1828-1829.
19. Roussel J: *Transfusion of human blood by the method of Roussel.* Guinness CHC translator. London: Churchill, 1877.
20. Higginson A: Report of seven cases of the transfusion of blood; with a description of the instrument invented by the author. *Liverpool Medico-Chirurgical Journal* 1: 102-10, 1851.
21. Waller C: On transfusion of blood. Its history and application in cases of severe haemorrhage. *Transactions of the Obstetrical Society of London* 1: 61-73, 1859.
22. Kuhns WJ: Blood transfusions in the Civil War. *Transfusion* 5: 92-4, 1965.
23. Roussel J: Nouvel Instrument pour la transfusion du sang. *Gazette des hopitaux* 2: 549, 1867.
24. Aveling JH: Successful case of immediate transfusion. *Lancet* 2: 147-8, 1872.
25. Gesellius F: *Die Transfusion des Blutes. Eire historische, kritische und physiologische Studie.* Leipzig: Wagner 1873.
26. Hasse O: *Die Lammblut-Transfusion beim Menschen.* St. Petersburg: Hoppe, 1874.
27. Ponfick E: Experimentelle Beitrage zur Lehre von die Transfusion. *Berl klin W II;* 333-6, 1874.
28. Landois L. *Die Transfusion des Blutes*. Leipzig: Vogel, 1875.
29. Thomas TG: The intravenous injection of milk as a substitute for the transfusion of blood; illustrated by seven operations. *New York Medical Journal* 27: 449-65, 1878.
30. Crowe S: *Halsted of Johns Hopkins. The Man and his Men*. Springfield: Thomas, 1957.
31. Crile G ed: *George Crile, An autobiography.* Philadelphia: Lipppincott, 1947.
32. Crile GW: *Hemorrhage and Transfusion. An experimental and clinical research.* New York: Appleton, 1909.
33. Landsteiner K: Ueber Agglutinations-erscheinungen normalen menschlichen Blutes. *Wiener klinische Wochenschrift* 14: 1132-4, 1901.
34. Decastello AV, Sturli A: Über die Isoagglutinine und Serum gesunder und kranker Menschen. *München medizinische Wochenschrift* 49: 1090-5, 1902.
35. Jansky J: Haematologische studien u psychotik. (Etudes hématologiques, dans les maladies mentales). *Praha* 8: 85-139, 1907.
36. Moss WL: Studies on iso-agglutinins and iso-hemolysins. *Johns Hopkins Bulleting* 21: 63-70, 1910.
37. Landsteiner K: Individual differences in human blood. *Science* 73: 403-9, 1931.
38. Oehleker F: *Die Bluttransfusion.* Berlin: Urban Schwarzenberg, 1933.
39. Hewson W: *Experimental inquiries. Part the first containing an inquiry into the properties of blood. With remarks on some of its morbid appearances*. London: Johnson, 1774.
40. Dieffenbach JF: *Die Transfusion des Blutes.* Berlin: Enslin, 1828.
41. Moss WL: A simple method of the indirect transfusion of blood. *American Journal of Medical Sciences* 147: 698-703, 1914.
42. Kimpton AR, Brown JH: A new and simple method of transfusion. *Journal of the American Medical Association* 6: 117-8, 1913.
43. Hustin A: Principe d'une nouvelle méthode de transfusion mugueuse. *Journal Médecine Bruxelles* 19: 436-9, 1914.

44. Reinhold H, Bernard-Dichstein C: The origins of today's stored blood transfusion practice: the contribution of Albert Hustin. In: Atkinson RS, Boulton TB, eds: *The History of Anaesthesia.* International Congress Series 134. London: Royal Society of Medicine, 433-40, 1989.
45. Hicks JB: On transfusion and a new mode of management. *British Medical Journal* 2: 151 and 203, 1868.
46. Hicks JB: Cases of transfusion with some remarks on a new method of performing the operation. *Guy's Hospital reports* 14: 1-14, 1869.
47. Arhus M, Pages C: Nouvelle théorie clinique de la coagulation du sang. *Archives Physiologie Normale et Pathalogique* 2: 739-46, 1890.
48. Thomas KB: *Curare. Its History and Usage.* Philadelphia: Lippincott, 1963.
49. Rendell-Baker L: The development and function of anaesthesia breathing systems. In: Atkinson RS, Boulton, TB, eds: *the History of Anaesthesia.* International Congress and Symposium Series 134. London: Royal Society of Medicine, 301-19, 1989.
50. Marshall G: The administration of anaesthetics at the front. *British Medical Journal* 1: 722-5, 1917.
51. Obituary. Sir Geoffrey Marshall. *British Medical Journal* 285: 567, 1982.
52. Boulton TB: Classical File. Sir Geoffrey Marshall, shock and nitrous oxide. *Survey of Anesthesiology* 36: 40-51, 1992.
53. Evans B: A doctor in the Great War. An interview with Sir Geoffrey Marshall. *British Medical Journal* 285: 1780-3, 1982.
54. Taylor DC: Note on gas oxygen and local anaesthesia for gunshot wounds of the abdomen. In: Crile GW, Lower WE, eds: *Surgical Shock and the Shockless Operation through Anoci-Association.* 2nd ed. Philadelphia: Saunders, 152-5, 1920.
55. Keynes G. *The Gates of memory.* Oxford: University Press, 1983.
56. Guiou NM: Blood transfusion in a field ambulance. *British Medical Journal* 1: 695-6, 1918.
57. Rous P, Turner JR: The preservation of living red blood cells in vitro. *Journal of Experimental Medicine* 23: 219-48, 1916.
58. Robertson OH: Transfusion with preserved red cells. *British Medical Journal* 1: 691-3, 1918.
59. Laurie RD: An apparatus for indicating the rate of flow of saline solution in subcutaneous and rectal administration. *Lancet* 1: 248, 1909.
60. Obituary. Sir Geoffrey Keynes. *British Medical Journal* 285: 299, 1982.
61. Marriott HL, Kekwick A: A continuous drip blood transfusion; with case records of very large transfusions. *Lancet* 1: 977-81, 1935.
62. Whitby L: Blood Transfusion. In: Cope Z, ed: *Surgery.* London: Her Majesty's Stationery Office, 1953: 46-57.

RICHARD DOUGLAS SANDERS, M.D.
Anesthesiologist, Inventor, Painter
(1906–1977)

JOSEPH J. BUCKLEY
Emeritus Professor and Head
Department of Anesthesiology
University of Minnesota Medical School
Minneapolis, Minnesota USA

Doug Sanders (Fig. 1) was an imposing figure of a man, well over six feet tall, with a long, chiseled face and lantern jaw. His shoulders were slightly stooped, and his long arms and massive hands seemed to reach almost to his knees. In his leather-elbowed jacket and bow tie, he resembled a Norman Rockwell sketch of the country doctor. Indeed he *was* a product of the country, for he traced his ancestry through three generations of hardy Tennessee mountain people. And he exuded that air of quiet dignity and self-confidence we have come to associate with the pioneers of that era.

Sanders was born in 1906 in the tiny village of Erin, Tennessee. His father was a dentist who also administered anesthetics. His mother was a professional whistler! Through exposure to his father's anesthetic practice, Doug was inspired to become a physician and earned his M.D. at the University of Louisville in 1928. After interning, he practiced family medicine in Kentucky during the difficult years of the Great Depression, supplementing a meager income by administering inhalation anesthesia for dental surgery. His aptitude as a clinical anesthetist soon earned him membership on the medical staffs of several Louisville hospitals, and by 1937 he had decided to devote himself full-time to anesthesiology. Thereafter, his reputation and practice flourished until, in 1942, he was inducted into the U.S. Army. Recognizing his experience as an anesthetist, the Army immediately appointed him Chief of the Anesthesiology and O.R. Section of its Valley Forge General Hospital. At that time, Valley Forge was the Army's primary center for facial reconstruction of soldiers wounded in WWII combat. The formidable challenges of intubating and

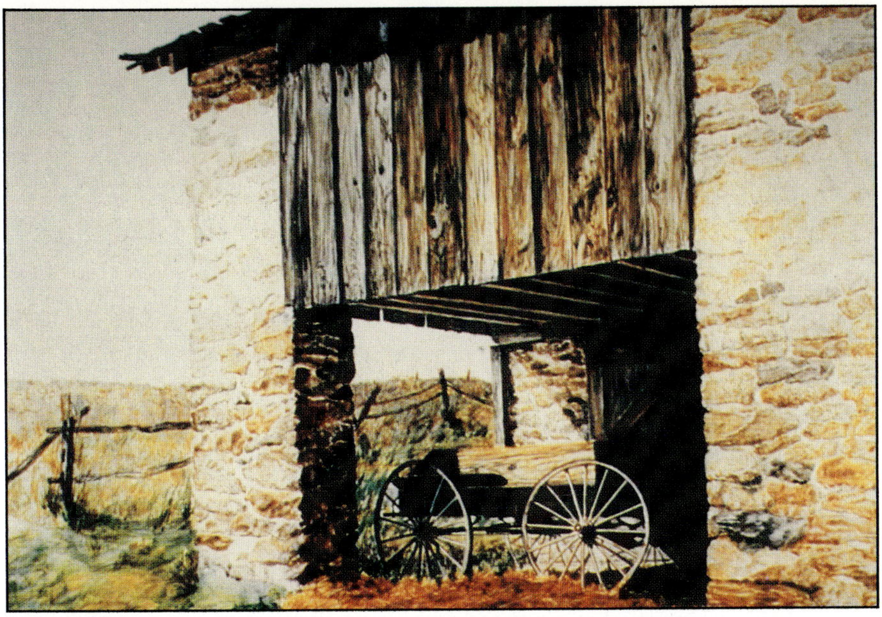

Fig. A.
Sanders'
rendition of
Pennsylvania
barnyard
(watercolor).

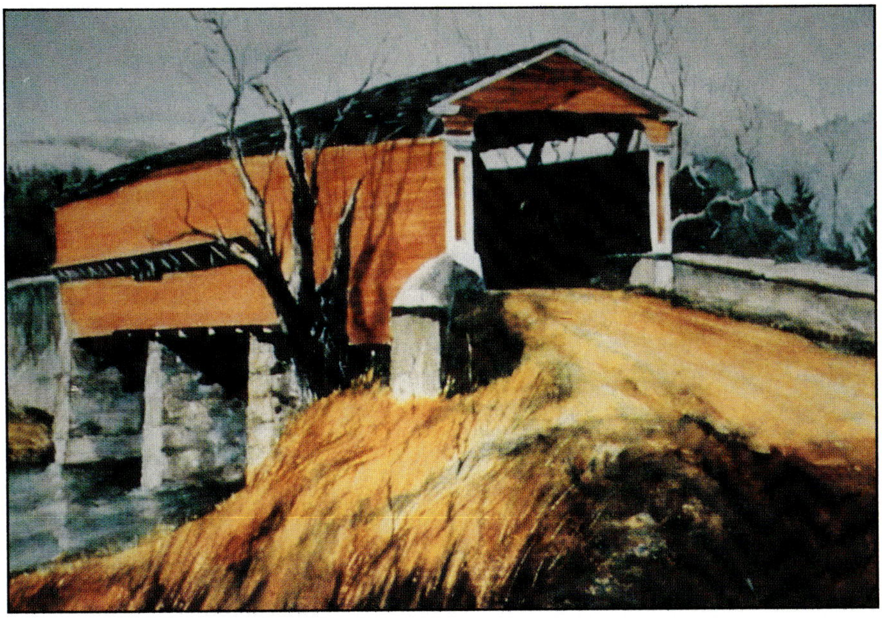

Fig. B.
Sanders'
wooden bridge
in Delaware
backcountry
(watercolor).

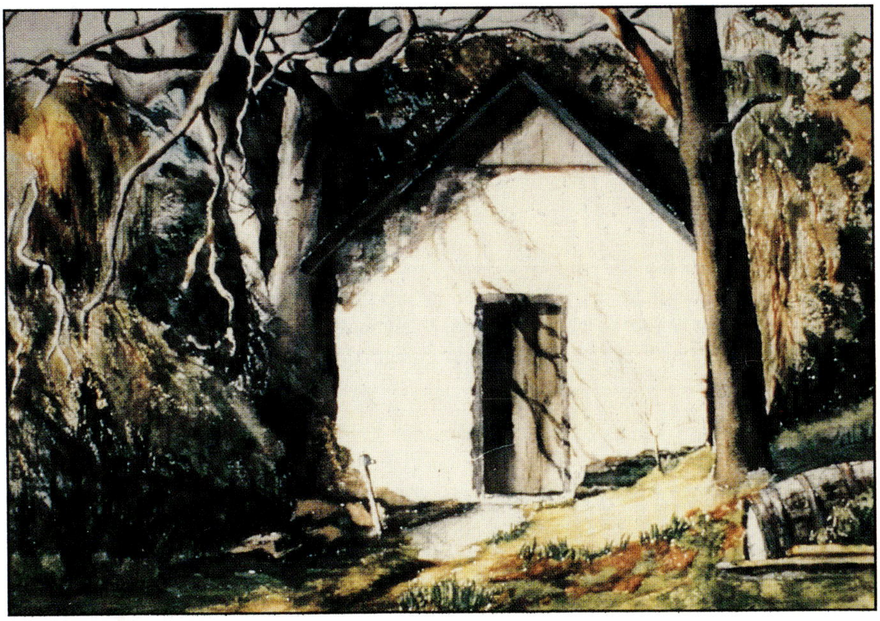

Fig. C.
Sanders'
storehouse
below the hill
(egg tempera).

Figs. A, B and C:
Besides his continuous pursuit of solutions to clinical problems, R. Douglas Sanders became an ardent painter of landscapes with an emphasis on Americana. Three of his works are depicted on the other side of this tip-in. For more information regarding his paintings, see pages 76 and 77.

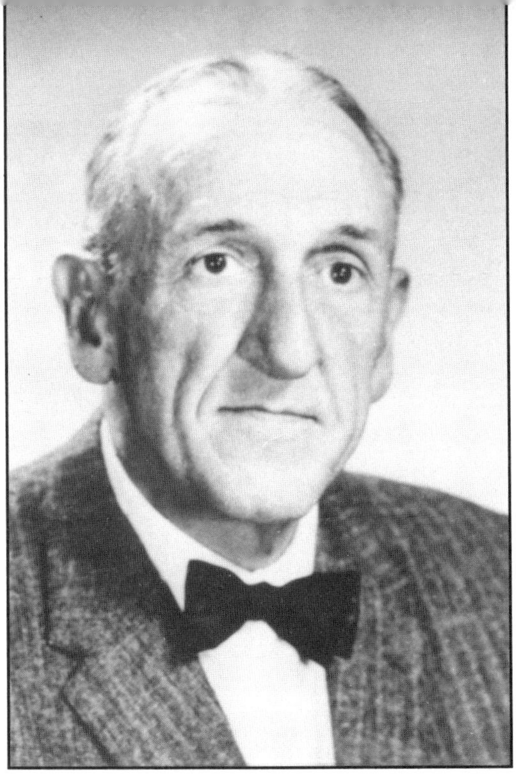

Fig. 1. R. Douglas Sanders, *circa* 1970.

maintaining airway integrity of those patients through long hours of maxillofacial surgery spurred Sanders to develop his earliest innovative device, the armored latex endotracheal tube, which will be described more fully below. He also modified the traditional Jackson laryngoscope, flattening its tubular blade for better tongue control and adding a battery compartment and light carrier to facilitate its use outside the operating room.

It is important to recognize that these early professional accomplishments were achieved despite the fact that Sanders had no formal training in anesthesiology. Yet, through persistent study and frequent visits to teaching departments, he eventually gained sufficient knowledge and skills to be certified as a Diplomate of the American Board of Anesthesiology in 1944. Upon discharge from military, Sanders became Director of Anesthesia at the Delaware Hospital in Wilmington, Delaware. As such, he was the first full-time anesthesiologist in the State of Delaware. He soon established a School of Anesthesia at Delaware Hospital, recruited a staff of dedicated anesthesiologists, and arranged an affiliation with Jefferson Medical College so that medical students could spend time in a private practice setting.

But Sanders was not simply an accomplished anesthetist and effective administrator. Rather, he was a true renaissance man, with interest and knowledge in such diverse subjects as metallurgy, navigation, rubber fabrication, physics, landscape painting, and proper use of the English language! But clearly, his most remarkable talent was conceptualizing new devices to solve common problems. An example is the endotracheal tube he designed during his military duty (Fig. 2). It was the first completely flexible, non-compressible rubber tube, made so by a monofilament nylon spiral embedded within its latex wall.[1] To make this tube, Sanders had to master the art of molding and dipping raw latex. Sanders then undertook to produce a cuff which could be applied to his new endotracheal catheter. At that time (late 1940's) most anesthetists used gauze mouth packs or oversized uncuffed tubes to effect a tracheal seal. After numerous unsuccessful trials, he finally managed to fabricate an inflatable latex rubber cuff on a handmade

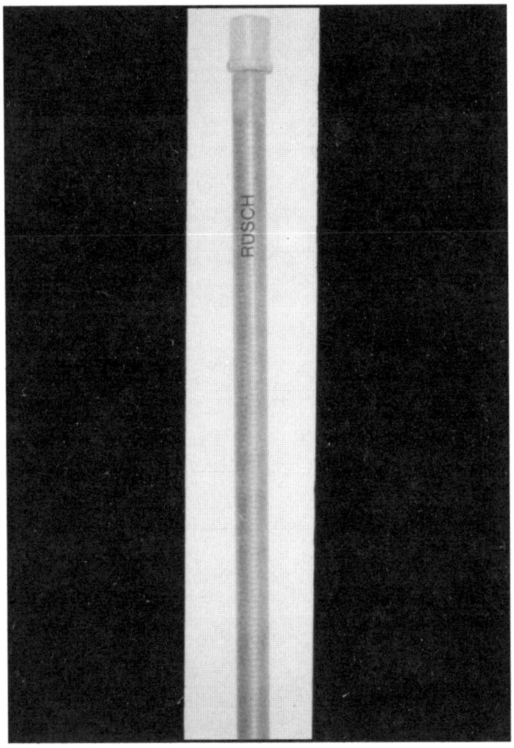

Fig. 2. Latex armored (nylon spiral) endotracheal tube.

aluminum mold. The process required repeated manual dipping and drying steps to produce a cuff which was soft yet durable. To simplify this tedious task he built an ingenious overhead rail from which the molds were suspended; this motorized rail sloped down at one point to immerse the molds in the bath of molten latex, then rose again to carry them into a drying oven a few feet farther along. Doug got the inspiration for this dipping/drying conveyor system during an idea-seeking visit he made to a condom factory!! Such was the diversity of his talents that he even did the necessary toxicity and tissue tolerance studies on these latex products, using tissue cell cultures obtained from friends at the Alfred I. DuPont Institute in Wilmington.

Never one to be secretive about his ideas or inventions, he gave prototype tubes and cuffs for trial by colleagues and friends and soon began to receive orders from anesthesiologists all over the country. Demand became so great that he relocated the molding-conveyor system from his basement laboratory to a technician's shop, much to the relief of his wife, Flora, who found the constant smell of hot latex oppressive! In contrast to the tenacity he showed in creating the tube and cuff, Sanders had little patience for the mundane tasks of marketing and distribution of his products and soon relinquished those functions to commercial firms. Although he had personally financed all of the studies, materials and equipment required to develop the tube and cuff, he never tried to patent the devices or to seek reimbursement or royalties from their subsequent commercial production.

It was not long before Sanders' creativity outgrew his pocketbook and his productivity thus was threatened. But his resourcefulness once again provided a solution which allowed him to pursue further research. Thus, in 1965, under the aegis of the Delaware Academy of Medicine, he founded the Anesthesia Research Foundation and recruited a number of generous private and corporate benefactors. As the Foundation's first president, he handled the administrative and legal responsibilities associated with its operation, and personally scrutinized and endorsed all requests for funding. Despite its designation as an *anesthesia* research organ, Sanders structured the Foundation's charter broadly enough that, presently, it funded research in such diverse areas as nutrition and advanced pulmonary disease, and it administered a loan fund for needy Delaware medical students, sponsored a lecture program for local physicians on new developments in various fields of medicine, and underwrote the expense of educating medical students in a private practice setting of Delaware Hospital.

In retrospect, it is apparent that this Foundation provided Sanders with the means to undertake his crowning inventive achievement. Several months after setting up the organization, he set out to solve a shortcoming of clinical medicine that had troubled him for years, namely, the lack of a safe, effective method of general anesthesia for bronchoscopic examination of the airways. Local (topical) anesthesia, as promoted by Chevalier Jackson, was the prevalent method at that time (1966). But bronchoscopy under local anesthesia, while quite safe, often was such a stressful experience that many patients refused to submit to it, especially if they had suffered through a previous awake endoscopic examination. A number of general anesthesia methods were in use at that time, but none provided consistently adequate anesthesia *and ventilation,* and most seriously impeded the endoscopist's ability to make an unhurried, thorough examination of the airways.

To solve this problem, Sanders seized upon an old principle of physics formulated by Daniel Bernoulli in 1738,[2] which states that when fluid flows through a tube, there is a direct relationship between the pressure and velocity of the fluid: the higher the pressure, the greater the speed at which the fluid flows. Further, if the tube is narrowed at some point, the velocity of flow increases while the pressure of the fluid decreases. Sanders recognized that Bernoulli's Principle could be applied to effect positive pressure ventilation through a bronchoscope. When he directed a jet of fast-flowing gas down and parallel to the long axis of the bronchoscope, a zone of negative pressure was created in the area just proximal to the jet which, in turn, caused room air to be entrained in the wake of the jet (the well-known Venturi tube effect). The total amount of gas that emerged from the distal end of the bronchoscope thus was the sum of the volume of gas from the jet plus the volume of the air entrained. Depending upon the diameter of the jet, the driving pressure applied to the jet, and the diameter of the bronchoscope, a predictable *inflation pressure* was achieved which was independent of the lung volume or compliance; on the other hand, the *volume* of gas actually delivered to the lung was directly proportional to the inflation pressure and inversely proportional to the lung/chest wall compliance.

Sanders fashioned his first "jet injector" by hand from a steel intravenous needle to which he soldered a simple clip to attach the injector to the proximal end of the Jackson bronchoscope (Fig. 3). Once he was satisfied that the method worked, he designed and fabricated a variety of injectors for the Hollinger and Negus bronchoscopes (Figs. 4,5,6) and placed a simple toggle valve in the pressure line to permit on-off cycling of pulmonary ventilation. He also conducted countless in vitro studies to establish the relationship of jet driving pressure and bronchoscope size to the maximum inflation pressure achieved.

The first public demonstration of his Ventilating Attachment was made by Dr. Sanders on September 27, 1966, at the annual meeting of the Academy of Anesthesiology; his earliest scientific paper describing the device appeared the following July in a regional professional publication, the Delaware Medical Journal.[3] Colleagues quickly recognized the importance of Sanders' innovation and clamored to have a jet injector for their own use. Again, he generously provided prototypes for trial by clinicians at various institutions. There followed several publications favorably comparing the injector technique to other established anesthetic methods of bronchoscopy[4,5,6], and an assortment of variations/improvements were described.[7,8]

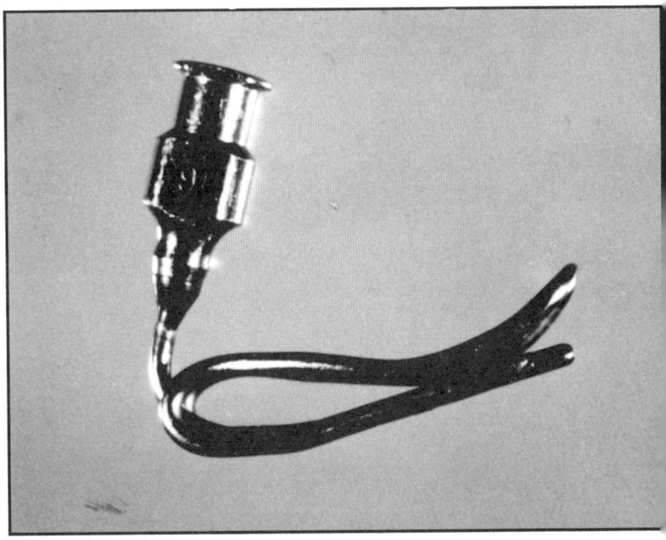

Fig. 3. Original handmade jet injector attachment for Jackson bronchoscope; intravenous needle is jet tube, clip provides attachment to 'scope.

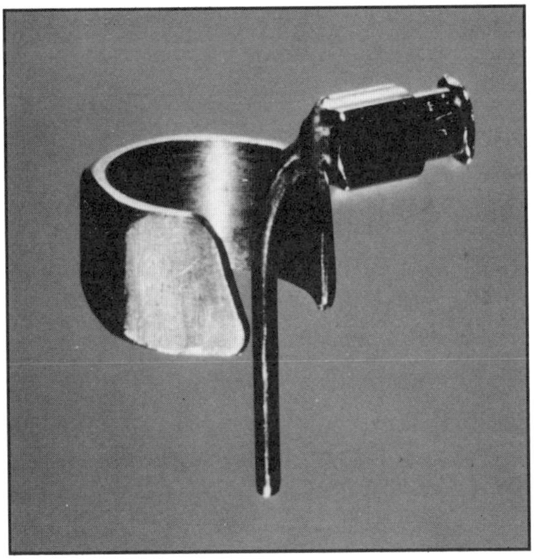

Fig. 4. Original injector for Hollinger bronchoscope; collar tapered to fit proximal neck of 'scope.

Sanders' ingenious innovation not only revolutionized anesthesia for bronchoscopy, but also spawned a variety of other techniques which employed the jet principle. In 1971, Spoerel[9] described a transcutaneous method in which a plastic intravenous catheter, inserted through the cricothyroid membrane, served as the jet tube for ventilation in emergency upper

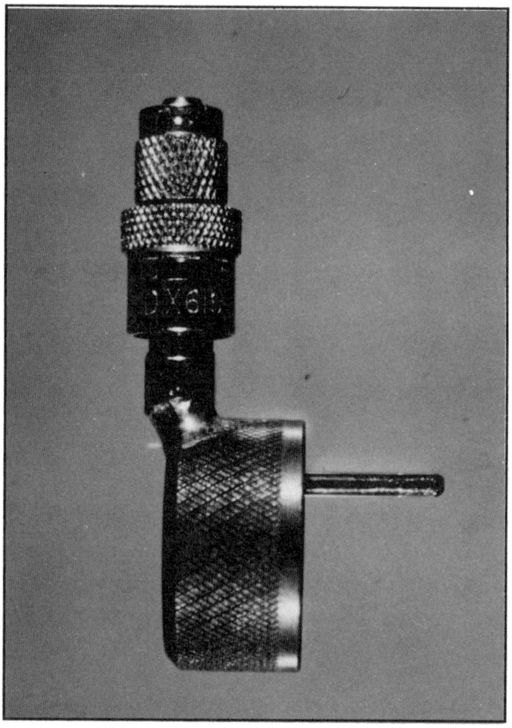

Fig. 5. Improved injector for Hollinger bronchoscope, with machined injector ring and Luer-Lok connector to accept O_2 pressure line.

Fig. 6. Early commercial injector attachment for Negus bronchoscope; Luer-Lok at left provides connection to O_2 pressure line.

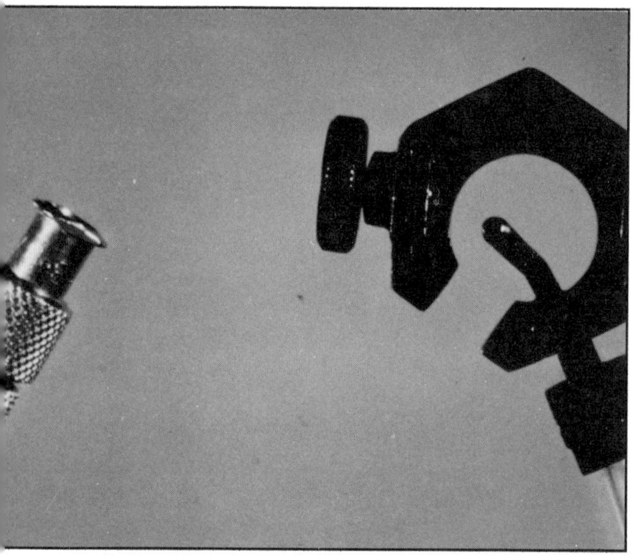

airway obstruction. Soon thereafter, several publications described how the jet injector technique could be adapted for suspension laryngoscopy.[10,11] And Carden[12] introduced another clever modification for microlaryngeal surgery which employed a short endotracheal tube onto which was molded a jet injector tube; this assembly was placed *below* the vocal cords and held in position by an inflatable cuff.

Within a decade after Sanders demonstrated that conventional positive pressure ventilation could be achieved via the jet principle, the potential of *high frequency jet ventilation* (HFJV) was recognized and explored by Sjostrand et al.[13] Subsequently, a variety of clinical applications of HFJV were developed for neonatal, surgical and intensive care situations.[14,15] Clearly, Sanders had discovered a modality which had widespread applicability.

Despite his continuous pursuit of solutions to clinical problems, Doug Sanders had many other secular interests. He loved the sea and the science of navigation and regularly sailed his Alden 38 on Chesapeake Bay. For a time he became intrigued with still photography and even dabbled in movie making when he thought it might be helpful in promoting his ventilating attachment. But his strongest recreational interest was landscape painting, and it became his passion during the last 20 years of his life. He was introduced to that hobby quite fortuitously in the early 1950's while he was under treatment for peptic ulcer disease. A pediatrician colleague brought a painting by Andrew Wyeth to his hospital room to enhance his recovery. Not only did the painting speed Sanders' convalescence, it also sparked in him an eagerness to try his own hand with the brush. As might have been predicted, he tackled the new hobby with the same enthusiasm he applied in his professional ventures, and it was soon evident that he had considerable artistic talent. He painted mostly outdoor scenes with emphasis on Americana, which he found in abundance in the lovely countryside of Pennsylvania and Delaware (Fig. A). His style quite obviously was influenced by Wyeth, his friend and neighbor. It was at Wyeth's suggestion that each summer Sanders vacationed on the coast of

Maine where he produced a number of excellent canvasses depicting that beautiful shore and environs. His early works were in watercolor or acrylic (Fig. B), but his preferred medium was egg tempera (Fig. C). This interest in painting led inevitably to Sanders' long and active participation on the ASA Committee on Art Exhibits. He frequently exhibited works and garnered ribbons at the ASA's Annual Meetings. Sanders' canvasses hang today in the Delaware Art Museum and Wilmington's Hotel DuPont.

Skilled anesthesiologist, imaginative inventor, master fabricator, talented artist—Doug Sanders was the embodiment of each of these identities. Few of his contemporaries can claim to have contributed so much of practical use to anesthesiology, and even fewer can match his artistic talent. The breadth of his creativity, and the fact that his contributions were achieved wholly through innate genius, unfailing self-reliance and personal financial sacrifice, surely place R. Douglas Sanders among America's outstanding medical innovators.

Acknowledgments

I am most grateful to Gerald J. Savage, M.D., James P. Aikens, M.D., and Ms. Geraldine Damiecki, CRNA, all former colleagues of Dr. Sanders; Mrs. Theodore C. Austin, Dr. Sanders' daughter; and Kumar G. Belani, M.D., Associate Professor of Anesthesiology, University of Minnesota Medical School, for their invaluable assistance in compiling this sketch.

References

1. Sanders RD. New endotracheal instruments. Anesthesiology 8:57-61, 1947.
2. Bernoulli D. In: Macintosh R, Mushin WW and Epstein HG, *Physics for the Anaesthetist,* F.A. Davis Co., 3rd Ed., p. 223, Phila., 1963.
3. Sanders RD. Two ventilating attachments for bronchoscopes. Delaware Med. J. 39:170-6, 1967.
4. Pender JE, Winchester LW, Jamplis RW, Lillington GA, McClenahan JB. The effects of anesthesia on ventilation during bronchoscopy. Anesth Analg 47:415-22, 1968.
5. Morales GA, Epstein BS, Cinco B, Adkins PC, Coakley CS. Ventilation during general anesthesia for bronchoscopy. J Thorac Cardiovasc Surg 57:873-8, 1969.
6. Duvall AJ, Johnsen AF, Buckley JJ. Bronchoscopy under general anesthesia using the Sanders ventilation attachment. Ann. Otol. Rhinol. and Laryngol. 78:490-9, 1969.
7. Carden E, Oulton J, Trapp W. A new and simple method for ventilating patients undergoing bronchoscopy. Anesthesiology 33:454-8, 1970.
8. Carden E. Positive pressure ventilation during anesthesia for bronchoscopy: a laboratory evaluation of two recent advances. Anesth Analg 52:402-6, 1973.
9. Spoerel WD, Narayanan PS, Singh NP. Transtracheal ventilation. B J Anaesth 43:932-9, 1971.
10. Oulton JL, Donald DM. A ventilating laryngoscope. Anesthesiology 35:540-2, 1971.
11. Albert SN, Shibuya J, Albert CA. Ventilation with an oxygen injector for suspension laryngoscopy under general anesthesia. Anesth Analg 51:866-70, 1972.
12. Carden E, Crutchfield W. Anaesthesia for microsurgery of the larynx. Can Anaesth Soc J 20:378-89, 1973.
13. Sjostrand U (Ed): Experimental and clinical evaluation of high-frequency positive pressure ventilation, HFPPV. Acta Anaesth Scand (Suppl 64) 1977.
14. Perel A, Segal E. The intraoperative use of high-frequency ventilation. Anesthesiology 61:37-45, 1988.
15. Froese DB, Bryan AC. High-frequency ventilation. Am Rev Resp Dis 135:1363-1375, 1987.

NOTE: Figs. A, B and C appear on the tip-in following page 72.

MEDICAL PRACTICE IN RURAL GEORGIA IN THE 1840'S

JAMES W. BURLESON
Atlanta, Georgia
USA

Medical practice has always reflected national culture. Nowhere was this more evident than in rural Georgia in the 1840's. The National culture in the United States was that of a frontier mentality, and this was reflected in concurrent medical practice. This period is known to American Historians as the "Jacksonian" or "Age of the Common Man" Egalitarian ideals led to the unsettling of many American institutions, medicine being only one. The spirit of freedom led to the rescinding of licensing laws, and every man was held to be free to practice medicine or to choose his practitioner from diverse groups. As Harvey Young has succinctly summarized it: "In the atmosphere of Jacksonian Democracy.... the common man sought common relief for his common ailments."[1]

In Georgia, this was manifest by repealing the "physicians' law." The Georgia legislature had passed this law in 1825 to license properly trained physicians. But in 1836 the legislature repealed this law to allow "irregular" practitioners to practice in Georgia as "necessary for the health of the people." The theory was that the masses could not appreciate superior training in any field and, when the common people came into political power, they were apt to ignore all training standards. All business, they thought, should be open to unrestricted competition. Why should "medical business" be any different from the others? By 1839, Georgia was inundated by a wave of these "irregular" practitioners.[2]

Irregular Practitioners

The first to take advantage of the growing criticism of regular medical practitioners was a man named Samuel Thomson. He had no formal training, but became a "doctor" who gained a reputation as a traveling "herbal practitioner," using roots and herbs exclusively in his treatments. His regular regimen included steam baths and botanical remedies, and he gradually concocted his own peculiar medical "system." He declared there was only one disease, and it was the result of cold. The only remedy then was heat. He recommended steam baths, followed by what he called "hot botanicals," such as cayenne pepper.

Explaining that the digestive system was like a "clogged stovepipe" which occasionally became filled with soot, he used botanic emetics, purgatives, diuretics, and sudorifics to "clean out the system." In his constant denouncements of the regular medical profession, he claimed that their training was designed to "see how much poison could be given without causing death." He loudly opposed everything they advocated, especially all mineral drugs.[3]

The second irregular practice to intrude into Georgia health care was homeopathy. It was begun by a German physician named Samuel Hahnemann. This man was unlike Thomson in that he was a well educated physician who had studied medicine in Leipzig and Vienna. But for 25 years or more he had done little else but travel around the world, writing and translating, but practicing only a minimum of medicine. His main fault, many physicians complained, was that he strayed too often from all conventional thought and spoke out against everything other practitioners advocated. He began to push the idea of "public and personal hygiene, exercise, good diet and fresh air." These things, he claimed, would prevent *all* communicable diseases.[4]

When homeopathy began to lose favor, however, it received a lift from another new cult called the "eclectic school of medicine," founded by Wooster Beach. Dr. Beach, like Hahnemann, had received a legitimate medical education, but he tended to follow the Thomsonian beliefs and emphasized botanical remedies. The believers in the two movements began to join forces, and eventually eliminated the Thomsonians completely.[5]

Still another group of cultists who were growing in favor about the same time were the Hydropaths. These practitioners believed in "internal and external applications of water" to treat the sick. They used what they called "pure water" or water that contained no minerals. Hydropathy (or hydrotherapy, as legitimate physicians called it) had long been recognized as a treatment for *some* patients, but it remained for a Silesian peasant named Vincent Priesnitz to come forward and make it a public cause for almost every ailment that attacked mankind.[6]

Two other cults that gained favor with the public during the same period were Mesmerism and Phrenology. Some surgeons experimented with Mesmerism, but it was not widely accepted. On the other hand, Phrenology, or the study of the "conformations of the skull as they affected mental faculties and character traits," became a social game for a while, but did not gain the acceptance of other off-beat methods of treating patients.[7]

Yet, as divergent as they were, all irregulars had but one thing in common: their enmity toward orthodox physicians. All of them claimed that the latter were "dangerous to the people and ineffective at best." They questioned the training and practices of regular physicians, and passed their distrust to anyone who would listen. In 1847, the Georgia legislature placed these cultists on an equal basis with orthodox physicians by the passage of an act to establish a Botanico Medical Board of physicians "for the better regulation of the Botanic or Thomsonian practice of medicine." Although, at the same time, regular physicians were able to have revised and sustained the 1825 act to regulate the licensing of physicians, the licentiates of the Botanico Medical Board were "fully exempted from said act."[8] This, then, was the milieu in which regular practitioners, such as Crawford Long, sought to practice medicine in rural Georgia in the 1840's.

Rural Medical Practice

Georgia was primarily a rural state in the 1840's. Although Athens, Augusta, Milledgeville, Columbus and Macon were growing, Savannah was the only large city in Georgia at this time.[9]

Rural practice was primarily bedside practice. Thus, rural distances played an important part in medical practice. The weather and horses, and the need to have both on one's side, is a constant motif in physicians' writing.

A Mississippi rural practitioner of this time writes of the missed turns, the soaking rain, the endless conversations with himself, all leading up to a late arrival at the patient's home, and his sense that "this practice of medicine is next to the soldier's life for vexation and discomfort. Can an equivalent for its toils and anxieties ever be rendered in money? I doubt it." Rural distances affected not only the practitioner's degree of comfort or the timeliness of his arrival, but also his opportunities for meaningful consultations, for acquiring new knowledge and colleagues at regional medical meetings, and for spending time with his family.[10]

Not only the rural distances, but the close-knit communities that sparsely populated them, loom large in physicians' accounts of their work. The doctor worked among relationships that were multiple and intimate. A patient might be new to an established practitioner's care, but there was little chance that the patient would be completely unknown to him. If the patient were a slave, this in itself would give him an identity in the white community of which the physician was a part. In this way, the country doctor did not know that nemesis of modern medicine, the anonymous patient. He treated people he knew: his landlord, his neighbor's wife, his creditors and debtors. As physicians stepped back from the bedside a bit, they gave accounts that revealed complex community values. Inadvertently or not, they became the bearers of secrets. Because they missed church to treat a patient, they found out who else was not there, and why not; they learned who drank too much and who was dependent on drugs; they learned whose children were healthy and whose abused; they knew who suffered in silence and who was hypochondriacal; they saw the variety in how much slave owners were willing to spend on the health of their slaves. In terms of obstetrics, the doctor's role as bearer of secrets is nowhere better seen than when he learned something of the sexual lives and attitudes of his neighbors, and thus encountered the community's values at an especially sensitive point.[11]

William Buchan's "Domestic Medicine" was revised and adapted to the diseases and climate of the United States of America by Samuel Powell Griffitts in 1809, and became an extremely popular medical guide for laymen in the nineteenth century. This book was especially popular with southern plantations owners, who used it as a basis for treatment of themselves, their families and their slaves. Thus, the country doctor was frequently called upon to *only* write the prescriptions called for in the book, but not actually treat the patient, and they usually simply sent the medicine requested.[12]

Most practitioners appear to have done relatively little obstetrical work at this time. Account books suggest that country doctors typically attended only five to eight obstetrical cases a year. Other types of surgical work, such as reducing fractures or suturing wounds, were far more common. Pulling teeth was almost a daily surgical task; and compared to this and to the constant routine of prescribing drugs for various ills, childbirth was an uncommon event in a physician's daily work. Nor was obstetrical practice particularly lucrative. Throughout the years we are discussing, physician's fees remained fairly constant: typically, one to three dollars for a routine medical call and prescription. The fees for childbirth—typically eight to fifteen dollars—reflect the time devoted to the case, not a higher rate. Thus, in the context of a general practice, obstetrical work typically yielded neither a substantial portion of the practitioner's income nor sufficient clinical experience to sharpen his technique or develop his professional self-confidence.[13]

Conclusion

This, then, is the picture of the typical medical practitioner in rural Georgia in the 1840's. With the formation of "The Medical Society of the State of Georgia" in 1849, following the guidelines of the American Medical Association (organized in 1847), legitimate physicians began to move to the forefront of medical practice in Georgia. It was, however, many years before the irregular practice of medicine in Georgia ceased.

References

1. Breiger GH, Editor. The Medical Profession. *Medical America in the Nineteenth Century: Readings from the Literature.* Baltimore: The Johns Hopkins Press, 1972:59.
2. Gay EW. *The Medical Profession in Georgia 1733-1983.* Atlanta: Auxiliary to The Medical Association of Georgia, 1983:186.
3. Ibid.: 186-8.
4. Ibid.: 189.
5. Ibid.: 189-190.
6. Ibid.: 191-92.
7. Ibid.: 192-93.
8. Ibid.: 193-94.
9. Ward, J. The Decade of the 1840s in Georgia. *Third International Symposium the History of Anesthesia.* Atlanta: 1992 Proceedings
10. Stowe SM. Obstetrics and the Work of Doctoring in the Mid-Nineteenth Century American South. *Bulletin of the History of Medicine. 64:558-9, 1990.*
11. Ibid.: 559.
12. Rothstein WG. *American Physicians in the Nineteenth Century: from Sects to Science.* Baltimore: The Johns Hopkins University Press, 1972:43.
13. Stowe SM. Obstetrics and the Work of Doctoring in the Mid-Nineteenth Century American South. *Bulletin of the History of Medicine.* 64:548, 1990.

ANESTHESIA NEAR THE CENTER OF THE "STORM"

ROD K. CALVERLEY
University of California, San Diego, California, USA

The medical support that assembled to care for the Coalition Forces of the 1991 Gulf War was extraordinary in its size and complexity. By 24 February 19,000 surgical and medical beds were prepared for casualties. By that date three times as many physicians had been deployed to the Persian Gulf as served in any year in Vietnam. This remarkable achievement had been completed within three months of the President's decision to prepare a land offensive. While no individual physician viewed the full scope of Operation Desert Storm, I was privileged to witness some of the activities of U.S. Army medical hospitals in the Kuwait Theater of Operations. This presentation is a participant's view of the anesthesia support provided by the men and women of several nations in that area. When a final medical history is developed, unintended errors may be found in this text for which I apologize, but ask the reader to accept this as a personal perspective of a great enterprise in military anesthesia, the international response to the challenge of Operation Desert Storm.

In late July, 1990 many of the anesthesia personnel who would meet again in the desert had attended the first (and we anticipated last) meeting of NATO anesthetists in London, England. At that time of relaxed international tension, the care of military casualties seemed an historical concern. As we discussed anesthesia techniques, methods of ventilation and aeromedical evacuation, we anticipated that this information would find its next application in disaster relief. Ten days after we exchanged farewells and had returned to our homes, an unexpected event occurred which was to bring us together again just eight months later.

The Scenario

Iraq conquered Kuwait on August 2, 1990. Despite international condemnation, the invaders refused to negotiate a peaceful solution and instead brutally repressed all Kuwaiti resistance. When the leaders of Saudi Arabia recognized these acts as a threat to their own security, they requested American military support to forestall further aggression. As the summer of 1990 ended, the crisis continued to intensify. An anti-Iraq coalition evolved as other nations joined the United States in dispatching naval, land and air forces. The first troops to arrive were combat forces who remained dependent upon host-nation facilities for medical care until Army and Air Force as well as ship- and shore-based Navy hospitals became operations. For reasons of security, the first military hospitals were positioned well behind the projected line of battle as our defensive forces might have been obliged to yield ground if Iraq had launched a major attack.

In November, when Iraq remained obdurate, Coalition Forces were instructed to plan a land offensive to free Kuwait. Because the Iraq Army ranked among the world's largest and had been battle-hardened by eight years of war with Iran, military strategists anticipated a fierce campaign. They calculated that tens of thousands of allied soldiers might be wounded by mines, small arms and artillery fire, aerial or armored assault, as well as suffer additional injury from chemical and nuclear weapons or be incapacitated by biological agents. While the first priority was given to the movement of additional combat forces, our commanders realized that hospitals would be vital to the ground war. They initiated a rapid and unprecedented call-up of medical reserves. There was no time to enlist civilian volunteers. It became a "come as you are" war with reliance on existing active duty and reserve forces. Even after "Operation Desert Storm" commenced on January 16, our leaders prudently limited Coalition Force offensive actions to aerial assaults with only limited ground-based reconnaissance until a sufficient number of forward medical hospitals were positioned to receive casualties.

Medical Preparations

After deployment hospital teams prepared rapidly. On New Years Day, 1991 there had been only two U.S. Army Evacuation hospitals in position near the projected line of attack. By 20 February, 93 U.S. Army, Navy and Air Force Hospitals were ready to receive casualties. The ground offensive began four days later.

Other nations joined with us to dispatch forward military hospitals to Saudi Arabia in a display of international medical cooperation unrivalled since the Korean conflict and World War II. The British, Canadians, Norwegians and Swedes erected Field Hospitals. The British and French also had forward anesthesia facilities in Field Ambulance Units. While I did not have an opportunity to assess the forward hospital faculties of our Syrian, Egyptian, Saudi and Omani allies or the Polish hospital ship positions in the Gulf, informal visits to the tent hospitals of our Canadian and European partners featured demonstrations of models of lightweight, rugged and versatile anesthetic and resuscitative equipment not yet incorporated in the American inventory. Some of the lessons learned by the French in Chad, by the British in the Falklands and by the Norwegians, whose equipment has been fielded in Arctic and desert environments, will be considered in the design of units planned for new facilities of our Medical Force 2000.

American contributions by the Army, Navy and Air Force featured a massive fielding of the tent hospitals of Deployable Medical Systems (DEPMEDS)-equipped facilities. The largest of these were the 500 bed U.S. Navy Fleet Hospital and the 400 bed Army Evacuation Hospital, which were staffed to support all surgical specialties. Anesthesiologists and nurse anesthetists also served in the Army's 200 bed Combat Support Hospitals (CSH), and 60 bed Mobile Army Surgical Hospitals (MASH). U.S. Navy Surgical Support Companies also had anesthesia services near the line of battle. Neither the Navy nor the Army routinely placed anesthesia personnel in their very mobile Battalion Aid Stations or Casualty Clearing Companies, both of which were only equipped to provide a very limited degree of emergency service. While the preparatory and clinical experiences described in this account are based on my view of Army facilities,they reflect comparable experiences of fellow Navy anesthesiologists.

DEPMEDS equipment is designed to be carried by sea or land transportation in Milvans, metal cargo containers from which double-walled Temper tents and all supplies are withdrawn. Special purpose Isoshelter cargo containers are created for the Operating Room (OR), Radiology, Laboratory and Central Medical Supply modules. Their rigid walls are designed to pivot outwards providing a floor area twice or three times greater than that of the transported container. All anesthesia and surgical supplies are carried within the OR Isoshelter. The Ohmeda 885A anesthesia machine and the portable operating table may be disassembled in sturdy metal containers, but several other pieces of equipment, including ventilators and monitoring equipment, were difficult to repack securely.

When we first opened our Milvans, which had been stored in Europe or on the island of Diego Garcia for many years, the experience resembled that of entering a time capsule. A second frustration came in completing an inventory as the anesthesia equipment, drugs and supplies were intermingled with OR material. Items, such as Magill forceps, might be misplaced for several days until discovered in a surgical tray. Only after every item had been examined were shortfalls evident. Large EKGs were our only standard monitor. Few ventilators were available. Many drugs were not to be found. Curare was the only relaxant; diazapam, the sole tranquilizer. Narcotics were often in distressingly short supply. No pediatric equipment was stocked except for what we brought in our baggage. One hospital lacked cuffed endotracheal tubes. As a consequence anesthesia teams engaged in very spirited trading. Those with abundant supplies of oxygen traded their surplus for isoflurane or halothane. Fortunately, most shortfalls were corrected by late-arriving supplies, but, while the Theater Commanders knew the timetable for the attack, subordinate units did not know how much time they would be granted to complete preparations before our troops were committed to battle.

The operating room environment was adequate, but had limitations. Two side-by-side OR tables crowded the facility. The floor, which was supported on jacks, trembled with the impact of distant bombardments. Dust freely penetrated the OR. As the free entry of sand served as a warning of the potential for penetration by nerve or mustard gas if chemical shells were to fall nearby, protective masks were always at hand. When the M-17 mask was worn, stethoscopes were useless. As the ORs were very noisy, instruments with aural alarms had little utility. It may have seemed inappropriate for those asked to practice in an austere field environment to call for visual-display NIBP devices, oximeters and multi-function monitors, but they were essential to the mission. Other shortfalls were effective patient warming devices, blood warmers and high-volume water irrigation for contaminated wounds. The staff of each hospital was obliged to address its problems independently. Many concerns could have been rectified by a central direction of anesthesia support.

Clinical Notes

During the phase before the offensive, stress might have been manifested to an erosive degree, but I noted only one consistent concern. For anesthesia providers, it was not due to frustration over life in the field or apprehension over any personal hazard, stress was only expressed as: "Will we be able to do our job?" "Will we be able to overcome any shortcomings of supply and give good care?" While our hospital convoy remained "up-loaded" during its slow journey into Iraq throughout the 100 hour war, but for each hospital that received casualties, the answer was an emphatic, "Yes. They did a fine job!" However, despite our limited casualty experience, we all realized that the future may not treat our forces so kindly. The rapid forward movement of our forces outpaced our hospital elements. Had large numbers been wounded when storms made aeromedical evacuation impossible, our wounded would have been denied care. We all recognize a great obligation to improve and to update repeatedly our anesthesia inventory so that American anesthesia personnel serving in a future conflict or civilian disaster will have good resources with which to perform their duty.

After returning from Iraq we were able to give assistance at the Evacuation Hospitals and later were to learn of the experiences of other anesthetists that had cared for the wounded. Each team reported that, among the providentially few American casualties, injuries of the extremities caused by multiple shrapnel wounds were the predominant battle wound sustained by those who survived to reach a hospital. All agreed that body armor and helmets provided an excellent form of preventive medicine.

While members of every surgical discipline saw cases, orthopedists attended more than 50% of our wounded. The anesthesia techniques employed varied with the surgical injury. Regional blocks were used regularly. From the first day of the ground campaign, U.S. hospitals received and treated more enemy prisoners of war than Americans or allies. The care of these men, many of whom had been left on the desert for days before being found by our troops, taught an important lesson. We learned again that injured men who have survived days of abandonment will not have occult injuries demanding immediate surgery. If severely wounded, they would have expired long before their hospitalization. Instead, it was essential to give attention to fluid resuscitation before subjecting patients to the further stresses of anesthesia and surgery.

In the following weeks the care of refugees occupied several MASH facilities. Only a small number of civilians had been displaced by the 100 hour war, most sought sanctuary with American forces after elements of the Iraq army attacked villages suspected of harboring individuals who opposed their regime. Many children were wounded and some killed by their own country's soldiers. The children's care demanded pediatric equipment not previously thought essential to a military mission.

Those who served the Coalition Forces in Kuwait City after the liberation also witnessed war's cruelty. We learned of the seemingly mindless destruction inflicted upon the civilian population and the devastation brought by looting. Nowhere was this more evident than in the pillaging of the medical school where laboratories, classrooms and the library had been ransacked. The clinical facilities of the hospitals sustained less physical damage, perhaps because the occupying forces had anticipated their own need to care.

At the Mubarak Hospital I met four physician anaesthetists who had performed courageously under daily threats to their safety. These men had stayed at their posts and continued to care for patients after 18 members of the department had fled. Despite great hazard they even accepted the risk of attending wounded Kuwaiti guerrillas which, if discovered, would have brought summary execution. The freedom fighters were cared for in a ward marked, *"Infectious Disease!! Risk of AIDS!! Keep Out!!"* which discouraged inspection by the patrolling soldiers. Surgery was performed after midnight. The casualties were wheeled to and from the OR past the sleeping guards. These actions by the anaesthetists, surgeons and nurses of Kuwait were in the very best tradition of selfless service given without consideration of personal risk.

An After-Action Assessment

Throughout the campaign anesthesiologists and nurse anesthetists of the U.S. forces and those of our allies served thousands of patients most of whom were citizens of Iraq, the country with which we had been in conflict. These experiences, when completely collected and evaluated, will have future applications, both in terms of the development of equipment and the training of anesthesia personnel. That we did not encounter hundreds of Americans wounded is a point of great thankfulness to us all. Our nation was spared a great toll of injured and killed in 1991, but we cannot have confidence of a similar outcome in the future. Even if our medical teams had returned from Desert Storm without having attended a single wounded soldier, sailor, or marine, they would still have given their nation good service. They acted in the role of firemen, individuals ready to respond immediately should disaster strike, but whose duty is honorable even if there is not a great conflagration during their period of duty.

Among the lessons learned are these:

1. At this time we need airmobile surgical units which could be brought forward to a position close to our casualties. A prototype has been developed by members of the anesthesia team attached to the 82nd Airborne Division. This unit employs oxygen concentrators, versatile drawer-over PAC anesthesia vaporizers as well as battery-powered suction devices and ventilators.

2. The time to prepare equipment and to stock supplies for use in a military conflict or major civilian disaster is beforehand. The pace of mobilization denies us an opportunity for deliberate preparation. If we fail to give due attention to maintaining a current inventory of drugs and supplies, serious deficiencies in patient care will follow.

3. The national experience of Desert Shield/Desert Storm demonstrates our dependence upon a well-trained and disciplined reserve force. More than 75% of military medical personnel are civilians who serve in the Reserves or National Guard. Anesthesia personnel perform a vital function in each of those forces. If they are to work effectively, however, they must be prepared to train during periods of peace so that there will be no difficulty in adapting to the arduous environment of field medicine. I encourage all those who are in good physical condition to consider service. I also urge the civilian associates of Reservists and members of the Guard to recognize that their colleagues need adequate time for military leave from their civilian work for field training. All members of the active duty forces, reserves and National Guard know that the coming period of history may bring us to war again. If there is war, the survival of our sons and grandsons, as well as our daughters and granddaughters, may depend upon the actions and foresight of those in military service today.

HOW MARCH 30TH CAME TO BE DOCTORS' DAY

ROD K. CALVERLEY
University of California, San Diego, California, USA

Anesthesiologists feel a proprietary attachment to March 30, Doctors' Day, because they have learned that the date was selected in recognition of Crawford W. Long's first use of diethyl ether as a surgical anesthetic in 1842. Since the time of the first public salute to doctors by the ladies of Barrow County Medical Auxiliary on that date in 1933, Doctors' Day has become a national event and is now gaining even broader interest. On the 150th anniversary of Long's first surgical anesthetic, Emory University, The Medical College of Georgia, the Georgia and Greater Atlanta Societies of Anesthesiologists and the Anesthesia History Association will welcome physicians and historians from several countries to The Third International Symposium on the History of Anesthesia (TISHA) in Atlanta, Georgia March 27-31, 1992. Because anesthesiologists attending the symposium from other regions will have historical interests focused on the origins of our specialty, they may not immediately appreciate the high regard for Dr. Long's character that has been maintained for more than a century in the southeastern United States. Last year I sensed how deeply the memory of Dr. Long is revered by southern physicians during a social evening in an unusual setting — a palace in Kuwait more than 7,000 miles from Long's native state of Georgia.

On March 30, 1991 a Kuwaiti family invited five doctors of the 377th Combat Support Hospital of Chattanooga, Tennessee, to their home to celebrate "futur," the evening feast which follows a day of fasting during Ramadan. After dinner the quintet of stocking-footed, battle-dress-uniformed doctors joined the elegantly robed men and women of the family on couches which circled a lavishly decorated room. Servants silently served beverages. After toasts were exchanged to recognize the leaders of the United States and Kuwait, our orthopedist proposed that, as this was Doctors' Day, we salute Crawford W. Long. When called on by our host to explain why Crawford Long should be remembered, the orthopedic surgeon responded by describing not only Long's achievements, but also his selflessness, patriotism and generosity. He told the Kuwaitis that in southern grade schools all children of his generation had learned of Crawford W. Long and that the doctor was widely revered as a man of noble character. The conversation in Kuwait excited my curiosity. I wanted to learn more of the nature of the anesthesiologist who was so respected.

After we returned to America, my telephone calls to southern libraries brought convincing evidence that Crawford Long remains an object of great regional pride. While librarians often display a professional objectivity in replying to questions regarding archival information, in several instances their initial response was the forceful assertion: "Crawford Long was a good and caring doctor who was a fine southern gentleman, Sir." Their declaration taught this northern questioner that Long is respected for his character as well as his achievements.

The Crawford W. Long Museum, Jefferson, Georgia

The life and times of Crawford Long are well demonstrated in the exhibits of the Crawford W. Long Museum located on the site of Long's office on College Street in Jefferson, Georgia. While delegates to TISHA will travel together to view this fine collection, all anesthesiologists travelling north of Atlanta on Interstate Highway 85 are encouraged to visit Jefferson to see the community and its nationally-known museum. Many fine old buildings grace this quiet town. A few residents even boast: "In 1842 Crawford Long not only put James Venable to sleep, he anesthetized the whole town and some parts have never awakened yet."

A sense of the spirit of antebellum life in this area begins while driving along Highway 129 toward Jefferson. Doctors in practice now may consider how different and difficult every element of a physician's life would have been 150 years ago. How laborious travel would have been before railroads or all-weather roads served the countryside. How isolated doctors would have felt without an opportunity to transfer a critically ill patient to a metropolitan hospital. How hard life would have been for a dedicated physician such as Long who was so respected as a surgeon that he was often called by colleagues to ride great distances to operate upon their injured patients.

The Crawford W. Long Museum has been expanded to capture the spirit of Long's life and historical period as well as to present exhibits of the history of anesthesia since 1842. Visitors will be pleased to meet the executive director, Ms. Susan B. Deaver. She enjoys sharing her expert knowledge of the life of Dr. Long who was born in 1815 in nearby Danielsville, GA. His family encouraged a good education for him at Franklin College (now the University of Georgia). After studying medicine informally with Dr. Grant of Jefferson, he entered the medical school at Transylvania, Kentucky, but later transferred to the University of Pennsylvania and then "walked the wards" of New York hospitals before returning to Jefferson to begin his practice. While many have become familiar with Long's documented use of ether on eight occasions before 1846, as well as his reticence in publishing his discovery and of the Congressional contentions that followed, the story of Crawford Long has other facets.

Susan Deaver, James Harvey Young and other scholars have continued to study the life of this man who has been consistently regarded as an exemplary physician and citizen. Despite being nearly impoverished after the devastating war of 1861-65 that is remembered in Georgia as "The War of Northern Aggression," Long, at that time practicing in Athens, Georgia, satisfied his debts at great personal cost yet, when he died in Athens, GA in 1878, scores of his professional accounts remained unpaid. He was also remembered as a compassionate physician who had remained in practice until his last illness. A report exists that while he was attending a woman in labor, he collapsed from a stroke. He insisted that attention be given to the mother and newborn infant before anyone aided him. Sixty-four years later, at the time of the Long Centennial celebration in Jefferson, a lady stated that she had been that infant and that the story was verified by her family. Personal accounts such as these by patients, friends and family members contributed to the development of an intense regional pride in the noble character of Dr. Long.

Whether these stories are accurate remain points of conjecture, but it is certain that few other physicians have been as enthusiastically supported by their contemporaries or by succeeding generations as has been Crawford W. Long. In 1877 a leading surgeon, J. Marion Sims, wrote a strongly worded essay supporting Long's achievement. In the decades to follow memorials were erected at locations associated with his career.

Long's Statue in the National Capitol

In 1864 the U.S. Congress invited each state to present statues of two of its distinguished citizens who were "worthy of this national commemoration" to be placed in the Capitol. Most states did not respond until this century. Crawford Long's name was selected in 1910. After the sculptor's commission was paid by a public subscription, the statute was dedicated on March 30, 1926. There was a delay in selecting the name of the second Georgian deemed worthy of national honor. Georgia finally settled on Alexander H. Stephens, who may have been Long's roommate at Franklin College and who had been the Vicepresident of the Confederacy, to be their second permanent representative in the Capitol.

Anesthesiologists who tour the Capitol will find that Long is the only figure representing their specialty. They will also count seven times as many statues of lawyers (44) as there are doctors (6). Of the six physicians honored, three are not recognized for their service as clinicians. John McLoughlin was the chief administrator of Oregon before that territory was claimed by the United States. John Gorrie developed refrigeration in Apalachicola, Florida, with the initial aim of cooling the rooms of fever patients, but left practice as he sought wider commercial applications of his patents for the making of ice. Florence Sabin is remembered by Colorado for her work in embryology and public health; she is the only 20th Century physician of the six. Of the six physicians honored, only three, Crawford Long, Ephraim McDowell, and Marcus Whitman attended the sick until the end of their careers.

Dr. Long has received other significant tributes. Visitors to Georgia who travel between Savannah and Florida are encouraged to drive slowly as they enjoy the rural scenery of his namesake, Long County. In 1930 his name was given to the Crawford W. Long Hospital in Atlanta when that institution became public. The Long Museum in that hospital's lobby warrants an hour of study. In 1940 Long became the first pioneer of anesthesiology to have his portrait presented on an American postage stamp. An eponymous lectureship has been maintained by Emory University for 26 years. Films such as the 1953 TV movie, "Bless the Man," have reviewed his career. One year ago his name was selected as a charter inductee to the Atlanta "Walk of Fame." This month Long's pioneering use of ether will be a focus of the Third International Symposium on the History of Anesthesia. His contributions will also be a featured part of Doctors' Day observances in all corners of the nation on Monday, March 30, 1992.

The Origin of Doctors' Day

For many years doctors in our southeastern states have been presented with red carnations on the occasion of Doctors' Day. The custom was first recommended by the Southern Medical Association Auxiliary in 1935. They had voted to pass a motion presented by the Georgia State Medical Auxiliary who had endorsed a resolution prepared in 1933 by their Barrow County members which read: *"Whereas, the Auxiliary to the Barrow County Medical Society wishes to pay lasting tribute to her Doctors, therefore, be it resolved by the Auxiliary to the Barrow County Medical Society, that March 30, the day that famous Georgian Dr. Crawford W. Long first used ether anesthesia in surgery, be adopted as 'Doctors' Day,' the object to be the well-being and honor of the profession, its observance demanding some act of kindness, gift or tribute in remembrance of the Doctors."* Perhaps some of the enthusiasm for the selection of March 30 may have been related to the publication of a popular biography, "Crawford W. Long and the Discovery of Ether Anesthesia," written in 1928 by his daughter, Frances Long Taylor.

The custom spread gradually to other areas. In 1958, the U.S. House of Representatives passed a resolution recognizing Doctors' Day. More recently, the U.S. Congress again considered the issue in 1990 in the form of Resolution 366 under the sponsorship of members of the Mississippi delegation, Senator Thad Cochran and Congressmen Michael Parker and J.V. "Sunny" Montgomery. The Bill was considered and passed the House of Representatives on "Ether Day," October 16 which, by coincidence was the occasion of the 144th anniversary of W.T.G. Morton's first public anesthetic. President George Bush signed Public Law 101-473 on October 30, 1990 to designate March 30, 1991, as "National Doctors Day."

Because most actions of historical significance arise in the mind of an individual, I've been curious to learn, "Who first thought of naming a day to honor doctors? What events motivated that person?" The first answer can be found on a bronze marker placed in 1989 by the Southern Medical Association (SMA) Auxiliary near the courthouse in Winder, Georgia, the county seat of Barrow County. Beside a picturesque representation of a carnation the inscription reads, *"To Honor Mrs. Charles B. Almond, Originator of Doctors' Day March 30, 1933."*

The SMA Auxiliary also published "The History and Handbook of Doctors' Day" which describes the lady's motivation. From the time of her early childhood in rural Ft. Lamar, GA, Eudora Brown had admired the gentle kindness of her family doctor. In 1920 Eudora married Dr. Charles B. Almond and, believing that healing the sick was man's greatest profession, became convinced that medical practitioners deserved a day of recognition. She selected March 30 to honor the man she considered Georgia's most famous son as she knew his first anesthetics had been administered in nearby Jefferson. After her resolution was passed by the County Auxiliary, the day was marked by mailing commemorative cards to the county's physicians and their wives, laying flowers on the graves of Crawford Long and other doctors and by a formal dinner. During the meal several toasts were offered to encourage the continued observance of Doctors' Day.

It is unlikely that Eudora Brown Almond or any of the other guests who saluted the first Doctors' Day in the residence of Dr. and Mrs. William Randolph could have imagined the consequences of her action. I doubt that they would have forecast its extraordinary growth. It is unlikely that they would have anticipated that the President of the United States would sign an Act to establish a National Doctors Day and that on the day of its first observance after the law was enacted, a toast to Crawford Long and Doctors' Day would be offered during a sumptuous dinner in Kuwait. Her kind action will be remembered again on March 30, 1992 at the Crawford W. Long Memorial Lecture on the occasion of the sesquicentennial of the first documented ether anesthetic, an event that will be commemorated during the Third International Symposium on the History of Anesthesia.

AN EARLY ETHER VAPORIZER DESIGNED BY JOHN SNOW
A Treasure of the Wood Library-Museum of Anesthesiology

ROD K. CALVERLEY
University of California, San Diego, California, USA

The achievements of John Snow (1813-1858) are respected by anesthesiologists of all countries. His publications, particularly the 88-page monograph "On the Inhalation of the Vapour of Ether in Surgical Operations," first published in September 1847, are regularly reprinted and are now more widely read than are the works of any other 19th-century pioneer of anesthesiology. Scholars are deeply impressed by the broad scope and rapid development of his scientific observations. Clinicians admire Snow's ability to relate his research to clinical practice. Distinguished investigators believe that John Snow's understanding of the scientific foundations of anesthesia were unequaled for almost a century.

An example of Snow's skill in intermingling practical concern and scientific observation is his ether inhaler, shown on page 17 of his 1847 monograph (Figure 1). As the accompanying text reveals, he selected its components carefully. For example, he chose a breathing tube which ". . . ought to be so capacious as to offer no impediment to the most rapid inspiration; and to meet this requirement it must be wider than the trachea. . . ."[1] Although recent reconstructions of this device are on display in British museums, originals are not. A fortuitous discovery was recently made in the United States at the American Society of Anesthesiologists' Wood Library-Museum (WLM), Park Ridge, Illinois. A previously unappreciated instrument has been identified as an authentic inhaler of John Snow's design. It now ranks among the most prized objects of the WLM collection.

Visitors to the WLM marvel that a prototype of Snow's inhaler could have been designed, introduced in the medical literature and marketed commercially within a month of Snow's first having witnessed ether anesthesia. From the moment when the inhaler was identified, I have been curious to learn the history of its development. How could Snow have prepared it so quickly? Did he create an original design or did he re-assemble components

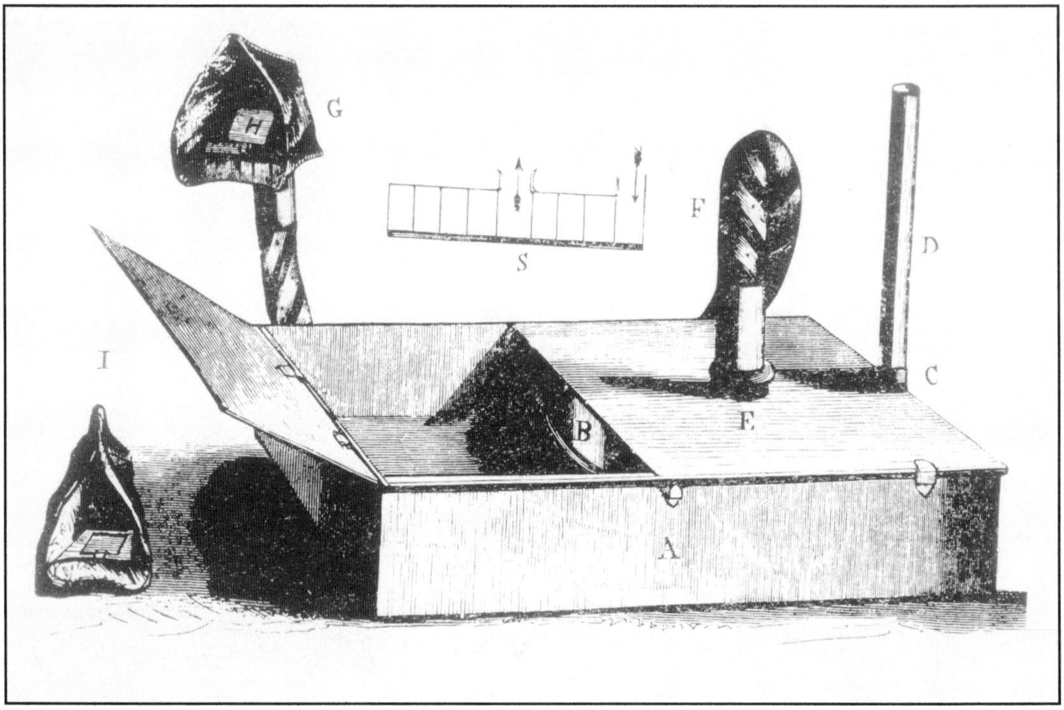

Fig. 1. John Snow's Final Modification of his Ether Inhaler.

devised for other applications? If so, what was their original purpose?These questions reflected my ignorance of 19th-century technology, a deficiency compounded by a lack of access to journals of that period. Recent opportunities to correspond with British scholars and to visit historical libraries in Britain, have given me a better understanding of the origins of the vaporizer's components. For readers who, like me, enjoy resolving historical puzzles, I would like to describe my "path of discovery" chronologically from when I first saw this intriguing device.

Identification of the Anesthesia Inhaler

In 1979 the Trustees of the WLM purchased an "Anaesthesia Inhaler" from Simon Kay, a London antique dealer for £540. Its provenance was, and still remains, unknown. For many years thereafter it rested undisturbed in its finely crafted wooden box on a shelf in the WLM rare book room. It came to attention again when Dr. Garth Huston showed the WLM Trustees some valuable books that had been recently purchased for the library. As he surveyed the shelves, he saw the box and casually placed it on a table with the comment that it was believed to be an early nitrous oxide inhaler.

While the group moved on to inspect other objects, I opened the box. The largest objects within it were a coiled tube and a black metal tin. A cursory examination showed that the small, circular and rather shallow tin, about 5 inches in diameter and 2-1/2 inches deep, could not have been constructed to contain a gas; it had to have been designed to receive a liquid, which from the volume contained was likely to be ether. Although slightly rusted, the metal tin showed no marks of use. With a clinician's curiosity, I assembled the components; a round metal vaporizing chamber, a brass quadrant valve which could be turned to allow the inspired vapor to be diluted with room air, a 28-inch-long flexible tube with an internal diameter of 5/8 of an inch, a wooden T-piece connector and a glass mouthpiece. Without deliberate thought, I reflexively tested my newly assembled circuit by placing the mouthpiece against my lips and inhaling. To my chagrin, I immediately drew the dust of decades deep into my lungs provoking a violent cough. As the exhaled dust flew from the distal arm of the T-piece, I heard the lick of a valve closing, a sound which excited greater curiosity. I disassembled the T-piece and found that it contained two wooden spheres of 5/8-inch in diameter positioned as caged inspiratory and expiratory valves. Until that moment I had not appreciated that valves very similar in concept to the non-rebreathing valves of mid-200th-century construction had been used many decades earlier.

As I continued my examination, I was caught up in admiration for the utility of the vaporizer's design and searched for any information that would identify its gifted designer. The wooden box was unlabeled, but a small brass plate on the vaporizer read:

"Ferguson
221, Giltspur Street"

The WLM librarian, Patrick Sim, and I were unable to find a reference to Ferguson in K. Bryn Thomas' "The Development of Anaesthetic Apparatus" or other British and American historical texts. We did, however, find Ferguson of Giltspur Street, London, among the manufacturers listed in a copy of Elisabeth Bennion's catalog, "Antique Medical Instruments," but did not find a vaporizer among her illustrations of Ferguson's equipment. From Bennion's history of the Ferguson company, we were able to derive the period of its manufacture as follows: Ferguson had relocated to Giltspur Street in 1828; the firm's name changed to Ferguson & Son in 1851; therefore, our vaporizer must have been manufactured before 1851 and after December 1846 when the news of ether anesthesia crossed the Atlantic to Britain.

Some time later I unexpectedly found an appreciation of Ferguson's work when reading the papers of Dr. Alexander Wood, the Edinburgh pioneer of subcutaneous injection. Wood incorporated into his ingenious development of the syringe and hollow needle.[2] In 1965 Faulconer and Keys expressed the opinion that Wood's complete apparatus was manufactured by Ferguson.[3] The WLM inhaler was produced by a leading British manufacturer of the period, but the identity of its designer remained a mystery.

This problem resolved unexpectedly when Dr. Samuel Tirer sent me a manuscript to review along with photocopies of pages from the *Lancet* of 1847. Fortuitously, even though it was not the topic of his research, my friend included an illustration which riveted my attention because it depicted an inhaler almost identical to that in the WLM collection. The accompanying text reported the January 23, 1847, meeting of the Westminster Medical Society. The first sentence began, "Dr. Snow placed on the table an apparatus for the inhaling of the vapour of ether.[4] The WLM Trustees were soon delighted to learn that the vaporizer, which had rested in obscurity in our museum, was a product of John Snow's genius!

The *Lancet* diagram included details of the vaporizer's construction. Although the device Snow demonstrated in January 1847 lacked the quadrant valve to permit the mixing of ether with room air, it was otherwise very similar to the WLM vaporizer. The article included a schematic internal view which revealed a spiral plate within the vaporizing chamber similar to that shown in Snow's monograph. The accompanying description revealed Snow's awareness of the advantages provided by the water bath. He stated:

> When used, the inhaler was to be put in a hand-basin of water, mixed to a particular temperature, corresponding to the proportion of vapour that the operator might desire to give; and the caps being removed, and the mouth-tube attached, when the patient began to inhale, the air would gain the desired temperature in passing through the metal pipe; it would then come upon the surface of the ether, where it would have to wind round three or four times before entering the tube going to the mouth-piece, thus ensuring its full saturation, and preserving it at the desired temperature. There was no valve, or any

other obstruction to the air, till it reached the mouth-piece, which was of the kind used in other inhalers, and contained the valves necessary to prevent the return of the expired air into the apparatus.[5]

A review of the *London Medical Gazette* of 1847 revealed an article of March 19, 1847 in which Snow described a vaporizer which featured a quadrant valve that had been designed for Snow by Ferguson to permit the introduction of air without the requirement of removing the mouthpiece.[6] This was the WLM vaporizer (Figure 2). Two weeks later on April 3, 1847, Snow described a portable ether vaporizer for which no illustration was provided.[7] The final version was the model incorporating the rectangular metal tin described in the monograph. I have recently learned that Dr. Richard Ellis has catalogued Snow's ether vaporizers chronologically as Mark I - January 23, Mark II - March 19, Mark III - April 3, Mark IV - September, 1847.[8] The WLM is, in Dr. Ellis' classification, a Mark II device.

At the first opportunity, I compared the WLM vaporizer with the text and illustrations of Snow's September 1847 monograph. The WLM vaporizer was the second prototype of the well-known Snow ether vaporizer which we find illustrated within its rectangular metal water bath. I could now follow the evolution of his vaporizer from its original version as illustrated in January, 1847 in *Lancet* through the intermediary modification in the WLM collection and then to its final form in the Snow September 1847 monograph. The text of the monograph served as a guide to the factors which had motivated Snow's responses to deficiencies in his early vaporizers. The most striking of these were the addition of the metal waterbath to house the vaporizer and the substitution of a face mask incorporating inspiratory and expiratory flap valves for the mouthpiece.

Snow explained his motivation for designing a malleable facemask as follows:

"For the first three months I used a mouth-piece which did not include the nostrils; consequently they had to be closed, and the patient was obliged to breathe entirely by the mouth. This plan always succeeded (except, perhaps, in one instance), and generally very well, but sometimes not without difficulty; for some

Fig. 2. Snow's Modified Ether Vaporizer (as illustrated in the London Medical Gazette p 501, March 19, 1847).

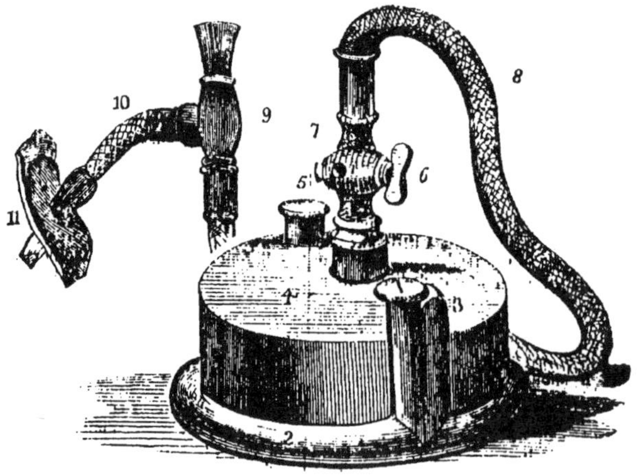

1, Cap which unscrews to admit the air to
2, Metal pipe.
3, Entrance of ditto into
4, Spial chamber.
5, Star closing aperture for putting in or pouring out ether.
6, Two-way tap.
7, External opening of ditto.
8, Flexible tube.
9, Ebony tube, containing ball valves of cedar wood.
10, Portion of flexible tube to admit change of position of
11, Mouth-piece, with soft cushion, &c.

of the adult patients, after they lost their consciousness, made such strong instinctive efforts to breathe by the nostrils, that the air was forced through the lachrymal ducts, and occasionally they held the breath altogether for a short time, and were getting purple in the face, when the nostrils had to be liberated, for a short time, to allow respiration of the external air, and thus a delay was occasioned. I was therefore ready to adopt a face-piece invented by Mr. Sibson, of the General Hospital, Nottingham, which permitted inhalation by the nostrils as well as by the mouth. This face-piece. . . was the foundation of that I now use, which has been altered. . . to allow of the introduction of valves into it. . ."[9]

Snow explained his preference for the low resistance flap valves over the brass quadrant valve of the WLM model by stating:

> "I have contrived the expiratory valve to turn on a pivot, so as to allow of the admission of external air, and to supersede the use of a ferrule or two-way tap. . . When a stop-cock with graduated openings is used. . . the air passes through the external opening in preference to the more circuitous route over the ether; and when the respiration is gentle, the whole of the air the patient breathes may enter by an outward opening that would only admit a third part of what he inspires when the respiration is forcible."[10]

In a remarkably short time Snow had achieved several very practical improvements.

Snow stated that the rectangular metal box was added to serve ". . .as a waterbath when the apparatus is in use, and at other times containing the elastic tube and face-pieces."[11] I performed a simulated trial which revealed another important, but unstated, advantage of the covered rectangular water bath; the lid held the vaporizer in a stable position. My test showed that earlier models, designed to float unrestrained in a basin of water, could tip unexpectedly if the patient should turn his head or the anesthetist shift position. A tug along the flexible tube might overturn the vaporizer which brought the risk of liquid anesthetic entering the tube. The concentration of anesthetic would then vary erratically with the potential of an even greater hazard — liquid ether flowing along the breathing tube to the patient. Snow not only pioneered the use of water bath to ensure that the anesthetic vapor pressure was constant but, by fixing the vaporizer in a horizontal position, also overcame the risk of erratic variations in anesthetic concentration precipitated by movement of the vaporizer.

The monograph also provided a point of information which may explain why the WLM's unused vaporizer may be the only existing representative of its type. Snow commented, "This part of the apparatus (the vaporizer) was at first made of tinned iron, but it was found occasionally to become rusty by use."[12] Because even the better grades of ether available in 1847 were contaminated by water, it is probable that every Snow vaporizer put in service to deliver anesthetics was destroyed by corrosion. Our WLM model may have survived only because it had never been used for anesthesia.

Snow also described the origins of the components of the vaporizer. In January 1847 he had commented only that, "In the interior (of the inhaler) was a spiral plate of tin, soldered to the top, and reaching almost to touch the bottom. . . When the patient began to inhale, the air. . . would have to wind round three or four times before entering the tube going to the mouth-piece, thus insuring full saturation (with ether vapor)."[13] In September he reported in the monograph that, "This spiral arrangement is adopted from the inhaler of Mr. Julius Jeffreys for aquerous vapour."[14] Because no footnote or reference was provided, a new element was added to the mystery. Who was Jeffreys? Snow's acknowledgment did make clear, however, that the spiral platc was not of his own design.

The Jeffreys Inhaler

I learned no more about Jeffreys until I studied medical journals of 1840-1850 in Britain. The first entry that caught my eye was a February 1847 illustration of a Jeffreys inhaler with an unsigned commentary posing the question: "By a remarkable coincidence we find that an instrument identical in principle with that invented by Dr. Snow, was invented some years ago by Mr. Jeffrey (sic) as an inhaler. The circumstance reminds us of the case of the new planet, in which two rival discoverers are in the field."[15] (Neptune was first observed on September 23, 1846 in a position which had been independently predicted by two mathematicians, John Adams and Urbain Le Verrier.)

Although we do not know who challenged Snow for failing to credit Jeffreys' prior preparation of a coiled inhaler, an earlier entry in the literature revealed that Snow had previously recognized Jeffreys' claim. Any contemporary accusation that Snow plagiarized was refuted by Snow's first commentary on anaesthesia in which he identified his inhaler as being modeled on Jeffreys'. The *London Medical Gazette* recorded the meeting of the Westminster Medical Society of January 16, 1847, a session held seven days before Snow demonstrated his first vaporizer. The secretary reported: "He (Snow) was getting an instrument made which would enable the surgeon... to administer an atmosphere (of ether) of any strength he wished... The instrument... was on the plan of the inhaler of Mr. Jeffreys, with some alterations and additions."[16] At the first opportunity Snow had acknowledged Jeffreys' invention.

Who was Jeffreys? A review of the *London Medical Gazette* led to a multi-part article, "On artificial climates and the restoration and preservation of health," published in 1842 by Mr. Julius Jeffreys (1801-1877).[17] Jeffreys' thesis was that, based on his personal experience as a surgeon in India, the humidification and warming of air was of advantage both in the treatment of respiratory disease and in the prevention in cold climates of losses of heat and moisture in the exhaled breath. Jeffreys reported that the motivation for his invention came from a concern for his sister who was debilitated by paroxysms of severe coughing. He created an instrument that would warm and humidify the air she inhaled. The Jeffreys inhaler contained an internal coil positioned so that, as the patient inhaled, the inspired air could not simply traverse the short distance across the radius of the vessel but was channeled a longer distance to become fully humidified. This concept was incorporated later by Snow.[18]

Although it may appear that Jeffreys' device represents only an eccentricity of Victorian medicine, a well-researched biography of Julius Jeffreys by Dr. David Zuck presents a different perspective. Dr. Zuck recognized that Jeffreys' concept of humidification had a modern application. Jeffreys marketed a portable humidifier which he called a "Respirator," a term which Dr. Zuck points out that the Editors of the Oxford Dictionary conclude was coined by Jeffreys. Jeffreys' "Respirator" consisted of a plate of finely soldered metal grids which formed a latticework within a frame that could be worn over the lower face in cold weather. Dr. Zuck described its function as follows: "During exhalation warmth would pass from the breath to the lattices, and moisture would condense on them. During inspiration the cold air would be warmed, and humidified."[19] A patient's testimonial read that the "Respirator" had the property of making all the air that goes down one's throat as warm as summer air. Jeffreys patented the "Respirator" and gained royalties from the sale of several thousand. Dr. Zuck was the first to realize that Jeffreys had prepared a humidifier identical in principle to the heat and moisture exchanger (HME) of Swedish design now often positioned between the endotracheal tube connector and the Wye-piece of an anesthesia circuit.

Read's Valves

While I now understood the history of the vaporizer, the origin of the non-rebreathing valves remained a mystery. Snow's phrasing that the valves were of the sort "in ordinary use" suggested that he had not invented them, but other questions remained: When had they been first designed and for what purpose? Had Snow been the first to use the valves in an anesthetic circuit? No one with whom I corresponded could answer the questions, but visits to British museums brought progress.

The rich collections of 19th-century medical devices in the Science Museums in Oxford and London featured two ether vaporizers, both of which antedated Snow's first inhaler. The Science Museum in Oxford had a reconstruction of Peter Squire's inhaler, which had been employed by his nephew, William, for the first public demonstration of ether in England on December 21, 1846, when Sir Robert Liston amputated a coachman's leg. Squire's inhaler featured a non-rebreathing valve, one closely resembling the valve of Snow's vaporizer. The Science Museum in London had an original Tracy's inhaler. It was an impractical design, having a narrow and elongated glass vaporizing chamber shaped like the bowl of a large Meerschaum pipe, but Tracy had precluded rebreathing by incorporating valves of the same type. Since the valve design used by Snow had also been selected by Squire and Tracy, it was certainly "in ordinary use," but who had used it first?

The published descriptions of the vaporizers on display in Oxford and London gave more information. In a letter written January 18, 1947, for the *London Medical Gazette*, S. J. Tracy of St. Bartholomew's Hospital reported that his Tracy inhaler had been prepared by Mr. Ferguson of Giltspur Street, soon to be Snow's manufacturer also, and that, by the date of the letter, Tracy had already administered 20 anesthetics with it. He referred to the non-rebreathing mechanism as a "double-valved mouthpiece of the description in ordinary use."[20] While two of Ferguson's clients, Tracy and Snow, failed to identify the designer of the valves, a witness's account of Squire's first use of an inhaler on December 21, 1846, brought the answer. The reporter of the London Medical Gazette commented, "It (Squire's inhaler) consisted of a Nooth's Apparatus. . . and one of Read's flexible inhaling tubes. . ."[21] Once again, I had learned a name, Read, but knew nothing of the original purpose or history of the invention. Certainly, Read's valve must have been in regular use because it had been chosen not only by Snow and Tracy but also by Squire. I was soon to learn that other anaesthetists had also selected Read's valve.

On January 13, 1847, 23 days after Squire's first public anesthetic and only a few days before Snow's first vaporizer was marketed, the Pharmaceutical Society of London held an extraordinary meeting in which models of seven ether inhalers were displayed by their inventors. Five of these featured Read's valves. Mr. Squire was joined by Messers. Hooper, Clendon, Bell, and Gilbertson, all of whom shared in a spirited debate over the merit of their devices. The Society's secretary noted, "Some discussion arose about priority of invention, caveats, patents, registration, etc. which the Chairman very properly cut short, as being foreign to the objects of the meeting."[22] Read's valves had such utility that they had been chosen by five of Britain's first anesthetists at least seven days before Snow's first inhaler was marketed.

For some time my search was handicapped by too narrow a focus of interest. Because I had learned of Read's valve through its medical application in inhalers, I attempted to find references to Read by searching among articles published by physicians of the period to identify the disease or diseases which a Doctor Read might have attempted to remedy by creating a non-rebreathing valve for inhalation therapy. The search remained unsuccessful even when British friends extended it to include alternate spellings of Read. Fortunately, I directed a request to Dr. Ghislaine Lawrence, the Assistant Keeper of the Science Museum in London, who initiated a broader search of the technical literature. To my good fortune, her associates came upon a remarkable document — Read's patent. The patent (#4484) was awarded on July 11, 1820, to a Mr. John Read (1761-1847) for "An Improvement in Syringes." The accompanying diagram showed that spherical valves within the chamber of a syringe provided unidirectional flow which permitted the syringe to be used as a pump. Read prepared pamphlets to describe the sizes of his valved syringes and their applications in activities which ranged from horticulture (spraying fruit trees) through veterinary medicine (medicating horses and cattle) to clinical practice (pumping the stomach or applying an enema). The anesthetists of 1847 had certainly been correct in describing Read's valves as being "in ordinary use."

I searched the medical literature for references to Read's valves and found three. The first was written by a distinguished London surgeon, Sir Astley Cooper. The latter two were citations by a then little-known but now highly regarded physician of Soho, John Snow.

My literature search had begun with the first volume of *Lancet* when the journal was first published in 1823. Fortuitously, Reid's (sic) syringe was cited in the Index. The relevant account described an experiment supervised by Sir Astley Cooper on Friday, November 21, 1823 in the operating theater of Guy's Hospital. That afternoon, opium in water had been poured down the throat of a restrained dog. After an interval of 33 minutes, when the animal showed effects of the narcotic, the stomach was evacuated by Read's pump syringe. The reporter continued, "The instrument succeeded very well in the dog, which appeared to be little worse for the experiment. Mr. Reed (sic) was in the theatre during the whole of the time, and superintended the use of the instrument; on quitting he received the unanimous applause of those present."[23]

While lecturing at St. Thomas's Hospital the following Wednesday, Cooper lauded Read by stating: "This experiment, Gentlemen, delighted me; I do not know that I have ever experienced greater pleasure in my life than I felt in going home from the Hospital on that day. With respect to antidotes against the effects of poison, it is well known that they are, in a great degree, useless. . . . A few weeks ago, a nurse in this Hospital died in consequence of having swallowed opium. No relief was administered to her; but can it be said, after what we saw on Friday; that no relief could have been administered to her?"[24] Soon thereafter, Read's priority to the invention was challenged, but his claim prevailed.

While John Read's stomach pump was a significant contribution to the general practice of medicine, two other applications of his equipment were reported by John Snow. Both papers suggested a cordial interactions between the two men and, on Snow's part, a respect for Mr. Read, who at 80 years of age, was still actively designing equipment. In December, 1841 Snow read a paper, "On paracentesis of the thorax" to the Westminster Medical Society, in which he discussed the risk of the uncontrolled entry of air into the pleural space via a canula during paracentesis. To reduce this hazard, Snow added a stopcock to the canula. He remarked that the canula he had designed was one which "any member can get made by his own instrument maker" and added "It has since been manufactured, under my directions, with great accuracy, by Mr. Read of Regent Circus."[25]

The introduction of the stopcock was the second collaboration on instrument design recorded between Snow and Read. The first occurred earlier the same year. On October 16, 1841, precisely five years before Morton demonstrated ether's anesthetic action, Snow read a paper before the Westminster Medical Society, "On asphyxia, and on the resuscitation of still-born children." In that paper, which may be Snow's first work relevant to anesthesiology, Snow recommended three actions now considered fundamental elements of resuscitation. These actions were: using supplemental oxygen, suctioning the airway and performing mechanical ventilation. Snow related that in 1838 John Read had prepared a syringe to ventilate adults. Quoting Snow, "So the matter rested, until a short time ago, when Mr. Read, knowing I took an interest in the subject, called to show me an improvement in his apparatus. . . . I then suggested that he should make a little instrument on exactly the same plan, adapted to the size of new-born children. It consists of two syringes, one of which, by a tube adapted to the mouth, and closing it, withdraws air from the lungs, and the other syringe returns the same quantity of fresh air through a tube fitted to the nostrils."[26] Read's valves were essential to the action of the syringes. Five years later Snow again selected Read's valves for his ether vaporizers and, in so doing, designed the first of a series of vaporizers that were the most functional of that historical period.

The single surviving Snow vaporizer will be on public display in the new Wood Library-Museum of Anesthesiology. All anesthesiologists who view it as it lies shielded behind walls of glass will be impressed by its attractive and functional design. For me it has been more than a museum-piece, it has been as magical as Aladdin's lamp for it has led me on a study of the technology employed in the era in which anesthesia was discovered. By touching the vaporizer I have been led to a new appreciation of the skills of John Snow. When I first assembled and breathed through the inhaler, I could not have anticipated that my dust-driven cough would provoke a study of the components incorporated by John Snow in his first ether vaporizers.

Acknowledgements

I wish to express my appreciation to Mr. Patrick Sim, Librarian of the Wood Library-Museum, Park Ridge, Illinois. Many British historians, particularly Dr. Barbara Duncum, Dr. Richard Ellis and the late J. Alfred Lee gave invaluable advice. Dr. Ghislaine Lawrence and her colleagues at the Science Museum, London provided generous assistance. I wish to thank the Burroughs Wellcome Fund for the financial support provided by a Wellcome Research Travel Grant.

References

1. Snow, J: On the inhalation of the vapour of ether, p 20, London, J. Churchill, 1847.
2. Wood A: New method of treating neuralgia by the direct application of opiates to the painful points. Edinburgh Medical and Surgical J: 82:265, 1855.
3. Faulconer A. Keys, TE: Foundations of anesthesiology, p 1022. Springfield, Illinois, Charles C. Thomas, 1965.
4. Anonymous: Westminster Medical Society: report of meeting on 23 January 1847. Lancet i:120-21, 1847.
5. Anonymous: Lancet i:121, 1847.
6. Snow J: On the inhalation of the vapour of ether. Lond Med Gaz: 39: 498-502, 1847.
7. Anonymous: Westminster Medical Society: report of meeting on April 3, 1847, Lond Med Gaz: 39: 646-47, 1847.
8. Ellis RH: The inhalers of Dr. John Snow: his marks and his score. Proceedings of the History of Anaesthesia Society, London. 8b: 81, 1990.
9. Snow J: On the inhalation of the vapour of ether. p 22.
10. Snow J: On the inhalation of the vapour of ether. p 23.
11. Snow J: On the inhalation of the vapour of ether. p 16.
12. Snow J: On the inhalation of the vapour of ether. p 20.
13. Anonymous: Lancet i: 121, 1847.
14. Snow J: On the inhalation of the vapour of ether. p 19.
15. Anonymous: Apparatus for inhaling ether. Medical Times February 20, 1847.
16. Anonymous: Westminster Medical Society: report of a meeting of January 16, 1847. Lond Med Gaz: 39: 156.
17. Jeffreys J: On artificial climates for the restoration and preservation of health. Lond Med Gaz: 29: 814-22 et seq.
18. Jeffreys J: On artificial climates for the restoration and preservation of health, Lond Med Gaz: p 821.
19. Zuck D: Julius Jeffreys - pioneer of humidification. Proceedings of the History of Anaesthesia Society. London 8b: 70-80, 1990.
20. Tracy J: Apparatus for the respiration of ether vapour. Lond Med Gaz: 39: 167, 1847.
21. Anonymous: Lond Med Gaz: 39: 38.
22. Anonymous: Transactions of the pharmaceutical society meeting of Wednesday, January 13, 1847. Pharm J 6: 353, 1847.
23. Anonymous: Guy's Hospital Report, Lancet i: 275-277, 1823.
24. Cooper A: Surgical Lecture November 26, 1823. Lancet i: 299, 1823.
25. Snow J: On paracentesis of the thorax. Lond Med Gaz: 29: 707, 1842.
26. Snow J: On asphyxia, and on the resuscitation of still-born children. Lond Med Gaz: 29: 225, 1841.

THE END OF ETHER ANESTHESIA IN THE USA

CHRISTER CARLSSON
JONAS P. KARLSSON
FELICIA B. DANIELS
ROBERT D. HARWICK
Departments of Anesthesiology and Surgery, Temple University Medical School, Philadelphia, Pennsylvania, USA

From an historical perspective, significant efforts are spent on documenting the beginning of various techniques[1] and their early development. Less often, the end of the use of a special technique is described. This is probably due to the more difficult task of defining the end unless such a one is posed by regulations.

Ether anesthesia has been credited to Crawford W. Long for his use of this anesthetic for the surgical removal of a neck tumor in 1842; credit has also been given to William T.G. Morton, who in 1846 gave the same type of anesthesia for a procedure.

From that time ether anesthesia became widely used, and within one year almost 200 publications describing other cases appeared.[2] For more than 100 years ether anesthesia was popular, but introduction of other gases and intravenous agents offered alternatives. Development of surgical techniques, surgical equipments, and need of modern approach to anesthesia made ether anesthesia less useful. The final straw came with strict regulations on safety in operating rooms to avoid fire and explosion. Thus, ether anesthesia in the USA was last given on October 20, 1982, at Temple University Hospital, Philadelphia.[3] The following is a presentation of the last years of ether anesthesia from that institution.

Clinical Material

One of the authors (RDH) had a preference for ether anesthesia with spontaneous respiration for head-neck cancer procedures. Therefore, all his 541 surgical cases done from 1975 to 1982 were reviewed retrospectively. Of the 541 patients, 332 were done under ether anesthesia; 243 were men and 89 women, with an age distribution of 69 ± 10 years, respectively.

Since preoperative workup and postoperative followup varied over the eight year period, this study concentrated on a limited number of variables so as to give a brief summary. We have therefor collected data on ASA physical status, diagnosis, surgical procedures, anesthesia time, survival during hospitalization, type of induction of anesthesia, level of monitoring, and early intraoperative hemodynamic changes.

Results

Ether anesthesia was a preferred anesthetic technique until 1979, at which time its use decreased to about 25 percent of cases until the last one in which it was employed. It is interesting to report that several patients received multiple ether anesthetics. Thus, one patient received five anesthetics, four patients four, 14 patients three, and 34 patients two anesthetics. The patients' physical status, according to the ASA classification, were 10 patients in class I, 186 class II, 125 class III and 11 class IV. There was no death intraoperatively; six patients did not survive the hospitalization period (2 percent). The total anesthesia time averaged 5.7 ± 2.2 hours.

In most patients, induction was done with a short-acting barbiturate (Pentothal[R]), but other intravenous agents were also used as a supplement for the induction. Nineteen patients were induced with inhalation technique (18 with cyclopropane, one with ether) and then continued as an ether anesthetic. Ether was supplemented with nitrous oxide in 319 cases, and with narcotics (most often fentanyl) in 24 cases

Patients were always monitored with EKG and manual blood pressure readings. In all patients but six, normal sinus rhythm was noted; atrial contractions and sinus tachycardia (three patients) were recorded. After 1978, more advanced monitoring was employed (19 patients with urine output, 18 patients with an arterial line and eight patients with central venous pressure monitoring).

Blood pressure changes and pulse rate changes were studied over the first 90 minutes as an indication of the stability provided by the anesthetic technique. The systolic blood pressure recorded before anesthesia for all patients was 126 ± 22 mm Hg. This varied to a highest value of 148 ± 20 and a lowest of 96 ± 22 during the studied time period. Pulse rate was initially 86 ± 15 and varied to a highest of 105 ± 14 and to a lowest 68 ± 23.

Discussion

Ether anesthesia has always been quoted as a "safe" anesthetic [4], with wide safety margins and a low rate of severe complications. Our retrospective study of 332 ether anesthetics in very sick patients supports such a statement. Only ten patients were considered healthy prior to the surgery; 311 of the patients had either mild or severe systemic disease, and 11 patients were in fact classified as having incapacitating systemic disease. Moreover, they underwent almost six hours of surgery.

With this in mind, a mortality during hospitalization of two percent must be considered acceptable.

In 19 patients the anesthesia was a true inhalation technique. The other patients were induced with intravenous agents, intubated and then exposed to the ether vapor. Most of the patients also had nitrous oxide and in some patients narcotics were given as an adjuvant.

Up till 1978 all patients scheduled for head and neck cancer surgery by RDH were done under ether anesthesia. After this period, the frequency went down because of introduction of other inhalation anesthetics, but also because of too costly maintenance of Operating Room floors to provide safe conditions.

It is of interest to note that both systolic blood pressure and pulse rate varied significantly during the first 90 minutes of the procedure. This can be explained by stimulation from intubation, surgical incision, bleeding, etc. It is possible that a pure inhalation anesthetic technique would have provided a better steady-state situation since the induction would have been slower with higher tissue concentrations of ether.

Finally, the 3:1 relationship of men to women clearly indicates that smoking was an important causative factor for the cancer.

TABLE I:
Ether anesthetics 1975 – 1982 in head and neck cancer cases.

Year	1975	1976	1977	1978	1979	1980	1981	1982
Number of cases	61	69	64	79	73	67	73	55
Ether anesth. number	61	69	64	68	19	20	19	12
percent	100	100	100	86	26	30	26	22

References

1. Secher O; Forty-six "first anaesthetics" in the world. Acta Anaesth Scand, 34: 552-6, 1990.
2. Wright AJ: How it all began. Anesthesia History Newsletter, 10: 2-16, 1992.
3. Carlesson C, Cooper, SC; 136 years of ether anesthesia. Anesth Analg; 70: 339-40, 1990.
4. Dodd, RB; Diethyl Ether: Its effects in the human body. Thomas Publisher, 1962, 72-78.

PAUL ZWEIFEL
An Early Contributor to Obstetric Anesthesia

DONALD CATON
Professor of Anesthesiology and Obstetrics and Gynecology
Department of Anesthesiology
University of Florida College of Medicine
Gainesville, Florida, USA

Paul Zweifel, a Swiss-born obstetrician, made two observations important to obstetric anesthesia. He was the first to demonstrate, unequivocally, that drugs given to the mother during labor cross the placenta to the fetus. He also demonstrated that umbilical arterial and venous blood differ in oxygen content. With this observation he established that the fetus consumes oxygen in utero, a deceptively simple point, but one that had been in contention for almost half a century.

Zweifel was born in 1848 in Hongg, a suburb of Zurich. Both his father and grandfather had been physicians practicing in that city. Zweifel was educated in Zurich. After graduating from medical school he volunteered for service as a military physician in the Franco-Prussian War. When he returned he studied obstetrics and gynecology in Zurich under Adolph Gusserow, who was a leader in obstetrics.[1,2] Gusserow, who was born in Berlin and educated in Berlin, Würzburg and Prague, was appointed in 1872 to the chair in Strasburg, Alsace Lorraine.[3] Zweifel went with him.

Gusserow's appointment was a direct consequence of the outcome of the Franco-Prussian war, which was the creation of Bismarck, the Iron Chancellor. The Kaiser's troops soundly defeated Napoleon the Third and occupied the often disputed territory of Alsace Lorraine. In the aftermath of the war, Bismarck staffed the medical school with some of the best talent available. Among those chosen with Gusserow was Felix Hoppe-Seyler, who is generally regarded as a founding father of the discipline of physiological chemistry, or biochemistry as it now is known. In 1870 he already was well established in his career and had started a journal of biochemistry.

For Zweifel, the opportunity to work with Gusserow and Hoppe-Seyler was propitious. Zweifel performed the decisive work, but he

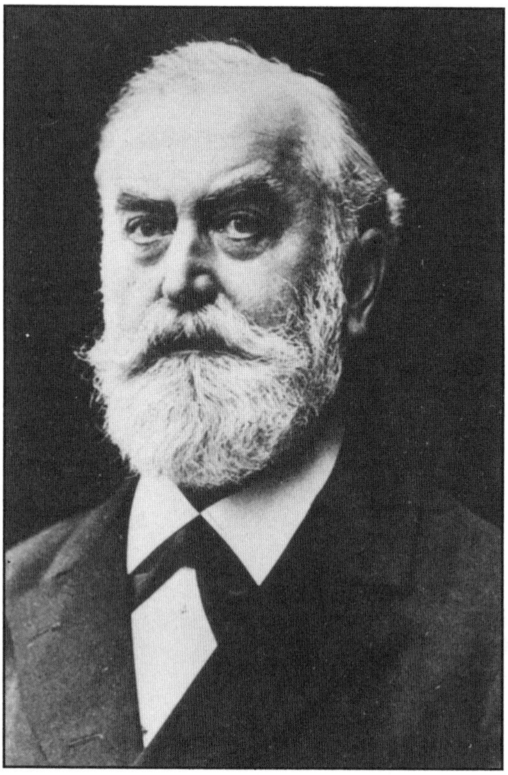

Fig. 1. Paul Zweifel (1848-1927).

answered questions posed by Gusserow. Moreover, he was able to perform the work in Hoppe-Seyler laboratory and used many procedures developed by him. Gusserow's primary interest was the metabolism of the fetus. What does it need to grow? How does it obtain what it needs? Does the fetus carry out its own metabolism or is this done for it by the mother? The questions, centuries old, had never been resolved. Since the early part of the century many believed that the mother carried out all metabolic processes for the fetus and that the fetus was nourished by swallowing amniotic fluid. Physicians at that time had no concept of fetal oxygen needs and little understanding of the role of the placenta and umbilical circulation as organs of respiration and nourishment. Shortly after the move to Strasburg, Gusserow published a long and thoughtful paper discussing the problem.[4]

Gusserow saw a way to attack these problems experimentally by studying the transmission of drugs from mother to fetus. In effect, he proposed a pharmacologic method to study a physiologic problem. His paper included his own observations of children whose mothers had been given potassium iodide during the course of pregnancy. Gusserow found increased amounts of potassium oidide in the amniotic fluid and urine of their children and concluded that it had been transmitted. Though this clearly established the existence of transmission, his paper left open the question of the time course of the process since the women had received the salt for days or weeks before labor.

Zweifel's first paper was an outgrowth of a clinical observation. He had noticed a yellow tint to the urine of infants whose mothers had been given chloroform during labor. He knew the drug could cause jaundice and speculated that it also might be a factor in the etiology of icterus neonatorum. For this to occur, however, the drug would have to cross the placenta rapidly enough to build up a significant concentration in the infant during the course of labor. To settle the question he studied two groups of neonates, one group exposed and the other not exposed to chloroform. Using a reducing agent, he tested for chloroform in urine obtained by catheterization or in freshly delivered placenta, blotted free of maternal blood. Tests for chloroform were uniformly positive in samples from exposed infants and negative in those from controls.

Zweifel published his results in a short paper in *Klinische Wochenschrift*[5] in 1874, which was widely read and accepted by most. An exception was an obstetrician named Fehling.[6] He challenged Zweifel on two points. First, he described experiments of his own in which he anesthetized pregnant dogs and then gave them curare. The dogs stopped moving, but the fetuses did not. He assumed that the curare did not cross the placenta. From this he reasoned that, if curare could not cross the placenta, neither could chloroform. Fehling also suggested that the positive tests for chloroform in the placenta were a technical error, the result of contamination from maternal blood not completely removed by blotting.

Fehling's criticism stimulated Zweifel to publish a second, much longer paper.[7] In it he presented a long review of the subject of fetal nutrition. Proceeding to a criticism of Fehling's argument, Zweifel gave all recent evidence as part of a rebuttal. He ended with a description of two experiments that he performed to support his own claim. In the first experiment, Zweifel demonstrated chloroform in fetal blood by mixing it with phenylalanine in the presence of heat and potassium hydroxide. The mixture forms phenycargamine, which has a very characteristic, pungent odor. It was, therefore, a qualitative test. The experiments were not without technical difficulties. The major problem he had was freeing chloroform gas from fetal blood. He finally accomplished this by chopping the clots and heating them. He even tried eluting chloroform by passing a stream of coal gas, but the mixture exploded and destroyed his glass apparatus. Helping Zweifel with these experiments was another young physician from the psychiatric clinic named von Mering, subsequently to become famous as a discoverer of the pharmacologic properties of barbituric acid. In the last part of his paper, Zweifel describes a second set of experiments in which he demonstrates that the urine and blood of newborns contained salicylic acid. This may seem a trivial point, but at that time obstetricians used salicylic acid often to relive labor pain.

Zweifel published another paper in 1876[8], which described his use of a light absorption technique to demonstrate a difference of oxygen content in the blood of intact umbilical vessels. He showed that no difference occurred when mothers became hypoxic. With this experiment he showed that oxygen crosses the placenta, that it does so rapidly — during one passage of blood through the placenta, and that the fetus consumes oxygen.

Zweifel's papers had a tremendous impact on the medical profession. Revolutionizing thinking about fetal pharmacology and physiology, they were discussed widely at obstetric meetings throughout Europe and the United States. Never again did anyone question the existence of fetal metabolic activity or need for oxygen. Since then, physiologists have sought to determine the magnitude of the need and the factors that regulate the availability. His experiments also stimulated widespread studies of morphologic and pharmacologic factors that influence the rate of transfer of compounds between mother and fetus.

Zweifel had a long and distinguished career in obstetrics and gynecology. At age 28 he was appointed to a post in Erlangen. Within 10 years he succeeded another famous obstetrician, Crede, to the chair in Leipzig, where he worked for the remainder of his career. Zweifel published more than 160 scientific papers. After he left Strasburg, most of them dealt with problems in gynecologic surgery. He also wrote several books, one of them co-authored with a son, also an obstetrician. Zweifel died in 1927, at age 79. Obituaries by his colleagues are effusive.

Bibliography

1. Füth P: Paul Zweifel. Deutsche medizinische Wochenschrift 53:1198, 1927.
2. Doderlein A: Zum Gedächtnis P. Zweifels. Arch für Gynaekologie 131:1-8, 1927.
3. Nagel W: Adolf Gusserow. Deutsche medizinische Wochenschrift, March 15, 1906, p 11.
4. Gusserow A: Zur Lehre vom Stoffwechsel des Foetus. Arch für Gynaekologie 3:241-270, 1871.
5. Zweifel P: Einfluss der Chloroformnarcose Kreissender auf den Fötus. Klinische Wochenschrift 21:1-3, 1874.
6. Fehling H: Zur Lehre von Stoffwechsel zwischen Mutter und Kind. Arch für Gynaekologie 9:313-318, 1876.
7. Zweifel P: Der Uebergang von Chloroform und Salicylsäure in die Placenta. Archiv für Gynaekologie 12:235-257, 1877.
8. Zweifel P: Die Respiration des Fötus. Archiv für Gynaekologie 9:291-305, 1876.

FROM FANNY TO FERNAND
Consumerism in Pain Control during the Birth Process

RICHARD B. CLARK, and CYNTHIA D. PITCOCK
Division of Medical Humanities
and the Departments of Anesthesiology
and Obstetrics/Gynecology
University of Arkansas for Medical Sciences
Little Rock, Arkansas, USA

Published in part in the
"American Journal of Obstetrics and Gynecology"

The first obstetric anesthesia administered in the United States was given to Fanny Appleton Longfellow, on April 7, 1847, in Cambridge, Massachusetts. (Fig. 1) Her physician was Dr. Nathan Cooley Keep, and he and her husband, the famous poet Henry Wadsworth Longfellow, held the ether-soaked handkerchief over Fanny's face.[1] Dr.Keep had heard of the demonstration in the ether dome in Boston the previous October and had used ether in dental cases, but this was the first time he utilized it for obstetrics. He advised the Longfellows of the experimental nature of the procedure, and the Longfellows agreed on its use. Thus, the first example of obstetric anesthesia also provides us with the first example of consumerism associated with obstetric anesthesia. The experiment was a success, as mother and child did well. Fanny was enthusiastic and vocal. Controversy arose as to whether the relief of obstetric pain was theologically and medically acceptable, as exemplified by the debates of Channing, Charles Meigs of Philadelphia, James Y. Simpson, and the Scottish clergy.[2] As this audience knows, the controversy was quieted in 1853 when Queen Victoria requested chloroform for the birth of her eighth child, Prince Leopold.[3] John Snow was the anaesthetist.[4] Both Fanny Longfellow and Queen Victoria praised the technique, and patient demand heightened.

For the next several decades inhalation analgesia/anesthesia was the only feasible means of relieving labor pain. In 1853 Alexander Wood of Edinburgh invented the

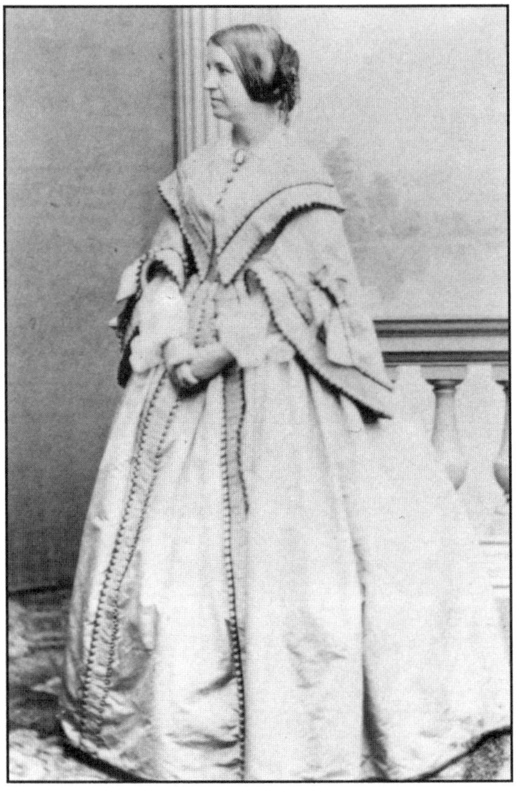

Fig. 1. Fanny Appleton Longfellow (1817-1861). Courtesy of the National Park Service, Longfellow National Historic Site, Cambridge, Massachusetts.

hypodermic syringe and needle, and the way was prepared for injectable analgesia.

Morphine was isolated and described by Serturner in 1803 and hyoscine in 1871. The stage was now set for "Dämmerschlaf" or twilight sleep, described by Von Steinbuchel, of Graz in 1902.[5] Carl J. Gauss of Freiburg popularized the method and reported 1000 cases in 1906.[6] This method became very popular, and women came from all over Europe, and indeed, from America to be delivered at the famous Frauenklinik in Freiburg.

The activities in Freiburg attracted the attention of the press, and two reporters from *McClure's Magazine,* a popular American magazine of the day, visited the clinic and reported their experience in the June, 1914, issue of the magazine.[7] Another reporter, Mary Boyd, delivered in Freiburg and reported her experience in the October, 1914, issue of McClure's.[8] Tracy and Boyd also published a book, "Painless Childbirth" which appeared in 1915.[9] As zealous advocates of the method they published several pictures of children delivered with Dämmerschlaf, and their bright, alert appearance testified to the safety of the method.

Twilight sleep became popular in America and the *National Twilight Sleep Association* was founded in order to bring the message to the women of America.[10] "Ordinary women," as well as "Club women" were to be alerted, and meetings and rallies were held, even in department stores.[11] The rally in this instance at Gimbels was held "between the marked-down suits and the table linens." The medical profession was generally opposed to twilight sleep at this time, and one prominent lay leader displayed her healthy twilight sleep infant to the audience, intoning "if you women want it (Twilight sleep), you will have to fight for it." Does that not sound familiar?

Twilight sleep began as a medical treatment, but the cause was taken up by non-physicians who institutionalized it, linked it to women's rights and who became militant and dogmatic. As a consumer group, they pressured the medical profession to utilize their progressive beliefs.

As time passed, the depressant effects on the neonate became apparent, and the death of one of the most visible leaders, Mrs. Francis X. Carmody, in childbirth, in 1916, had a devastating effect. The family of Mrs. Carmody claimed publicly that her demise was unrelated to twilight sleep, yet the blow fell upon the associations and damaged them fatally.

The next step in this story was taken by Dr. Grantly Dick-Read, a London obstetrician in the 1930's. His belief was that birth was a natural process and should not hurt any more than digestion. Pain accompanying labor and delivery is an illusion and the result of cultural conditioning, which he called the "fear-tension-pain syndrome."[12] A woman's learned fear of childbirth produces pain, but the normal contraction of the uterus should not be interpreted as painful.

The "natural" childbirth method centered upon a patient education effort. Women were instructed in the physical process of giving birth; they were re-educated concerning the anticipation of pain. Like Simpson several decades earlier, they interpreted labor as work rather than suffering. The "natural" childbirth movement, in contrast to Twilight Sleep, gave parturients the role of active participation in labor and delivery. Grantly Dick-Read developed a regimen of relaxation designed to reduce muscular tension during labor. As his method became popular, he developed antenatal classes including lectures on pregnancy, labor and delivery. His training, an effort to reprogram patients' concept of pain, included breathing and muscular exercises.

Experiments along the line of psychological preparation, education and reconditioning were launched in the Soviet Union by Velvosky and Nicolaiev whose early work employed hypnosis for pain relief.[13]

Velvosky's work, based upon science, but also upon trial and error, formed a basic theoretical agreement with Simpson and Channing, namely, that pain had no essential function in childbirth. Although he differed from Grantly Dick-Read who saw pain as an illusion, Velvosky agreed with him that a fundamental cause of pain was fear. This fear, he believed, was a generator of unfavorable reflexes. The brain, correctly preconditioned, could *distract* the pain-reflex by a series of breathing exercises which would then minimize pressure of the diaphragm upon the uterus. Thus, the Soviet method relieved pain by means in part of accelerated breathing and by providing additional oxygen.

This was the method which Dr. Fernand Lamaze observed when he visited Nicolaiev's Leningrad clinic in 1951. Lamaze, impressed with the painless deliveries he witnessed, decided to introduce the Soviet system at his clinic in Paris. (Fig. 2) He was the director of the Metal-Workers Lying-In Hospital, and within a year, he had instituted a system which resembled the one he had observed in Russia.[14] It is worthy of note that Lamaze modified the method for cultural rather than scientific reasons, adapting it to the urbane French woman as he understood her.

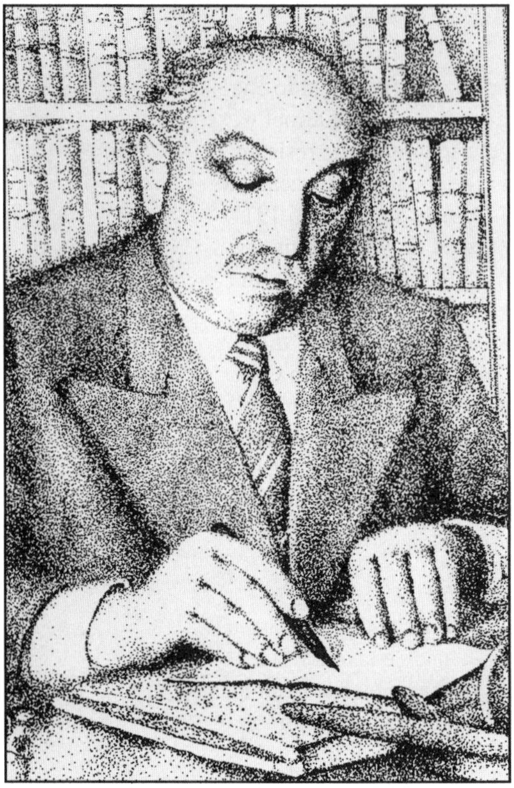

Fig. 2. Dr. Fernand Lamaze (1890-1957). Sketched from a photograph.

The Lamaze Method became popular throughout France within the year of its introduction to the wives of the metal workers in Paris. Lamaze himself became a celebrity; indeed a film was soon made about his efforts to establish "*accouchement sans douleur.*" The method was brought to the United States by a woman who, living in Paris temporarily, became Lamaze's patient. She was a resident of New York when she became pregnant a second time and, seeking a physician who would cooperate with her newly-learned pain relief techniques, she became frustrated. Marjorie Karmel reported her experience in the *Ladies Home Journal* in the early 1950's, and the Lamaze Movement was launched on this side of the Atlantic. Like her Twilight Sleep antecedents, Karmel side-stepped medical literature and sought popular support. She published a book in 1959 which enjoyed enormous success. (*"Thank you Dr. Lamaze"*)[15] This account was dramatic and readable and was designed to extol the

Lamaze Method and to encourage consumerism among patients. Karmel was vivid in her descriptions of the resistant medical community as she sought obstetrical care in New York.

Once again, as in 1914, physicians were accused of withholding medical innovation. Karmel joined forces with Elizabeth Bing, a former adherent of the Dick-Read school, and together they formed the American Society for Psychoprophylaxis in Obstetrics. The rapid acceptance of the Lamaze Method in the United States may be attributable to the efforts of Karmel and Bing, to their organization which promoted the teachings of Lamaze, and to Bing's own best seller which soon followed. (*Six Practical Lessons for an Easier Childbirth*).[16]

Significantly, the attitudes of obstetricians must also be taken into account. Although the media cast physicians in the role of obstructionists concerning psychoprophylaxis, this was not uniformly the case. Physicians in fact encouraged the use of what has been called "non-interventionist" methods. The Lamaze Method readily assumed the lead in the United States ahead of other methods which used psychological methods to ameliorate labor pain. In spite of a controversial history, psychoprophylaxis became part of the contemporary obstetrical practice in the 1960's, and the ultimate triumph of Lamaze was in part the genius of organization and timing.

In addition to the consistent flow of popular literature (Lamaze's own book was published in 1958, "Painless Childbirth"), a cadre of trainers furthered the Lamaze method. Their instruction of patients in small groups consisted of three elements: (1) information concerning pregnancy, labor and delivery; (2) training in relaxation; and (3) breathing techniques. The instructors, always female, served as an emotional back-up for the parturients, and they solicited feedback concerning the labor and delivery experience of each patient. Within a decade, 180 instructors were coaching 8,500 women annually, and by 1975, 2,500 instructors were training 190,000 per year. A powerful client-base became the vehicle for the Lamaze marketing success.

Significantly, the timing of Karmel's book coincided with a developing interest by obstetricians in psychological rather than chemical pain relief for labor and delivery. The Dick-Read method had been introduced and had been widely publicized in the United States. The weakness of his overall approach was his insistence that birth was a painless phenomenon. Lamaze incorporated elements of the systems he knew — both Velvoski and Dick-Read at a time when the women's movement in the United States embraced childbirth as a social issue.

As with the Twilight Sleep movement fifty years earlier, women sought greater control over their parturition, and the Lamaze Method offered an uncomplicated means. This time, however, in the context of the 1960's, control meant drug-free delivery rather than the use of scopolamine and morphine. Feminist rhetoric again assailed the medical profession to change its ways concerning pregnancy, labor and delivery. The instructional approach of Lamaze trainers was frankly adversarial concerning physicians. This attitude was central to another method which was developed in the 1960's by Robert Bradley. His *Husband-Coached Childbirth* instructional material listed the medical profession as "obstacle one" to be overcome by patients planning natural childbirth. "Most doctors are egocentric," he warned.[17] Patients were encouraged to keep looking until they found an "educated doctor, usually a younger one." Supported by a national association, the Bradley Method borrowed from Dick-Read and Lamaze but never achieved the widespread popularity of these movements.

In the postfeminist period, Lamaze rhetoric has mellowed concerning the question of anesthesia. Widespread experience has shown that a majority of women receiving Lamaze training ask for pharmacologic analgesia or regional block during labor. A new *synthesis* appears to be taking shape, combining Lamaze and epidural anesthesia. Some women felt that Lamaze preparation resembled training for an athletic contest.[18] Hospital administrators, as in the days of Twilight Sleep have added birthing suites, birthing rooms, and even labor, birthing and recovery rooms to meet the demand of patients. In the contest for control, the setting of labor and delivery takes on great importance. Thus, to answer an impulse for home deliveries, medical centers have altered their facilities to respond quite blatantly to consumerism. In no other area of medicine are the demands of the patient (now called consumers) so recognized. Patients of the 90's assume a role for which their grandmothers prepared them. They demand the right to make decisions concerning pregnancy, labor and delivery, and in this stance, they may or may not share responsibility with their physicians for the outcome.

References

1. Pittinger CB: Anesthetization of Fanny Longfellow for childbirth on April 7, 1847. *Anesth Analg* 66:367-74, 1987.
2. Simpson WG, ed: *The works of James Young Simpson, Edinburgh Scotland.* Adam and Charles Black, 177: 1971.
3. Weintraub S: *Queen Victoria, an intimate biography.* NY: E.P. Dutton, 224: 1987.
4. Snow J: *On chloroform and other anesthetics:* London, England. John Churchill, 1858.
5. Von Steinbuchel H: *Vorläufige Mittheilung über die Anwendung von Skopolamin-Morphium Injektionen in der Geburtshilfe.* Z. Geburtsh Gynaek 26:1304, 1902.
6. Gauss CJ: *Geburten im künstlichen Dämmerschlaf.* Arch f Gynäk 78:579, 1906.
7. Tracy M, Leupp C: Painless childbirth. *McClure's Magazine* 43:37-51, 1914.
8. Boyd M, Tracy M: More about painless childbirth. *McClure's Magazine* 43:55-69, 1914.
9. Tracy M, Boyd M: *Painless Childbirth.* Frederich A. Stokes Co., New York, 1915.
10. Leavitt JW; Birthing and anesthesia: the debate over twilight sleep. In: Leavitt JW, ed. *Women and Health in America.* Madison: University of Wisconsin Press, 177, 1984.
11. "Mothers Discuss Twilight Sleep." *New York Times,* November 18, 1914.
12. Dick-Read G: *Childbirth without fear.* NY: Harper & Brothers, 1944.
13. Velvovsky I, Platonov K, Polticher V, Shugom E, eds: *Painless childbirth psychoprophylaxis.* Moscow, USSR: Foreign Language Publishing House, 1960.
14. Lamaze F: *Painless childbirth,* Celestin LR, trans. London, England: Burke, 12-13, 1958.
15. Karmel M: *Thank you Dr. Lamaze.* Doubleday, New York, 1959.
16. Bing E, *Six Practical Lessons for an Easier Childbirth.* NY: Harper and Rowe, 1965.
17. Bradley RA: *Husband-coached childbirth.* NY: Harper and Rowe, 194-98, 1965.
18. Ephron N: "Having a baby after 35." *New York Times,* Dec. 26, 1978.

THE INTERNATIONAL MEDICAL CONGRESS OF 1912, WORLD WAR I AND THE TRANSATLANTIC TRIANGLE

DORIS K. COPE
Associate Professor of Anesthesiology and Physiology
University of South Alabama, Mobile, Alabama, USA

This research was supported by the American Society of Anesthesiologists Wood Library-Museum Fellowship, 1990-91

At the turn of the twentieth century in New York City at the New York Skin and Cancer Hospital, a dermatology intern, James Tayloe Gwathmey, described anesthesia as slapping an "unknown quantity of ether" on a patient's face, with straps and orderlies holding the patient down. Oxygen enrichment of air was unknown and vaporizers were used only for special academic demonstrations.

Gwathmey soon demonstrated such facility in modifying and using anesthetic equipment that he abandoned entirely the practice of dermatology to become one of the first American private practice anesthesiologists. He was continually borrowing ideas from his colleagues and adapting them to his lucrative clinical practice. For example, as a house officer he reported his improvement in the Bennett's inhaler, reducing the weight and bulk of the apparatus by over one-half. He then contracted with Kay-Scherer & Co. of New York City to produce and manufacture this device. In 1907, he collaborated with Richard von Foregger to combine Foregger's Oxygen-Generator with an ether-oxygen outfit which also could administer chloroform. He then demonstrated in cats that the lethal doses of chloroform, ether, and anesthol were higher with the addition of oxygen. He also used the heat from von Foregger's exothermic reaction to warm the anesthetic vapors, which he believed increased safety while also serving the practical purpose of preventing nitrous oxide, then not as pure and dry as now, from freezing the valves. Interestingly, explosions were not reported as a by-product of heating the anesthetic vapors.

A major problem with anesthesia equipment at this time was that the dose of anesthesia

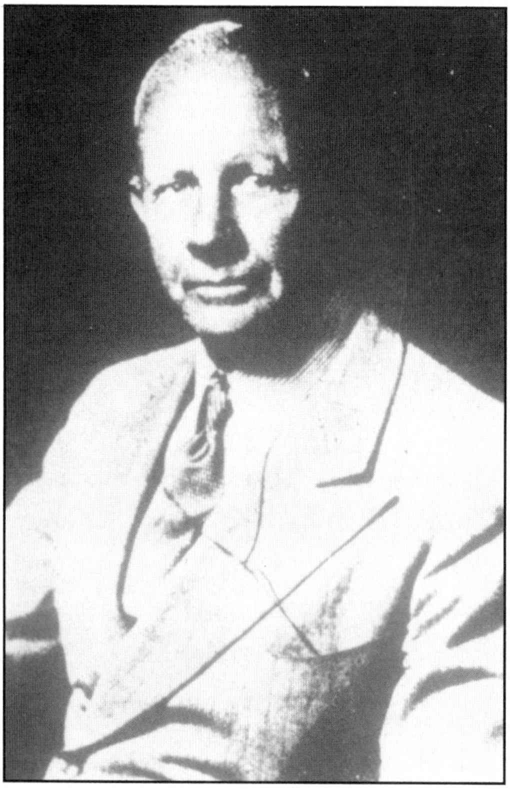

Fig. 1. James Tayloe Gwathmey.

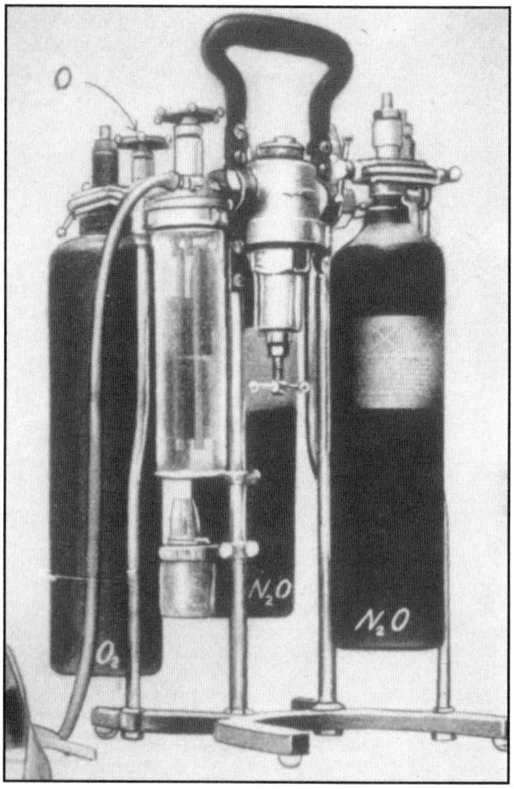

Fig. 2. Gwathmey nitrous oxide oxygen apparatus.

was at best an approximation, with guesswork adjustment of gas flow based on experience. The patient's response was the end-point in dosage. In 1905, Gwathmey demonstrated a vapor inhaler that attempted to control the concentration of vapor inhaled by the apparatus, which consisted of four graduated lengths of tubing. The longest one reached the bottom of the bottle, supplying approximately 1 percent chloroform, while the shortest barely penetrated the stopper, delivering a 0.1 percent concentration.

Thereafter, Walter Boothby and Frederick Jay Cotton introduced an anesthetic apparatus with reducing valves for both nitrous oxide and oxygen and a sight-feed apparatus to estimate the amount of each anesthetic delivered. Later, Gwathmey modified this bulky 50-pound apparatus to an anesthesia machine weight 14.5 pounds that he demonstrated in 1912 in Minneapolis. The gas supply in the Gwathmey-Woolsey nitrous oxide-oxygen apparatus was furnished by two one-hundred gallon tanks of nitrous oxide and one forty gallon tank of oxygen, providing approximately two hours of anesthesia. Later models, Fig. 2, included a pressure reducing valve for nitrous oxide invented by an instrument maker, J. Langsdorff. Regulating valves for N_2O and O_2 were present, as well as an adjustable alcohol lamp under the apparatus to warm the anesthesia gases. The unique feature of this apparatus, as seen in Fig. 2, is the incorporation of a "sight-feed apparatus" developed first by Cotton and Boothby, which consisted of a nickel partition dividing a warm water bath to "quantitate" N_2O and O_2 flowing through the water. A three bottle version for the administration of chloroform and ether, as well as nitrous oxide and oxygen, was subsequently developed from this early model. An exit tube connected the anesthetic bag and mask to the patient. A photograph demonstrating Dr. Gwathmey using this apparatus, as seen in Fig. 3, was published in his 1914 textbook, which was the most comprehensive and only American textbook of anesthesiology at the time.[1]

In 1912, as the first president of the American Association of Anesthetists, the first national organization for the specialty practice of anesthesiology, founded largely by his own efforts within the American Medical Association, James Tayloe Gwathmey presented a paper at the 17th International Congress of Medicine in London controversially entitled "Oil-ether Anaesthesia: An Attempt to Abolish Inhalation Anaesthesia." This paper, describing Gwathmey's collaborative work in the animal laboratory with the pharmacologist, Professor Wallace of Bellevue Hospital, extols the benefits of oil-ether rectal anesthesia over inhalation or intravenous anesthesia. After his presentation, followed by unsuccessful attempts to reproduce his methods resulting in death from anesthesia overdose, intense criticism and opposition to rectal anesthesia followed. However, at the same meeting, Gwathmey also participated in a symposium on nitrous oxide-oxygen anesthesia with Drs. Crile and Teter, demonstrating his new portable sight-feed apparatus to Dr. H.E.G. Boyle, who was present at the time.

Unlike his attempts to popularize rectal anesthesia, his anesthesia apparatus and experiences encouraging the private practice of anesthesiology were embraced enthusiastically by Dr. Boyle, who five years later wrote:

> My own interest in the matter is due entirely to Dr. James T. Gwathmey, of New York, whom I met at the Congress in 1912. He persuaded me to get a machine and try for myself, and I have not regretted it.[2]

In England, prior to the use of nitrous oxide-oxygen anesthesia at St. Bartholomew's Hospital, a medical student, Charles F. Hadfield, described the preponderance of chloroform anesthesia for all but the shortest operations. At that time it was believed that:

> Anaesthesia was in a static condition, was tacitly assumed to have reached its zenith, and no further improvements were expected or even sought. Conditions remained much the same until shortly before the first war period.[3]

From this encounter, Boyle persuaded the governors of the 1st London General Hospital to import two Gwathmey machines, which he adapted with washers and connectors to fit

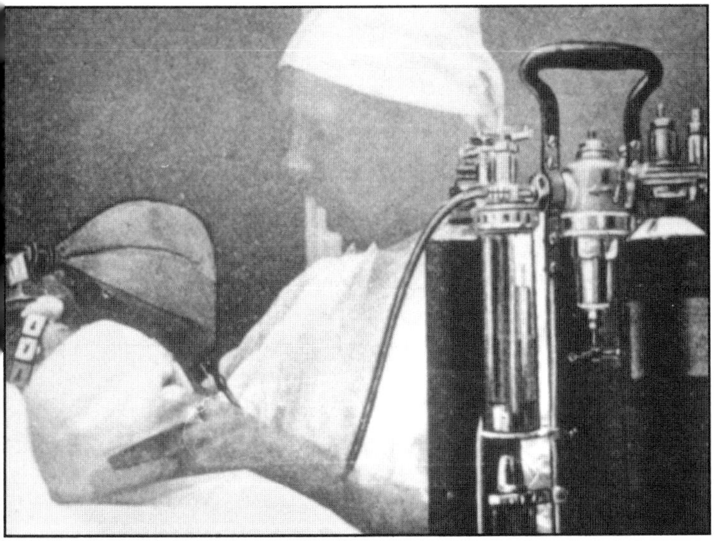

Fig. 3. Gwathmey administering anesthesia with his own apparatus.

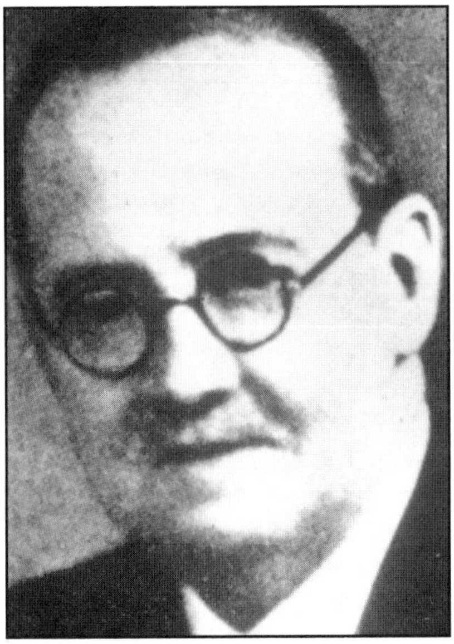

Fig. 4. H.E.G. Boyle.

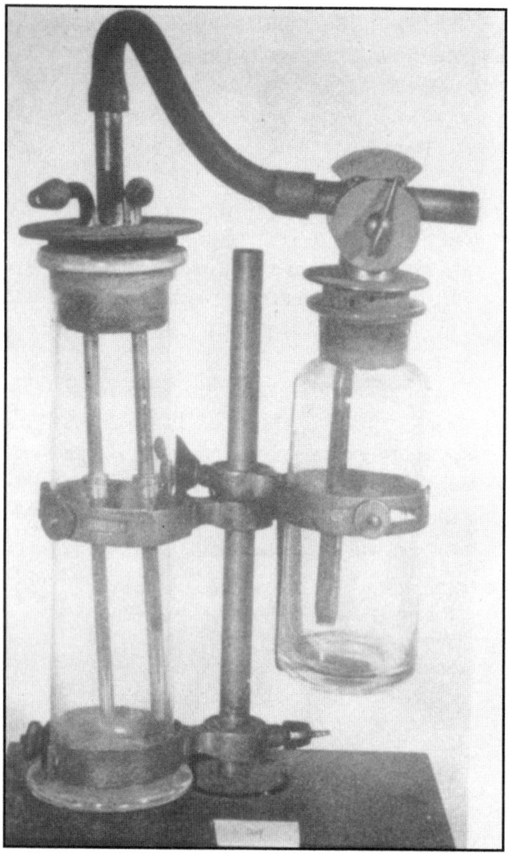

Fig. 5. Boyle apparatus.

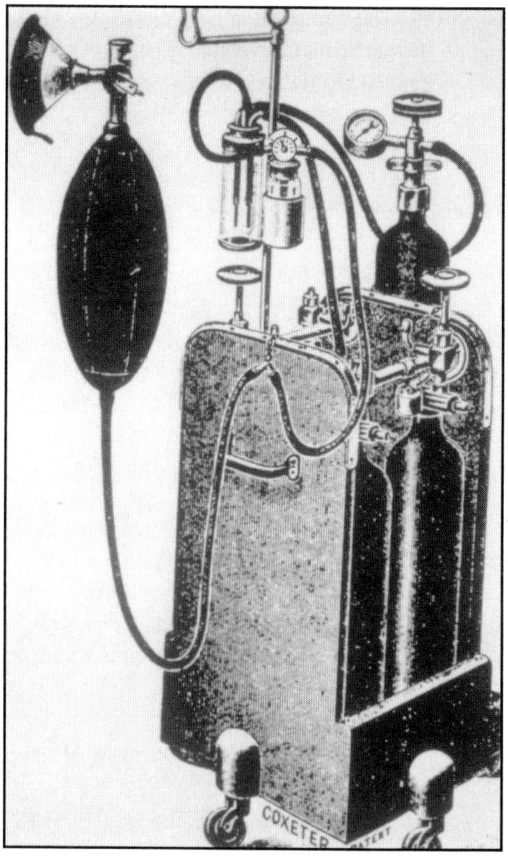

Fig. 6. Boyle apparatus packaged for military use.

British canisters for use in his own very busy private practice and later during World War I. By 1917 he had reported his experience using this equipment for 711 cases, 550 in which he himself had administered the anesthesia. His early equipment included an ether head and separate bottle for N_2O and O_2, shown in Fig. 5. He then wrote a proposal to the Coxeter Manufacturing Company to produce the Gwathmey anesthesia machine adapted to British oxygen and nitrous oxide canisters, packed in a heavy wooden box for military use, which is shown in Fig. 6. In this model the four cylinders had reducing valves and the gas mixture was directed through a Cattlin bag.

In 1915, James Tayloe Gwathmey's only son, William, a 22 year old student, sold his books, guns and even clothing to enlist in the Allied cause. Two years later, James T. Gwathmey visited his wounded son and stayed to serve in the U.S. Army Medical Corps on the Western front in France. There, he tried to streamline anesthesia care by experimental arrangements of the operating theater. At the No. 17 Casualty Clearing Station in France, in 1917, Gwathmey inspired a young British physician, Geoffrey Marshall from Guy's Hospital, to try his bubble-through apparatus. Marshall liked the American machine and subsequently designed a similar portable machine, seen in Fig. 8, enlisting a tinsmith to build the apparatus in the trenches. Sir Anthony Bowlby, a surgeon who also knew Boyle from St. Bartholomew's Hospital, urged Marshall to persuade an English manufacturer to produce the machine, and a prototype was eventually produced by Coxeter. The curved tubes in the bubble bottle were characteristic of Marshall's apparatus. The complete apparatus, shown in Fig. 9, had no reducing valves and the gas mixture was piped through a Cattlin rebreathing bag. In his 1920 recounting of this apparatus he stated:

> We must have apparatus that is light, simple and compact. . . The general principles of this outfit are similar to that of Dr. Gwathmey and others[4]

However, before Marshall was able to publish any account of his apparatus, Boyle, still a Captain in the Royal Army Medical Corps, formally described the nitrous oxide-oxygen-ether outfit in the *British Medical Journal* in 1919 and in the St. Bartholomew's Hospital Journal later in the same year. His continuing upgrading of the original anesthesia apparatus resulted in the design of a head unit recognizable as the immediate forerunner of the modern anesthesia machine. His dedication to teaching helped establish a tradition that "a Bart's man could always be relied upon to give a decent anaesthetic."[3] Thereafter, Boyle's name became indelibly linked with the modified Gwathmey apparatus, later upgraded with a Coxeter dry flowmeter. Sir Geoffrey Marshall, advised that there was no future in anesthesia, became the most Senior and revered Internist at Guy's Hospital after the War.

References

1. Gwathmey JT: *Anesthesia.* New York: Appleton, 1914.
2. Boyle HEG: *Lancet.* i:226, 1917.
3. Hadfield CF: *Brit J Anaesth* 22: 107-117, 1950.
4. Marshall G: *Proc Roy Soc Med* III: 16-18, 1920.

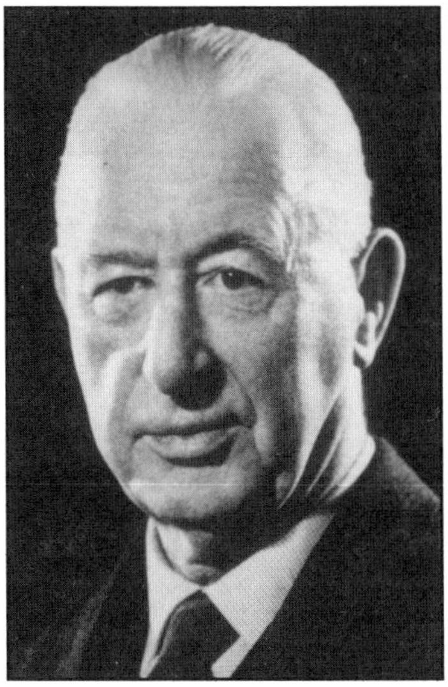

Fig. 7. Sir Geoffrey Marshall.

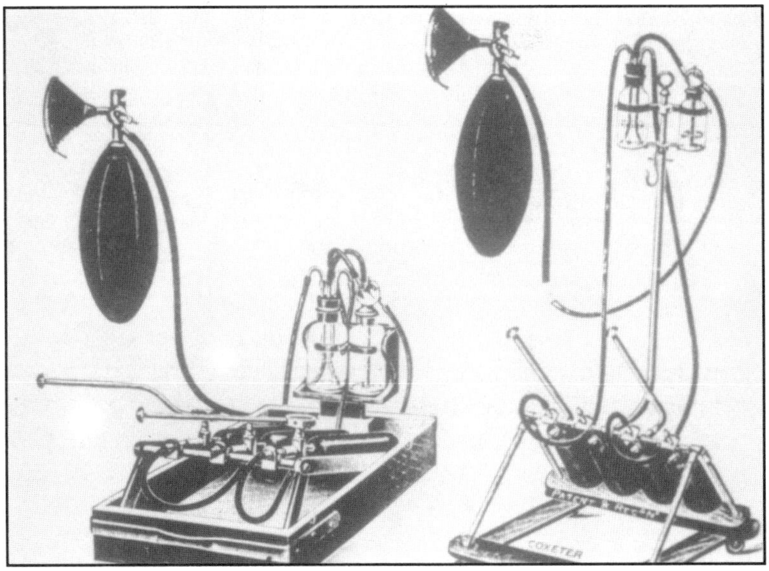

Fig. 9. Portable Marshall Apparatus.

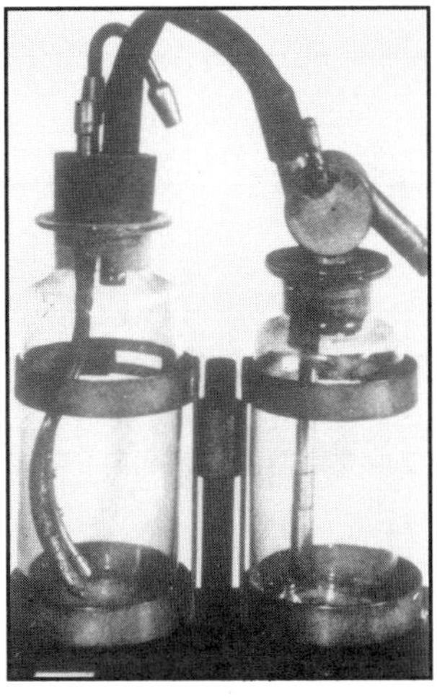

Fig. 8. Marshall Apparatus.

THE FIRST ETHER ANAESTHETIC OUTSIDE OF AMERICA AND EUROPE

JOHN L. COUPER
Medunsa South Africa

In a paper read at the fourth South African Medical Congress in Grahamstown in 1897, Dr. William Guybon Atherstone stated his administration of ether to Frederick Carlisle for the amputation of the leg at the lower third of the thigh "was its first use out of America and Europe."[1] This took place on Wednesday, 16 June 1847, and was reported in the *Graham's Town Journal* of Saturday, 19 June, under the heading, "Painless operation by means of ether."[2] Atherstone had been invited to talk at the Congress in honour of being the first person to administer ether outside America and Europe fifty years previously.

In the late 1950's, Schmidt studied Cape Town newspapers and found a report in *De Verzamelaar, id est The Gleaner* of 20 April, 1847, of the successful use of ether by Alfred Raymond for the extraction of two teeth from one gentleman and one tooth from another.[3] Schmidt considered this and two subsequent reports of the use of ether by Raymond with skepticism.[4] He made no attempt to find out anything about Raymond or how the news of ether could have reached Cape Town.

Research presented at the Second International Symposium on the History of Anaesthesia clearly showed that Alfred Raymond had used ether in Cape Town on at least four occasions before its use by Atherstone,[5] and had given a demonstration of ether at one of the Rev. Mr. Brown's series of lectures on the Pathology and Structure of the Human Frame to the Cape Town Institute for the Diffusion of Useful Knowledge.[6]

Raymond's use of ether followed soon after the arrival in Table Bay of the steamship *Pekin,* which was the first ship to bring newspapers and journals with accounts of painless surgery by means of the inhalation of ether.[5] Probably more important than the arrival of newspapers in the spread of the news of ether was the presence of the ship's surgeon, Dr. T. Bell, who had published a case report in the *London Medical Gazette* in January of his administration of ether for the amputation of the leg of a pregnant woman.[7] No reports of Dr. Bell's visit to Cape Town could be found, but it is inconceivable that he did not make contact with the medical fraternity while the *Pekin* spent a week in Table Bay and tell them of ether and the inhaler he used. Dr. Bell administered ether on 28 April, 1847, for the amputation of the arm of a lascar seaman, using an inhaler made by Mr. Hooper of Pall Mall while the *Pekin* was in Mauritius.[8]

Dr. Gwen Wilson has made an extensive study of how the news of ether reached Australia. There were two routes by which mail from England reached the Antipodes — the Cape route and the overland route.[9] The Cape route was across the Atlantic to Buenos Aires, then direct to Australia without calling at the Cape of Good Hope, but sailing further south and taking advantage of the roaring forties to be blown straight to Australia. By this route the news of ether reached Australia via the *Mountstuart Elphinstone* in 127 days, having left England on 23 December, 1846, and arriving in Sydney on 28 April, 1847. Dr. Belisario used ether in Sydney for teeth extraction in May. The first surgical operation in Australia under ether, given by Dr. William Russ Pugh, was a St. John's Hospital, Launceston, Tasmania on 7 June, the news having been carried by the *Lady Howden,* which berthed at Hobart on 27 May after a voyage of 128 days from England.

The overland route was quicker and it took approximately 100 days for newspapers and mail to reach Australia. The ships sailed from England through the Mediterranean sea to Alexandria, where passengers and mail re-embarked on barges through the Mahmoudien canal, then transferred to Nile steamer to Cairo. They then went overland for 3 days to Suez, where they boarded one of the two large P&O steamers, *Hindostan* or *Beatnick,* for Point de Galle in Ceylon, where they were transferred to the *Braganza* or the *Lady Mary Wood* to Singapore, and once more transferred there to the *Lightning* for passage around western Australia to Melbourne and Sydney. The larger steamers continued from Galle to Madras and Calcutta.

It is not surprising that news of ether reached places *en route* to Australia, and in fact ether was used by Mr. A.J. Ratton, the assistant surgeon at Malacca in the old Straits Settlements, for the amputation of the arm of a Malay Iascar on 28 April, 1847 [10]. All the documented evidence so far points to Cape Town being the first place outside America or Europe where ether was administered. Indeed, in the list of forty-six first anaesthetics in the world compiled by Dr. Ole Secher, Cape Town gets the credit of the first ether use outside Europe.[11]

Studying the overland route, one would have expected that India would have known of ether before the Straits Settlement and Australia, and even before the news reached South Africa. The British East India Company was the leading power in India by the mid 1700's and there were large English settlements and British troops throughout India, particularly in the major coastal cities. The P&O steamers in the 1840's went on to Madras and Calcutta after calling at Galle.

In the report in the *Graham's Town Journal,* 19 June 1847, headed, "Painless Operations by means of Ether," we find the following paragraph after the announcement that Atherstone had used ether:

> This discovery seems to give an entirely new character to the surgical art, and to open a door for further research, the ultimate extent, importance and value of which to mankind it is impossible to calculate. The same practice has, we learn from late papers, been introduced into medical practice in British India, where for some time the subject of mesmerism had excited a good deal of attention. It is now thought that the two processes may be employed with equal success, and which does not appear improbable, judging from the following case which we have taken from the *Madras Crescent* of 20 February.[2]

There followed a case report of the use of mesmerism. Could the *Madras Crescent* of 20 February, 1847, have carried reports of the use of ether in India? Or were the reports or ether from later newspapers? Lee suggests that the news of ether reached Malacca by late February or early March, and this is some considerable distance from major Indian ports.[10]

My attention was now drawn to India as being the first country outside America and Europe that saw the administration of ether for painless surgery. A chance remark by Professor Diviker of Bombay led me to the *Englishman* (Later the *Statesman*) of Calcutta of Monday 22 March, 1847, and this report clearly put the use of ether in Calcutta on 20 March, 28 days ahead of its first reported use in Cape Town.[12] The report is as follows:

> Our reporter furnished us on Saturday with a notice of an operation performed on that day at the College Hospital, on a man under the influence of the vapour of ether. A gentleman who was present, has since supplied us with some further particulars. The operation was performed by Mr. Richard O'Shaughnessy, with his usual skill. The patient had received severe injuries from the accidental bursting of a gun; besides a compound fracture of both bones of the left leg, for which immediate amputation was necessary. On being brought into the Hospital, the pain he was suffering was so intense that he could not draw a full breath, nor bear the slightest movement. His countenance was anxious, and had a general appearance of irritability and suffering. He was made to inhale sulphuric ether from a Mooth's apparatus, exactly as described in Mr. Liston's operation. He became rapidly affected by it to a partial extent, so as to be evidently less conscious of suffering, although by no means insensible. His pulse at that time was quick and tolerably full. The operation was immediately performed, without removing him from the bed on which he had been first placed. The result was very gratifying to the spectators. The patient required no holding, and continued smoking from the apparatus with greater energy than before. He groaned a little while the principal artery was tied and when the limb was shaken. He afterwards said that he felt the shaking of the limb which was a good deal inflamed, but that he did not feel the cutting. His countenance became calm, and he expressed his thankfulness for being relieved from very great suffering. The cheerfulness of his countenance, similar to that of mesmerized patients, was remarked. The ether used was not particularly good, or it is probable that complete insensibility would have occurred.
>
> This case demonstrates the easy application of ether in accidents or other cases requiring immediate surgical operations, and with those previously reported in England and America, puts an end to the doubts of the profession as to the impossibility of *painless surgery*. If partial or perfect insensibility to pain can be produced by ether, then why not by mesmerism? We have two remedial agents instead of one, and others may be discovered possessing advantages not common to those now known. There will be a choice for the professional attendant according to circumstances, and he may avail himself of which he judges most suitable to the particular case before him. We think, too, that we shall hear no more of the *utility* of pain to the sufferer. The Surgeons will not again tell us that the agonies of an operation have a curative tendency. So long as mesmerism alone could sooth pain, in their vehement opposition to it, they took up the Stoical doctrine: they may not safely abandon it with equal advantage to their patients and themselves.

A couple of questions arise from this report. Had ether been used previously in Calcutta? Twice in the report the use of ether for immediate surgery was mentioned — that immediate amputation was necessary and later that the case demonstrates the easy application of ether in cases requiring immediate surgical operations. This gives the impression that ether might have been used previously for planned procedures. Further support is the statement that the ether used was not particularly good. Had the doctors experimented or even used ether in a planned manner when they would have had time to prepare a better quality ether?

Dr. Atherstone claimed that he had no details of apparatus when he used ether, and he made a contrivance for his administration of ether based on the Turkish narghili or hubble-bubble.[1] Did Atherstone see this account of the patient continuing smoking from the apparatus and did this report of "smoking" the ether give him the idea of contriving a hubble-bubble apparatus? Because Bombay and Madras are even nearer London than Calcutta, it is likely that reports of ether's use before O'Shaughnessy's may be found.

Henry Bigelow's remark on 16 October, 1846, "I have seen something today that will go round the world" was true prophecy indeed, and it is gratifying to find how quickly the news did spread to far off places, and that ether was used outside of America and Europe earlier than was thought.

References

1. Atherstone WG: Reminiscences of medical practice in South Africa fifty years ago. S. Afr med J. 4:243-247, 1897.
2. Painless operation by means of ether. Graham's Town Journal, p3 col 2, 19 June 1847.
3. De Verzamelaar, p2 col 2, Cape Town 20 April 1847.
4. Schmidt HJ: A history of anaesthesia in South Africa. S. Afr Med J., 32:244-251, 1958.
5. Couper JL: Putting the record straight — the first ether administration in South Africa. In the History of Anaesthesia Eds Atkinson RS, Boulton TB. Royal Society of Medicine, London, 149-153, 1989.
6. Cape Town Mail, p4 col 4, 19 June 1847.
7. Bell T: Amputation performed on a pregnant female under the influence of ether. The London Medical Gazette, New Series, 4:319-320, 1847.
8. Montgomery A: Application of ether. De Zuid Afrikaan p3 col 2-3, May 1847.
9. Wilson G: The news spreads along the trade routes of the British Empire. In The History of Anaesthesia, Eds Atkinson RS, Boulton TB. Royal Society of Medicine, London, 149-153, 1989.
10. Lee YK: The first anaesthetic in the Straits Settlements — 1847. Br J Anaes, 44:408-411, 1972.
11. Secher O: Forty six "first anaesthetics" in the world. Acta Anaesthesiol Scand, 34:552-556, 1990.
12. The Englishman, p2 col 2-3, Calcutta, 22 March 1847.

NEW LIGHT ON ALFRED RAYMOND WHO ADMINISTERED THE FIRST ETHER IN SOUTH AFRICA

JOHN L. COUPER
Medunsa, South Africa

It has been firmly established that the first recorded use of ether in South Africa was on 17 April, 1847, when Alfred Raymond administered ether for the extraction of two teeth from one gentleman and one tooth from another.[1] That this was not the first use of ether out of America and Europe, as commonly believed, has been revealed in a prior paper.

When I became interested in Alfred Raymond about ten years ago, there was nothing in contemporary works about Raymond beyond mere mention of the reports of his use of ether, and an account of the suffering of the Rector of the Grey Institute at the hands of Mr. Raymond. The Rector needed a tooth extracted and "Mr. Raymond, managed to extract two, together with a portion of the gum and a portion of the haw."[2]

An attempt was made to find out something about Raymond, who described himself as a Surgeon Dentist of the University of Paris,[3] by reading Cape Town newspapers from 1842 when he settled in that city; Grahamstown and Port Elizabeth newspapers when he moved to the Eastern Cape; searching State Archives in Cape Town and Mauritius; writing to every Raymond listed in the various telephone directories of South Africa; searching church records of the period; perusing other documents in historical libraries in Cape Town, Grahamstown and Port Elizabeth; shipping intelligence and requests in letters to the Editors columns of contemporary newspapers for anyone with any information on Alfred to get in touch with me. As a result of these sources, I was able to construct a family tree of sorts and receive accounts of anecdotal stories, but very little else. So I have tried to construct a picture of the man from these sources and from advertisements that he inserted into newspapers during the early years of his practice in South Africa.

Jean Victor Paul Alfred Raymond was born in Mauritius on 18 April, 1813. The Archival records in Mauritius are largely non-existent or in a very poor state, but it appears his father had the title doctor. No records could be found of his schooling and, although he called himself a

Surgeon Dentist of the Faculty of Medicine of Paris of the University of Paris, no record exists of his attendance there. There are, however, records of certificates awarded to Pierre Joseph Victor Raymond who was born in Mauritius on 13 September, 1807.

The earliest advertisement was in *Le Cernéen* on 25 September, 1838, shortly after his return to Mauritius from Cape Town, where he had married Catherine Sophie Cauvin on 9 July, 1839, and was merely an announcement of his hours of attendance and the site of his consulting rooms.

In 1839, an indication of a particular interest appears that of the teething of children "to promote the regularity of the teeth and prevent those pains which often proceed from neglect or inattention." This theme appears throughout his notices.

The Raymonds moved from Mauritius in 1842, and his first announcement from Cape Town appeared on 15 February, stating that he had had ten years practice in Mauritius and Paris where he was attached during 6 months to one of the best Hospitals. Four days later he informed the public that natural and artificial sets of teeth could be fixed, as well as every other operation in that line.

A month later an advertisement advertised his tooth powder, using an extract from an editorial of the *Mauritien,* "which gives a perfect whiteness and stops putrefaction and gives the breath an agreeable perfume." He later advertised that the tooth powder and a tincture would keep the teeth firm in the sockets. It is interesting to note that his first notices gave limited hours of attendance, but by mid-year he stated he may be consulted at any time of the day and during the night on personal application to him or a note requesting his attendance.

His advertisements in Port Elizabeth newspapers in early 1859 stated he had for the last 25 years paid particular attention to the too often neglected dentition of children, and one series of advertisements stated that children's teeth would be regulated in a new *modus operandi* of his own adopted by most of the eminent Dentists in France. Other dentists at the time were adding various qualifications after their names, and soon after Alfred started doing the same instead of merely stating surgeon dentist of the Faculty of Medicine of Paris or other claims. In his advertisements and notices over the years he used sixteen different titles and sources. With the denial by the Archivist of the University of Paris that he ever attended that institution, this leads one to presume that these were all fictitious titles or titles he had seen in advertisements by other dentists. Registration of dentists in South Africa only came into being in 1891; before, anyone could call himself dentist even without training. Dental studies at the University of Paris had to be pursued in the Faculty of Medicine until the founding of the dental school in the 1890's. The question arises, did Raymond receive any formal training in dentistry? The evidence seems to indicate he did not. His advertisement stated that he was attached for 6 months in one of the best hospitals in Paris. Would he have been allowed to practice dentistry, even been permitted to observe proceedings, if he was not a registered student at the University? Probably not. His elder brother did study medicine and his father had the title doctor (but I have not been able to find out any more details) so he could have been apprenticed to them and polished his apprenticeship at a hospital in Paris. The fact that he used 16 different titles seems to indicate he was not *au fait* with academic institutions and titles of the time.

That he must have had a strong, perhaps forceful, personality is reflected in two notices inserted in newspapers. In 1861 he stated that he "works only in gold — a sound durable, and therefore, cheap material. No work performed in any other material will be repaired by him." And in 1862, calling himself a Lecturer on Dentistry, "he requests those patients who may want his professional services NOT TO DELAY as constant employment is the only way to secure PERMANENTLY the services of a competent Dentist in this town." A month later he advertised himself as Dentist and oculist, and six months later "that he will in future devote his attention solely to the operations of the Mouth and Teeth and to disease of the Eyes." This advertisement of 28 November, 1862, was the last I could find, although he is listed in directories as living in Port Elizabeth until 1883.

In 1861 when he lived in Grahamstown, he advertised: "French taught by a Frenchman. Mons. A. Raymond B A of the Sorbonne, Paris has opened an Evening Class for Gentlemen willing to learn French. Heads of families will also find Mons. R. disposed to instruct, during his leisure hours and at their *own* residences, young ladies in the above language. . . ." It is the only occasion when he used the degree of B A.

Family Tree

The original family tree that I constructed was based on a letter from a great great grandson, Trevor Gary Raymond, who could give me no information about Alfred except his relationship. Trevor's grandfather (Alfred's grandson), Alfred Albert, was an alcoholic and as a result contact with the rest of the family was minimal.

More information was obtained as a result of letters requesting information published in Eastern Cape newspapers. Through this means I made contact with Rita Raymond Treherne (born Pullen) who is a great granddaughter through Alfred's fourth child — Josephine Estelle, who married John Arthur Pullen in 1864. Contact with the descendents of nine of her aunts and uncles (Josephine had ten children) has revealed only confirmation of Rita's anecdotes. Rita has a fairly moth-eaten photograph of Alfred, whom she knew as Paul. She said Alfred went to live with daughter Josephine on her farm in the Grahamstown district in 1883 when he would have been about 70 years old and likely to give up practice. Rita recollects that her mother spoke of her grandfather Alfred with affection and some amusement, and said he was a fiery old Frenchman (a cousin said a peppery short-tempered man) who had helped her with her French lessons whenever she came on holiday from boarding school. He was very fussy as far as personal cleanliness and hygiene was concerned. He had beautiful soft hands and always kept a piece of lemon next to the hand basin to use when he washed his hands.

By all accounts Alfred became eccentric, and when he went to live on the farm Josephine would not allow him into the house because she "couldn't have him there with the young children." So he lived in a room away from the house, on his own, and his food was taken to him there. Some family members even said the reason was that he molested the children. Alfred's wife died in March, 1863, after a long and protracted illness. One wonders whether this tendency to "molest" did not arise before Catherine's death when he advertised he would give French lessons to young ladies in their homes, and also that as a dentist he would be happy to call upon ladies in their own residences if requested.

One of Rita's cousins stated that by all accounts it would appear that Alfred Raymond "received somewhat cavalier treatment." A family story is that Alfred was so bitter against the Pullens (his daughter and son-in-law) that he put a curse upon them before he died — and they lost everything as a result and had to sell the farm. His daughter Josephine was a "grand dame," very proper and took no nonsense — could their personalities have been very similar and did this lead to this apparent clash between father and daughter? Josephine married at the age of 17, a year after her mother died, ostensibly to get out of the house away from her father.

One of the family's stories is that Alfred was a doctor, but was unable to get his papers from Paris because of a war, so he practiced as a dentist. At the time he arrived in Cape Town there existed a body in Cape Town called The Supreme Medical committee that was empowered to examine anyone who claimed to have a medical qualification and to register such a person as a medical practitioner if they thought fit. Alfred never applied to them for registration. Is this claim to have been a physician further indication that Alfred did not have a medical qualification and reflect his frustration because his brother and seemingly his father were qualified medical practitioners?

Alfred Raymond even seems to have been eccentric with his religious affiliation. He was married in the Dutch Reformed Church in Cape Town. No record of the birth and baptism of his eldest child could be found. His second child was baptized in the Anglican (Episcopalian) church in Cape Town and the next three in the Roman Catholic Church, of which he was a member. On moving to Port Elizabeth he appears to have had no church connection, although his wife was buried in an Anglican rite. Nor are there any records of affiliation with any church when he went to live on his daughter's farm. The family recollect that they were told that he said his matins alone in his room each morning as he was a devout Catholic.

This study has been an attempt to place on record something about Alfred Raymond, who was the first person to administer ether anaesthesia in South Africa.

References

1. Couper JL: Putting the record straight — the first ether Anaesthesia. Eds Atkinson RS, Boulton TB. Royal Society of Medicine, London 149-153, 1989.
2. Grobler V: The history of dentistry in South Africa 1652-1900. HAUM Pretoria, 30-32, 1977.
3. Raymond A: Dental Physiology. Cape Town Medical Gazette 1:19-20, 1847.

Titles Used in Connection with Raymond

1. Surgeon Dentist.
2. Surgeon Dentist of the Faculty of Medicine of Paris.
3. Surgeon Dentist of the "University of Paris."
4. DR RAYMOND.
5. Graduate of the Academy of Medicine of Paris.
6. Of the "Faculty of Medicine of Paris."
7. M C S P.
8. Graduate of the Faculty of Medicine of Paris.
9. B.A. of the Shorbonne.
10. M I C S P.
11. Of the Imperial School of Surgeons, Paris.
12. Lecturer on "Dentistry" etc.
13. Member of the College of Surgeons of Paris.
14. Member of the Imperial College of Surgeons of Paris.
15. Surgeon and Mechanical Dentist.
16. Surgeon and Practice Dentist.

HENRY HILL HICKMAN
Unsung Discoverer of Inhalation Anesthesia

DAVID A. CROSS
Clinical Professor
Department of Anesthesiology
The University of South Alabama Medical Center
Mobile, Alabama, USA

. . . If one grain of knowledge can be added to the general fund,
to obtain a means for the relief of pain,
then the labours of the author will be amply rewarded.
Henry Hill Hickman, 1842[1]

In the late 18th and early 19th centuries, England was captivated by the technologic advancements of the day, with little regard for the improvement of the accompanying human plight. Industrial accidents were common, and there was little compensation or job security for injured workers.[2] Adding to their suffering, surgery was barbaric by today's standards. Performing his art with neither anesthesia nor antisepsis, the surgeon based his proficiency and reputation on his speed and effective cauterization. Suppuration, not pain relief, was his primary concern.[3]

Henry Hill Hickman was born the son of John and Sarah (Hill) Hickman on January 27, 1800, at Lady Halton, a farmhouse in the parish of Bromfield, Shropshire, England, near Ludlow. There is some confusion as to whether he was born in the farmhouse or the cottage,[4] but it is known that his father farmed land which was owned by the Earl of Plymouth's estate.[5] At the turn of the century, Ludlow boasted a population of some 4,000 and was a noted aristocratic, agricultural, and glove-making center. The population was divided mostly between the decisively rich and the decisively poor. The aristocratic nature of the area gave rise to an abundance of transient gentry, whose need for a number of "services" gave rise to a like abundance of "pretty ladies." A high percentage of women held jobs. In 1815, some 90 percent of the glove-making work force was

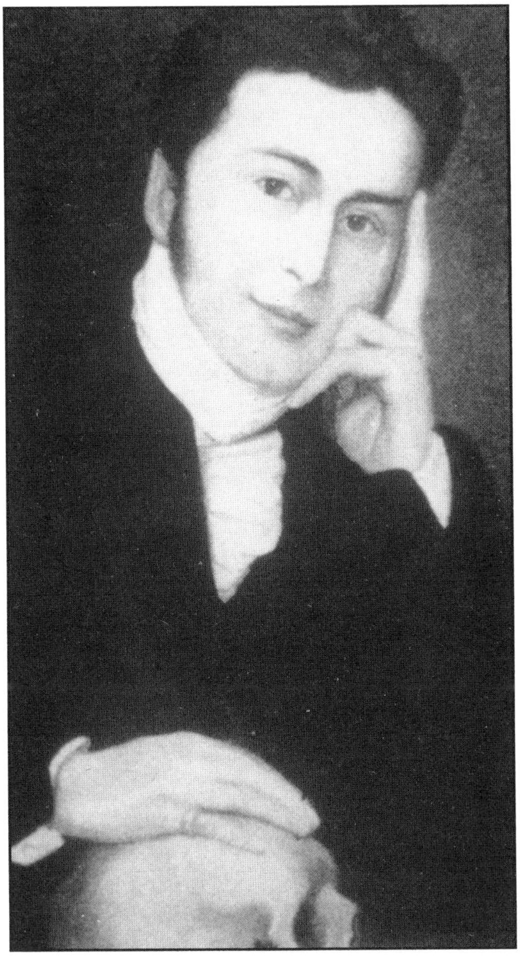

Fig. 1. Henry Hill Hickman (1800-1830).

women and children. Interestingly, there was apparently also a female surgeon practicing in Ludlow in mid-18th century.[6]

While Hickman's childhood is lost to history, we do know that he matriculated into the medical college at Edinburgh in late 1819, and attended the term of 1819-1820. He applied and was accepted into the Royal Medical Society of Edinburgh shortly after his matriculation. There is no evidence of his having ever graduated,[5] but he returned to Ludlow in early 1820 to begin his career in medicine as a country practitioner.[7] He obtained membership in The Royal College of Surgeons of London in May, 1820.

Hickman was appalled by the agonies suffered by surgical patients, and began to experiment with methods of alleviating their pain. He produced a state of "suspended animation" in animals by enclosing them in airtight containers and exposing them to carbonic acid (and their own exhaled carbon dioxide and unrecognized hypoxia, as well). Probably between March and April of 1823,[8] Hickman performed a series of experiments in which small animals (kittens, dogs, a mouse, and a rabbit), after exposure to the carbonic acid, were taken to a state of "apparent lifelessness," and ears or limbs were amputated without obvious pain, hemorrhage, or infection. The "suspended animation" was reversed almost immediately on re-exposure of the animals to "atmospheric air," and all animals recovered.[1] In experiment #5, Hickman relates:

> In this experiment animation was suspended during seventeen minutes, allowing respiration occasionally to intervene by means of inflating instruments."

In his discussion, Hickman wrote:

> I used inflating instruments in one experiment only, and therefore am not prepared to say to what extent such may be used with advantage; but I think it probable that those and the Galvanic fluid would operate in restoring animation in some cases. I was prepared to employ the Galvanic fluid if any case had occurred to render the operation of any stimulant necessary, but all the subjects recovered by being simply exposed to the open air;. . .

It is not known what experience Hickman had with resuscitation by the use of either respiratory assist devices or electricity. However, the Royal Humane Society in 1806 formally endorsed a valved bellows and a series of tubes for tracheal cannulation which might be attached to the bellows.[9] In addition, three papers were published just prior to his performing his experiments which may have influenced him. The first was anonymous, titled, "A

Popular treatise on Accidents, etc. for the use of Persons Residing at a Distance from Medical Assistance," Glasgow, 1823. It describes the necessity of inflating the lungs of drowned persons by what is now termed "mouth-to-mouth resuscitation." The second was Orfilia's "Secours à donner aux personnes empoisonnées ou asphyxiées; suivis des moyens propres à reconnaître les poisons et les vins frelatés, et à distinguer la mort réelle de la mort apparente," Paris, 1818. This paper describes intubation of the larynx with a Chaussier tube. The third paper is by Reece, titled, "The Medical Guide. . .," London, 1820. This 13th edition describes the use of the Persile Galvanic Pile over the heart for resuscitation, used in conjunction with laryngeal cannulation.[10]

Hickman was convinced that his "suspended animation" could be performed on human patients. Feeling unqualified to undertake such a step, he attempted to enlist the support of The Royal Society. The President of the Society at the time was Sir Humphray Davy, who had also been Superintendent of Beddoe's Pneumatic Medical Institution in Bristol. Davy was a personal friend of a Mr. T.A. Knight, a Squire and horticulturist residing at Downton Castle near Ludlow,[11-14] who was also a member of The Royal Society. Hickman wrote to Knight outlining his experiments, and requested that they be ". . .laid before the Royal Society;. . ." By then, Hickman had moved from Ludlow to Shifnal for reasons which are not readily apparent, but may have had something to do with better economic prospects.[15] Hickman heard no reply from Knight, and some six months later published an open letter to Knight which similarly outlined his experiments and request.[1] This time Hickman waited three years without public acknowledgement from either Knight or Davy.[11] The reasons are not known, nor is the extent of private conversations between the parties. Several factors may have been responsible for a seeming lack of interest. First, neither Davy nor Knight were physicians. Davy was a chemist and Knight was a horticulturist. Second, although Davy had investigated numerous gases at the Pneumatic Institute, the major emphasis was on the therapy of diseases with gases, primarily consumption, and not the relief of surgical pain.[3] One would think that, had Knight mentioned Hickman's work, Davy would surely have suggested nitrous oxide. There is no record of such a suggestion, or any indication that Hickman was even aware of Davy's work with the gas.[12] Davy completed most of those experiments just prior to Hickman's birth, and Davy himself overlooked the potential importance of a role for nitrous oxide in the relief of surgical pain. By this time, Davy's health was failing,[4] and he died in May, 1829.[14] Third, there was an increasing outcry against animal cruelty in medical experimentation in England at the time. These concerns had caused the rejection of Dr. Andrew Wilson Philip for membership in The Royal Society. He had been presented for membership by Knight, and Knight may not have wanted to risk being associated with another potential case of "animal cruelty."[15] The only public recognition of Hickman's letters to Knight was a letter in *Lancet* in 1826 titled, "Surgical Humbug," and signed only by "Antiquack." However, there is evidence that its author had access to Hickman's public pamphlet prior to Hickman's deletion of the line which claimed it had been read before the Society by Davy.[14]

Failing to enlist support in England, Hickman went to Paris in 1828 to petition King Charles X of France to allow him to present his work in the king's presence. The king, instead, formed a committee of the Académie Royale de Médecine to evaluate his experiments.[2-4,8,14,15] The Committee heard Hickman but, except for one member, the Committee rejected Hickman's work. The lone exception was Baron Dominique-Jean Larrey, a famous French surgeon.

Dominique-Jean Larrey served under Napoleon in numerous campaigns. His contributions to battlefield medicine were near legendary at the time, and included institution of the battlefield "flying ambulance" for early withdrawal of wounded to rear positions, and early amputation of wounded extremities (a view contrary to the popular medical treatments in the late 18th century.) After Waterloo, Larrey barely escaped death at the hands of the Germans and again at the hands of the French royalists. Even though he escaped death, the royalists stripped him of all titles and commissions. From 1815 to 1818, his only means of support was performing surgery on private patients. Some of his titles and commissions were restored in 1819, and in his will Napoleon awarded Larrey some 100,000 francs. Larrey died in 1842, having served some 40 years in the army and participated in some 26 military campaigns, including those in Austria, Prussia, Saxony, and Poland.[16,17] It is stated,[12] but not proven (WDA Smith, personal communication) that Larrey had witnessed painless amputations among wounded troops in very cold climates, which accounted for his singular interest in Hickman's work. However, Larrey was outvoted and allowed the matter to drop.

A broken Hickman returned to England in late 1828 and established a practice at Tenbury, where he died in 1830. He is buried at the church cemetery in Bromfield, Shropshire.

An irony of history is that Hickman may have been heard before the wrong French Academy. At the time, the French Academy of Medicine and the French Academy of Sciences were two separate organizations. In 1821, the French Academy of Sciences sponsored a prize competition on the causes of animal heat. The purpose of the competition was to defend Lavoisier's theory of combustion against the phlogiston theory. Changing standards of precision and sabotage by anonymous entrants, who refused to accept the Academy's definition of the question, caused the effort to fail. The result made Lavoisier's theory more dubious than ever in the eyes of many members of the Academy.[18] However, had Hickman been heard before the Academy of Sciences, he may have found an audience more interested in carbon dioxide.

Following the introduction of ether by Morton, the controversy that surrounded the designation of the founder of inhalation anesthesia prompted Thomas Dudley, a friend of Hickman's, to write the *Lancet* on March 27, 1847, calling attention to Hickman's work. The significance of Hickman's work was acknowledged by the French Academy of Medicine later in 1847. After Dudley again wrote the *Lancet* on March 27, 1947, the *Medical Times* finally acknowledged Hickman as the true originator on July 31, 1847, quoting from the printed reports from the French Academy of Medicine.[19] However, a search of the records of The Royal Society failed to find any reference to Hickman's work, and he is not mentioned in Garrison's *An Introduction to the History of Medicine*.[11] Of those few historians who have acknowledged Hickman's work, at least one credits his experiments to nitrous oxide.[20] Other investigators have independently "discovered" the anesthetic properties of carbon dioxide, including Charles Ozanam,[21] Paul Bert,[22] and Sir Benjamin W. Richardson.[23] Ozanam was the first to report the use of carbon dioxide as an anesthetic agent in a human in 1858, but did not mention Hickman and did not follow up on the study. Bert does not acknowledge Hickman's work or suggest further studies in humans or animals. Richardson incorrectly credits the originator of the anesthetic use of carbon dioxide to John Snow in 1848.

Thanks largely to the efforts of Sir Henry Wellcome[1] and two publications by Leake and Waters in 1928[24] and 1929,[25] Hickman was recognized by the Section of Anaesthetics of The Royal Society of Medicine in 1930,[3] which placed a plaque in his honor at Bromfield church. Since 1935, The Royal Society of Medicine has presented a medal in Hickman's name for excellence in anesthesia.[2]

References

1. Hickman HH: A letter on suspended animation, addressed to T.A. Knight, Esq. Printed at the office of W. Smith, Ironbridge, 1824.
2. Bloch H: Henry Hill Hickman (1800-1830): Country doctor and discoverer of inhalation anesthesia. South Med J; 80:1168-70, 1987.
3. Mettler CC: *History of Medicine*. Birmingham, Alabama, Gryphon Editions, Ltd., 1983, p 864-929.
4. Smith WDA: A history of nitrous oxide and oxygen anaesthesia, Part IV: Hickman and the "introduction of certain gases into the lungs." Br J Anaesth; 38:58-72, 1966.

5. Smith WDA: A history of nitrous oxide and oxygen anaesthesia, Part IVA: Further light on Hickman and his times. Br J Anaesth; 42:347-53, 1970.
6. Wright S: Holding up the sky: Women and their occupations in eighteenth-century Ludlow. Midland Hist (Gr Brit); 14:53-74, 1989.
7. Smith WDA: A history of nitrous oxide and oxygen anaesthesia, Part IVD: Further light on Hickman and his times. Br J Anaesth; 50:623-7, 1978.
8. Keys TE: Historical vignettes: Henry Hill Hickman. Anesth Analg; 51:349, 1972.
9. Mushin WW, Rendell-Baker L (eds): *The Origins of Thoracic Anesthesia.* The Wood Library-Museum of Anesthesiology, Park Ridge, 1991, p 32.
10. *Resuscitation, An Historical Perspective.* The Wood Library-Museum of Anesthesiology, Park Ridge, 1976, p 26-7.
11. Nuland SB (Ed): *The Origins of Anesthesia.* Birmingham, Alabama, Gryphon Editions, Ltd., 1983, p 33-7.
12. Sykes WAS: *Essays on the First Hundred Years of Anaesthesia, Vol. I.* Churchill Livingstone, Edinburgh, 1982, p 117-9.
13. McQuaker M: Henry Hill Hickman. Anesth Analg; 8:, 1929.
14. Smith WDA: A history of nitrous oxide and oxygen anesthesia. Part IVB: Further light on Hickman and his times. Br J Anaesth; 42:445-58, 1979.
15. Smith WDA: A history of nitrous oxide and oxygen anaesthesia, Part IVE: Henry Hill Hickman in his time. Br J Anaesth; 50:853-61, 1978.
16. Vess DM: French military surgery during the campaigns of 1792-1795. J Alabama Acad Sci; 37:303-8, 1966.
17. Wangensteen OH, Wangensteen SD, Klinger CF: Wound management of Amroise Pare and Dominique Larrey, great French military surgeons of the 18th and 19th centuries. Bull Hist Med; 46:207-34, 1972.
18. Kremer RL: Defending Lavoisier: The French academy's prize competition of 1821. His Phil Life Sci; 8:41-65, 1986.
19. Thompson CJS: Henry Hill Hickman. Br Med J; 1:843-5, 1912.
20. Mettler CC: *History of Medicine.* Birmingham, Alabama, Gryphon Editions, Ltd., 1983, p 218.
21. Ozanam C: De l'acide carbonique en inhalations comme agent anesthésique efficace et sans danger pendant les opérations chirurgicales. Comptes rendus hebdomadaires des séances de l'Académie des Sciences; 54:1154-5, 1858.
22. Bert P: *La Pression Barométrique.* Paris, 1878. Reprinted by Hitchcock MA and Hitchcock FA. Columbus, Ohio, College Book Company, 1943, -921-4.
23. Richardson BW: A synopsis of anaesthetics. The Asclepiad ii:257-77, 1885.
24. Leake CD, Waters RM: The anesthetic properties of carbon dioxide. J. Pharmacol Exp Therap; 33:280-1, 1928.
25. Leake CD, Waters RM: The anesthetic properties of carbon dioxide. Anesth Analg; 8:17-9, 1929.

THE HISTORICAL ROLE OF CARBOGEN INHALATION IN THE TREATMENT OF PSYCHONEUROSES

DAVID A. CROSS
Clinical Professor
Department of Anesthesiology
The University of South Alabama
Mobile, Alabama, USA

In 1928, Dr. A.S. Loevenhart, in conjunction with Dr. W.F. Lorenz, was studying various methods of cerebral stimulation at the University of Wisconsin. Loevenhart was an energetic and prolific Professor of Pharmacology and Toxicology at The University of Wisconsin, and had a strong interest in studying numerous facets of the central nervous system. His interests included treatment of CNS syphilis,[1,2] the relationship between biologic oxidation and respiratory functions[3] and the use of sodium cyanide for stimulation of respiration in cases of increased intracranial pressure.[4]

It was during the pursuit of this latter interest in 1916 that a transient improvement in mental status of a patient with dementia praecox was noted. However, it was not until 1928 that the aspect of the study was reinvestigated. Results were disappointing, but some temporary, fleeting improvement was noted in the study patients. Because it was felt that the poor results were due to the use of the wrong stimulant, and because of the toxicity of cyanide, another form of cerebral stimulation was sought. The investigators turned to various inhaled mixtures of carbon dioxide and oxygen.

Because of their lack of familiarity with the equipment and the techniques of administration of these agents, they enlisted the assistance of Dr. Ralph Waters. Their collaboration produced the first results of their experiments in 1929.[3] Improvement in the mental status of their patients was noted for as long as 25 minutes after cessation of the carbogen. They felt that 30 percent CO_2 was as high as was needed to effect a result and be "safe." Dr. Loevenhart died about one month following publication of the paper,[1] but not before he asked Drs. Chauncey, Leake, Arthur Guedel and Mary Botsford of the Department of Pharmacology and the Division of Anesthesia of the Department of Surgery at The University of California at San Francisco, to attempt to repeat their work. Leake, Guedel and Botsford did so, and published their work later in 1929.[5] Again, the safety of the technique was stressed, although Leake, Guedel and Botsford recommended only a 20 percent CO_2 concentration be inhaled, and suggested that multiple treatments daily might give improved longevity of the improvement in mental status.

It should be noted that these attempts were on patients suffering from PSYCHOTIC abnormalities. Interestingly, Drs. Leake and Waters had published two previous papers together in 1928[6] and 1929,[7] acknowledging and repeating the Work of Henry Hill Hickman in 1824,[8] but added human subjects. However, at that time, Leake and Waters recommended that CO_2 anesthesia be administered for only short periods of time in human subjects because of the probability of seizures.

Meanwhile, in 1934, Dr. L.J. Meduna, a psychiatrist in Budapest, Hungary, was investigating methods of producing improvement in catatonia by cerebral stimulation. Unable to understand, read, or write English, he heard only garbled reports of the work of Loevenhart, Lorenz and Waters, which he understood to involve the cisternal injection of oxygen. His attempts to repeat this experiment achieved no beneficial results. Finally, in 1937, he was correctly informed about these experiments by a visiting English physician, and undertook to correctly repeat them. His results were similar to those of the original investigators, with beneficial results lasting 30 minutes at most. He discontinued further experimentation. Meduna learned English and moved to the United States in the early 1940s, locating at the Illinois Psychiatric Institute. He continued his experiments in the use of intravenous cyanide in an attempt, as Loevenhart, Malone and Martin[4] had done previously, to improve the mental status of catatonic patients. His results were also unsuccessful. However, some patients who were given electrically-induced convulsions did recover.

He then examined the characteristics of the two different types of convulsions. He reasoned that cyanide convulsions were due to an inactivation of cortical integration and inhibition of the deeper motor centers, while the electric convulsions involved generalized cerebral cortical stimulation accompanied by a downward discharge from the cortex. He then developed his theory of reverberating circuits. Psychotic processes, he reasoned, are due to biochemical disturbances of the lower structures which upset or distort the emotional values formed in the cortex. He then thought that better results might be produced by using his cyanide injections on NEUROTIC patients, rather than the PSYCHOTIC patients. However, he was reluctant to use such a toxic agent in a mass experiment, and remembered the work of Loevenhart, Lorenz and Waters.

After much trial and error, he developed a technique of CO_2 coma produced by the inhalation of 30 percent CO_2 in 70 percent O_2. His selection of this mixture was influenced somewhat by the fact that a higher concentration of CO_2 would still be a maximum of 30 percent concentration. Patients inhaling this mixture would show the now-expected signs of hyperventilation, mild sympathetic discharge, CNS excitability, progressing to seizures and anesthesia.

On withdrawal of the mixture, the patients recovered rapidly, recounting a wide variety of experiences while "asleep," which were called *presque vu* by Dr. Meduna, and which were attributed to dreams or hallucinations.[9] His experiments led to his first publication on the subject in 1947.[10] The stated indications for treatment included conversion reactions, pseudopsychotic symptoms, faulty control of emergency reactions, sense of guilt or inadequacy, irritability and anxiety neuroses, and personality maladjustments. Obsessive compulsives, neurasthenic syndromes, and hypochondriac neuroses were contraindications.

Over the next twelve years, numerous reports confirming and refining Meduna's technique were reported.[11-29] MacRae[12] recommended the technique for the treatment of psychoneuroses during pregnancy, and recommended continuing the technique during delivery as the "safest" anesthesia for both mother and baby. Jackman and Schorr[16] presented a different theory. They felt CO_2 caused a chemical lobotomy of the frontal lobes, and thought that their theory could easily be integrated with that of Meduna. Fay published two papers[17-18] describing marked improvement in athetoid and muscular hypertonus patients following carbogen inhalation therapy. LaVerne[19] described a rapid coma technique using 70 percent CO_2 in 30 percent O_2 mixed in a breathing bag with some degree of inaccuracy, as no flowmeters were used. The patient was administered one breath of this mixture and the mask was then removed. The treatment was brief, but coma was induced rapidly with a prompt recover. He described a "favorable" clinical response. Peck[20] and Frank[21] appealed for standardization of the treatments.

There was numerous problems associated with the treatment methodology and reporting of data. Techniques were not standardized, the equipment was unfamiliar to most practicing psychiatrists, and many therapists were anxious about the occasional unpredictable response of the patient to treatment. Meduna tended to dismiss both failures and concerns alike to a lack of proper education to the process or insufficient numbers of treatments.[9,23]

However, several facts and reports tended to discredit the technique in ways which Meduna found difficult to refute. Smith,[30] in a brief report in 1953, reported a 33 percent benefit rate, no cures. Harris [31] compared the technique to psychotherapy alone. He showed no difference in overall success rate, with both groups showing a 62 percent improvement. However, there was a strong patient preference for psychotherapy. In 1954, Hargrove, Bennett and Steele[32] showed poorer results with carbogen treatments than with psychotherapy alone. They also noticed a preference among patients for psychotherapy because the sudden, almost explosive confrontation of the patient with his repressed dependency, aggressive, or sexual conflicts was terrifying.

Repeated treatments did not lead to alleviation of symptoms, but rather led to a flight from treatment. Freedman[33] reported twelve of fourteen patients showed poor or no improvement with carbogen treatments. Frank and McGraw,[34] while acknowledging that carbogen therapy might be of value, stated that its place seemed to lie in a wide armamentarium of treatments available to psychoneurotic patients because of the 60-70 percent success rate of nearly all investigators supporting the therapy was consistent with the overall response of psychoneurotic patients to any therapy. Carbogen could not, therefore, be regarded as "specific." In 1956, Hawkings and Tibbetts[35] showed no difference between patients receiving carbogen and compressed air. Both had a 50 percent improvement rate.

In addition, two separate reviews of the treatment of neuroses in 1955[36] and 1956[37] failed to mention carbogen therapy at all. The final factor in the treatment's falling from favor was the advent of better psychotherapeutic drugs during the same era.[38-46]

However, the use of carbogen therapy has not altogether disappeared from the psychiatric literature even today. LaVerne and Morris, in 1953,[47] and more recently LaVerne, in 1973,[48,49] have advocated carbogen inhalation as a treatment of addiction and alcoholism, accompanied by an appeal for further investigation from Chauncey Leake.[50] Even more recently, numerous authors have advocated carbogen inhalation as both a precipitator and a treatment for anxiety disorders and panic attacks.[51-63] These reports are, however, sporadic in the literature, and the future role of carbogen in the treatment of these disorders has yet to be fully determined.

References

1. "Death Notices:" JAMA; 92:1467, 1929.
2. Leake CD: A note on the scientific work of Professor A.S. Loevenhart. Wisconsin Med J; 28:277-8, 1929.
3. Loevenhart AS, Lorenz WF, Waters RM: Cerebral stimulation. JAMA; 92:880-3, 1929.
4. Loevenhart AS, Malone JY, Martin HG: Studies on stimulation of the respiration: The action of respiratory stimulants upon the respiration when depressed by increased intracranial pressure with special reference to sodium cyanide. J Pharm Exp Therap; 19:13-47, 1922.

5. Leake CD, Guedel AE, Botsford ME: The stimulating effect of carbon dioxide inhalations in dementia praecox catatonia. Calif West Med; 31:20-3, 1929.
6. Leake CD, Waters RM: The anesthetic properties of carbon dioxide. J. Pharmacol Exp Therap; 33:280-1, 1928.
7. Leake CD, Waters RM: The anesthetic properties of carbon dioxide. Anesth Analg; 8:17-9, 1929.
8. Hickman HH: A letter on suspended animation. Addressed to T.A. Knight, Esq. Printed at the office of W. Smith, Ironbridge, 1824.
9. Meduna LJ: The carbon dioxide treatment: A review. J Clin Exp Psychopath; 15:325-54, 1954.
10. Meduna LJ: Pharmaco-dynamic treatment of psychoneuroses: (A preliminary report.) Dis Nerv Sys; 8:37-40, 1949.
11. Liest LJ: Personality mutation following carbon dioxide inhalation. Dis Nerv Sys; 10:333-8, 1949.
12. MacRae LD: Carbon dioxide in obstetrics: (A preliminary report.) Dis Nerv Sys; 12:486-8, 1951.
13. Silver GA: Carbon dioxide therapy. N Carolina Med J; 12:486-8, 1951.
14. Weaver OM, Peterson DB, Anderson WH: Carbon dioxide therapy of psychoneuroses. Dis Nerv Sys; 12:355-61, 1951.
15. Peterson AL: Experience with carbon-dioxide therapy in psychiatric outpatients. Arch Neurol Psychiat; 67:699-701, 1952.
16. Jackman AJ, Schorr CA: Evaluation of carbon dioxide therapy of the neuroses. J Clin Exper Psychopath; 13:17-30, 1952.
17. Fay T: Effects of carbon dioxide (20 percent) and oxygen (80 percent) inhalations on movements and muscular hypertonus in athetoids. Am J Physical Med; 32:338-41, 1953.
18. Fay T: Twenty percent carbon dioxide inhalation in muscular rigidity: Indications and contraindications. JAMA; 152:1623-26, 1953.
19. LaVerne AA: Rapid coma technique of carbon dioxide inhalation therapy. Dis Nerv Sys; 14:141-9, 1953.
20. Peck RE: Standardization of carbon dioxide treatment. Dis Nerv Sys; 14:240-3, 1953.
21. Frank JA: A critical evaluation of carbon dioxide oxygen inhalation therapy in mental disorders. Am J Psychiat; 110:93-103, 1953.
22. Simon W, Hopkins GW: Autonomic nervous system tests in carbon dioxide inhalation therapy. J Clin Exper Psychopath; 14:176-83, 1953.
23. Meduna LJ, Jackman AI: Carbon dioxide inhalation therapy. A Res Nerv Men Dis, Proc (1951). 31:280-6, 1953.
24. Moriarty JD: Evaluation of carbon dioxide inhalation therapy. Am J Psychiat; 110:785-9, 1954.
25. Quarti C, Renaud J: La carbonarcose. Thérapeutique biologique des maladies fonctionnelles. Anesth Analg (Fr); 12:286-305, 1955.
26. Stiller R: Carbon dioxide as a useful tool in the treatment of neurotic disturbances. Illinois Med J; 14:243-6, 1957.
27. Moriarty JD: Appraisal of failures with CO_2 therapy. Dis Nerv Sys; 19:209-14, 1958.
28. Wilcox PH: CO_2 therapy in broad spectrum psychiatric treatment. Dis Nerv Sys; 20:97-101, 1959.
29. Singh K: Carbon dioxide treatment in psychoneurosis: A study of 238 cases in India. J Neuropsychiat; 2:167-71, 1960.
30. Smith JA: An evaluation of the results of treatment of 33 patients with carbon dioxide inhalations. Am J Psychiat; 104:626-49, 1953.
31. Harris A: A comparative study of results in neurotic patients treated by two different methods. J Ment Sci; 100:718-21, 1954.
32. Hargrove EA, Bennett AE, Steele M: An investigation of carbon dioxide as an adjunct to psychotherapy in some neuroses. Am J Psychiat; 110:844-7, 1954.
33. Freedman A: Observations on the treatment situation in carbon dioxide therapy. J Nerv Ment Dis; 121:359-66, 1955.
34. Frank JA, McGraw RB: Carbon dioxide therapy: A clinical evaluation of 200 patients. J Nerv Ment Dis; 123:563-7, 1956.
35. Hawkings JR, Tibbetts RW: Carbon dioxide therapy inhalation therapy in neurosis: A controlled clinical trial. J Ment Sci; 102:52-9, 1956.
36. Eitinger L: Studies in neuroses. Acta Psychiat Neurol Scan; Supp 101:1-47, 1955.
37. Terhune WB: Re-education in the treatment of psychoneuroses. J Med Assoc Georgia; 45:3-7, 1956.
38. Schlan LS, Unna KR: Some effects of myanesin in psychiatric patients. JAMA; 140:672-3, 1949.
39. Hoch PH: Evaluation of newer pharmacodynamic therapies. A Res Nerv Ment Dis, Proc (1951); 31:239-44, 1953.

40. Bower WH: Chlorpromazine in psychiatric illness. NEWJM; 251:689-92, 1954.
41. Parsons EH: New chemical agents in psychiatry. Postgrad Med; 18:193-8, 1955.
42. Barsa JA, Kline NS: Use of meprobamate in the treatment of psychotic patients. Am J Psychiat; 112:1023, 1956.
43. Ravina A: Une nouvelle médication de l'anxiété et des psychoses. Presse Méd (Fr); 63:1233, 1955.
44. Winkelman NW: Chlorpromazine in the treatment of neuropsychiatric disorders. JAMA; 155:18-21, 1954.
45. Arnot R: The place of sedatives in the treatment of psychoneuroses. Am J Psychiat; 113:10-5, 1958.
46. Brown SG: Chlordiazepoxide: An effective adjunct to psychotherapy of the neurotic states. AM J Psychiat; 119:774-5, 1963.
48. LaVerne AA: Carbon dioxide therapy (CDT) of heroin, methadone, addictions, and alcoholism. Behav Neuropsychiat; 4:13-28, 1973.
49. Critique: Carbon dioxide therapy (CDT) of heroin, methadone, addictions, and alcoholism. Behav Neuropsychiat; 4:1-8, 1973.
50. Leake CD: Prologue and epilogue of carbon dioxide therapy. Behav Neuropsychiat, 4:10-2, 1973.
51. Slater SL, Leavy A: The effects of inhaling a 35 percent CO_2 - 65 percent O_2 mixture upon anxiety level in neurotic patients. Behav Res Therapy; 4:309-16, 1966.
52. Orwin A: Augmented respiratory relief. Brit J Psychiat; 122:171-173, 1973.
53. Haslam MT: The relationship between the effect of lactate infusion on anxiety states, and their amelioration by carbon dioxide inhalation. Brit J Psychiat; 125:88-90, 1974.
54. Latimer P: Carbon dioxide as reciprocal inhibitor in the treatment of neurosis. J Behav Ther Exp Psychiat; 8:83-5, 1977.
55. Griez E, van den Hout MA: Treatment of phobophobia by exposure to CO_2-induced anxiety symptoms. J Nerv Ment Dis; 171:506-8, 1983.
56. Gorman JM, Askanazi J, Liebowitz MR, et al: Response to hyperventilation in a group of patients with panic disorder. Am J Psychiat; 141:857-61, 1984.
57. Backon J: Carbon dioxide inhalation therapy for anxiety; effectiveness due to increased prostacyclin and decreased thromboxane biosyntheses? Re-evaluation of a neglected technique. Med Hypotheses; 20:351-6, 1986.
58. Volpe J: Carbon dioxide inhalation treatments of neurotic anxiety: An overview. J Nerv Ment Dis; 175:129-33, 1987.
59. Fyer MR, Uy J, Martinez J, et al: CO_2 challenge of patients with panic disorder. Am J Psychiat; 144:1080-2, 1987.
60. Gorman JM, Fyer MR, Goetz R, et al: Ventilatory physiology of patients with panic disorder. Arch Gen Psychiatry; 45:31-9, 1988.
61. Papp LA, Goetz R, Cole R, et al: Hypersensitivity to carbon dioxide in panic disorder. Am J Psychiat; 146:779-81, 1989.
62. Harrison WM, Sandberg D, Gorman JM, et al: Provocation of panic with carbon dioxide inhalation in patients with premenstrual dysphoria. Psychiat Res; 27:183-93, 1989.
63. Griez E, de Loof C, Pols H, et al: Specific sensitivity of patients with panic attacks to carbon dioxide inhalation. Psychiat Res; 31:193-9, 1989.

JEFFERSON, GEORGIA IN THE 1840's

SUSAN B. DEAVER
Executive Director
Crawford W. Long Museum
Jefferson, Georgia, USA

Crawford Williamson Long was born in Danielsville, Madison County, Georgia, on 1 November 1815. However, it was in adjoining Jackson County in the town of Jefferson that Long began his medical career, first studying with a preceptor. Dr. George R. Grant, and then, after his formal training, establishing his medical practice. On 30 March 1842, Dr. Crawford Long made medical history, performing the first surgical operation using sulphuric ether. Although the standard sources on his life cite no reason, there are several factors which might explain why it was in Jefferson and not his hometown where Long made his discovery of anesthesia.

Jefferson's history begins in 1784 when Franklin County was created after the Creek and Cherokee Indians ceded lands in the northeast piedmont region to the state of Georgia. To entice settlers into the area, land was given free to Georgians under the bounty grant or headright grant systems. Others migrated from the states to the north — Virginia, the Carolinas or Pennsylvania. These people were mainly Scotch-Irish, eager for new land to cultivate. Crawford W. Long's grandfathers both came from Pennsylvania to northeast Georgia at this time, settling by 1790 in what would later become Madison County.

As settlement increased, Franklin County began to be carved up to form new counties. Jackson County was created in 1796 with a population of 350 hardy pioneers and covered an area of 1,800 square miles. The first seat of government was in Clarkesboro, which lost its central location when Clarke County was cut away from south Jackson in 1801. Citizens chose the village of Thomocoggan as the new county seat and moved the government there in 1803, renaming the town in honor of President Thomas Jefferson.

The selection of the site at Jefferson was partially due to the ample water supply from Curry Creek and four freely flowing springs.

Springs were so important in those days that, when the General Assembly enacted legislation in 1806 to regulate the town, they included a clause charging the commissioners with the responsibility of preserving the public springs. A town plan was drawn up consisting of thirty lots surrounding a public square; the configuration is labeled a Sparta subtype of Georgia's courthouse town plans. Later, Jefferson's limits would be at three-fourths of a mile in every direction from the center of the square.

Nestled in the northeast Georgia piedmont, Jackson County's abundant water supply, rolling terrain and red clay soil make for fertile land. Situated along the migration route and one the edge of the frontier, the county grew rapidly. The U.S. census records for 1800 show a county population of 7,147 and an increase to over 10,500 in 1810. With the creation of four counties — including Madison in 1811 — in the next decade taking some of Jackson's land and people, the 1820 population total fell to 8,343. In this year the census enumerator reported:

> Jackson County is about 20 miles square. The town of Jefferson in the center of the county contains about twenty houses including the Lord's and the courthouse and out houses, eight stores, three public houses, three saddlery shops, two blacksmith shops, one tin manufactory, and one shoe-maker shop. The town of Jefferson stands about equal distance between Athens and Hall courthouse.

In another twenty years, Jackson County's population would show a small increase to 8,529, with the ratio of whites to black remaining a fairly constant 70 to 30 percent. No census figures are available for the number of citizens residing within Jefferson's city limits until 1880. However, Frary Elrod, in his *Historical Notes on Jackson County, Georgia* (Jefferson, 1967), gives the population as 63 persons in 1796 when the county was founded, and 287 when Jefferson was incorporated as the county seat. The U.S. census for 1860 provides a means for calculating the number of Jefferson area residents, for in this census the population was counted by militia districts. There were 115 households in the Jefferson Militia District, totaling 655 white and free colored persons; the figure for black slaves has not been tallied. Through cross referencing names, it can be estimated that about 500 people were living in and around Jefferson in the 1840's.

Madison County was created in 1811 from portions of existing Jackson, Oglethorpe, Franklin and Elbert counties. In 1820 the population was recorded at 3,735 people, with an increase to 4,514 in 1840; black slaves accounted for about 30 percent. Although Madison County grew proportionately, her total population was continually only half that of Jackson. There are no numbers available for the town of Danielsville, established as the county seat in 1812.

Another comparison between the counties can be made with figures from 1820 showing the number of heads of households engaged in different pursuits.

Jackson		Madison	
28	Commerce	7	(1 of whom was Long's father)
150	Manufacturing	65	
2520	Agriculture	1217	

Thus, in all likelihood, one reason Crawford Long went to Jefferson is that it was an older and larger town than Danielsville, and Jackson a more progressive county. Other plausible reasons are the scarcity of physicians in Madison County at the time and the willingness of Dr. George R. Grant to take in medical students. Grant was enumerated in the 1830 Jackson County census as a physician, listed near others known to reside in Jefferson at that time. He had completed his medical training a few years before and by 1835 was sufficiently established in practice to purchase Jefferson town lots 22, 24 and one-half of 23 for $1000. Whether or not he advertised for students, and notwithstanding any unknown connection between him and the Long family, Dr. Grant agreed to serve as Crawford's preceptor after the young man's graduation from Franklin

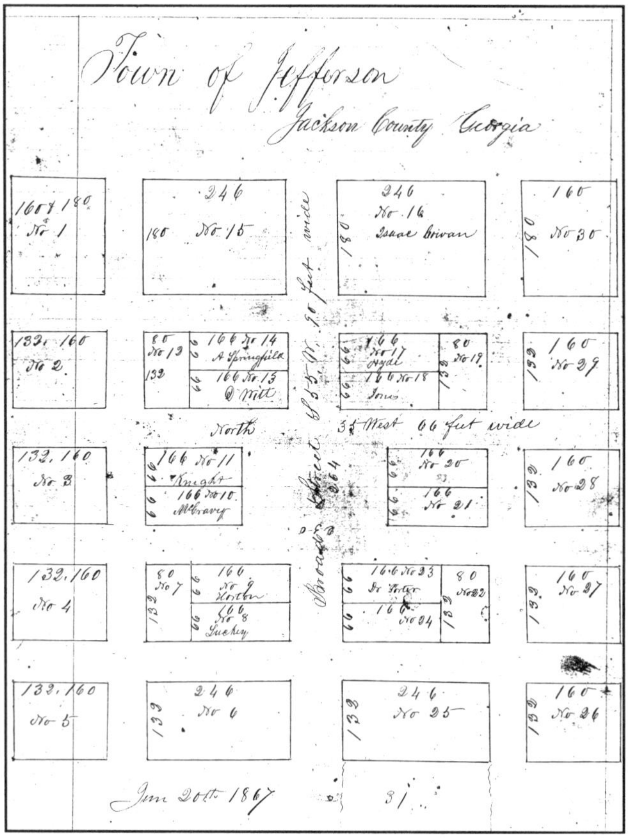

Figs. 1 and 2:
showing plots in the town of Jefferson dated June 20, 1867.

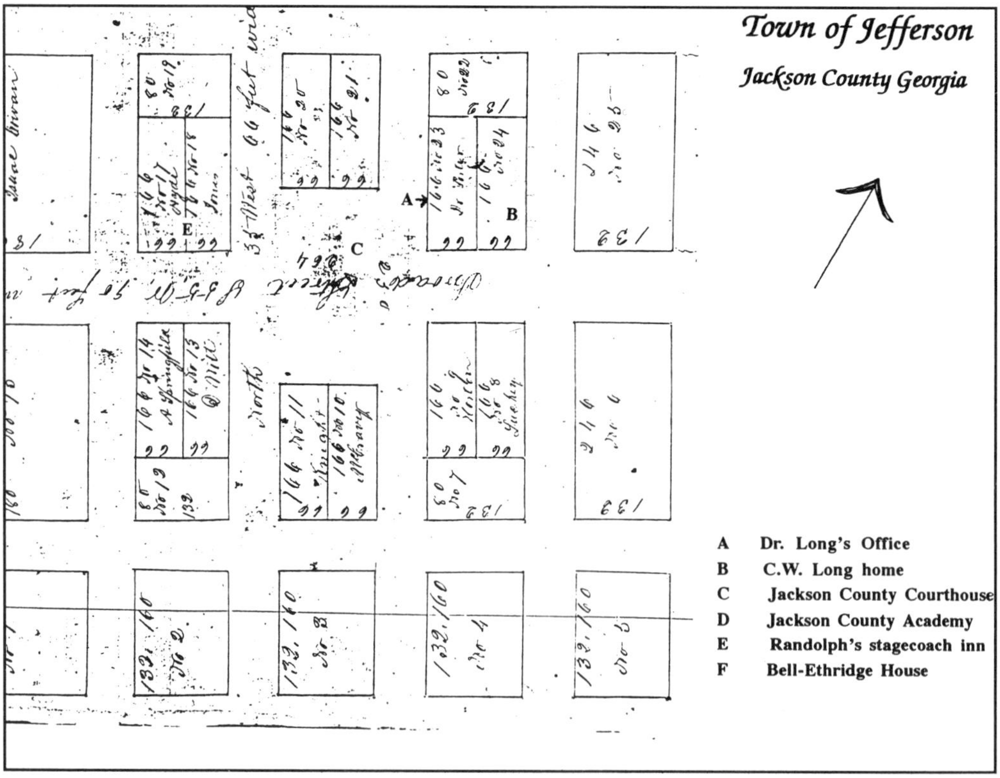

College, now the University of Georgia.

Long worked with Grant during 1835 and 1836. There are no details of this apprenticeship, but it is known that Long lived with his sister, Sarah Ann Elinor, and her husband, Giles Mitchell, while studying with Dr. Grant; their house still stands on Lawrenceville Avenue. Sarah and Giles were married in October 1835, and Mitchell's law office was located on the same lot as Dr. Grant's on the "downtown" square. James Long, Crawford's father, supported his son's desire to study medicine, but was reluctant to have him travel off to medical school at his young age. Therefore, the situation available in Jefferson was ideal.

Although extensive research has been conducted, a complete picture of Jefferson and her residents during the 1840's has not been definitively established. However, much is known. The town plat in Figure 1, showing 30 lots around a town square, was found in Deed Book O, page 751. It is dated 20 June 1867, but some names are for people who had either died or moved away long before this date. Deed research, though incomplete, has turned up transactions regarding named and numbered town lots, some as early as 1809, where the line of ownership is consistent with early property holders. Consequently, it is believed to be a representation of the original plan.

In addition, the original showed no north arrow, so for many years researchers who discovered it were reluctant to conclude it depicted Jefferson. It is only by rotating the plan counterclockwise ninety degrees that the plat matches the town layout. Compare the rotated plan (Fig. 2) with the aerial view of Jefferson taken in 1950 (Fig. 3). Figure 2 has been marked to show locations important in Crawford Long's time. Note that the town lies on an northeast/southwest axis.

In the 1840's, the town center was dominated by a two-storey courthouse (C), built in 1817 from locally made bricks. (This structure was dismantled and the bricks used for a new courthouse building erected a block away in 1879). Wooden buildings occupied the perimeter of the square and lined the roads leading into and out of town. The present brick structures on the square were built between 1890 and 1910 on the same property lines as the originals.

Although the railroad was built into Athens by 1841, Jefferson did not have rail service until the 1880's. Still, the town was a stop on the trade route between Augusta, Athens and the north Georgia mountains, and had a bustling commercial center. Of the 20 or so stores in Jackson County in 1840, 11 belonged to Jefferson residents and likely were located in the county seat. Known store locations were on Lots 8, 9, 10, 13, 14, 18, 21, 23 and 25.

Among the other tradespeople were two blacksmiths, two millwrights, three carriage or wagonmakers, a tanner and a tailor. At least one lawyer, Giles Mitchell, had his office on the square, occupying a portion of Lot 23 along with Dr. George R. Grant. There were several other lawyers and two more physicians in Jefferson. A hotel known as the "White House" sat on Lot 20. Across from it was the stagecoach inn Joshua Randolph began after 1835 on Lots 17 and 18 (E). (This large two-storied building can be seen in Figure 3. The property passed down through the family, finally being known as the Harrison Hotel. Figure 4 is another view taken in the 1950's before it was demolished.)

There being no navigable rivers in the county, transportation was over wagon roads. These led in all directions, connecting Jefferson with surrounding county seats. Another bisected the county from northwest to southeast. The Federal Road, passing four miles west of Jefferson, was begun in 1803 when the U.S. government received permission from the Cherokees to construct a road through their nation. Andrew Jackson blazed the trail, completed finally in 1815.

By the 1830's Athens was the commercial and industrial center of northeast Georgia. Her rapid growth was due to more than being the location of the state university. Several large cotton factories and a number of other manufactories were thriving, and it was a transportation center as well. Rail service was an early concern of business leaders. Their

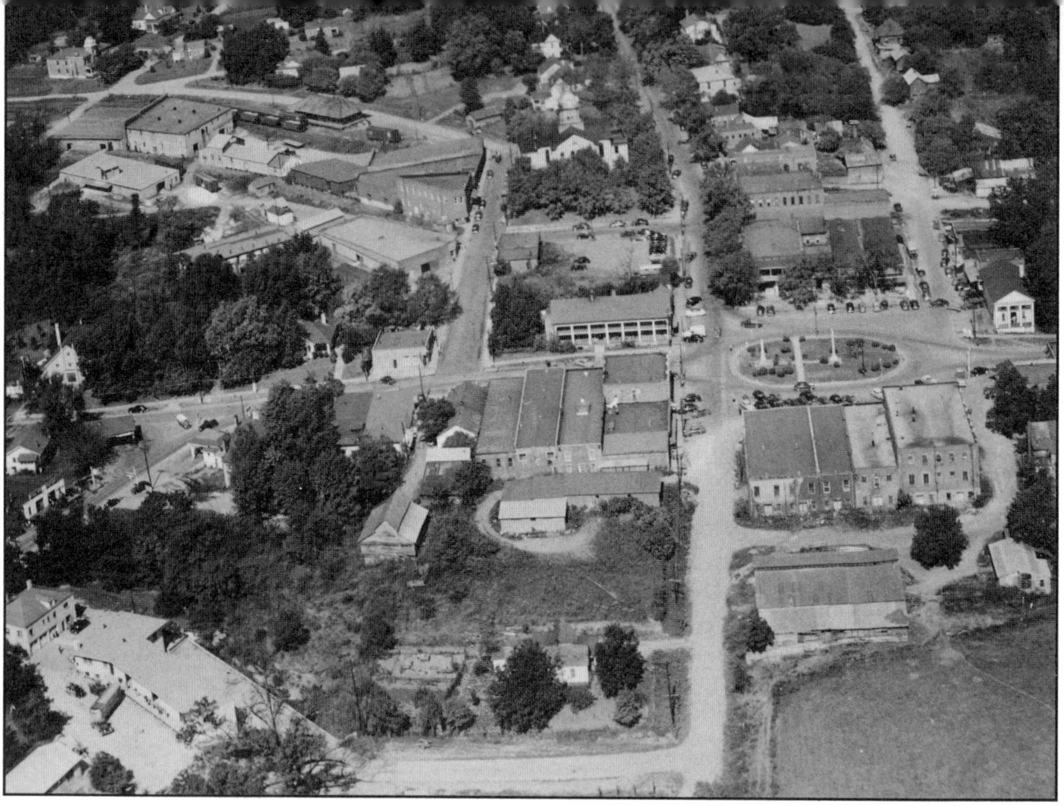

Fig. 3. Aerial view of Jefferson taken in 1950.

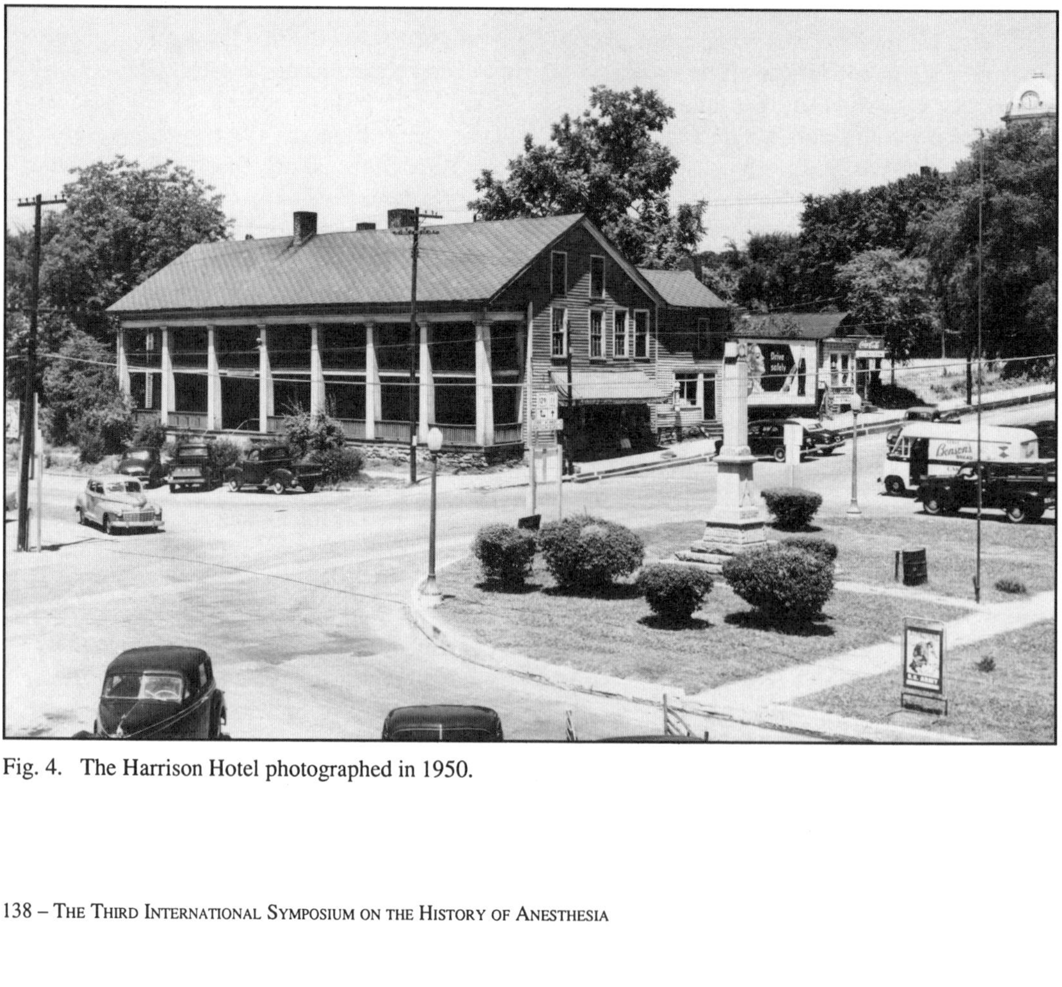

Fig. 4. The Harrison Hotel photographed in 1950.

dream was realized in 1841 when the Georgia Railroad connected Athens with Augusta, and later Atlanta.

Athens was as close as rail passengers could come to the gold region in the north Georgia mountains. From there, they went by stagecoach which took them through Jefferson. An 1845 advertisement touted one day service to Gainesville, leaving Athens after the arrival of rail cars from Augusta. Passage back on alternate days promised arrival in Athens prior to the train leaving for points south. This stagecoach to rail connection provided Jeffersonians with a link to ship travel as well.

The stagecoach brought mail, newspapers and literary journals to town. Athens papers served as the legal organ for Jackson County since newspapers were not printed here until 1875. Also arriving were family and friends who came to visit for a day, a month, or longer.

Social gatherings included school commencements, militia musters and court sessions, and perhaps a visit to the mineral springs on the Reverend Mr. Harrison's property north of Jefferson. Celebrations took place on the Fourth of July, Washington's Birthday and Thanksgiving. Weddings and funerals, or communal work activities such as house raisings, log rollings, and corn shuckings, also brought people together. It is possible that some Jeffersonians took advantage of the public lectures given in Athens. Topics were many and varied, including such things as phrenology, mesmerism, poetry, elocution, astronomy, diseases, and the poetry of the Bible. Traveling lecturers probably came this way — at least one who gave a laughing gas demonstration attended by some young men of the area.

Methodists, Baptists and Presbyterians held services and camp meetings in the area, although it is likely only the Methodists had their own sanctuary building in Jefferson at this time. It was situated on a hill in Woodbine, the city's cemetery, which is located just outside the original town plan to the south. Here the earliest grave dates from 1817.

Education of the town youth was not neglected. The Jackson County Academy was incorporated by the state in 1818, but it had begun operation earlier; a deed of purchase dated July 1813 refers to "the present Academy building." Alternately called the Jefferson Academy, by the 1840's it was located on Lot 26 (d), an easy walk for the young men eager for another "ether frolic" at Dr. Long's office. James Venable was a student here, as were Andrew Thurmond and Edmund Rawls, witnesses to the historic surgery on 30 March 1842. William Thurmond, Andrew's older brother, was principal of the Academy that year, and it was he who assisted Dr. Long with the operation. The school figures prominently in Jefferson's history as it later became one of the country's first privately endowed schools through a bequest of Georgia Railroad and Banking stock from William Duncan Martin in 1854.

Town lots had to be big enough to accommodate the many outbuildings necessary to maintain a household: smoke house, carriage, house, stable or bar, kitchen, privy, and the like. Most houses had vegetable and flower gardens, and yards were fenced to keep out roaming animals. The lots surrounding the Jefferson square were one-quarter acre in size, and those on the perimeter of the original 30 lot plan were one-half, two-thirds, three-quarters or one full acre.

Jefferson houses in the 1840's were of wood, mostly one-storey, although some had two stories. Foundations were stacked stone piers. Roofs were typically gabled, not hipped, and covered with hand-split shingles; the exterior-end chimneys were of clay or masonry. Interior walls were most likely not plaster, but random-width board made from heart pine. Furnishings were simple and probably locally made.

The smaller houses contained one or two rooms, falling into one of the following architectural types: Single Pen (one square or rectangular room); Double Pen (two square rooms, each with their own exterior door); Hall and Parlor (two unequal sized rooms); Saddlebag (two rooms around a central chimney); or Central Hallway (two rooms opening off a central hallway). Sometimes the central hallway would be open at the front and back, creating a breezeway between the two rooms; this type is called a Dogtrot house. Sheathed in clapboard or constructed of log, these simple structures often were encapsulated into larger houses as family size increased. The Georgian Cottage was another type of one-storey house built in this time period. It consists of a central hallway with two rooms on either side. In this house type, chimneys were most often built in the interior of the house, between each pair of rooms.

The type of dwelling Crawford Long shared with the Mitchells is called an "I-house." This term is applied to a residence one room deep, two rooms wide and two stories high, creating a two-over-two room configuration. The front facade was usually symmetrical, although the interior might have two unequal sized rooms in a Hall and Parlor type plan instead of a central hallway like the Mitchells' house did. I-Houses sometimes were built with one-storey shed rooms on the rear creating a two-over-four plan. This type of house is known as "Plantation Plain."

Both of these house types lent themselves to stylistic embellishments. Usually Greek Revival elements were added which were manifested in a trabeated (post and lintel) doorway with transom and sidelights, dentil mouldings or two-storey colossal columns. Still standing in Jefferson is a fine example of the I-House type, the Bell-Ethridge House (F), constructed c. 1836.

Crawford W. Long's boyhood home in Danielsville is a Plantation Plain type dwelling. Built c. 1817, the photographer (Fig. 5) shows its rather rundown appearance in 1936. Listed in the National Register of Historic Places, the privately owned house is undergoing rehabilitation. The shed porch has been removed and plans are to restore the original Federal pedimented porch. The description which follows was taken from the National Register nomination form (1977).

> The interior of the house is indicative of an imported eastern taste transferred into the upper piedmont of Georgia. The wood

Fig. 5. Crawford Long's boyhood home in Danielsville. The house still stands and is listed in the National Register of Historic Places.

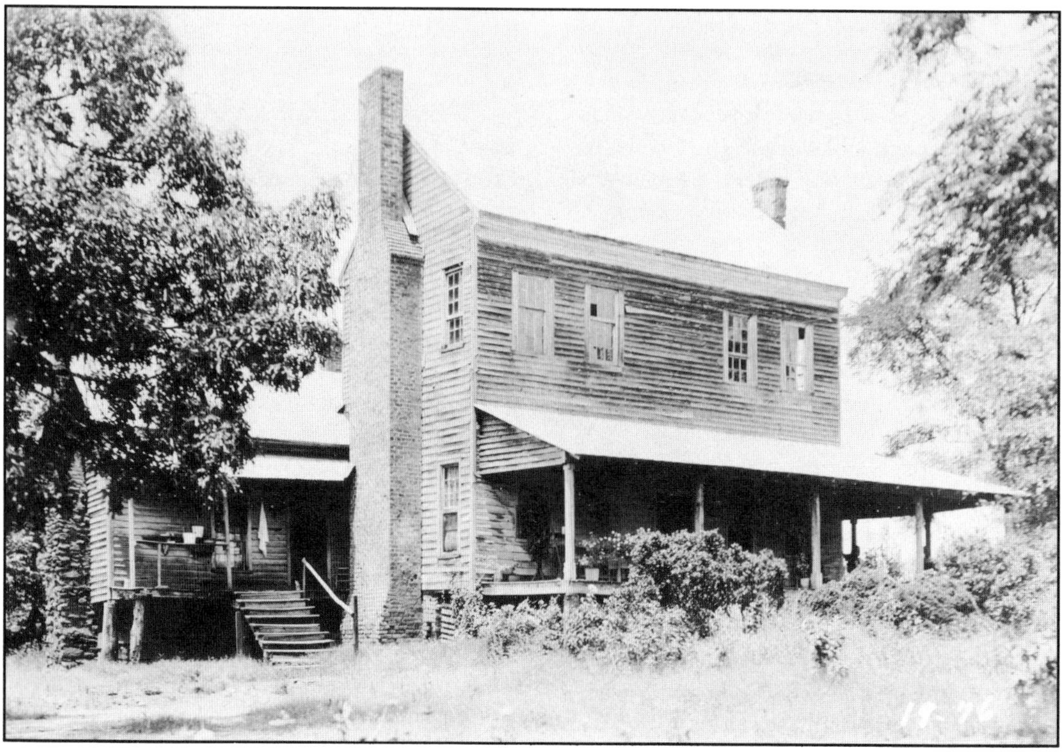

paneling and graining found in the formal rooms reflect quality craftsmanship and are a noteworthy accomplishment for the early date and time. The two second-story fireplace surrounds also convey a quality of craftsmanship. The smooth finishing of the interior wood indicates great care in construction as well. . . . It is a good architectural example of life on the early Georgia upper piedmont frontier.

After earning his medical degree at the University of Pennsylvania in 1839, Dr. Crawford W. Long spent some 18 months "walking the hospitals" in New York City. Urged to join the Navy as a surgeon, Long decided instead to return to Georgia. By this time he was already the owner of Town Lots 22, 24 and one-half of 23 as he had purchased his former preceptor's property in March 1840 for the price of $1000. Dr. Grant was moving on to Tennessee, so this was Long's opportunity to acquire an existing medical practice. Lot 23 has continuously been the site of a doctor's office and drugstore for the town since its 1806 incorporation.

Exactly where on Lot 23 Dr. Long's office building was located has not been definitely established. However, current thinking holds that it previously stood where the Crawford W. Long Museum's recreated 1840's Doctor's Office and Apothecary Shop exhibit is inside the Pendergreass Store building (a). Long's house was on Lot 24 (b), adjacent to his office; unfortunately, its appearance is undocumented. Crawford brought his bride Caroline there in August 1842.

Mary Caroline Swain was the daughter of a Jackson County planter and niece of a former governor of North Carolina. It is conceivable that a strong reason for Long choosing Jefferson was Mary Caroline, whom he had met prior to 1840. Their meeting and its effect on him is recounted in Frances Long Taylor's biography of her father (New York: Paul B. Hoeber Inc., 1928, p. 51).

> Although quiet and reserved the young doctor had a deep vein of sentiment, as was proved by his first and only love affair. After his graduation at Philadelphia during a brief visit to Jefferson he chanced to observe a graceful child of fourteen on the street and so impressed was he by her appearance he contrived to obtain a closer view of her. Her brilliant complexion, sparkling eyes, golden hair and vivacious manner captured his fancy completely and although ten years her senior he resolved then and there that he would marry her as soon as she should reach the marriageable age, which in that day was sweet sixteen.

Caroline obviously returned his interest as evidenced in a letter written to "Dr. Long, Sir" dated 25 April 1842. The original is part of the permanent collection at the Crawford W. Long Museum.

> You seemed to doubt whether your letters or presence would be welcome to me. I have never knowingly encouraged a tenderer feeling than friendship in the breast of gentleman merely for the gratification of a contemptible vanity. . . . If I had not confidence in you I should not have written this much, but it is impossible for me to be reserved towards one whose interesting letters causes me to look forward to the time when I shall enjoy the pleasure of conversing with their author. . . . You wished to know if any had succeeded in gaining my affections. I assure you I never loved a gentleman unless I do at present in my life and I believe you know it.

Crawford and Caroline's wedding took place on 11 August 1842 at Lebanon Methodist Church, which is in south Jackson County near her father's farm. They had an exceedingly happy marriage lasting almost 36 years, producing twelve children of which six survived both parents. Caroline kept a diary intermittently, and she wrote of their early years together.

> Yes, we had an earthly paradise — that of perfect love and harmony. . . . For his dear presence, fun and frolic, I lived. The laborious life of a village doctor with an extensive practice in the adjoining country

> and villages and towns, without railroads, is hard to conceive now. . . . During these earlier years of his practice the doctor was growing mentally in his chosen profession. His practice, already large, was extending; his fame as a surgeon acknowledged by the most eminent practitioners of that day; they often sending for him long distances to assist in difficult operations.

In answering the question why Dr. Long left Jefferson, one finds in Frances Long Taylor's biography on page 33: "This little town he considered only as a temporary home until a better opening in the South could be found." And on page 11:

> Crawford Long had long desired a wider field for the practice of his profession, and with his little family and faithful negro servants moved to Atlanta, where he remained one year. He soon had a flourishing practice, and made investments in what is now the business section of the city.

In January 1850, C.W. Long sold Lots 22, 24 and one-half of 23 to his cousin, Dr. John David Long, for $1230 and moved to Atlanta. However, in a year's time, the Longs would move again to Athens, where they remained for the rest of their lives.

On occasion, Dr. C.W. Long would return to Jefferson and Jackson County to treat family and friends.

In summary, the most plausible factors bringing Crawford Long to his destiny in Jefferson, Georgia, were: the town being older and more progressive than Danielsville; the availability of a preceptor in Dr. George R. Grant and later the opportunity to buy Grant's property and medical practice; and the chance to live with a family member.

What has been presented here delineates what is currently known, but research is by no means complete on Jefferson during Dr. Crawford W. Long's time.

References

Boland FK: The First Anesthetic: The Story of Crawford W. Long. Athens GA: The University of Georgia Press, 1950.

Curry JLM: Georgia in the 1840's. University Al: Confederate Publishing Co., 1980.

Deaver SB: Famous Georgians and Their Homes. Atlanta: Historic Preservation Section, Ga. Dept. of Natural Resources, 1985.

Deed records, Jackson County, Georgia.

Elrod LF: Historical Notes on Jackson County, Georgia. (Jefferson GA), 1967.

Georgia Department of Natural Resources. Georgia's Living Places: Historic Houses in Their Landscaped Settings. Atlanta: Historic Preservation Section, Ga. Dept. of Natural Resources, 1991.

Georgia Department of Natural Resources. National Register of Historic Places Nomination: Crawford W. Long Childhood Home. Atlanta:Historic Preservation Section, Ga. Dept. of Natural Resources, 1977.

Georgia Laws, 1806, 1812, 1872.

Hynds EC: Antebellum Athens and Clarke County. Athens: University of Georgia Press, 1974.

Jacobs J: Pharm. D. Dr. Crawford W. Long, the Distinguished Physician-Pharmacist. Atlanta, 1919. (Reprinted, 1992)

Linley J: The Georgia Catalog, Historic American Buildings Survey: A Guide to the Architecture of the State. Athens: University of Georgia Press, 1982.

Reap JK: Athens: A Pictorial History. Norfolk VA: Donning Company/Publishers, 1985.

Tabor P: History of Madison County, Georgia. Advocate Press, 1974.

Taylor FL: Crawford W. Long and the Discovery of Ether Anesthesia. New York: Paul B. Hoeber, 1928.

U.S. Mortality Schedule. Jackson County, Georgia, 1850.

U.S. Population Census. Jackson County, Georgia. 1820, 1830, 1840, 1850, 1860, 1880.

White WE, ed. The Early History of Jackson County, by G.J.N. Wilson. Atlanta: Foote and Davies Co., 1914.

ANESTHESIA IN THE WEHRMACHT (1939 – 1945)

R.J. DEFALQUE and A.J. WRIGHT
Dept. of Anesthesiology,
UAB School of Medicine, Birmingham, Alabama, USA

General Considerations

Two factors strongly shaped German military anesthesia in World War II:

1. Anesthesia's inferior status in pre-war Germany;[1,2] and 2. "Tactical-surgical" exigencies.[3,4]

1. Anesthesiology did not exist as a specialty in the Germany of 1939. German surgeons chose their anesthesia and closely supervised its administration by a nurse (in most hospitals) or a junior surgeon (in teaching centers). Training was practical and "on the job." Despite exciting discoveries by a brilliant pharmaceutical industry, German anesthesia had changed little since World War I, except for the resurgence of ether and spinal analgesia in the early 1930's. Ether was "open dropped," except in large hospitals where it was vaporized with a crude N_20-0_2 machine. Tracheal intubation, positive pressure ventilation, and rational fluid administration were largely ignored. Such rudimentary anesthesia had prevented the introduction in Germany of the great surgical advances made in the 1930's in the U.S. and Britain (especially in thoracic and abdominal surgery); German surgery was rapidly losing its world's supremacy. The problem was compounded by the political regime's intense chauvinism. The German Surgical Society and Ministry of Health rejected all efforts to create a specialty of anesthesiology in the later 1930's.[1,2]

2. To respond to the exigencies of a motorized war of rapid movement ("Blitzkrieg"), mass casualties, extensive wounds caused by new weapons, lack of surgical specialists and facilities, and to satisfy the army's demand for rapid return of the wounded to his unit, the new Wehrmacht's medical service had developed by 1939 a flexible plan for the surgical handling of the soldier wounded on the battlefield:

BATTALION	FRONT LINE	TRUPPENVERBANDPLATZ (TVP) (Battalion Dressing Station) General Medical Officer	Shock Pain Dressings, splints Hemostasis, airway, pneumothorax
DIVISION	4-6 kms	HAUPTVERBANDPLATZ (HVP) (Division Main Dressing Station) 2 general surgeons	As TVP (more complete) Moribunds to die Tracheostomies, amputations, chest wounds, vascular sutures
DIVISION	10-15 kms	FELDLAZARET (FL) (Div. Filed Hospital) 4 surgeons, 2 specialists 2-3 weeks recovery	Large wounds, spicas, amputations Abdominal, thoracic, vascular
ARMY	50-100 km Communication Zone	KRIEGSLAZARET (KL) Army Hospital All surgical specialists	Eye, ENT, CNS, Dental Major orthopedic, thoracic, abdomen
"KREIS"	Germany	RESERVELAZARET (RL) (Home Hospital) Large surgical staff	Definitive surgery Corrective surgery Rehabilitation

Overlap between each echelon and support from each upper group kept the system highly flexible and efficient. The emphasis was on treating the wounded for fast return to his unit or rapid and safe evacuation to a rear hospital for more extensive or definitive surgery, thus keeping the forward stations highly mobile and available for newer casualties. This favored the lightly wounded over the severely injured and allowed simple undemanding anesthetic techniques. The system worked well in the early campaigns (1939-1941) because of good weather, good communications, the proximity to the large German base hospitals, and especially the small number of casualties. But it failed abysmally in the Soviet Union and made impossible demands on the forward stations.[3] Surgery and anesthesia were refused to patients who would have survived in the Allied armies.

German Anesthetists[5-10]

Inexperienced physicians and drafted medical students were quickly trained on the job to administer anesthesia in most rear hospitals (KL,RL). Large base hospitals in Germany continued to employ their civilian nurses. In the FL and many KL, anesthesia was given by a surgeon, an internist, a dentist, or a medical orderly. Anesthesia was rarely needed in the TVP. Each HVP had at least two "narcotizers," medical orderlies who, among other O.R. duties, provided anesthesia under a surgeon's direction. They were NCOs selected for their intelligence, maturity and skill. Like the surgeons, they worked in two shifts of eight hours, but during the great Eastern battles many surgical teams worked for 20 hour spells, operating on 200-300 patients, sustained by caffeine, tobacco, and pervitin.

Many German surgeons after the war fondly remembered their "narkotizeurs" and had high praise for their skill and dedication. The inspectors' reports[5] agree that anesthetic accidents were rare despite the lack of training and the working conditions. They quickly acquired vast experience with a few simple techniques, and the speed of most surgical procedures, which only required an induction dose of anesthetic, probably contributed to that low morbidity. Great emphasis was placed on the observation of the pulse, the respiration, the color of the face, the eyes signs, and the symptoms of respiratory obstruction. The blood pressure was rarely monitored.

Anesthetic Techniques and Agents[8-10]

A few rapid, simple anesthetic techniques became popular as younger, hastily trained surgeons met an increasing number of casualties in the forward stations.

1. Local anesthesia:

a. Nerve blocks were rarely performed because of time exigencies and most surgeons' lack of experience with them. Older surgeons, especially in rear hospitals, used brachial plexus (Kuhlenkampf, Mulley), sciatic or distal extremity nerve blocks. Intercostal nerve blocks were frequently used for chest wall repairs, occasionally supplemented by i.v. anesthesia. Procaine 1-2 percent, usually with epinephrine, was used.

b. Local infiltration (0.5-1 percent) procaine with epinephrine) was rarely used at the front because of lack of time, the patients' poor emotional status, and the extent of the wounds, unless life-saving surgery was needed in a shocked patient. It was the technique of choice in face, neck, chest, head, and spine traumas.

c. Spinal anesthesia was rarely performed in the front stations because of lack of time, the surgeons' unfamiliarity with the technique, and the well-known danger of hypotension in shocked patients. A few older surgeons, especially in the rear, used it for surgery of the lower extremities or lower abdomen. Ephedrine was often given i.m.prophylactically. Procaine (50-100 mg) or tetracaine (8-10 mg), occasionally with epinephrine, were used.

d. Cocaine 2-10 percent was extensively used in ophthalmology, ENT, and urology.

2. I.V. anesthesia:

a. Skophedal (S.E.E.) weak (i.v.) or less often strong (i.m.) was extensively used to produce a deep twilight sleep:
   - many minor procedures were done with or without additional local anesthetic infiltration: wound debridements, vascular sutures, reductions.
   - evipan (see below) could be added to produce 10-15 minutes of deep anesthesia for amputations, extensive wound debridements, reduction and casting of major fractures, etc.
   - skophedal was also a common premedication for inhalation anesthesia after 1942.

b. Evipan (hexobarbital) became extremely popular because of its rapid and deep anesthetic action, simplicity of administration, quick emergence, and circulatory stability. Overdose with respiratory arrest was easily produced, requiring manual artificial ventilation and analeptics (lobelin, cormaine, picrotoxin). Evipan was used:
   - as only anesthetic, generally preceded by a heavy narcotic premedication, e.g. skophedal as described above,
   - as an induction agent for ether inhalation in frightened patients. Eunarcon, another i.v. barbiturate, was occasionally used after 1942 in the Soviet Union as it came premixed and did not freeze. It depressed the circulation more than evipan.

3. Inhalation agents:

a. Chloroform: despite the Inspector General's recommendation in 1939, chloroform was rarely used because of its circulatory depression in shocked patients and the younger surgeons' lack of experience with it. A few older surgeons used it in rear hospitals. A few drops of chloroform were often added to speed up or deepen an ether anesthesia.

2. Ethyl chloride "Rausch" was popular for mass casualties in the forward stations: 30 to 50 drops were poured from a spray bottle on a mask or piece of gauze while the patient inhaled deeply, counted, and kept an arm raised. Surgery was started as soon as the count stopped and the arm dropped; consciousness returned within a few minutes. Motor and autonomic responses were usual and expected. The Germans considered the "Rausch" an analgesic, preanesthetic stage, but it was in fact a short, light anesthesia. Ethyl chloride Rausch was also frequently used for induction of ether anesthesia.

3. Ether remained by far the favorite inhalation agent throughout the war because of its safety and simplicity of administration, despite its flammability, slow induction and recovery tying down physicians and orderlies, and its airway irritation. The patient's face was protected with vaseline, then covered with gauze, and after a few drops of Eau de Cologne ether was slowly dripped on a Schimmelbush mask while the patient was counting with the arm raised and inhaling deeply. Most often, however, induction was done with evipan or ethyl chloride. A generous premedication of narcotic and atropine was the rule. Some surgeons owned an Ambredanne's apparatus. In the large hospitals in Germany, ether was vaporized with a N_2O-O_2 gas machine. Positive pressure, if needed, was done with a bag and a tightly-fitting mask. In the field, some ingenious surgeons had had valves inserted on the German Army respirator to allow positive pressure.

Other Drugs

1. Narcotics and premedicants: German soldiers, even those in severe shock or with pneumothorax, received a generous dose of narcotics in the TVP (morphine, dilaudid, oxycodone or, after 1942, skophedal) Premedication (pantopon, morphine with atropine or skophedal was generally given before general anesthesia.

2. Fluids: unless the injury was immediately life-threatening, surgery, especially if general anesthesia was necessary, was postponed until the patient was out of shock. Shock was treated with quiet, heat, and fluids added with various cardiac stimulants (sympatol, strophantine, calcium, caffeine, camphorated oil) or analeptics (lobelin, coramine, picrotoxin). Volume expansion was done with saline (tutofusin, normasol), or glucone 5 percent solutions. In the last part of the war, periston (a PVP) was commonly used after severe hemorrhage when available. Blood was used sparingly: 250-500 ml in most wounded, rarely 1000 ml after massive bleeding. Transfusion reactions were frequent. Bank blood was rarely available at the front and most transfusions were done with a field apparatus (Tsank, Clemens, Braun) from "volunteers" (medical orderlies, lightly wounded patients). Plasma and dry plasma were produced towards the end of the war, but were rarely available in the field.

Conclusions

German military anesthesia in World War II was vastly inferior to its US-British counterpart. It was an important cause, though not the main one, of the poor surgical care of the German soldier wounded on the battlefield. The lessons of the war, however, were not lost and contributed to the rapid birth and vigorous development of anesthesiology in post-1945 Germany.

References

1. Killian H: Im Kampf gegen der Schmerz. Mein Abenteuer mit der Narkose. München, Kindler Verlag, 289-315, 1979.
2. Killian H: Plan zur Neuordnung des Narkosewesens in Deutschland. Schmerz-Narkose-Anaesthesie 14:73-87, 1941.
3. Ring F: Zur Geschichte der Militärmedizin in Deutschland. Berlin, Deutsche Militärverlag, 275-320, 1962.
4. Orator V: Leitfaden der Feldchirurgie im Bewegungskrieg. Leipzig, JA Barth, 3. Aufl. 1943.
5. Fischer H: Aus der Erfahrungsberichten der Beratenden Chirurgen im Krieg 1939-1945. Darmstadt, Wehr-und-Wissen Verlaggesellschaft, 48-55, 1963.
6. Haberer v.H: Kriegschirurgische Erfahrunden aus dem Osterfeldzug 1941. Münch Med Wschr 89:437-442, 1942.
7. Melzner E: Der Frontchirurg auf den Hauptverbandplätzen des Ostens. Dtsch Militärarzt 9:20-42, 1944.
8. Nestmann F: Narkoseerfahrungen im Felde. Med Klin 38:824-826, 1942.
9. Holle F: Praktische Erfahrungen über die Schmerzbekämpfung in der Kriegschirurgie des Hauptverbandplatzes und Feldlazarets. Dtsch Militärarzt 7:85-89, 1942.
10. Hesse F: Die operative Schmerzbekämpfung im Kriege. Dtsch Militärarzt 7:185-191, 1942.

ROBERT MORTIMER GLOVER (1816–1859), Another Anesthetic Tragedy

R.J. DEFALQUE and A.J. WRIGHT
UAB Dept. of Anesthesiology
Birmingham, Alabama, USA

Early Years

Little is known of Glover's early years. Entries in the records of his medical school and professional societies[1] show that he was born in Durham (N.E. England) but moved to Edinburgh at a young age. After a classical education he attended 13 quarters at Edinburgh School of Medicine, doing clerkships in the wards of the Royal Infirmary under James Y. Simpson, James Syme and John Reid. His famous teachers, in later testimonials,[2] remembered him fondly as a brilliant and hard-working student. He obtained his L.R.C.S. in 1837 and spent the next 18 months attending lectures and demonstrations at the Hotel Dieu, Charite, St. Louis, and other noted Parisian hospitals. He co-founded the Parisian Medical Society in 1837 and became its first vice-president. He returned to Edinburgh at the end of 1838 to continue his studies and on June 15, 1840, passed his M.D. examination with a thesis titled, "On the physiological and medicinal properties of bromine and its compounds," suggesting an early interest in pharmacologic research.

Newcastle Years

In the summer of 1839 Glover moved to Newcastle-upon-Tyne and became a physician at its Eastern Free Dispensary. He also taught chemistry, physics and toxicology at the Newcastle College of Medicine and Practical Sciences, a small school of 15 to 20 students, founded in 1834.[3] The position was unsalaried. His application for staff privileges at the Newcastle Infirmary was rejected, despite flattering recommendations by his famous Edinburgh teachers. He may have been accepted later since he worked in the late 1840's with John Fife who practiced surgery there. Glover must have continued his pharmacologic work soon after arriving in Newcastle since he published one research paper in 1841 and two in 1842. The 1842 papers on the physiologic effects of some halogenated compounds are of great interest: not only did they earn Glover the Harveian prize, but they also are the first demonstration of the anesthetic effects of chloroform.[4] Injecting respectively 1.8 and 3.6 ml of chloroform in the jugular vein of 2 large dogs, he produced unconsciousness, loss of corneal reflex, loss of response to pinching and pricking, and motor weakness, a state from which both quickly recovered. Two rabbits which received 3.6 ml of chloroform in the stomach or the peritoneal cavity showed the same symptoms, but died 20 minutes later. The autopsies of the animals showed intense pulmonary congestion and Glover concluded that chloroform was a potent pulmonary toxic. Unlike Flourens 5 years later, Glover missed the relevance of his findings for anesthesia. He was thus rather disingenuous when he claimed, soon after Simpson's discovery, that he had not recommended chloroform for anesthesia because of its pulmonary toxicity.[4]

From 1843 through 1849 Glover was chairman of the Department of Chemistry, then of Materia Medica and Therapeutics, lecturing on chemistry, toxicology, pharmacology, medical jurisprudence, and the philosophy of medicine. In October, 1849, he applied for, but was denied, the Chandos Chair of Medicine at St. Andrews, left vacant by John Reid's death. The denial came despite warm recommendations by his Edinburgh teachers and Newcastle colleagues and students, and after 10 years of a busy clinical and research career.[2]

After the clinical introduction of chloroform in 1847, Glover helped Newcastle surgeons give anesthesia, including T.N. Meggison, Hannah Greener's surgeon at the time of her death on January 28, 1848. Glover assisted Sir John Fife at her autopsy, and his bias about chloroform pulmonary toxicity may well have influenced Sir John's conclusion that her death was due to pulmonary congestion caused by chloroform.[4]

In December, 1850, Glover was elected a F.R.S.E., (Fellow of the Royal Society of Edinburgh) but he does not seem to have participated in the Society's activities after his nomination. Around that time he also became a Corresponding Fellow of the Medical Society of London.

Petty quarrels among the Newcastle College's 12 teachers reached a boiling point in the Spring of 1851 with the nomination of Dean Embleton's protégé as chief of surgery. Insults were exchanged, honors wounded, apologies refused, all of which led to the dissolution of the College in late August of 1851. Glover proved to be a spiteful and petulant partisan: he joined a colleague in a nightly raid on the College's museum to retrieve his pathology specimens, and refused to return the key of the building and the stolen material. He later joined the seceding minority to found a new medical school (Fife School) at the end of 1851. He taught there through 1852.[3]

London Years

Glover left Newcastle for unknown reasons in late 1853 or early 1854 and moved to London. On November 29, 1854, he was unanimously elected House Physician at the Royal Free Hospital, a famous London institution then primarily caring for outpatients. He promised to obtain his L.R.C.P. (License of the Royal College of Physicians) within 6 months.[5] The hospital Medical Board found Glover's work unsatisfactory and, after several complaints, they sent him on April 9, 1855 a formal letter of reprimand censoring him for neglecting his outpatients and failing to take his LRCP.[5] The causes of Glover's problems are unknown. He also seems to have given up his pharmacologic researches, as all his London publications address clinical or epidemiologic subjects.

On February 26, 1855, Glover resigned his hospital post and enlisted as Assistant Surgeon in the Army Medical Corps for service in Crimea.[5] He arrived in Scutari, the site of the three main British hospitals, in May or June, 1855, when 50 percent of the hospitalized British soldiers still died from infection, despite the reforms started by Miss Nightingale and the War Office. Glover seems to have contracted amebic dysentery in Scutari and he blamed it for his later abuse of opium and chloroform.[6-8] Glover's activities in the Crimea, the date of his return, and his initial professional work in

London are unknown. He resigned from the Royal Free Hospital and obtained his L.R.C.P. in 1856.[6,7] From 1856 through early 1859 he published a few articles, pamphlets, and books on clinical, epidemiologic, and medicolegal subjects.

The last year of Glover's life is well documented.[6-8] He at that time had become destitute, was supported financially by ex-colleagues, and took large amounts of opium, chloroform and camphor, sometimes to the point of stupor. He shared the lodgings of W.R. Rochfort, a druggist suspected of practicing medicine illegally under Glover's name and of providing him with his drugs.[6-8]

Six weeks before his death Glover married an escapee from the Colney Hatch Lunatic Asylum and lived with her in a hotel for indigents until her recapture one week later.

Glover's Death

On April 8, 1859, while being visited by his colleague F.J. Gant, Glover drank 2 to 5 ounces of chloroform over 2 hours and fell into a deep coma. Several friends and colleagues tried various inept treatments, but failed to revive him, and he died on April 9, 1859, between 7.30 and 8.00 p.m. An autopsy, done 44 hours later, found large amounts of chloroform-smelling bloody mucus throughout the whole gastrointestinal tract and mild fatty degeneration of the liver and kidneys. A judicial inquest, held on April 13, concluded that death had been due to an accidental overdose of chloroform drunk to produce intoxication.[8] Glover had no known relative and his burial site is unknown. No portrait has been found.

References

1. Records of: Edinburgh School of Medicine; Royal Society Edinburgh; Harveian Society; Royal College of Surgeons. (Edinburgh).
2. Testimonials in Favour of the Appointment of R.M. Glover to the Chandos Chair of Medicine at St. Andrews. Newcastle-upon-Tyne, GB Richardson, 1849.
3. Dale G, Miller FJW: Newcastle School of Medicine 1834-1984. Sesquicentennial Scrap-book. Faculty of Medicine, University of Newcastle. 1984:16-17.
4. Defalque RJ, Wright AJ: R(obert) Mortimer Glover and the first chloroform anesthesia. Anesthesiology 70:1033-1034, 1989.
5. Archives of the Royal Free Hospital, Hampstead, London.
6. Editorial. The Week. Br J Med 1:313-314, 1859.
7. Gant FJ: Letter to the Editor. Death of Dr. Glover. Lancet 1:425-426, 1859.
8. West London Observer, April 16th, 1859. Melancholy Death of Dr. Glover.

AMBULATORY ANESTHESIA IN 1929

H. de SOUSA
Department of Anesthesiology
SUNY Health Science Center
Syracuse, New York, USA

Contemporary ambulatory anesthesiologists may feel their specialty is more advanced now than ever. A society exists to promote and refine the practice of ambulatory anesthesia, currently dependent on expensive and immobile gas machines, compressed gases, potent intravenous drugs, and complex monitoring equipment. However, rarely mentioned is the fact that most anesthetics to date have been safely administered without the use of muscle relaxants, tracheal tubes, or electronic monitoring. One generation ago, truly ambulatory anesthesiologists were apparently at ease using techniques and skills that would terrify most and humble the rest of us.

A fortuitous discovery in a flea market of *Catalogue of Surgical Instruments & Appliances* of Down Brothers, Ltd., London 1929, provides insight into what equipment an ambulatory anesthesiologist required at the time. A 50 page section entitled "Anaesthetic Apparatus" begins by suggesting equipment to carry in Physicians' and Surgeons' Bags (wide-mouth, with removable sterilizable lining, in black or brown Cowhide, for approximately US$150 in today's currency). Listed is a choice of one each of the following:

> Mouth Wedge; Mouth Gag; Mouth Props; Air Way: Tongue Forceps; Mask for open Ether; Drop Bottle; Warm Ether and Chloroform Apparatus, Shipway's; Sponge Holding Forceps; Sterilized Sponges; Nitrous Oxide and Oxygen Apparatus; Cylinders of N20 and 0 (sic) with stand; Spinal Syringe for Anaesthesia; Emergency Tracheotomy set.

EARLY USE OF REGIONAL ANESTHESIA IN OBSTETRICS

H. de SOUSA
Department of Anesthesiology
SUNY Health Science Center
Syracuse, New York, USA

Historical references in obstetric anesthesia texts attribute the earliest use of regional anesthesia to the pioneers of spinal and caudal anesthesia working at the turn of this century. Even the 1903 edition of J.W. Williams' Obstetrics states the first publication on this subject, "Cocaine Anaesthesia — its employment at the time of labour" was by Kreis in August, 1900.

However, the July 3, 1886 editorial of *The Medical Record* — "A Weekly Journal of Medicine and Surgery" published by Wm. Wood & Co., was entitled "Suppression of Pain in Labor by the Local Application of Cocaine."

The earliest description of the use of cocaine for this indication, hitherto attributed to an American surgeon, Dr. William M. Polk, was currently being disputed by Dr. M.S. Jeannel, who indicated that the French surgeons Doleris and Dubois reported on January 17, 1885 the effective relief of labour pain in 6 of 8 parturients. (Note: this is only 4 months after Koller's original announcement of the use of cocaine for anesthesia). Polk used a paracervical injection of 4 minims (0.25 ml) of 4-percent cocaine (pg. 85 Cocaine in Gynecology and Obstetrics by W.M. Polk in *Cocaine and Its Use in Ophthalmic and General Surgery* by H. Knapp, M.D., published by G.P. Putnam's Sons 1885) whereas MM. Doleris and Dubois painted the cervix with a 4-percent solution of cocaine mixed with lard. (Analgesia of the Genital Passages Obtained by the Local Application of Cocaine During Labor. *J.A.M.A.* April 11, 1885) These were the first reports of the use of paracervical block for labour, a technique that regained popularity in the 1960's. Additional early reports of this effective technique were widespread — Dr. M.S. Jeannel, cited in the above issue of The Medical Record; G.H. Roque Dabbs, M.D., *British Medical Journal* 1885 and 1887, and Dr. Blodgett in a discussion on "Anaesthesia in Normal Labor" in the *Boston Medical and Surgical Journal* 1887, Page 457.

This discussion provides some insight as to why such an apparently effective and safe technique was not only abandoned but also forgotten within 15 years. Dr. Kingman, obviously an authority on the subject, having given a presentation on anesthesia for labor, was asked why he omitted this technique from consideration in his paper. He answered that it did not seem to him to be competitive with existing general anesthetics, and he had never used it because he "doubted its ability to relieve the highly complex pain of parturition." Surprisingly, the same speaker, when defending the humane use of ether over no anesthesia, says "Shall we refuse to use it simply because, so far, some have gotten along without it?" The entire innervation of the uterus is supplied by nerves in the paracervical area, a fact even Doleris was unfortunately unaware of ("the pains from this source (the uterus) are usually slight, and cannot be affected by cocaine.") Did lack of definite knowledge concerning the paths of afferent nerves of the uterus prevent the scientific application of regional anesthesia as an alternative to general anesthesia in obstetrics? Are effective alternate therapies often not considered or abandoned for lack of a known physiologic or anatomic basis?

JAMES ROBINSON
England's True Pioneer of Anaesthesia

RICHARD H. ELLIS
*The Royal Hospital of St. Bartholomew,
London, England, United Kingdom*

The discovery of anaesthesia, in Boston in 1846, was a precious, glorious and entirely American achievement, in which no other country had any part to play whatsoever. Paradoxically, however, its subsequent development, promotion and wider acceptance depended almost entirely on circumstances, on people and on events outside America, and especially in Britain. In essence, the Bostonians — in late 1846 — could only inform their influential friends and contacts outside America and hope that their miraculous invention could be insinuated into, and then accepted by, the minds of medical men the world over.

The American dentist William Thomas Greene Morton[1] was, arguably, the most famous and influential of all the early anaesthetists. Second only to Morton in this respect was the English physician Dr. John Snow[2] with his meticulous, logical and scientific approach — to which the recent publication of his largely unobserved early researches titled, "On Narcotism by the Inhalation of Vapours,"[3] is a most eloquent testament.

In Britain, however, there was a third man — another person who deserved recognition, who was active and influential from the very start, and well before Snow began to make his own unique contributions. This man was James Robinson, (Fig. 1) who was not only the true pioneer of anaesthesia in England, but was also a catalyst for its general acceptance in the United States. Hitherto, Morton's inventiveness and Snow's erudition have combined to eclipse the important part played by Robinson at the time of anaesthesia's introduction in late 1846 and early 1847. The third man, James Robinson, was a British dentist. He was a remarkable man by any yardstick and had enormous influence on anaesthesia at its formative, and therefore most vulnerable time. Until very recently, his contributions to early anaesthesia have been almost completely overlooked. This international symposium is an ideal occasion on which to give an account of these contributions.

From the historical point of view, the links

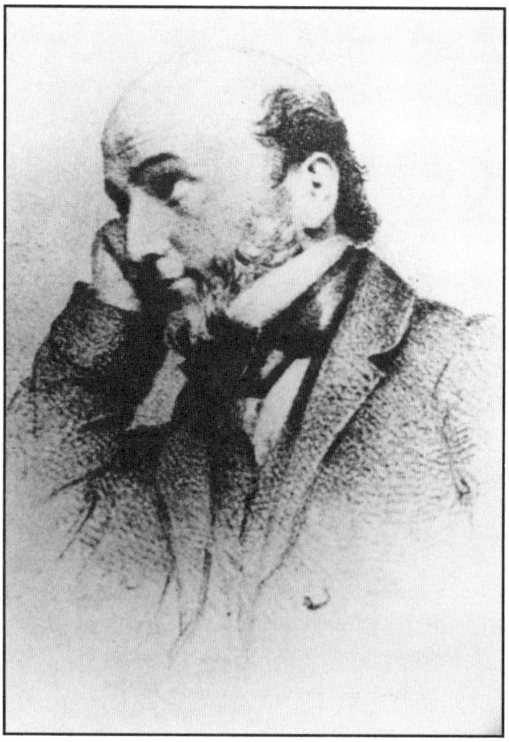

Fig. 1. James Robinson (1813-1862). Rarely has a person who has done so much been so overlooked by so many for so long.

between anaesthesia and dentistry in the late 1840's were extremely close. Indeed, it would be correct to say that anaesthesia would not have been introduced in the ways in which it was had it not been for dentists and dentistry. For in Boston, where the whole process effectively began (and in Britain as well), it was dentists who were the true pioneers of anaesthesia — even though dentistry at the time was held at arms length, and was disdained by the medical professions in both countries.

Anaesthesia began in Boston, and was introduced by the dentist William Morton who, on September 30, 1846, first used ether anaesthesia[1] for dental extraction in his own practice in Boston, Massachusetts. Two weeks later he gave the first public demonstration of ether for surgery.[4] It was this demonstration which established anaesthesia. It took place in Boston on the 16 October, 1846, at the Massachusetts General Hospital. For this present purpose it is enough to note that among those present,[1] in addition to Morton, were Professor John Collins Warren (the surgeon who performed the operation), George Hayward (Professor Warren's second-in-command at the Hospital) and Henry Jacob Bigelow, a young surgeon who had recently joined the staff of the Hospital. I will return to these three men a little later.

Initially, Morton — to gain financial advantage — attempted to conceal the true nature of the ether.[5] Despite the initial enthusiasm generated by his use of anaesthesia,the secrecy with which he surrounded his invention was repugnant to most people. Morton was vilified for attempting to restrict the use of his humanitarian discovery and to benefit financially from such restriction.[6] Morton's reputation was not the only casualty of this unfortunate approach, for his gauche attempt at secrecy was one of the principal factors which led to a more or less muted reaction to the introduction of ether in America, the very country in which anaesthesia had been born. In these circumstances, the response of the medical professions in other countries to the discovery of ether anaesthesia was to be a most important factor in fostering its general adoption during its earliest days. Essentially, this means the reaction of doctors in Europe — especially those in France and Britain. The initial reaction of French doctors to the news of anaesthesia's invention was lukewarm and dismissive,[7] and so it was the reaction of the British doctors which was to condition the acceptance of ether anaesthesia outside Boston.

It is convenient to gather together the threads of the story at the time of anaesthesia's introduction to Britain. The first anaesthetic ever given in England was administered in a small, private house in central London[8] which at the time was the home of Dr. Francis Boott, who was an expatriate American doctor.[9] It was Boott to whom the news of ether's introduction in Boston some two months earlier, had been sent. The house has since been demolished, but its site is commemorated by a plaque[10] which records that England's first anaesthetic was given on Saturday 19 December, 1846. The instigator of that historic event was undoubtedly the American Dr. Boott, but the first anaesthetic in England was actually given by the dentist James Robinson — who not only administered the anaesthetic but also performed the operation, namely, the extraction of a diseased molar tooth. The whole procedure was witnessed by Dr. Boott and his family. It was entirely successful, and was enthusiastically reported by Dr. Boott to the medical press.[9]

How James Robinson in particular — of all British dentists — came to be involved in the beginnings of British anaesthesia will emerge from an outline of his life and career as a dentist and of his contributions to the well-being of British Dentistry. James Robinson[11] was born into a naval family in Southampton in 1813. He was the youngest son of a Captain Charles Robinson of the Royal Navy who, in passing, served for a time aboard Nelson's flagship H.M.S. Victory.[12] Of James Robinson's childhood and schooldays nothing is known, save that he was educated "to fit him for any station in society."[11] He left school in 1827, at the age of 14, and immediately began his career in dentistry by becoming apprenticed to an established practitioner. The only surviving account of this period of Robinson's life recorded that he was apprenticed, in 1827, "to a gentleman who practised as a surgeon and a chemist in London, with whom he remained engaged in the usual routine of his profession till the expiration of his indentures."[11] This is a brief but most revealing account of his apprenticeship, and the words were probably written by Robinson himself, and were certainly approved by him, since they appeared in a later dental journal of which he was the Editor. At their very best, these lacklustre words hint dismally of uninspiring work with an uninspiring master, tolerated only because of the contract of apprenticeship.

We would do well to remember that in Britain, at the time of Robinson's apprenticeship the professions as we know them today had scarcely become organised or regulated,[13] and there was little or nothing to prevent untrained people dignifying themselves as surgeons, dentists or chemists before a virtually unprotected public. Robinson later became deeply committed to the creation of a proper and professional structure for dentistry. It may well have been during his apprenticeship with a man described as both a surgeon and a chemist — and who was quite likely to have been neither — that the need for the reform of his chosen profession first occurred to him.

In 1830, at the age of 17 and when his apprenticeship was completed, Robinson evidently thought that he could or should improve on his training, and he immediately enrolled as a student at Guy's Hospital, London for a period of some months.[14] On leaving Guy's, he enrolled for a while as a student at the London University.[15] On completion of these further studies he set up a small dental practice in central London, but later — as he became more successful — he moved to the larger premises at which he was to spend the rest of his working life.[16] The house (its present-day address is 14 Gower Street, London, WC2) was Robinson's principal residence during his most creative and influential years: it still stands today in virtually its original form, both inside and out.

At the time when Robinson entered dental practice, dentistry in Britain was unrecognisable as the profession which we know today.[17] The great majority of so-called dentists were unscrupulous charlatans who combined their dentistry with a whole variety of other occupations. The several contemporary accounts of dentistry at the time accord with Robinson's own recollection, when he later wrote that "Falstaff himself never possessed a more heterogeneous or nondescript army than those who now compose the majority of dentists in England."[18] A dental journal of 1844 described most contemporary British dentists as being ". . .low, vulgar and ignorant men who not only practise as dentists but do so publicly, drenching the papers with advertisements and hawking their valueless aid and worse goods with unblushing effrontery. . . ."[19] This dismal view is confirmed in the writings of Alfred Hill, the distinguished historian of British dentistry, who a few decades later recalled that "The overwhelming proportion of dentists at this time were mere tradesmen, and sadly lacking in scientific knowledge."[20] To emphasise this, it is possible to construct a list, from such sources, of some of the trades which so-called dentists then relied on, and to which their exodontia was just a useful additional source of income earned by crude and thoughtless care. These included chimney sweeps, chemists, blacksmiths, decayed tradesmen, quack doctors, failed doctors, old clothesmen, travelling showmen, cobblers, bakers, watchmakers, brewers' clerks, milkmen and itinerants (tramps).

But amidst this awful list was a leavening of inspired, thoughtful, and in every way excellent dental practitioners — determined to raise the status of their calling and to create a profession. One of this number, indeed head and shoulders above most others,[20,21] was James Robinson. As a result of the efforts of these few ethical and professional dentists was born the Reform Movement of British dentistry. Robinson was one of the most active of those involved in this movement, and he accomplished much in the name of dental reform and improvement. In 1842 he proposed the founding, in London, of the first British society at which ethical dentists could exchange professional knowledge and views.[22] This was open only to those who did not combine their dentistry with any other work and who did not advertise themselves. Understandably, attendances were sparse and the society did not prosper. In 1843 he founded and edited the first British journal devoted exclusively to dentistry, namely, the British Quarterly Journal of Dental Surgery.[23] This was short-lived, but in the following year the irrepressible Robinson produced another similar journal named "The Forceps."[24] This survived for some 15 months and then ceased publication, largely on account of the lack of interest among most other dentists. Later in his career, in 1856, Robinson was a founder member, and first President, of the short-lived College of Dentists.[20] This College disbanded soon after dentistry was incorporated into the Royal College of Surgeons of England in 1859.[25] One of the College of Dentists' activities was to found, in 1861, the National Dental Hospital in London. Robinson was instrumental in this hospital's creation and supported it enthusiastically.[22]

There were several other dental achievements and honours which Robinson obtained, and these attest to the leading place he occupied in British dentistry in the mid-1840's. In 1846 he was awarded an Honorary Doctorate of Dental Surgery by the Baltimore College of Dental Surgeons.[26] This was, at the time, the only proper society of dentists in the world.[27] Robinson had written a number of articles for their journal and was acknowledged to be an international authority on dentistry. In 1848 he was appointed Surgeon Dentist to the Royal Free Hospital[28] — one of the great teaching hospitals of London, and a year later he was appointed Surgeon Dentist to Queen Victoria's husband, His Royal Highness Prince Albert.[29] (Prince Albert made several visits to the house in which Robinson lived and worked, and each visit caused a flurry of excitement in the household and among Robinson's apprentices who also lived and worked there.)[30] Clearly, by the late 1840's, James Robinson had become one of the most prominent dentists in London, and was well-known and successful. He had a reputation as an eminent and progressive dentist, and was living and working at his house which was then numbered 7 Gower Street.

At precisely the same time, Dr. Francis Boott,[9] the expatriate American doctor who had retired from active medical practice, but who still kept in contact with medical colleagues in both Britain and America, was living a few hundred yards away from Robinson at number 24 Gower Street.[31] Thus, it is quite understandable that, when Francis Boott set out to arrange his own trial of ether anaesthesia, he should have turned to his near neighbour, the energetic and enthusiastic London dentist, James Robinson. As it happened, Francis Boott acted wisely when he chose James Robinson to help hm set up this trial,[8] which was to become the first use of anaesthesia outside the United

States of America, and also the catalyst to ether's widespread adoption. Together, Boott and Robinson considered how they could best organise their own trial of ether. They had several tasks, of which the most challenging was the creation of a suitable inhaler for the ether. Boott and Robinson only had a word-picture of Morton's original Boston inhaler,[4] and would obviously have needed to devise their own. Nonetheless, within a few hours they had improvised a rudimentary ether inhaler. It was part of a Nooth's Apparatus, which had been designed for the domestic manufacture of soda-water.[32] It had three glass chambers, and each of these could be separated from the others. Robinson and Boott at first only used the lowermost conical chamber, which suited their requirements perfectly.

Figure 2 shows the only illustration which exists of the original vapouriser,[33] and even this shows the first of the several modifications which Robinson and Boott made — in this instance — to the valve. Contemporary papers ascribe the apparatus to Robinson,[34,35] although he was undoubtedly aided and abetted by Dr. Boott. This simple vapouriser was used during

Fig. 2. The only illustration of the inhaler with which James Robinson (aided and abetted by the expatriate American Dr. Francis Boott) gave the first anaesthetic ever to be administered outside the United States of America.

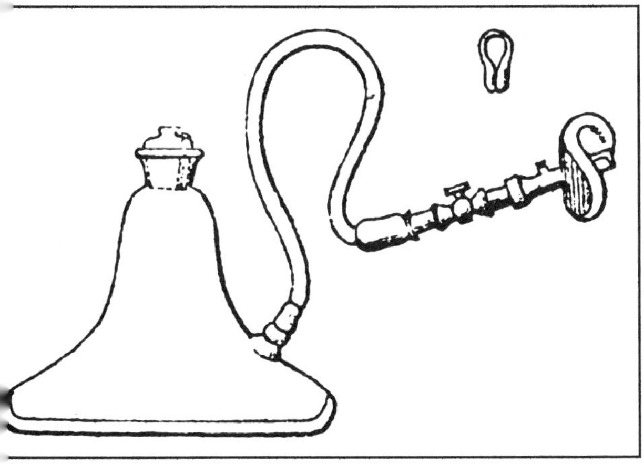

that first weekend for Boott and Robinson's earliest cases. That of their first patient — a Miss Lonsdale, whose molar tooth had been extracted[8] — was entirely satisfactory, and there was clearly no shortage of patients available to Robinson and Boott, for several more trials with ether were made by them at Boott's home during the weekend.

Robert Liston was — at the time — preeminent in the London surgical scene. He had been invited by Boott to see what was going on, and was sufficiently impressed with what he saw[36] to obtain a modification of Robinson's inhaler, and it was this modified version (known as Squire's Inhaler[37]) which was successfully used by a man named William Squire two days later for Liston's famous case, at London's University College Hospital, of amputation first performed under general anaesthesia,[8] a case which received enormous publicity in Britain, in America, and throughout the rest of the English-speaking world. Despite this initial success, however, the later results which were obtained with the Squire's ether inhaler were unpredictable and unsatisfactory.

Within a few days, Robinson further modified his inhaler and added the uppermost chamber of the Nooth's Apparatus, and also sponges to his own device.[38] This he did in order to provide anaesthesia for more prolonged surgical operations. Thereafter Robinson's inhaler, in competent hands, was reliable and produced satisfactory operating conditions. Armed with this modified, and now efficient inhaler, Robinson became adept at giving ether for dentistry and for prolonged surgical operations. He rapidly gained a reputation as the most skillful administrator of ether anaesthesia in Great Britain. This reputation is apparent from several medical journals of the time. For example, early in January, 1847, The Medical Times reported a horrendous story. "At University College Hospital Mr. Liston attempted the operation of amputation of the forearm with the assistance of Mr. Squire's apparatus; but after endeavoring to produce insensibility for 10 minutes without success the arm was amputated with the usual amount of pain."[39] (It was not only that Liston was impatient; it was mainly because, by this time, he was beginning to think that ether could not always produce insensibility.)[40] Again, at University College Hospital, we can read that "...a woman was to have a breast tumour removed by Mr. Liston. After inhaling the vapour of ether for upwards of twenty minutes without any sensible effect, the operation was performed with the usual amount of pain."[39] At this point, James Robinson was sent for as he had obviously and quickly established himself with a reputation as a successful anaesthetist. The journal then continued, "After this a woman was operated on for partial closure of the mouth. Mr. Robinson superintended the inhalation of the vapour using his own apparatus: the patient became insensible in two minutes and the operation was completed before she was aware that it had begun."

At the end of January, 1847, some six weeks after ether anaesthesia's first use in Britain, The Medical Times stated, "Mr. Robinson's success in inventing a most perfect apparatus cannot be questioned."[41] Other equally enthusiastic remarks make it clear that, at the time, some people in Britain thought that ether did not really produce insensibility, and they also emphasise the reassuring effect which James Robinson' anaesthetic expertise had on these doubters. "The results have now been witnessed by hundreds of the profession, and they have acknowledged that it really exerts the influence attributed to it by our American brethren, and that it may be employed without danger or difficulty."[42] At the end of January, 1847, The Medical Times described Robinson as "a gentleman who has had more experience in the administration of ether than any other in the kingdom."[43] Such unreserved enthusiasm for James Robinson, and for his innovative skill in administering the still strange and novel process of ether anaesthesia, was essential for its acceptance into Britain. Even Robert Liston himself — as we have seen — was on the point of abandoning its use[40] and reverting to his former methods because of the inability of his anaesthetists to regularly produce insensibility with ether. We can imagine the shambles, literally the shambles, he must have witnessed as he tried to operate during what we now know as the "stage of excitement" of unmodified ether anaesthesia. Anaesthesia, at this stage, was sustained virtually entirely by James Robinson's success in the administration of ether using the apparatus which he had perfected. This success Robinson could repeat time and time again.

But there was a "bandwagon" effect, and many others tried to imitate Robinson's work by hastily designing their own inhalers[44] and using them to try and produce unconsciousness. Almost all did more harm than good,[45] for only one man is reported to have succeeded in emulating Robinson's skill, and this man went on to lay the foundations of the speciality of anaesthesia upon the ground which James Robinson had prepared in those first six weeks. This man was Dr. John Snow.[2] John Snow's interest in anaesthesia was aroused very early and, some eight days after Robinson had first used ether in London, he called on Robinson at his Gower Street home to see the new-fangled process for himself. As a result, Robinson was able to write to a medical journal just before the end of December, 1846, and say that "I again operated this morning with the most perfect success, in the presence of my friends — Mr. Stocks, Mr. Snow, and Mr. Fenney."[38] In this way, in the house on Gower Street, and with James Robinson's help, John Snow began his renowned career as the world's first and most influential specialist physician anaesthetist.

Snow's approach was cautious, reasoned and scientific: Robinson's was pragmatic and empirical, but nonetheless effective. While Snow was pondering the subtleties of anaesthesia and had determined to put them on a scientific footing, Robinson, with his simple approach and (it must be said) no small amount of luck, was able to demonstrate anaesthesia's reliability and effectiveness to influential but sceptical doctors.

Within a matter of weeks, Snow supplanted Robinson as anaesthesia's champion,[40] but Robinson did not abandon his interest in the subject. He continued to be actively involved in its propagation, and remained aware of the developments which Snow, and others, were making. When, in November 1847, Simpson (in Edinburgh) introduced chloroform,[46] Robinson corresponded with Simpson about the agent[47] and began to use it in his own practice. Within four weeks (that is by mid-December 1847), Robinson had invented his own chloroform apparatus.[48] It was an effective inhaler in Robinson's hands, and the editor of The Lancet described it as being "remarkably ingenious."[48] John Snow himself drew attention to it when first writing up his own, more sophisticated chloroform vapouriser some four weeks later.[49]

On several occasions between 1849 and 1856, Snow went to Robinson's practice on Gower Street to give chloroform to patients while Robinson extracted teeth.[50] Clearly, the two men knew of each other, professionally if not socially, over a period of nine years. At one time Snow, who obviously had more than a nodding acquaintanceship with Robinson, recorded his high opinion of him in the following words, "Mr. Robinson has had great experience and deservedly earned a high reputation connected with the administration of ether and chloroform."[51] In due course, we will come to yet another appreciation by Snow of Robinson's achievements in anaesthesia.

During Robinson's very active and progressive period in anaesthesia — which lasted some 4 months — he was kept very busy indeed. His involvement with ether anaesthesia was considerable and, judging from the contemporary accounts which are still available, no one was more involved and committed to its welfare in those earliest days than James Robinson. Seemingly, every day Robinson demonstrated his skill with ether in his own practice in Gower Street. In addition, he administered ether anaesthesia before onlookers, who were arguably sceptical of the whole thing, at several London teaching hospitals, of which University College, King's College, Guy's, and the Westminster Hospitals were mentioned by name.[52] He also demonstrated ether at a number of private homes, including his own, Dr. Boott's and Lady Blessington's. The accounts of these demonstrations made at private homes in London are to be found in Robinson's own textbook of ether anaesthesia.

Although John Snow's famous work, "On the Inhalation of the Vapour of Ether,"[53] is the most renowned of all the early works on anaesthesia, it was not published until 7 months after the first textbook on the subject appeared. The first published textbook of anaesthesia was written by James Robinson and was entitled, "A Treatise on the Inhalation of the Vapour of Ether."[54] It was published in late February, 1847, and attracted encouraging reviews from medical journals of the time.[55,56] A facsimile edition of the work was published in 1983.[57] Robinson's original text is unique, for it provides the only lengthy account of the earliest days of anaesthesia in Britain to be written at the time when the events were actually happening, by one of those most closely involved. (Incidentally, Robinson was the first person in Britain to suggest the use of oxygen in association with anaesthesia.[58] This he did in a letter to The Lancet, in March, 1847, but his observation was too late for inclusion in his book.) In his book Robinson recorded only his simple and clinical observations. Having no scientific data to present in support of ether's importance, Robinson, somewhat naively, described how ether had been administered by him, not only to ordinary folk, but also to the social élite of London. Some of these aristocrats had seen the use of ether at Dr. Boott's home in Gower Street and in various London hospitals. A number of demonstrations were also made — by Robinson — early in January, 1847, at the fashionable London salon which was the home of Lady Marguerite, the Countess of Blessington. She was one of London's leading, and somewhat notorious, society hostesses of the time.[59] Several of her close friends took part in the so-called experiments with ether inhalation at Lady Blessington's home, of which Robinson made so much in his book. No surgery was performed during these episodes. (Those who inhaled there included, among others, Prince Napoleon Bonaparte,[60] who seems to have taken a very close interest in ether anaesthesia in England. He not only inhaled the ether on two occasions himself, from Robinson, but also witnessed its use at Boott's Gower Street home, at several London teaching hospitals, and at Gore House. At the time he was living in exile in London, but a few years later returned to France to be proclaimed Emperor Napoleon the Third.

In the later years of his life Robinson also had a house on the outskirts of London (in Kenton, Middlesex), and it was here that he died in March 1862.[61] He was then aged 48. The circumstances of his death will sound incredible to our ears today. Two days earlier, while walking in his garden, he had used a pocket-knife to prune a branch from a tree. As he did so, the knife slipped and accidentally punctured his femoral artery. There was not much external bleeding, but he retired to bed. During the next 36 hours or so — even though he was attended by two doctors who had been summoned by his wife — he slowly exsanguinated and died. No treatment other than the passive observation of haemorrhage seems to have been suggested. James Robinson left a widow; they had no children. Robinson's grave is in Highgate Cemetery in central London, and is in very poor condition being now completely overgrown.

There were fulsome obituaries of Robinson in the British Medical Journal,[62] The Lancet[63] and the dental journals in Britain[29,64] and America.[65] This must say something about the advances which had occurred in dentistry during Robinson's professional life. As we now know, many of these advances were brought about to no small extent by Robinson's own efforts. When he embarked on his professional career, it would have been inconceivable for a dentist who was not medically qualified to have merited an obituary in any medical journal whatsoever. Robinson, however, richly deserved such recognition, not only for his achievements in Dentistry, but also for all that he accomplished for Anaesthesia in its earliest days.

His most auspicious involvement with the specialty lasted from late December, 1846, until sometime towards the end of April, 1847. That is a period of some four months, beginning with the very introduction of ether anaesthesia. He administered the first anaesthetic ever given in England. He was instrumental — and was probably the guiding light — in devising the first anaesthetic apparatus ever used in England. He demonstrated the process of ether anaesthesia to William Squire and Robert Liston, and thereby ensured that a convincing demonstration of its use for major surgery would soon afterwards take place. Not being content with having given the first successful anaesthetic in England, Robinson went out of his way to gain more experience of ether anaesthesia. It would seem from contemporary journals that he lost no opportunity to show how genuine the new-fangled (and initially dubious) process was. In addition, on many occasions, he was called in by eminent medical men to give ether; he was obviously their preferred choice as an anaesthetist in these earliest days. He developed his apparatus into something which was, for a time, considered to be the most perfect device for administering ether anaesthesia. (It was superseded only by John Snow's apparatus, and by no other.)[56,66] He demonstrated ether anaesthesia to the leading doctors in London, and was the first person to show John Snow what happened during etherisation. He made simple, clinical observations of the events which occurred during anaesthesia and, drawing on these, suggested methods of administering ether safely and effectively. He was the first person in Britain to suggest the use of oxygen with anaesthesia.

He also ensured that anaesthesia was both widely and well publicised. He contributed articles in the medical press,[67,68,69] and similarly wrote articles or letters in the lay press.[70,71] The wider lay press coverage, important in maintaining the impetus of the discovery soon after its introduction, frequently referred to Robinson's pioneering work with ether anaesthesia. In addition, he demonstrated ether insensibility to leading members of London "society" whose support for the process would have carried no small weight with the general public.

Robinson also made a lengthy defence of ether anaesthesia when, a few months after its introduction, four deaths were attributed to its use during surgical operations. Robinson (anticipating John Snow's approach in later cases)[72] analysed each of the reports and was able to refute the criticism of ether by showing that the deaths were due to the surgical procedures themselves and not at all to the effects of the ether anaesthesia.[73] His views were published in Britain and — later — were given prominence in the United States.[73]

As if this was not enough, Robinson also wrote the world's first textbook on anaesthesia.[54] All these endeavours were performed in about four months, and in addition to Robinson's daily work as a dentist, since it was principally by his skill as a dentist that he had to earn his living.

Viewed with the perspective of history, the most important of all his many contributions to early anaesthesia was his ability to succeed with ether anaesthesia when others, and by that I mean a large number of others, had failed. It is difficult to underestimate the significance of Robinson's consistency and success in administering ether anaesthesia, especially where others had failed to do so. His expertise in this regard had a most reassuring effect on Robert Liston and others in Britain. As a result, Liston decided to persevere with the use of anaesthesia instead of following what may well have been his own inclinations and abandoning the process. That this effect on Liston was important for the acceptance of anaesthesia in Britain cannot be doubted.

It is not widely appreciated, however, that this was also an important consideration in America, where ether anaesthesia was not, at first, generally accepted outside Boston. When the news was received that ether had been enthusiastically adopted by leading surgeons in London, the faltering support for anaesthesia gained momentum in America, and the possibility that its use might be abandoned there, for a while at least, was removed. The evidence for this statement, which has not previously been widely publicised, can be found in the writings of three Americans and one Briton — each of whom had unquestionable authority for the views they put forward.

Professor John Collins Warren was, as we saw, the first surgeon in Boston to operate under ether anaesthesia. Warren dominated the American surgical scene[74] and was, at the time, excellently placed to tell of the beginnings of anaesthesia in the United States. He hinted at the problem when he wrote, "As is frequently the case in this country, the new home product was not received with the enthusiasm it would have been had the same emanated from one of the great European clinics."[7] George Hayward, who was Warren's second-in-command in Boston (and a few days after ether's first use succeeded Warren as Surgeon-in-Charge at the Massachusetts General Hospital),[75] was more precise, and proclaimed, "It is remarkable that the only spot in Christendom in which the discovery was received with coldness . . .was in our own country . . . The course of the scientific men of Europe was widely different."[75] Henry J. Bigelow was, as we saw at the beginning, a young surgeon newly on the staff of the Massachusetts General Hospital at the time of ether's introduction. later he achieved great eminence.[76] He was in a unique position to observe and record the events as they occurred. He wrote directly of the problem and said that, ". . . so soon as the discovery received the confirmation of European testimony . . . opposition rapidly subsided."[77] (To which it is only necessary to add that this confirmation came from Britain, rather than from any other European country.)

But the point was articulated most clearly by no less an authority than the meticulously observant Dr. John Snow — the world's first physician anaesthetist. Snow was thoroughly familiar with Robinson's work on anaesthesia, and kept himself informed of all the developments in America. He expressed his opinion in the following words, "Considerable opposition was made to the inhalation of ether in America, soon after its introduction, and it seemed likely to fall into disuse, when the news of its successful employment in the operations of Mr. Liston, and others in London, caused the practice of etherisation to revive. Mr. Robinson, dentist, gave much time and attention to the exhibition of ether in London on its first introduction, and was on the whole very successful. This was not generally the case, however, with other operators during the first six weeks of the new practice."[2]

Thus, James Robinson's efforts — judged by strictly impartial, authentic and impeccable contemporary accounts — sustained anaesthesia not only in Britain but, paradoxically, in the United States as well. I have no doubt that, without Robinson's intervention and energy, the early history of anaesthesia would have been very different indeed. My intention has not been to rewrite the history of the beginnings of anaesthesia in either Britain or America, nor to deny that credit which will always be due — and given — to other, and hitherto more famous names. I have wished only to highlight the crucially important part which James Robinson played in establishing anaesthesia, to reveal some overlooked pages in the history of its earliest days, and to explain why Robinson's pioneering achievements should be accorded due recognition.

James Robinson's life exemplified that most attractive notion — and arguably one of the most worthy, but elusive, of all personal qualities — the zeal of truly disinterested devotion to a cause. Rarely, I think, has a person who has done so much been so overlooked by so many for so long.

References

1. Rice N: *Trials of a public benefactor.* 1st edn. Boston: Pudney and Russell, New York, 1859.
2. Snow J: *On Chloroform and Other Anaesthetics (with a memoir of the author by Benjamin Ward Richardson).* London: Churchill, 1858.
3. Snow J: *On Narcotism by the Inhalation of Vapours (with an introductory essay by Richard H. Ellis).* London: Royal Society of Medicine, 1991.
4. Bigelow HJ: Insensibility during surgical operations produced by inhalation. *Boston Medical and Surgical Journal* 35: 309-17, 1846.
5. Jackson CT, Morton WTG: *Improvement in Surgical Operations.* United States' Patent Number 4848. 12 November 1846.
6. Morton WTG: *A Memoir to the Academy of Sciences at Paris on a New Use of Sulphuric Ether.* New York: Schuman, 1847.
7. Warren JC: *The Influence of Anaesthesia on the Surgery of the Nineteenth Century.* Privately printed: Boston, 1900.
8. Boott, F: Surgical operations performed during insensibility, produced by the inhalation of sulphuric ether. *Lancet* 1: 5-8, 1847.
9. Ellis RH: The introduction of ether anaesthesia to Great Britain. 2. A biographical sketch of Dr Francis Boott. *Anaesthesia* 32:197-208, 1977.
10. Annotation. A commemorative plaque for the site of the first anaesthetic given in England. *Anaesthesia* 39:84, 1984.
11. Annotation. Mr. Robinson. *The Forceps* 1:54, 1844.
12. O'Byrne W: *A naval biographical dictionary.* 1st edn. London: Murray, 1849.
13. Reader WJ: *Professional Men: the rise of the professional classes in nineteenth-century England.* 1st edn. London: Weidenfield and Nicolson, 1966.
14. Guy's Hospital, London. *General Entry of Pupils* 1823-1832. Folio 141, pupil number 478.
15. *The Registers of University College, London* 1829-1830.
16. *The Post Office London Director* 1846. London: Kelly.
17. Richards ND: Dentistry in England in the 1840s: the first indications of a movement towards professionalization. *Medical History* 12:137-52, 1968.
18. Robinson J: An Address to the Society of the Alumni of the Baltimore College of Dental Surgery. *American Journal of Dental Science* 10:225-56, 1850.
19. Editorial. *The Forceps* 1:230, 1844.
20. Hill A: *The History of the Reform Movement in the Dental Profession in England.* 1st edn. London: Trübner, 1877.
21. Editorial. *The Dental Review* 4:147-49, 1862.
22. Payne JL: Milestones in the History of British Dentistry, 1855-1860, 1877-1880, 1919 and After. *British Dental Journal* 45:137-42, 1924.
23. *The British Quarterly Journal of Dental Surgery* 1:1, 1843.

24. *The Forceps* 1:1, 1844.
25. Cope Z: *The Royal College of Surgeons of England: a History*. 1st edn. London, Anthony Blond, 1959.
26. Obituary. *The Dental Review* 4:189-91, 1862.
27. Annotation. The Baltimore College of Dental Surgery, *Boston Medical and Surgical Journal* 22:161, 1840.
28. *Management Committee Minutes of the Royal Free Hospital, London* 2:232, 1848.
29. Death of Mr. James Robinson. *British Journal of Dental Science* 5:146, 1862.
30. Donaldson A: *Personal communication.* Archives of the British Dental Association, London. 1988.
31. *The Post Office London Directory* 1846. London: Kelly. (as above).
32. Zuck D: Dr. Nooth and his Apparatus. *British Journal of Anaesthesia* 50:393-405, 1978.
33. Painless surgical operations: description of Robinson's inhaler. *the Medical Times* 15:290-91, 1847.
34. Medical Intelligence – Ether vapour apparatus. *London Medical Gazette* 4:167-68, 1847.
35. Annotation. Painless surgical operations. *The Medical Times* 15:271-73, 1847.
36. Squire W: On the introduction of ether inhalation as an anaesthetic in London. *Lancet* 2:1220-1, 1888.
37. Squire W: On the inhalation of the vapour of Ether, and the apparatus used for the purpose. *Pharmaceutical Journal and Transactions* 6:350-2, 1847.
38. Letter from Mr. J. Robinson. *The Medical Times* 15:273-4, 1847.
39. Editorial — Painless operations. *The Medical Times* 15:289-90, 1847.
40. Annotation. Operations without pain. *Lancet* 1:546, 1847.
41. Annotation. Painless surgical operations: description of Robinson's Inhaler. *The Medical Times* 15:290-91, 1847.
42. Correspondence. *The Medical Times* 15: 292, 1847.
43. Editorial. Painless operation. *The Medical Times* 15: 328, 1847.
44. Pharmaceutical Society Report. *Lancet* 1:73, 1847.
45. Westminster Medical Society Report. *Lancet,* 1:99-100, 1847.
46. Discovery of a new anaesthetic agent more efficient than sulphuric ether. *London Medical Gazette* 5: 934-7, 1847.
47. Robinson J: Practical remarks on the employment of chloroform in surgical operations. *Lancet* 1:135-6, 1848.
48. Annotation. Robinson's Inhaler. *Lancet* 2:655, 1847.
49. Snow J: On the inhalation of chloroform and ether. *Lancet* 1:177-80. 1848.
50. Snow J: *Three Manuscript Volumes of Casebooks* 1848-1858. London: The Royal College of Physicians.
51. Snow J: On narcotism by the inhalation of vapours, part 6. *London Medical Gazette* 7NS:614-9, 1848.
52. Annotation. Painless surgical operations. *The Medical Times* 15: 310-11, 1847.
53. Snow J: *On the Inhalation of the Vapour of Ether in Surgical Operations.* 1st edn. Churchill: London, 1847.
54. Robinson J: *A Treatise of the Inhalation of the Vapour of Ether.* 1st edn. Webster: London, 1847.
55. Review of A Treatise on the Inhalation of the Vapour of Ether by James Robinson. *London Medical Gazette* 4NS: 347, 1847.
56. Review of A Treatise on the Inhalation of the Vapour of Ether by James Robinson. *Lancet* 1:284, 1847.
57. Robinson J: *A Treatise on the Inhalation of the Vapour of Ether.* Facsimile edition, with an introductory essay by Richard H. Ellis. Eastbourne: Balliére Tindall, 1983.
58. Robinson J: Antidote for resuscitating patients after inhaling the vapour of ether. *London Medical Gazette* 4NS:610, 1847.
59. Sadleir M: *Blessington-D'Orsay: a Masquerade.* 1st edn. Constable: London. 1933.
60. Duffy D: *Eugenie and Napoleon III.* 1st edn. Collins: London, 1978.
61. The late Mr. James Robinson. *Lancet* 1:285-6, 1862.
62. Annotation. Death of Mr. James Robinson. *British Medical Journal* 1:269-70, 1862.
63. Obituary. *Lancet* 1:266, 1862.
64. Obituary – James Robinson. *The Dental Review* 4:189-91, 1862.
65. Dr. James Robinson. *The Dental Cosmos* 3:665-6, 1862.
66. Plomley F: Maidstone Ophthalmic Institution. *Lancet* 1:159, 1847.
67. Robinson J: Inhalation of aether in surgical operations. *Provincial Medical and Surgical Journal* 1:54, 1847.

68. Robinson J: Mode of employing ether vapour in surgical operations. *London Medical Gazette* 4NS:166-7, 1847.
69. Robinson J: On the inhalation of ether. *Lancet* 1:168-9, 1847.
70. *'The Observer.'* London: 3 January 1847.
71. *'The Morning Chronicle.'* London: 29 December 1846.
72. Snow J: On narcotism by the inhalation of vapours, part 6. *London Medical Gazette* 7NS:614-9, 1848.
73. Flagg JFB: *Ether and chloroform: their employment in surgery, dentistry, midwifery, therapeutics, etc.* 1st edn. Philadelphia: Lindsay and Blakiston, 1851.
74. Warren E: *The Life of John Collins Warren.* Boston: Ticknor and Fields, 1860.
75. Hayward G: *Surgical Reports and miscellaneous papers on medical subjects.* 1st edn. Boston: Phillips Sampson, 1855.
76. Bigelow WS: *A Memoir of Henry Jacob Bigelow.* Boston: Little Brown, 1900.
77. Bigelow HJ: *Surgical Anaesthesia: Addresses and other papers.* 1st edn. Boston: Little Brown, 1900.

TIMES OF THE SIGNS
The Origins of Charting

B. RAYMOND FINK
Department of Anesthesiology, University of Washington
Seattle, Washington, USA

We owe to Henry K. Beecher (1904-1973) our knowledge of the origin of the general anesthesia chart. He credited it to A.E. Codman, a physician at the Massachusetts General Hospital, to whom charting the patient's pulse rate during an operation was suggested in 1894 by his chief, Dr. F.B. Harrington. The practice was enthusiastically encouraged by a leading surgeon, none other than Harvey Cushing (1869-1939), and the first anesthesia record to be seen in public duly appeared in a paper by Cushing in 1902.[1] Beecher left open the larger question of the origin of medical charting in general. When did a graphic record of the vital signs become a routine part of a patient's daily care? The answer turns out to be especially interesting to anesthesiologists because it is bound up with a forerunner of the Cushing chart found in a long forgotten early clinical study of curare. The answer also has a broader significance, because charting implies measurement, and publication of systematically recorded measurements may be taken as marking the starting point of a natural science. By this criterion, the year 1902 saw the beginning of anesthesiology as a clinical science. But which was the birth date of scientific clinical medicine in general? There is no straightforward reply. Here is what my search has turned up.

I begin with a personal communication from R.J. Wolfe, which mentions that at the New England Hospital for Women and Children fever charts were part of the patients' records from 1872 onwards, but Wolfe does not find temperature charts, printed and called "clinical" charts, in the patients' records of the Massachusetts General Hospital until 1874; pulse and respiration charts were apparently not added until the early 1880s. However, these dates may merely reflect incomplete preservation of the archives, for Dr. Alan Van Poznak has sent me photocopied charts from patients' case notes from the New York Hospital dating back to 1866. One may surmise that these developments were in part the first-fruits of the revolution in nursing care which had begun at that time. The first school and home for "new style" nurses was established by Florence Nightingale (1820-1910) at St. Thomas's Hospital in London in 1860;[2] the first ones in the United States were opened in 1873.[3]

The next consideration is that measurement presupposes the existence of measuring instruments. For the present inquiry this means tracking the history of instruments for noninvasively determining patients' blood pressure, pulse and respiration rates, and temperature.

There is little difficulty in dating the non-invasive measurement of blood pressure. The first practical clinical instrument probably was the sphygmomanometer introduced by Samuel F. K. von Basch (1837-1905) in 1881 but it was unreliable, particularly when the blood pressure was low. The sphygmomanometer cuff, invented by Scipione Riva-Rocci (1863-1937) in 1896, enabled accurate detection of the systolic pressure during palpation of the pulse at the wrist, and this instrument was brought to the Massachusetts General Hospital by Cushing in 1898. The diastolic pressure became detectable with auscultation of the brachial artery at the elbow, as described by N.S. Korotkoff (1874-1920) in 1905.

Counting the pulse has a lengthier history, beginning with Johannes Kepler (1571-1630).[4] Galileo Galilei (1564-1642) discovered the isochronicity of the pendulum while still in his teens, by timing the large and small swings of a windblown lamp hanging in the cathedral of Pisa with his pulse. He put the discovery to work in his pulsilogon. This consisted of a weight suspended from the rim of a wheel by a string. The length of the string was adjusted by turning the wheel till the swing-time of the pendulum equaled the pulse interval; a pointer and scale indicated the pulse rate. Christiaan Huygens (1629-1695) contrived to regulate a weight-driven clock by a rod pendulum in 1656, and the spring-driven watch was in use before the end of the century. In 1707, Sir John Floyer (1649-1734) measured the pulse rate by counting its beats with a watch that ran for exactly 60 seconds and published his results in a classic book *The Physician's Pulse-Watch.* It seems that Floyer may have been the first ever to present observational data in the form of a table. A centered seconds hand was part of Harrison's fourth chronometer (1759) and a pocket watch with a seconds hand and a stop-start control goes back to 1780, but counting pulses could hardly become a medical or nursing routine before the advent of mass produced pocket watches, an American contribution of the 1840s. Timing the pulse by the watch was explicitly taught by Robert James Graves (1796-1853), of Dublin, in his *Clinical Lectures* of 1848.

The decisive developments in charting, however, were connected with the measurement and recording of body temperature. This, too, had been initiated by Galileo. His air thermometer consisted of a partially exhausted bulb that supported water in a graduated tube. When the bulb was placed in a person's mouth, the air expanded and changed the water level in the tube. Gabriel Daniel Fahrenheit (1686-1736) introduced the mercury thermometer in 1713, and Anders Celsius (1701-1744) the centigrade scale in 1742, but the thermometers of those days were nearly 30 cm (one foot) long and required five minutes to yield a measurement. A convenient clinical maximum-reading instrument was not designed until 1866, by Karl Ehrle (1843-1917).[5]

Surprisingly, almost as long delayed as the clinical thermometer was the practice of presenting measurements as a graph. Rectangular coordinates had been invented by René Descartes (1593-1650) but data continued to appear in tabular form for another two hundred years and graphs became popular only after the publication of Whewell's Book, "The Method of Curves" in 1840. Whewell advocated the use of graphs for the analysis of results and as a means of eliminating error and facilitating accurate deduction.[6] The very first medical publication containing a graph appears to have been a research article by Ludwig Traube (1818-1876), *Über Kristen und kritische Tage,* dated 1851/1852,[7] in which the course of fever was displayed as a twice daily record of temperature, but that practice probably did not become standard until 1868. In that year, for example, the doctoral thesis of Jeannot

Scheinesson, *Untersuchungen uber den Einfluss des Chloroforms auf die Warmeverhaltnisse des thierischen Organismus,* presented elaborate records of the temperature of numerous dogs, all in the form of tables. Again, the Edinburgh Medical Journal of 1868 contained an eleven-page article on Thermometric Observations on the Fevers of Children, by G. Stevenson Smith, a resident medical officer. It included no charts but presented the morning and evening temperatures for up to two weeks in 13 cases, exclusively in tables. The year 1868, however, also registered a major transition. E. Wegener of Stettin's article *zur Pathologie und Therapie des exanthemischen Typhus* displayed the daily temperature, pulse, and respiration rates both in individual tables and combined on six individual charts. That was the time when Louis Pasteur (1822-1895) was laying the foundations for the germ theory of communicable disease.

Carl August Wunderlich (1815-1877) published his famous book *On the Temperature in Diseases: a Manual of Medical Thermometry* in German in 1868 and an English translation appeared in 1871. Wunderlich began his studies of temperature in disease in 1853, but at the time these were ridiculed as useless subtlety,[7] and it was said of Wunderlich that his clinical visits were made more to the fever charts than to the patient. But the book did contain numerous temperature charts, and had a major influence on bedside practice. Wunderlich stressed that the patient's temperature should be recorded on a "ruled map" as a continuous line. He added that the frequency of the pulse and respirations should be similarly recorded but in different colours, and there should also be space for important notes.

Against this background, I wish to draw attention to a remarkable clinical study of curare by Voisin and Liouville,[8] dating from 1866. Curare was one of the first drugs to be the subject of a meticulous clinical study and report. Voisin and Liouville's investigation was published as a slender monograph, a fact that may help to explain why it remained virtually unnoticed. It described 10 cases of status epilepticus treated by subcutaneous injections of purified curare and included charts that graphed the pulse, temperature, and respirations of each patient at thirty minute intervals for eight hours, and twice daily thereafter for another five days. To historians of anesthesiology two points of particular interest are, first, that the study documented the safe clinical use of curare at the Hospice Bicêtre in Paris, 75 years before it was introduced into the operating room and second, that charting of the patients' vital signs in response to a drug antedated Codman and Cushing by thirty years. Incidentally, Cushing's initiative encountered so much resistance that he declared this to be "one of the most interesting illustrations on record against the introduction of an instrument of precision into clinical use. It is precisely what happened in the case of the thermometer, the stethoscope, the X-ray, indeed of the watch itself." The reason for the opposition? An editorial in the British Medical Journal spoke volumes: "by such methods we pauperize our senses and weaken clinical acuity."[9] How profoundly attitudes have changed.

But what effected the change? The short answer is the measurements themselves. For measurement is the beginning of science, and science has more than once transformed man's entire perspective of himself and his relation to the universe. It happened after Copernicus placed the sun at the center of the solar system, and again after Darwin proposed that the panoply of life arose from small inherited variations accumulated by natural selection. Anesthesiology, so named in 1939, probably uses measurement more intensively than any other field of clinical medicine.

References

1. Cushing HW: On the avoidance of shock in major amputations by cocainization of large nerve trunks preliminary to their division, with observations on blood-pressure changes in surgical cases. Annals Surg 36: 321-343, 1902.
2. Singer C: A Short History of Medicine. Oxford, Clarendon Press, p. 298, 1944.
3. Garrison FH: An Introduction to the History of Medicine. Philadelphia, WB Saunders, p. 653, 1913.
4. Fishman AP, Richards DW (Editors): Circulation of the Blood. New York, Oxford University Press, p. 77, 1964.
5. Diepgen P: Geschichte der Medizin. Berlin, de Gruyter, Vol. 2, part 2, p. 161, 1965.
6. Tilling R: Br J Hist Science 8: 193-212, 1975.
7. Ebstein E: Dreihundert Jahre klinischer Thermometrie. Klin Wochenschr 7: 950-953, 1928.
8. Voisin A, Liouville H: Études sur le curare. Paris, Masson, 17pp., 1866.
9. Major RH: The history of taking the blood pressure. Ann Medical Hist 2: 47-55, 1930.

THE FIRST "SPINAL" ANESTHESIA
A Lucky Failure

B. RAYMOND FINK
Department of Anesthesiology University of Washington
Seattle, Washington, USA

When J. Leonard Corning (1859-1930) unintentionally produced the first spinal – or perhaps epidural – anesthesia in 1885,[1] a kind providence must have been watching over his patient. His plan was to treat the patient's neurological complaint by an ingenious method he had invented for the occasion. Corning intended to apply medication locally to the spinal cord by depositing cocaine between the spines of two lower thoracic vertebrae, so that the venous drainage from the interspinous space would carry the drug into the cord. It was a clever if fallacious scheme, but he evidently thought that he had succeeded in carrying it out. This much is familiar.

What has gone generally unremarked is the lucky escape of the patient. The British Pharmacopeia of 1885 declared the maximum dose of cocaine hydrochlorate (sic) to be 1 grain (65 mg), without specifying a route of administration. Corning's patient received two injections, each of cocaine 55 mg, in the space of a few minutes, a total of 110 mg, but survived without suffering any of the dire consequences to which his physician's insouciance about dosage and spinal anatomy had exposed him. It is not as if Corning had not been cautioned. The New York Medical Journal, the journal which published Corning's report on October 31, 1885 had on December 6 of the previous year, ended its leading article "THE NEW ANESTHETIC" with the following wise warning:

> no doubt much yet remains to be done in the way of experiment and observation before the sphere of the new anesthetic may be defined, and it may be prudent for those who may undertake to furnish us with these data not to count too much on the innocuousness of the drug, for it should be noted that Dr. Hall (NYMJ Nov 21, 1884) experienced marked constitutional symptoms from an injection of thirty-two minims of a four-per-cent solution of the drug.

Corning's temerity contrasts strongly with the measured approach of August Bier (1869-1941), who performed the first deliberate spinal surgical anesthetic in 1898.[2] Bier, of course, had the benefit of using the lumbar puncture procedure devised by his colleague Heinrich Quincke (1842-1922) a few years earlier. Also, the then current German Pharmacopeia of 1890 specified that the maximum dose of cocaine hydrochloride was 50 mg. Bier instilled cocaine 15 mg into the subarachnoid space of his first case. He decreased the dose to 10 mg for patients 2, 3, and 5, and to 5 mg for patients 4 and 6 as well as for the experiment on his assistant Dr. Hildebrand, all with satisfactory effect.

Comparing the two reports, we may be thankful that Corning's series was limited to one. His anatomy was imaginative, the drug dosage was unsafe, and his injection technique could not tell him whether or not the needle-point was in a vein or even in the subarachnoid space. It is fortunate that his bright idea did not end in circulatory or respiratory arrest, for that could have delayed the advent of surgical spinal anesthesia for a long, long time.

References

1. Corning LJ: Spinal anesthesia and local medication of the cord. New York Med J 42:317-19 (Sept 19), 1885.
2. Bier A: Ueber einen neuen Weg Localanaesthesie an den Gliedmassen zu erzeugen. Arch klin Chirung 86:1007-1016, 1900.

DR. GEORGE MARTINE AND A BRONCHOTOME
St. Andrews 1730

A.L. FORREST
University Department of Anaesthesia
Dundee, Scotland

My interest in Dr. George Martine began a year ago when a plaque was erected in the old University town of St. Andrews to commemorate his life and work. He attended the University in 1715, obtaining his M.D. in 1725. He made interesting observations on the circulation of an animal, noting the altered dimensions of the blood vessels, in the velocity of the current, and the pressure of the blood, in a paper published in 1740, perhaps a forerunner of the fight or flight reaction. He did much research of the temperature, giving an admirable account of the early history of the thermometer, and he was familiar with the concept of absolute zero perhaps one hundred years before Kelvin.

Martine was also a skillful surgeon and in the "Philosophical Transactions" of 1730, he described the operation of bronchotome which he performed in St. Andrews to save the life of a young lad who was all of a sudden taken ill with a violent trouble in his throat. He presented with great pain, dyspnea, and an impossibility of swallowing either liquids or solids; everything returned forcibly by the mouth and nose when he made an effort to get it down. Martine was sure that the seat of the disease was in the larynx and the fibers common to it, and the top of the gullet. As far as he could see, there was nothing wrong with the tonsil or the other parts in view, and there was no external tumor of the larynx. The frequency and strength of the pulse was not considerably changed. Despite repeated bloodings, blistering between the shoulders and cupping, the patient asked for any experiment to save his life. And so Martine pierced his windpipe and inserted a leaden pipe, as was used for tapping in the dropsy. Within four days his breathing was perfectly easy, and his swallowing almost so, and the cannula was removed.

One can only speculate at the cause of this respiratory obstruction. The presentation of severe pain, dyspnea, and total dysphagia could fit in with epiglottitis. It is unlikely that Martine was able to view the larynx indirectly at that time. A cyst of the larynx must also be considered, but the cyst would have remained by the fourth day and interfered with unobstructed breathing. Alternatively, the pharynx or trachea can be affected by diphtheria without obvious infection of the fauces. Palatal palsy occurs about the tenth day with regurgitation of fluids through the nose. Diphtheritic involvement of the larynx can result in stridor or respiratory obstruction, but the patient would have been much more ill, often with a tachycardia and hypotension.

Of further interest was the fact that, when mucus blocked the cannula in the trachea, a layman proposed "to make the pipe double, or one within the other; that the instrument might safely and easily be taken out and cleaned when necessary, without any molestation to the patient." This was almost certainly the first description of an inner cannula accompanying a tracheotomy tube, although there is no proof that Martine used it in this case. It is clear that he was surprised by the secretions which derived from the trachea.

The word tracheotomy did not replace bronchotome until the early 19th century. Goodall records only 28 successful tracheotomies being performed before 1825. Though much had been written about the operation, few surgeons had actual experience of it or had achieved a successful outcome.

Clearly, Dr. Martine's operation, performed in St. Andrews all those years ago, was a landmark in the treatment of respiratory obstruction in a young patient.

THE STELLENBOSCH MACHINE
The Independent Design of an Anesthesia Machine

PATRICK A. FOSTER
Penn State University,
Hershey, Pennsylvania, USA

The chance to design, build and use successfully a major piece of anesthesia equipment independently of major producers is worth documenting, if only because anesthesia machine design is well ingrained in the annals of anesthesia, and since the product appeared to have anticipated many of the standard practices of today.

The opportunity arose in the early 1950's when the new University of Stellenbosch teaching hospital complex was planned in Cape Town. It was to be a 2000 bed hospital and the largest in the southern hemisphere under one roof, with 50 operating rooms, each having its own anesthesia induction room, along with altogether 250 recovery beds. A dental school and outpatient dental hospital were to be incorporated into the medical school.

It thus seemed feasible to amortize the cost of a revised anesthesia machine design in the anticipated order of well over 100 units. Colleagues in the local and regional branches of the South African Society of Anaesthetists were asked what they disliked or found lacking in existing equipment and for their suggestions for improvement.

A look at the 1950 state of the art Boyle's machine explains better than words the motivation. The thought of having to work with such equipment for the next 25 years — the usual life of a machine — was unthinkable; it was so disorganized. And it bore no resemblance to Boyle's original concept. Boyle was a London anesthesiologist who trained under Clover in the era when gases, if used at all, were "hand made." He helped lead British practice into the age of the gas and oxygen cylinder machine, using Gwathmey's original pattern as a starting point. His 1919 vintage "outfit" — simply cylinders and vaporizers on wheels, had an elegant simplicity that was retained when a dressing trolley with back bar was used to mount components. In fact, there had been little progress in design in the 25 years after Boyle's

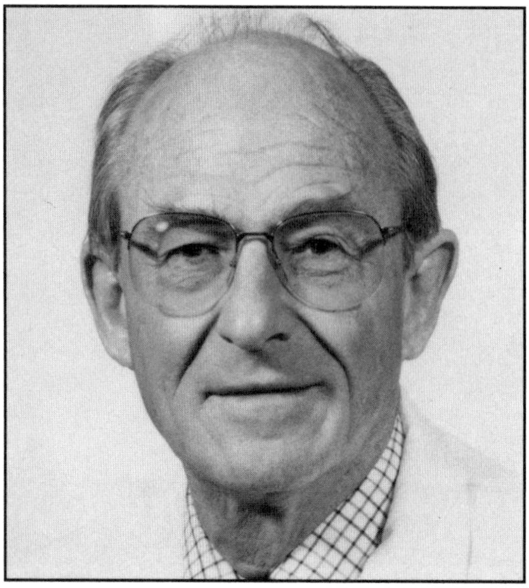

Fig. 1.

1925 model until the 1939 war changed priorities. This is beautifully depicted in a painting that hangs in the medical school of the University of Cape Town, done by a war artist in the western desert campaign about 1942, showing the continuing simplicity of basic anesthetic equipment.

By the late 1940's, the concept had become a disordered overload of components. The problems of the 1950 machine were not so much in the components as in the random clutter in which they were haphazardly scattered over a standard OR trolley. The pattern of this trolley dated from the previous century when the average stature of the common person was 6 to 9 inches shorter, and so its dimensions no longer applied. In fact, the evolution of the design seemed totally to have lost direction. This was perceived to be the consequence of the unrestrained input by engineers without insight into the anesthetic process or knowledge of the inside of a hospital. One could foresee that, if some design conventions were not soon established, as for instance apply in automobiles, the life support anesthesia machine could become a killing machine. The urgent need, it was decided, was for user input to tidy up the design by offering some ergonomically acceptable logic for the layout and general construction, if possible anticipating the important anesthesia technology then on the developmental horizon. Component design was considered a secondary goal: definition of function, not engineering detail, is the appropriate role for the user. Guidance in general layout principles came, amongst others, from the writings of Le Corbusier, the French architect who had reemphasized in his buildings and their furniture or their engines that the basic module must be man, reflected in the reach of an arm or the span of a hand, the height of a work surface when standing or sitting, or what a normal visual field can comfortably scan. The engineers had overlooked this.

In today's jargon, this was to be a *Rationale* for an *Anesthesia Work Station*, which can be roughly defined as a gas machine with ventilator which could incorporate any of the various monitors, data processors and recorders, infusion devices, and suction needed for routine anesthesia.

A number of "new" concepts were proposed. Some were labeled so "revolutionary" as to be unworkable (but they worked).

1. Considerably increased work surface areas were called for at correct heights; the prolongation of surgery had made the option of sitting as well as standing during anesthesia important (and would incidentally allow paraplegics to use the machine). The dimensions of the trolley were rewritten to stay within the floor area occupied by the Boyle's machine, with at least a quadrupling of the usable working surface. A writing surface was provided for the sitting person.
2. Boyle, being left-handed, had apparently designed his trolley model for left-handed use. The layout was reconfigured for the right-handed user, which implied that the machine should be positioned near the patient's right shoulder and the flowmeters repositioned to the right-hand back corner of the machine, as viewed from the front.
3. The machine was to be considered primarily as a gas delivery system that would provide accommodation for other

functions. Zones were allocated for these functions on the proposed machine trolley so that like functions with their relevant displays could be grouped together.

4. The principle of always placing displays above controls was accepted (so that you could see what you were doing was being accomplished). In turn, this led to the organization of a standardized gas delivery system display into a Dashboard: input gas pressures, flowmeters, and feedback information on circuit pressure and content. A standard layout for gas delivery controls was proposed that would allow the controls for 5 gases, 2 vaporizers, emergency oxygen and ventilator to be placed into the span of a hand. These controls were placed below the work surface so as to be usable sitting as well as standing.
5. All gas lines were color-coded, with their control knobs both touch and color-coded. There was at that time no accepted touch code standard, so that one was devised.
6. The machine frame was designed to be easily cleaned. Stainless steel side panels could be hosed down and all breathing circuit components, except the flowmeter head and reserve cylinders, were mounted inboard to allow this.
7. Entonox had recently been introduced and was accepted as the back-up pipeline should either the oxygen or nitrous oxide line fall, as it could supply an adequate concentration of either gas to continue safely. Back-up cylinders were mounted on the rear of the frame for easy changing during use, while the valve spindles were accessible to the user from the front.
8. A monitoring rack was provided above the flowmeter dashboard at standing eye level, and later inclined to improve visibility sitting. An area within the machine was allocated for back-up batteries and data processing.
9. Operation in darkness was catered for by beta-light illumination of flowmeters and elsewhere (these give a constant light output for 25 years). By placing the oxygen control in the right corner of the frame and the gas outlet in the left, one could quickly orient oneself to the machine in total darkness.

First prototypes of the machine were built by the hospital authority workshop and user tested. Thereafter, tenders were called from commercial producers. The first of these test models was received in 1968 for clinical trials. Final units were delivered from 1970 on and have been in use since with minor modifications. Altogether, about 100 units were supplied to the Stellenbosch and other teaching hospitals, and somewhere near 200 residents have trained with this machine.

Fig. 2. Proposed designated zones on anesthesia machine frame.

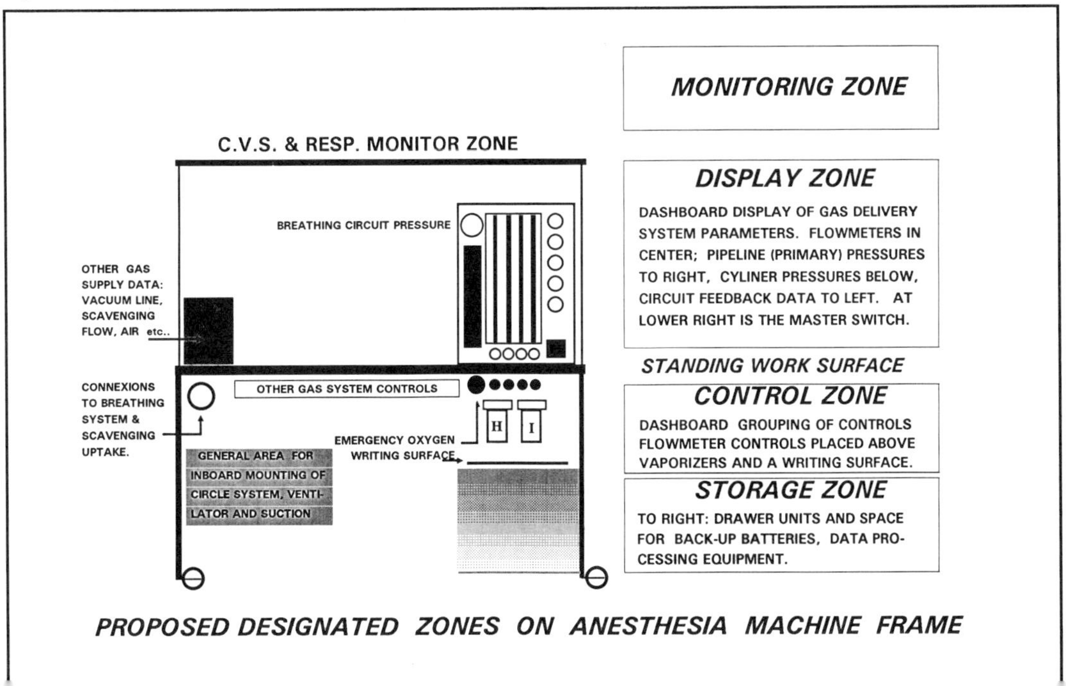

HOW QUALITY ASSURANCE INFLUENCED THE DEVELOPMENT OF ANESTHESIA IN 19TH CENTURY SCOTLAND

ELIZABETH A.M. FROST
Scarsdale, New York, USA

During the 50 years that followed its first public demonstration, anesthesia was administered by almost any medical or paramedical person —usually one with minimal or even no training. Calamities were not uncommon, but when one compared the risks of anesthesia in the hands of an untrained person to the horror of surgical pain, any anesthesia was usually selected.

A series of events in Glasgow towards the end of the 19th century focused the public attention on anesthetic administration. The presence at that time of an educator and clinician, Sir William Macewen, a man certainly not averse to making major public stands, was enough to launch what was probably the first organized survey of anesthetic teaching, administration, and operating room reporting. It was his concern for the safety of his patients that prompted a nationwide questionnaire analysis of the responses, and implementation of changes in daily operating room practice.

Several circumstances led up to the establishment of the committee that was to conduct this early quality assurance program. Professor Joseph Lister, the pioneer of antiseptic surgery, was University Professor of Surgery in Glasgow from 1860-9. During that time he wrote three papers on anesthesia.[1] He emphasized the dangers of chloroform administration, especially in the sitting position, and advocated monitoring of respiration rather than the pulse. In a letter to a fellow student, J. T. Clover, which is preserved in the archives of the University of Vancouver, he wrote: "With regard to giving chloroform, increasing experience has only served to give me increased confidence in the old way of the folded towel."

Professor Lister was vehemently opposed to the introduction of any anesthetic apparatus and to the emergence of specialist anesthetists. He strongly believed that his own clinical clerks were superior to any other trained chloroformists.[2] Shortly after his departure to

Edinburgh, one of his students, William Macewen, was appointed Surgeon in Charge of Wards at the Glasgow Royal Infirmary. Lister had already left Glasgow when Macewen graduated in Medicine in 1869. However, Macewen had contacts with Lister while he was a student dresser in Lister's department, and these contacts were a powerful influence on his choice of a surgical career and on many of his academic interests.[3] One might have thought that this influence would have extended also to the management of anesthesia, but the pupil had different ideas an priorities from the teacher.

Macewen had developed an early interest in the treatment of laryngeal obstruction and had devised a series of tubes that could be passed orally. On July 5, 1878, he intubated the trachea of a conscious patient prior to the induction of chloroform anesthesia. In 1879, at a meeting of the Glasgow Medico-Chirurgical Society, he delivered a paper on his work.[4] The case reports were published the following year in the British Medical Journal which was considered a more prestigious publication.[5]

Lister had emphasized the inherent dangers in anesthesia; Macewen stressed its importance and the solemn responsibility of the administrator. He differed from Lister by strenuously encouraging specialization. He insisted on training in anesthesia for all medical students assigned to his service and he gave systematic lectures and practical instruction. He awarded a certificate of proficiency after a written examination and practical test of 12 chloroform administrations given under his supervision. The lectures, practical instruction and certification process was a personal one mandated by Professor Macewen only for those who worked in his wards and was not generally required of all medical students. In fact, experience in the administration of anesthetics was not a requirement at all. In contrast, prior to graduation from the University of Glasgow, all students had to obtain a certificate of proficiency in vaccination!

Macewen's persistence in emphasizing the need for anesthetic training was repaid, and on October 9, 1882, Mr. McEwan, Chairman of the Glasgow Royal Infirmary Board of Governors, proposed at the quarterly meeting that the pathologist should deliver a course of lectures on anesthetics at the beginning of each winter session, and that all assistants should hold a certificate attesting to knowledge of this subject. The resolutions were amended by the omission of "pathologist" in November 1882.[6] The medical staff approved these minutes a few weeks later.

However, progress in the mandating of training in anesthesia was not rapid enough. Unfortunately, early in 1883, a resident (a term rather loosely used to denote either a medical student or recently graduated physician who lived in the hospital) administered chloroform to an elderly patient who died during the operation. Mr. McEwan wrote to the "Glasgow Herald" (the principal newspaper in Western Scotland), publicizing the case and he stated that, under no circumstances should residents untrained in anesthetic administration be permitted to administer chloroform.[7] Two days later, two members of the staff of the Royal Infirmary, Mr. James Morton and Dr. Leishman, replied in terms that cast severe doubt on McEwan's professional competence and even his right to exist. In defense of the institution, they argued that anesthetics had been safely administered to many by untrained personnel and that surgeons should not be hampered by petty rules and regulations requiring additional paper work. The bitter debate continued for several weeks, progressing to calumny, and was epitomized in a letter signed "Former Resident." — "Mr. McEwan has occupied the Director's Chair for twenty years and now feels able to sit in judgment on the relative merits of chloroform and ether. If he lives much longer, and his knowledge grows in the same ratio, he will soon be able to dispose of the surgical staff altogether."

A certain amount of bravery (or stupidity) was clearly demonstrated. Today, the chief executive officer of any hospital (let alone the major university hospital in the largest city of a country) would probably not publicly disclose such poor practices; staff physicians, who wished to remain as such, would not defame their employer; and most newspapers might be loath to print a frankly acrimonious exchange.

However, good came from this incident. A special committee of the Managers of the Glasgow Royal Infirmary was formed on March 1, 1883. Under the leadership of Professors W.T. Gairdner and John Cleland, and firmly supported by Sir William Macewen, a letter was sent on March 16, 1883 to medical superintendents of 40 hospitals and medical schools in the United Kingdom inquiring as to their practice in the administration of chloroform. A questionnaire, attached, sought information as to the existence of formal regulations governing the use and administration of anesthetics, availability of special instruction, the qualifications of persons administering anesthetics, and presence of specialist anesthetists. The institutions that responded are listed in Table I. The response rate was almost 50 percent (out of 40 hospitals surveyed) and was as follows:

1. *Are there formal regulations as to the use of chloroform?*
   Yes (8) No (10)
   (No regulations in Scotland)
2. *Is special instruction provided?*
   Yes (9) No (9)
   (Instruction was available in Edinburgh, Aberdeen, Leeds, Dublin and several of the London hospitals)
3. *Are resident medical and surgical clerks permitted to administer chloroform unsupervised?*
   Yes (16) No (2)
   (Only Dundee and Dublin required that anaesthetics be given only if one of the consultant staff was present)
4. *Are there resident medical officers?*
   Nine hospitals used assistants as chloroformists, 3 used principal officers, 4 allowed both and 2 did not answer the question
5. *Are resident medical officers legally qualified to practice medicine and surgery?*
   Yes (16) No response (2)
   Has instruction in anaesthesia been a requirement of qualification for appointment?
   No requirement (4) No response (2)
6. *Can assistants, not legally qualified in surgical wards give anaesthetics?*
   Yes (6) No (11)
   No response (1)
7. *Is a specialist appointed for the administration of anaesthetics?*
   Yes (4), including Aberdeen, Guy's St. Thomas' and King's College Hospital - the latter 3 in London
   No (11) No response (1)
8. *Have fatal accidents occurred?*
   In 13 hospitals, known fatalities had occurred.
   Have they modified the practice of anaesthetic administration?
   In no hospital was practice changed by untoward anaesthetic events.

After Tabulation of the results of the survey, the convenor, John Ure, recommended the following proposals to the managers of the Glasgow Royal Infirmary.

1. All new assistants shall be instructed by the Surgeon in anaesthetic administration and this instruction should include practical demonstrations.
2. Prior to appointment, assistants should demonstrate to the managers of the hospital evidence of anaesthetic instruction.
3. After satisfactory completion of the course of instruction, the Surgeon will give the assistant a certificate to be given to the hospital Superintendent.
4. No unqualified assistant (that is, house officers who have not satisfactorily completed a course in anaesthetics) can operate or administer anaesthesia unsupervised.
5. In the case of a dire emergency, any qualified assistant may act appropriately in the absence of the Surgeon. All such cases must be reviewed, however.
6. The Superintendent may act in the absence of the Physician or Surgeon in Charge.
7. All anaesthetics in the Surgeon's absence must be entered in the Operation Book.
8. Anaesthetic deaths are reportable and must be investigated.
9. An operating log must be kept which contains the names of patients, operations performed and results. This record should be completed immediately after the operation. Outpatient accident cases should also be recorded.

This resolution, which corresponded substantially with the original McEwan proposals, was adopted on March 7, 1883.[6]

Sir William Macewen immediately insisted that his previous teaching practices, which had been mandated only for his clerks, be required of all medical students. By 1884, at the beginning of each session, a week was devoted to systematic lectures on anesthetics, including a review of Macewen's experimental work.[7] Each student was required to administer at least 12 chloroform anesthetics under Macewen's direct supervision.[8] In so doing, he certainly disproved Silk's statement in 1892 that there was "no systematic instruction in anesthesia in Scotland, Ireland and the provinces."[9]

Although, as a result of this survey and the efforts of Sir William Macewen, anesthetic training was firmly established in Glasgow, it was not generally the case in the rest of Great Britain. In the remainder of the country the struggle, by the General Medical Council of Great Britain, to force compulsory training in anesthetics continued. It was not until 1911, thanks largely to the efforts of F.W. Hewitt, that all medical examining bodies demanded evidence of satisfactory instruction in anesthetics.[9]

In the United States, the situation was worse. Although the American Board of Anesthesiology was established in 1941, formal training for all medical students has been only slowly accepted and is still not universal. Even now, in many states, supervision of anesthetics administered by nurses may fall to a surgeon who is not required to have any anesthetic training at all.

I gratefully acknowledge the assistance of Dr. Derek Dow, Archivist, University of Glasgow, in the preparation of this paper.

TABLE I

Of the 40 hospitals surveyed, responses were received from 18.

Scotland	Edinburgh Royal Infirmary Glasgow Western Infirmary Dundee Royal Infirmary Aberdeen Royal Infirmary Perth Infirmary Greennock Royal Infirmary
London	St. Thomas' Hospital Guy's Hospital Westminster Hospital King's College Hospital University College Hospital St. Mary's Hospital
Rest of England	Manchester Royal Infirmary Liverpool Royal Infirmary Leeds General Infirmary Bristol Royal Infirmary Sheffield Royal Infirmary
Ireland	St. Vincent's Hospital, Dublin

Hospitals responding to the questionnaire sent out from the Board of the Glasgow Royal Infirmary.

References

1. Lister J: On Anaesthetics. Part 1, 1861; Part 2, 1870; Part 3, 1882. Holmer's System of Surgery. Volume 3, 3rd edition, London 1883.
2. Watt OM: Glasgow Anaesthetists 1846-1946. James Pender, Clydebank. 1962, pp 15-17.
3. Miller JD: William Macewen: Master of Surgery. Virginia Medical 106:363-8, 1979.
4. Macewen W: The introduction of tubes into the larynx through the mouth instead of tracheotomy and laryngotomy. Glasgow Med J; 9:72-4; and 12:218-21, 1879.
5. Macewen W: Clinical observations on the introduction of tracheal tubes by the mouth instead of performing tracheotomy or laryngotomy. Br Med J; 2-122-4, (July 24), 163-265, (July 25), 1880.
6. Board of Managers Reports, Glasgow Royal Infirmary 1882-83, Archives, University of Glasgow.
7. Watt OM: Glasgow Anaesthetics 1846-1946. Clydebank: James Pender, 1962,; 15.
8. Macewen W: Presidential introduction to a discussion on anesthesia. Glasgow Med J: 34:321, 1890.
9. James CDT: Sir William Macewen and anaesthesia. Anaesthesia; 29:743-53, 1974.

REMINISCENCES ABOUT ARTHUR LÄWEN
An Extraordinary Pioneer in Anesthesia

M. GOERIG, and J. SCHULTE am ESCH
Department of Anaesthesiology
University Hamburg, Germany

The young Läwen already in 1901 had with curarization, intubation and artificial respiration the keys for modern anesthesiology in his hands." With these words in an obituary, the surgeon, Professor K.H. Bauer (1890-1978) of Heidelberg, praised only a few of his colleague's contributions to anesthesiology.[1] "Läwen was in many ways a man before his time." Bauer's appraisal is true even today. One needs to consider the medical accomplishments of Arthur Läwen and in particular his pain alleviating methods of local anesthesia. It is nearly impossible to present fully the range of his anesthesia investigations and developments. One can only attempt a brief presentation of a few of the more important contributions of an anesthesiologist who always had the patient in mind.

Biography

Arthur Läwen was born on February 6, 1876, in the German city of Waldheim in the county of Saxonia (Fig. 1).[2] Having studied medicine in Rostock, Freiburg, Munich and Leipzig, he received his medical license in 1900.[3,4] In the same year he began his surgical training at the Lutheran Hospital of Leipzig, where his teacher was Heinrich Braun (1862-1934), a pioneer of local anesthesia worldwide.

Realizing the talent of his young assistant, Braun arranged a residency for him under Friedrich von Trendelenburg (1844-1924), who was at that time head of the department of surgery at the Leipzig University clinic. Both Trendelenburg and Braun, who were renowned for their contributions to the development of anesthesiology, awoke in the young Läwen curiosity for the unsolved questions of this specialty. (Fig. 2, 3a, 3b)[2,5,6,7] It is therefore not surprising that many of his publications appeared in the years of his residency, paving the way for his future direction.[8-15] After having specialized in 1908, he was nominated professor and a few years later, in 1913, was appointed as the head of surgery to the newly built St. George Hospital in Leipzig.[2]

During the first world war, he had surgical experience as a military officer of the German

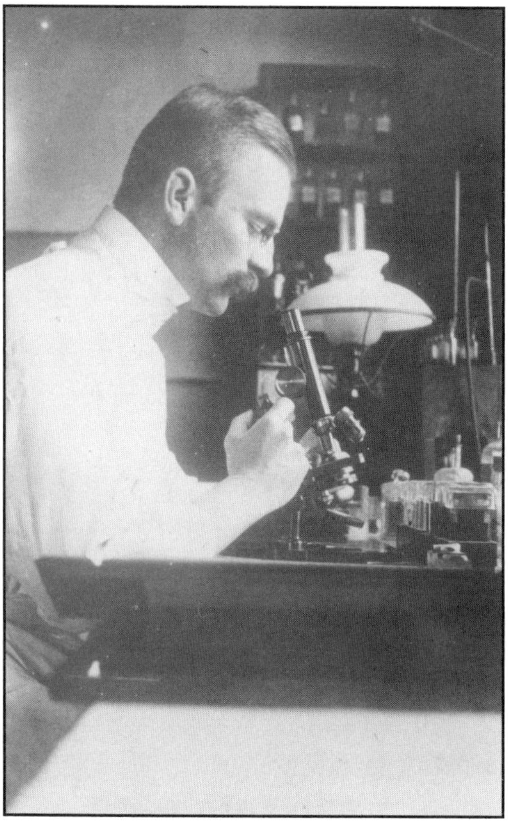

Fig. 1. Arthur Läwen (1876-1958).[2]

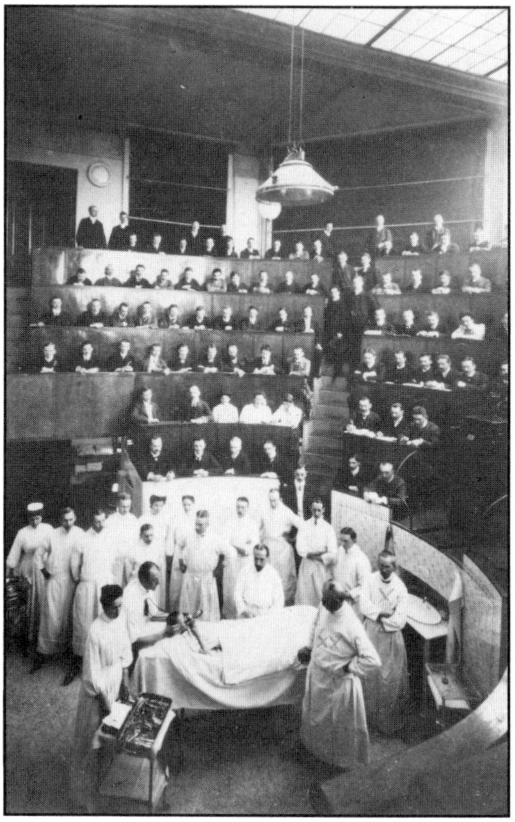

Fig. 2. Arthur Läwen * in the operating theater of the Surgical Department of the University Clinic Leipzig: Please note: (in front) Professor Friedrich von Trendelenburg**, ca 1912.[37]

Fig. 3a. Certificate of Heinrich Braun for Arthur Läwen, 26.12.1909.[2]

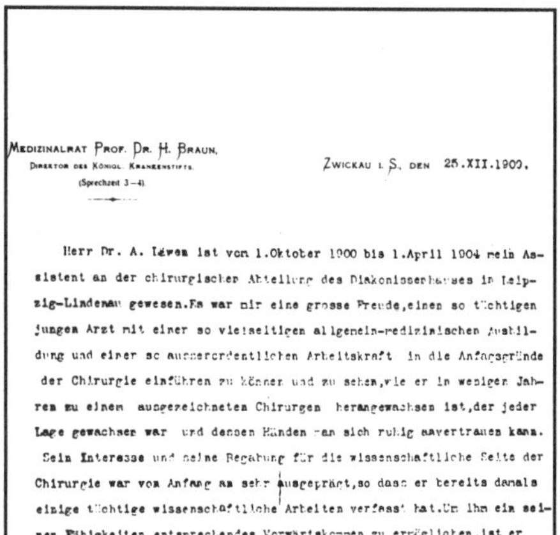

MEDIZINALRAT PROF. DR. H. BRAUN,
DIREKTOR DES KÖNIGL. KRANKENSTIFTS.
(Sprechzeit 3–4)

ZWICKAU I. S., DEN 25.XII.1909.

Herr Dr. A. Läwen ist vom 1.Oktober 1900 bis 1.April 1904 mein Assistent an der chirurgischen Abteilung des Diakonissenhauses in Leipzig-Lindenau gewesen. Es war mir eine grosse Freude, einen so tüchtigen jungen Arzt mit einer so vielseitigen allgemein-medizinischen Ausbildung und einer so ausserordentlichen Arbeitskraft in die Anfangsgründe der Chirurgie einführen zu können und zu sehen, wie er in wenigen Jahren zu einem ausgezeichneten Chirurgen herangewachsen ist, der jeder Lage gewachsen war und dessen Händen man sich ruhig anvertrauen kann. Sein Interesse und seine Begabung für die wissenschaftliche Seite der Chirurgie war von Anfang an sehr ausgeprägt, so dass er bereits damals einige tüchtige wissenschaftliche Arbeiten verfasst hat. Um ihm ein seinen Fähigkeiten entsprechendes Vorwärtskommen zu ermöglichen, ist er im Jahre 1904 auf mein Betreiben und auf meine Empfehlung in der chirurgischen Universitätsklinik in Leipzig als Assistenzarzt angestellt worden.

Prof. H. Braun

Fig. 3b. Certificate of Friedric von Trendelenburg for Arthur Läwen, 6.2.1911.[2]

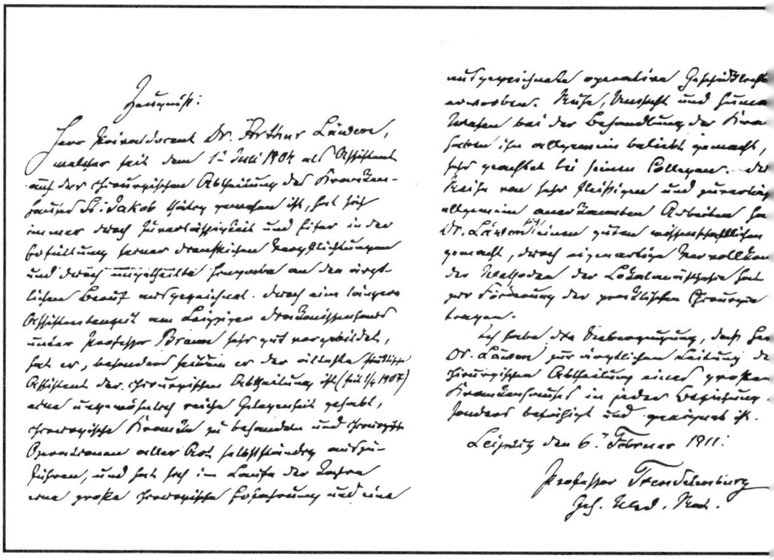

Zeugnis:

Herr Privatdozent Dr. Arthur Läwen, welcher seit dem 1. Juli 1904 als Assistent auf der chirurgischen Abteilung des Krankenhauses St. Jakob tätig gewesen ist, ...

Leipzig den 6. Februar 1911.

Professor Trendelenburg
Geh. Med. Rat.

Medical Corps and later wrote a chapter in a standard textbook on the topic of war wounds (Fig. 4).[2,16,17] In 1920, he became Professor of surgery at the Marburg University, where he remained until 1928 when he moved to Königsberg.[18] Fleeing from the invading Russian troops in February, 1945, he settled in the home of his daughter who lived in the West German Lüneburger Heide. Shortly before his death, the German Surgical Society nominated him as an honorary member, a recognition which he claimed to be the highlight of his life (Fig. 5).[2] Arthur Läwen died on January 30, 1958, a living shadow of the great scientist he had been some years earlier.[2,4]

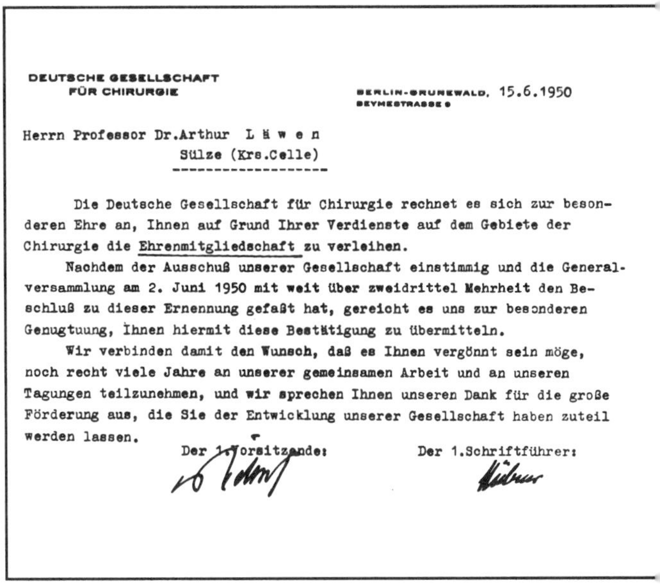

DEUTSCHE GESELLSCHAFT
FÜR CHIRURGIE

BERLIN-GRUNEWALD, 15.6.1950
BEYMESTRASSE 9

Herrn Professor Dr.Arthur L ä w e n
Sülze (Krs.Celle)

Die Deutsche Gesellschaft für Chirurgie rechnet es sich zur besonderen Ehre an, Ihnen auf Grund Ihrer Verdienste auf dem Gebiete der Chirurgie die Ehrenmitgliedschaft zu verleihen.

Nachdem der Ausschuß unserer Gesellschaft einstimmig und die Generalversammlung am 2. Juni 1950 mit weit über zweidrittel Mehrheit den Beschluß zu dieser Ernennung gefaßt hat, gereicht es uns zur besonderen Genugtuung, Ihnen hiermit diese Bestätigung zu übermitteln.

Wir verbinden damit den Wunsch, daß es Ihnen vergönnt sein möge, noch recht viele Jahre an unserer gemeinsamen Arbeit und an unseren Tagungen teilzunehmen, und wir sprechen Ihnen unseren Dank für die große Förderung aus, die Sie der Entwicklung unserer Gesellschaft haben zuteil werden lassen.

Der 1.Vorsitzende:

Der 1.Schriftführer:

Fig. 5. Honorary Membership of the German Surgical Society in 1950.[2]

Läwen's Contributions to the Development of Local Anesthesia

As soon as Läwen became a resident to the Braun led surgical department of the Lutheran hospital, general anesthesia was almost replaced with the various new techniques of local anesthesia. As a result of American contributions to the development of local anesthesia, and especially of conduction anesthesia, and its promotion by the Berlin surgeon, Carl Ludwig Schleich (1859-1922) and his French colleague Paul Reclus (1847-1914), the new methods of local anesthesia became generally accepted in Germany.[19] This acceptance was increased with Heinrich Braun's 1904 introduction of novocaine and its

Fig. 4. Arthur Läwen as surgeon at the "West-Front" during the World War I, ca 1916.[2]

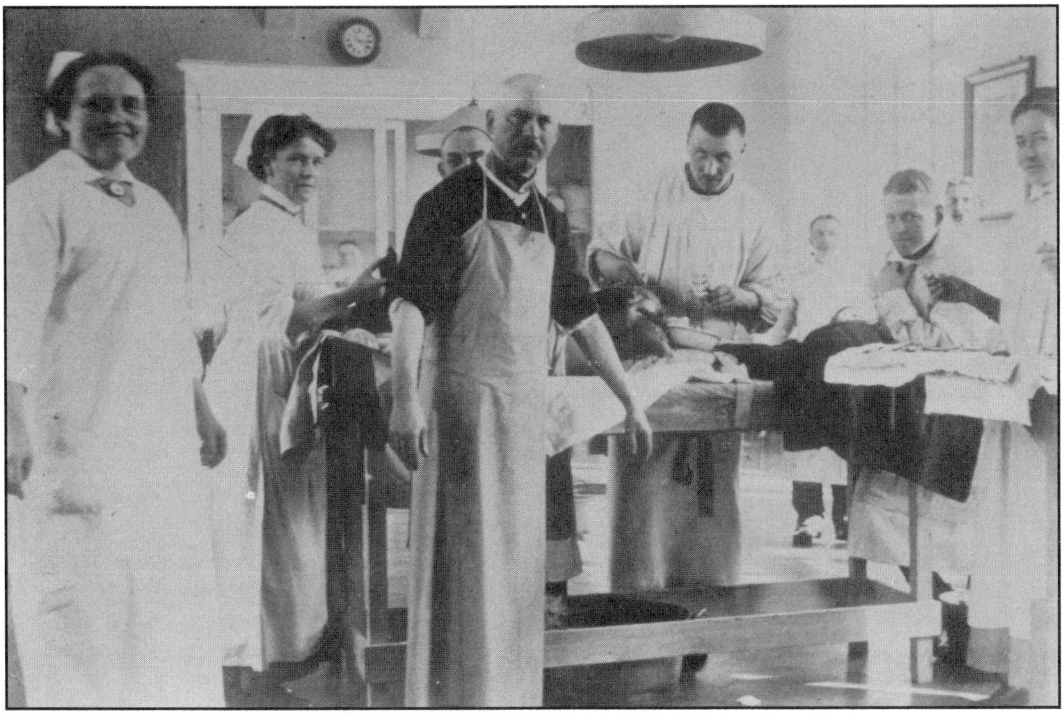

advantageous combination with vasoconstrictors like Suprarenin.[5] It came as no surprise that Läwen, also preoccupied with technically improving the methods of local anesthesia, made great contributions to the development of this field. Above all, his interest was the development of sacral and paravertebral anesthesia.[20-29]

In 1901, the French surgeon Cathelin was the first to report an epidural drug injection through the sacral hiatus.[30] A year later Cathelin published a monograph concerning the indications and risks of the method, also discussing its possible analgesic indications in the field of surgery.[31] Nevertheless, his assessment of the method was rather skeptical since he had primarily injected cocaine, which had only decreased and did not entirely alleviate the pain. Similarly skeptical was the German obstetrician Walter Stöckel (1871-1961), who had attempted to use epidural injections in order to achieve painless child-bearing.[32,33] Cathelin had been the first to use the term "sacral anesthesia," a term which Läwen later used in describing his results after injecting the newly available drug novocaine instead of cocaine.

Läwen injected sodium bicarbonate to alkalinize novocaine chloride so as to improve the quality of the preparation by increasing the rate, onset and duration of its initial effects.[34] Thus, the attained quality of sensory as well as motor paralysis of the nerves was markedly improved. Using his special solution, Läwen was able to recommend the injection of up to 25 cc of a 0.5 percent alkalinized novocaine preparation without risks of an intoxication.[34] It is worth mentioning that Läwen injected the local anesthetic in the sitting patient, a technique different to that of Cathélin and Stöckel, who had favored the lateral position.[25] Due to these modifications, Läwen was able to report a high success rate with the technique. In later publications, Läwen renamed the method, "Extradural Anesthesia," and it became an important part of the regimen of anesthesia for operative obstetric surgery that it is today.[25]

Oskar Gros (1877-1947), of the Leipzig Pharmacological Institute, had called Läwen's attention to the improved analgesic quality of the alkalinized novocaine solution, and this was the reason Läwen had first researched and later had applied, as well as analyzed, the validity of this claim.[34-38] In the last few years, many articles have been published concerning the various effects of alkalinized local anesthetic drugs and have confirmed Läwen's analyses made 70 years ago.[39]

The consequence of the newly available drug was that a broader application of novocaine in various local anesthetic methods became possible.[20,22] Furthermore, due to the reduced risks of toxicity, new indications for the sacral anesthesia technique were noted by Läwen in the following years when he discussed the new technique in several articles.[20,22,24] He later reported similar advantageous applications of his bicarbonated novocaine in other fields of surgery.[25] Nevertheless, his preparation did not receive the success it deserved. There was often a loss of efficacy which was proportional to the length of time the already prepared bicarbonate solution was stored. 40 Years later, the Hoechst Company produced a buffered basic novocaine solution with a pH of 7.8-8, thus circumventing the problem of bicarbonate instability.[41] In the thirties, this drug preparation became the preferred local anesthetic in dentistry in Germany when the abuse of cocaine had dramatically increased, a consequence of its wide use by wounded men after world war I.[42]

Paravertebral Techniques and Analgetic Concepts

Like the improvements in sacral anesthesia, Läwen also contributed to the development of paravertebral anesthesia. The German obstetrician, Hugo Sellheim (1871-1936), first reported the advantageous use of paravertebral conduction block in 1905, but had discontinued the method because of its technical difficulties.[43] Moreover, the method was often complicated by toxic reactions as a consequence of the doses used. Läwen began by improving the technical aspects of the method by aiming the block at the lower thoracic and lumbar nerves, which had enabled not only painless inguinal hernia but also kidney surgery.[23] After an extensive study of its segmental distribution in the internal organs, the German surgeon Max Kappis (1881-1938) further developed Läwen's method into one which could be applied to differential diagnosis of acute intra-abdominal illness.[44] He also noted its pain alleviating attributes, applying it as an effective and safe method for postoperative pain relief, such as after cholecystectomy, gastrectomy, or any kind of kidney surgery. Kappis also considered the paravertebral techniques as an effective prophylaxis against postoperative pneumonia, a topic which Läwen had extensively presented in a report in 1906.[45] Outside of aspiration intraoperatively, he saw the other main cause of this serious complication to be pain limiting adequate ventilation and causing infrequent expectoration. Even today, these circumstances are often blamed for these problems in the elderly, high risk patient. Bearing in mind these complications, Läwen in 1911 had advocated the routine warming of the inhaled anesthetic in long operations, developing a special device for this purpose.[45] Thus, any cooling of the patient's body temperature would be prevented, so that any disposition for pneumonia would be excluded as much as possible.

At the time of his surgical residency, Läwen did much of his research in collaboration with the already mentioned Institute of Pharmacology of the University of Leipzig.[37] Consequently, he published numerous articles concerning the pharmacologic attributes of local anesthetics such as alypin, novocaine and stovaine.[8,12,13,15] These preparations, promoted primarily as ideal substitutes for cocaine, were with time noted to have toxic side-effects, and thus became an additional reason for Läwen to scrutinize and compare them.[15] Läwen warned that, especially the concentrated solutions of stovaine, should not be applied to patients to avoid the possibility of directly damaging the nerve fibers.[15] He considered novocaine to be a dependable and useful anesthetic with a relatively low toxicity, and one which showed no toxicity to connective and other tissues. Furthermore, "the combination of the vasoactive substance like suprarenin and novocaine can be sterilized without decreasing its effectiveness, making novocaine a worthy competitor of cocaine.[15] Proof that this assessment was indeed true is seen in the use of novocaine as a local anesthetic in the following decades. Läwen continued his pharmacologic research and, for example, in 1930 he examined the effect of general and local anesthetics on the physiologic tone of striated muscle fibers.[46] After 1933, Läwen was responsible for the publication of Heinrich Braun's well-known textbook titled, "Local Anesthesia, Its Scientific Basis and Its Practical Application."[40] In 1951, he was the editor of the last revised, updated and expanded edition of this standard textbook, which is worth reading even today.[47]

The Application of Curare in the Field of Surgery and its Use in the Therapy of Tetanus

As a resident of the surgery department of the University of Leipzig, Läwen was involved with the therapeutic possibilities of curare.[9] He conducted his animal experiments at the Institute of Pharmacology, which was at that time led by professor Rudolf Böhm (1844-1926). Läwen's interest in curare is not surprising since Böhm's specialty was research concerning this drug.[48] He was renowned as an outstanding researcher of this muscle relaxant, having in 1895 published an extensive monograph concerning its chemical and pharmacologic properties.[49,50] Some years previously, in 1884, another surgical resident of the clinic in Leipzig, Dr. Karg, had reported on the use of curare in tetanus.[51] He had prophylactically tracheotomized and artificially breathed for patients previously treated with curare, but unfortunately without definitive success. Nevertheless, mitigation of the symptoms were observed so that the author requested further experimentation in this matter.[51]

Years later, in 1906, Läwen advocated the use of curare for the symptomatic therapy of tetanus after extensive animal experimentation.[9] He expressly noted the necessity of removing septic foci and of using high doses of antitoxin. He recommended the dose of curare to be 5-8 mg which, in the case of paroxysms, could be supplemented with intravenous injections. In any case, the patients were to be tracheotomized and artificially ventilated. Of interest is Läwen mentioning that the use of the drug characteristically caused a twitching of the lower jaw muscles, an increase in saliva secretion, and hiccough, well-known effects that are unique for muscle relaxants.

A Respirator for the Curarisized Patient

Six years later, Läwen discussed the possibilities of using curare for strychnine poisoning.[52,53] As with tetanus, he suggested the use of artificial respiration after a tracheotomy and included a detailed description of his newly designed respirator. The vital capacity could be preferentially set and the respiratory rate adjusted between 16-20 respirations per minute. This device had successfully ventilated a patient with an apnea due to an increased cerebral pressure for many hours. The electrically powered apparatus could be used also for resuscitations, such as caused by an intoxication or even during an operation, as its combination with any anesthetic vapor was possible. In the same article, Läwen vehemently opposed Sauerbruch's categorical denial of the use of any form of positive pressure ventilation. This judgment was supported by the fact that all of the patients undergoing positive pressure ventilation had been observed to retain a stable circulation. Furthermore, there had been no changes in the postmortem histology of the lung tissue, even after undergoing 8 hours of artificial respiration with the above apparatus. After describing the respirator, Läwen also listed the surgical indications for curare.

Successful Use of Curare in Abdominal Surgery

It was a logical step that Läwen was the first physician to intentionally use curare as a muscle relaxant.[24,54] In 1912 for the first time he discussed the surgical indications for this drug in his article titled, "Of the connection between local anesthesia and general narcosis of upper extradural anesthesia and of epidural injections of anesthetic solutions for tabetic crisis."[24] Often, towards the end of an intraabdominal operation, the anesthesia during the suturing would be so deep that the patient was seriously in danger of losing his life. With the application of a 2 percent curare to a total dose of 0.8 mg, Läwen intended to weaken the motor nerve impulses and, with his epidural injections of a bicarbonated local anesthetic like novocaine, intended to maximally block the sensory nerve impulses. At the end of his article, he mentioned the advantages of an intravenous curare injection, but was sorry that he could not continue these investigations because of the impurities of the preparation. Läwen especially praised the exceptionally good "somatic state" of the anesthesized patients, even during longer operations. Thus, Läwen was the first surgeon to use curare in an operation, a determination which resulted in its use today as an integral part of most intubation anesthesias. He did not continue his research with curare in the following years. One possible reason was his accepting the post as a head of surgery of the newly built St. George Hospital in Leipzig.[2]

At the end of the 1920's, however, again committed himself to the symptomatic therapy of tetanus. At that time, the new rectally applied narcotic avertin was the topic of discussion in many surgical sub-specialties.[55] Läwen was the first to administer avertin for tetanus, and in 1927 he reported a 13 day therapy of a patient, having used a total of 154.4 grams of the drug.[56,57] In Läwen's opinion, the patient only survived the illness because of a concurrent high dose of antitoxin. For this reason, he requested that an experimental study of the value of curare-avertin combined therapy for tetanus be made by a colleague of his clinic. As a result, a synergistic increase in the effectiveness of both drugs was observed, allowing Läwen to advocate tetanus as a further indication for the concurrent use of avertin and curare. With this combination therapy of sedation and curarization, Läwen had created a concept which has become an integral part of today's tetanus therapy.

Läwen lived to witness the successful worldwide use of another of his prophetic combination concepts in the late 1940's, namely, that of artificial respiration with the application of muscle relaxants.[58-60] Asked by one of his surgical colleagues in the beginning of the 1950's why he thought the surgical use of curare had not taken place sooner in Germany, Läwen answered tersely, "Sauerbruch was against it."[2] Unfortunately, that was not all that Ferdinand Sauerbruch (1875-1951) was against. He had also delayed the use of the intubation technique in the operating room with his great influence within the German Surgical Society. Although he made many contributions to the field of surgery, he had truly hindered the modernization of anesthesiology.[61]

In reports of the advantageous intraoperative use of curare in the 1940's, Läwen's earlier pioneering work in this field was never mentioned.[58-60] On the other hand, this promotion of the use of curare never gained any popularity and this is probably the reason it was not taken into consideration.

If one were to summarize Arthur Läwen's numerous publications relevant to anesthesia and his contributions to this specialty, the words of the Heidelberg surgeon would be the most suitable: "In many ways, Läwen was a man before his time."[1] The precise manner in which Arthur Läwen conducted his investigations can only be summed up with the following quote from the famous French research scientist, Claude Barnard: "Man can learn nothing unless he proceeds from the known to the unknown."

References

1. Bauer KH: Die Wandlungen der Anaesthesie vom Standpunkt des Operateurs. Langenbeck's Arch f klin Chir 282:162, 1955.
2. Brammer L: (daughter of A. Läwen) personal communications Oct. 1989, Dec. 1990, May 1991.
3. Borasch Fr: Arthur Läwen. Dtsch Ges f Chir 2:3, 1976.
4. Erb Arthur Läwen. Chirurg 5:239, 1958.
5. Braun H: Die Bedeutung des Adrenalin für die Lokalanaesthesie. Langenbecks Arch klin Chir 69:150, 1903.
6. Braun H: Die örtliche Betäubung, ihre wissenschaftlichen Grundlagen und praktische Anwendung. 8th edition. Verlag von Johann Ambrosius Barth, Leipzig 1905.
7. Braun H: Ueber einige neue örtliche Anaesthetica. (Stovain, Alypin, Novocain). Dtsch med Wochenschr 42:1667, 1902.
8. Läwen A: Experimentelle Untersuchungen über dic Gcfässwirkung von Suprarenin in Verbindung mit örtlich anästhesierenden Mitteln Dtsch Zschr f Chir 74:163, 1904.
9. Läwen A: Experimentelle Untersuchungen über die Möglichkeit den Tetanus mit Curarin zu behandeln. Mitt Grenzgeb Med u Chir 16:803, 1906.
10. Läwen A: Vergleichende Untersuchungen über die örtliche Wirkung von Kokain, Novokain, Alypin und Stovain auf motorische Nervenstämme. Arch f Exper Pathol u Pharmakol 56:138, 1906.
11. Läwen A: Ueber Lungenkomplikationen nach Bauchoperationen. Bruns Beitr z klin Chir 50:501, 1906.
12. Läwen A: Vergleichende experimentelle Untersuchungen über die örtliche Wirkung einiger neuer Lokalanästhetika (Stovain, Novocain und Alypin) auf motorische Nervenstämme. Bruns Beitr f klin Chir 50:621, 1906.
13. Läwen A: Erfahrungen über Lumbalanästhesie mit Stovain, und Novokain mit besonderer Berücksichtigung der Neben- und Nachwirkungen. Bruns Beitr f klin Chir 50:632, 1906.
14. Heinicke H, Läwen A: Experimentelle Untersuchungen und klinische Erfahrungen über die Verwertbarkeit von Novokain für die örtliche Anästhesie. Dtsch Zschr f Chir 80:180, 1905.
15. Heinecke H, Läwen A: Erfahrungen über Lumbalanästhesie mit Stovain und Novokain mit besonderer Berücksightigung der Neben- und Nachwirkungen. Bruns Beitr z klin Chir 50:632, 1906.
16. Läwen A: Schmerz, seine Beseitigung und Verhütung. In: Schjening: Handbuch der ärztlichen Erfahrung im Weltkriege. Berlin, 1920.
17. Läwen A: Anästhesierungsverfahren im Felde. Ergeb Chir Ortho 11:365, 1919.
18. Anonymus Der Letzte. Die Chirurgische Universitätsklinik Königsberg in Preussen 1935-1935. Ostpreussen-Rundbrief 1961.
19. Darmstaedter E: Begründung und Ausbau der Cocain-Localanästhesie. Schmerz, Narkose, Anästhesie 10:196, 1938.

20. Läwen A: Über Extraduralanästhesie für chirurgische Operationen. Dtsch Zschr f Chir 20:108, 1910.
21. Läwen A: Über die Verwertung der Sakralanästhesie für chirurgische Operationen. Dtsch Zschr f Chir 20:708, 1910.
22. Läwen A: Über Leitungsanästhesie an der unteren Extremität, mit Bemerkungen über die Technik von Injektionen an den Nervus ischiadicus bei der Behandlung der Ischias. Dtsch Zschr f Chir 111:252, 1911.
23. Läwen A: Lokalanästhesie für Nierenoperationen. Münch med Wochenschr 26:1390, 1911.
24. Läwen A: Ueber die Verbindung der Lokalanästhesie mit der Narkose, über hohe Extraduralanästhesie und epidurale Injektionen anästhesierender Lösungen bei tabischen Magenkrisen. Bruns Beitr f klin Chir 80:168, 1912.
25. Läwen A, von Gaza W: Die Extraduralanästhesie. Ergeb der Chir u Orthopäd 5:38, 1913.
26. Läwen A: paravertebrale Novokaininjektionen zur Differentialdiagnose intraabdomineller Erkrankungen. Münch med Wochenschr 1423, 1922.
27. Läwen A: Weitere Beiträge zur Sakralanästhesie und zur paravertebralanästhesie für diagnostische und operative Zwecke Münch med Wochenschr 35:1449, 1925.
28. Läwen A: Über Paravertebralanästhesie zur Operation von Leisten und Schenkelhernien. Schmerz 4:289, 1928.
29. Läwen A: Sakralanästhesie und transsakrale Anästhesie Abl f Chir 1933.
30. Cathelin F: Une nouvelle voie d'injection rachidienne. Méthode des injections épidurales par le procédé du canal sacré. Comptes rendus des Séances et Mémoires de la Societé de Biologie. 53:452, 1901.
31. Cathelin F: Les injections épidurales par ponction du canal sacré. Paris 1903.
32. Stöckel W: Über sakrale Anästhesie. Abl f Gyn 33:1, 1903.
33. Doughty A: Walter Stöckel (1871-1961). A pioneer in regional analgesia in obstetrics. The History of Anesthesia Society, Vol. 5, Proceedings of February 1989 Meeting - Mayday Hospital Croydon, 25.
34. Läwen A: Ueber die Verwendung des Novokains in Natriumbikarbonat-Kochsalzlösungen zur lokalen Anästhesie. Münch med Wochenschr 39:2044, 1910.
35. Gros O: Über eine Methode, die anästhesierende Wirkung der Kokalanästhetika zu steigern. Münch med Wochenschr 39:2042, 1910.
36. Gelbke N: Die geschichtliche Entwicklung des Pharmakologischen Instituts der Leipziger Universität unter besonderer Berücksichtigung der Gründerjahre. med. Dissertation, Universität Leipzig, 1955.
37. Kestner I: (c/o Institute for the History of Medicine of the University of Leipzig), personal communication concerning A. Läwen, summer 1989.
38. Kestner I, Thom A: 575 Jahre Mediznische Fakultät der Universität Leipzig. Johann Ambrosius Barth, Leipzig 1990.
39. Hilgier M; Alkalinization of bupivacaine for brachial plexus block. Reg Anesth 10:59, 1985.
40. Läwen A: Die örtliche Betäubung, ihre wissenschaftlichen Grundlagen und praktische Anwendung. 8th edition. Verlag von Johann Ambrosius Barth, Leipzig 1933.
41. Hoechst-Company, personal information concerning alkalinized novocaine solutions. Feb. 1989.
42. Goerig M, Beck H: Natriumbicarbonat-Zusatz zum Lokalanaesthetikum-Schon einmal vor 80 Jahren. Anaesthestist Supplement 1, 38, 1989.
43. Sellheim H; Die Herabsetzung der Empfindlichkeit der Bauchdecken und des Peritoneum parietale durch perineurale Injektionen anästhesierender Lösungen an die Stämme der Nn. intercostales, des subcostalis, des Ilihypogastricus und des Ileoinguinalis. Verh Dtsch Ges f Gyn 1906, 1905.
44. Kappis M; Sensibilität der Bauchhöle Mitt. Grenzgeb. Med u Chir 26.
45. Läwen A: Uber die Vorwärmung von Aether - und Chloroformdämpfen für die Narkose. Münch med Wochenschr 40:2097, 1911.
46. Läwen A: Über den Einfluss von allgemeiner und örtlicher Betäubung auf den physiologischen Tonus der quergestreiften Muskulatur des Menschen. Bruns Beitr f klin Chir 148:323, 1930.
47. Läwen A: Die örtliche Betäubung, ihre wissenschaftlichen Grundlagen und praktische Anwendung. 9th edition. Verlag von Johann Ambrosius Barth, Leipzig 1951.
48. Boehm R: Das Südamerikanische Pfeilgift Curare in Chemischer und Pharmakologischer Beziehung. Hirzel Verlag, Leipzig 1895.
49. Boehm R: Ueber Curarin und Curaril. Ther d Gegenw 489, 1904.

50. Boehm R: Handbuch der experimentellen Pharmakologie. Springer Verlag, Berlin 1920.
51. Karg: Die Behandlung des Tetanus mit Curare. Arch f klin Chir 29:338, 1883.
52. Läwen A, Sievers R: Zur praktischen Anwendung der instrumentellen künstlichen Respiration am Menschen. Münch med Wochenschr 41:2221, 1910.
53. Goerig M, Schulte am Esch J: Arthur Läwen-Wegbereiter der maschinellen Beatmung des relaxierten Patienten. Anaesthesist, Supplementum 1 39:94, 1990.
54. Goerig M; Letter to the editor (Anesthesiology) Pioneering Curare in Anesthesia. Anesthesiology 30:172, 1990.
55. Goerig M: The Avertin-Story. 3. International Symposium on the History of Anesthesia. Atlanta 1992.
56. Läwen A: Avertin zur Behandlung des Tetanus. Zbl f Chir 238:2370, 1927.
57. Läwen A: Weitere Erfahrungen über die symptomatische Behandlung des Tetanus mit Avertin. Zbl f Chir 4:194, 1928.
58. Griffith HR, Johnson GE: The use of curare in general anesthesia. Anesthesiology 3:418, 1942.
59. Cullen SC: The use of curare for the improvement of abdominal muscle relaxation during inhalation anesthesia. Surg. 14:261, 1943.
60. Gray TC, Halton B: A milestone in Anaesthesia. Proc Roy Soc Med 39:400, 1946.
61. Nissen R: Erlebtes aus der Thoraxchirurgie. Thieme Verlag, Stuttgart 1955.

AUGUST HILDEBRANDT
The Man Beside August Bier

M. GOERIG and H. BECK
Department of Anaesthesiology,
University Hamburg, Germany

If one were to look into the history of spinal anesthesia, he would find two physicians described in one tale: the surgeon, August Bier (Fig. 1), and his medical assistant, August Hildebrandt (Fig. 2).[1] Both worked in the same Academic Hospital of the Royal Clinic of Surgery at Kiel.[2] Bier (1861-1949) was senior physician to the surgical department which was led by Friedrich von Esmarch (1823-1908) (Fig. 3).[3] Esmarch had already given up everyday clinical activities, allowing his energetic senior physician to take over these responsibilities.[2]

The internist Heinrich Quincke (1842-1922), worked in the same hospital, and in 1878 had already used a spinal tap for diagnostic reasons.[4,5] Years later, in 1890, Quincke began to use lumbar puncture as a means of therapy.[4] He reported in many articles and congresses the possibility of treatment through drug injection into the subarachnoid cavaity.[5] Bier grabbed at "the idea of invasive therapy, a technique that Esmarch did not agree with, but nevertheless did not hinder." In short, these were the circumstances that led the senior physician, Bier, and his assistant Hildebrandt, to their first attempts at spinal anesthesia on August 15, 1898.[1] The observations and descriptions of the effects, as well as the side effects of spinal anesthesia, published by August Bier in 1899, are well-known. Bier wrote explicitly of Hildebrandt's helpful assistance in these self-experiments. Nevertheless, it seems that Hildebrandt was not considered a partner in the experimentation and for a short time disappeared from the scene.

Two years later, in 1901, Bier reported on his practice of spinal anesthesia at the German Surgical Congress in Berlin. At that time, Bier had become the Chairman of the Surgical Department of the University of Greifswald, where he had conducted 1200 spinal anesthesias, of which he made a comprehensive report.[6,7] At the end of his review, Bier discussed the topic of who was first responsible for the development of this technique. He mentioned James Leonard Corning (1855-1925), who at that time claimed to have developed the concept of spinal anesthesia in

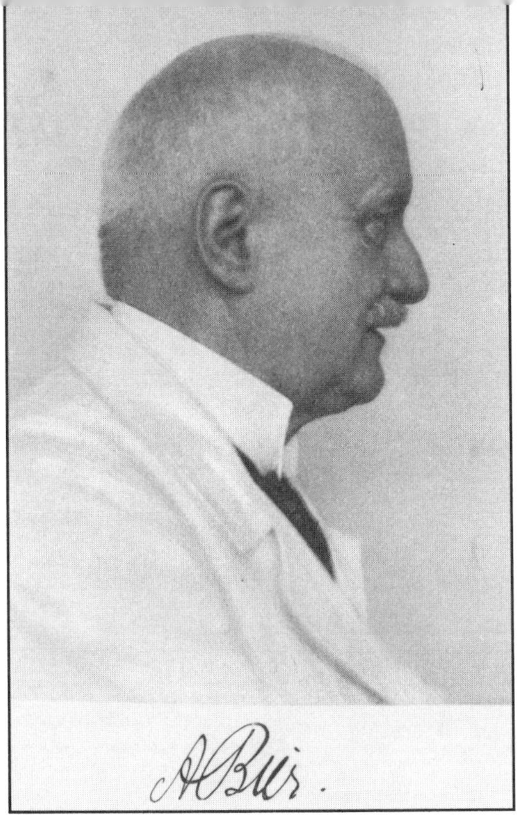

Fig. 1. August Bier (1861-1949).[47]

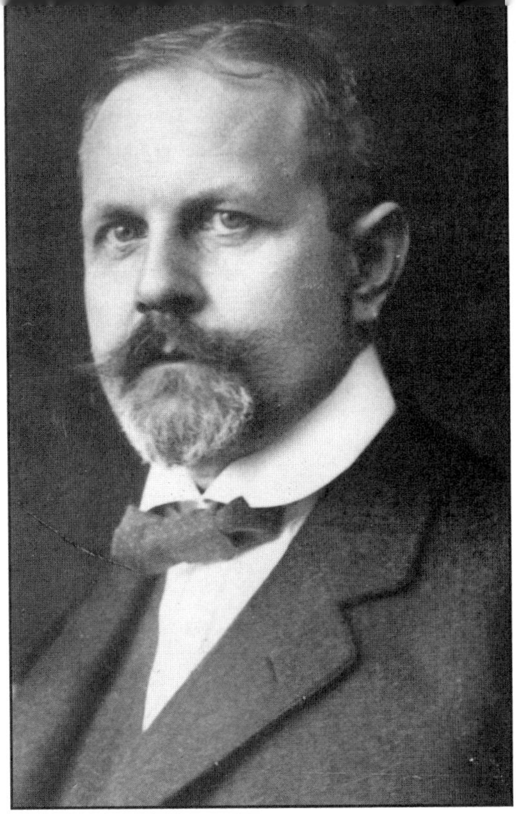

Fig. 2. August Hildebrandt (1868-1954).[13]

1885.[8-12] Bier briefly described that he had heard of Corning's "experiments."[6] But he expressly denied any experimentation with spinal anesthesia. It is reasonable to believe that Bier was telling the truth. But where was Hildebrandt and what became of him?

Hildebrandt's Biography

August Hildebrandt was born in Wittingen, a small town in the area of Lüneburger Heide, on May 20, 1868.[2,13] Studying medicine at the Universities of Kiel, Böttingen and Munich, he received his medical license in 1892. In the same year, he wrote his dissertation in the specialty ophthalmology at the Ludwig Maximillian's University in Munich. He worked as a general practitioner in Lüneburg for four years before he moved to Berlin. Here he was employed by the Institute for Microbiology, which was conducted by Robert Koch (1843-1910) at that time. Moving to Kiel in 1896, he accepted a residency at the Royal Surgical Clinic, where he was employed until his withdrawal in 1899. He then became an active medical officer and as such became a member of the German Red Cross, where he was ordered to participate in the Boer Wars of South Africa (Fig. 4).[13,14] He published several reports in which he described his experiences during his few months' participation.[15] He returned to Germany, was promoted and sent to China, where the Boxer Revolt had begun in the years 1900-1901. Back in Germany, he accepted a job at the University Anatomy Institute in Berlin. In 1903, he again changed his place of work, this time accepting a medical residency in the Surgical Department of the Charité Hospital. The Chief surgeon was at that time Franz König (1832-1910).[13] In 1905, Hildebrandt specialized in surgery and published an exhaustive study of military surgical experience with war injuries.[13,16] In the years 1905-1907, he published his acclaimed two volume monograph of "Modern Warfare Missile Wounds." It is worth mentioning that he never published any anesthesia-related articles.

In the spring of 1907, Hildebrandt was nominated professor just before Bier took the place of Ernst von Bergmann (1836-1907) as the surgical Chairman of the Royal Clinic of Surgery in Berlin.[13,17,18] In 1913, Hildebrandt went on another Red Cross expedition during

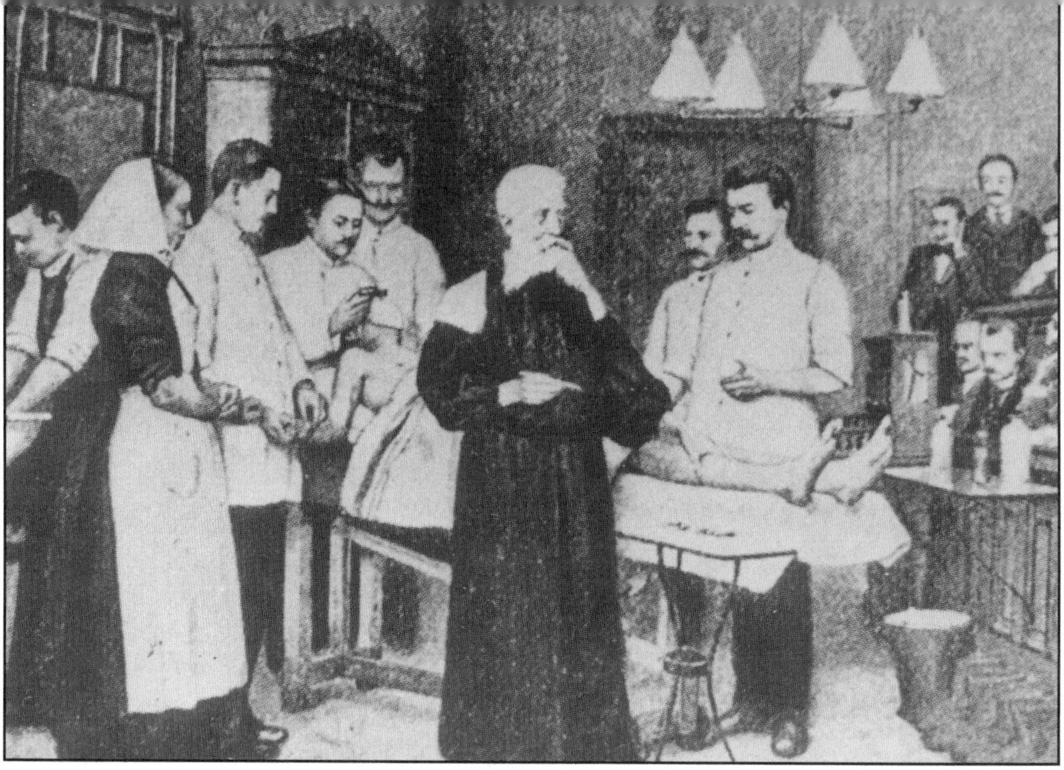

Fig. 3. Friedrich von Esmarch in his "black-operation-robe" (1823-1908).[46]

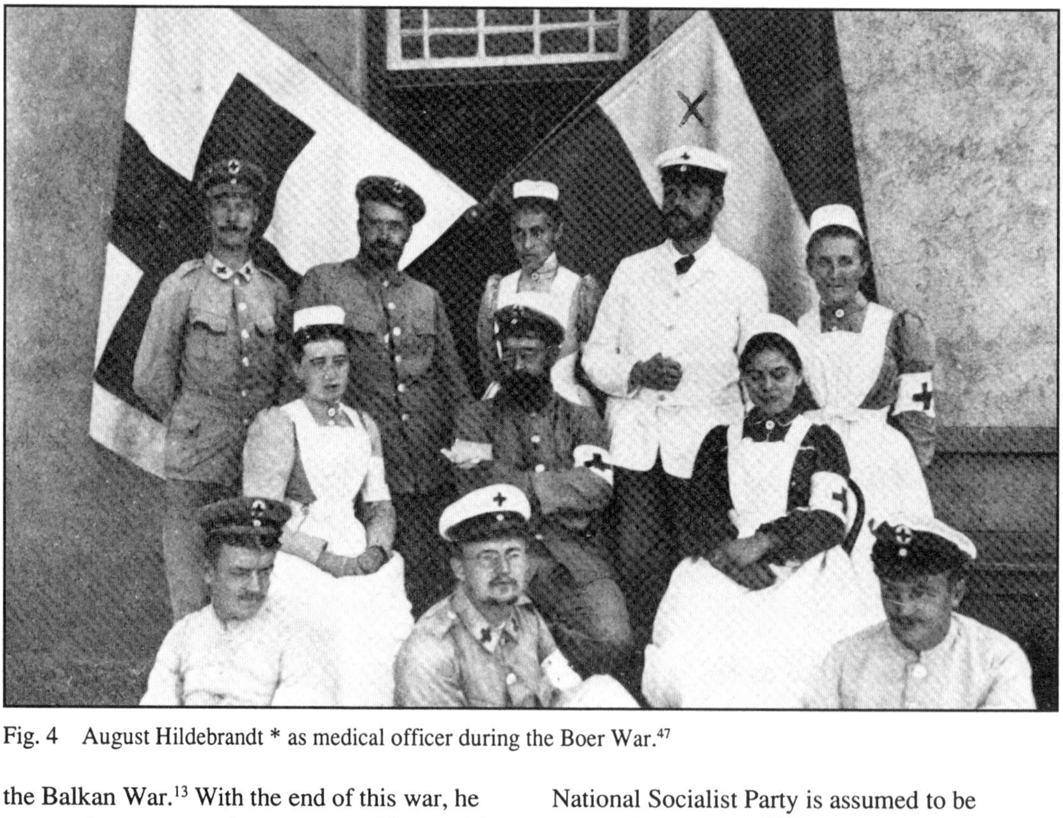

Fig. 4 August Hildebrandt * as medical officer during the Boer War.[47]

the Balkan War.[13] With the end of this war, he accepted a post as senior surgeon at Eberswalde Hospital, 45 km to the North of Berlin, working there until his dismissal in 1934, for which the National Socialist Party is assumed to be responsible (Fig. 5).[19,20] With a colleague, Hildebrandt founded a "Surgical Orthopedic Sanatorium" in Berlin, where he worked until

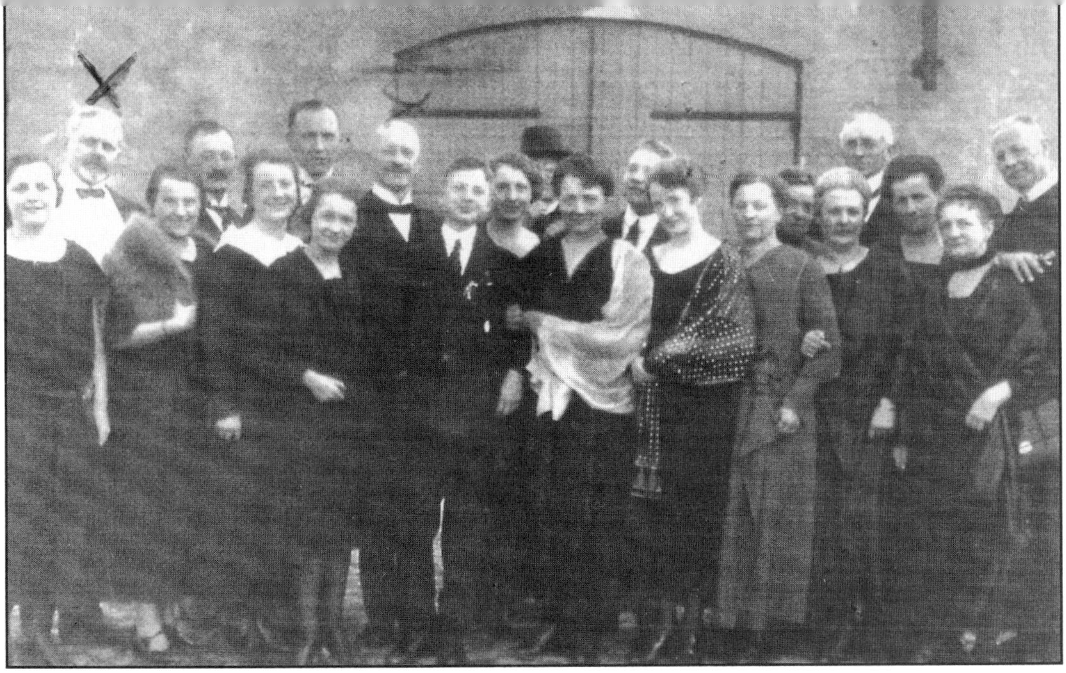

Fig. 5. August Hildebrandt * at the Eberswalde Hospital, *circa* 1926.[20]

1943.[13] In order to avoid the bombing of Berlin, Hildebrandt moved to Holstein in the northern part of Germany, where he opened a general practice in Süderhasted, near Hamburg.[21] Later, he fled to Bad Reichenhall, then to Fürstenfeldbruck, and finally ended up in Munich where he passed away on August 15, 1954.[13]

Hildebrandt's Personality

If we are to believe an interview with one of his nurses, Hildebrandt was certainly an imposing figure (Fig. 6).[22,23] He evidently had an irascible temperament, being ever distrustful and "constantly bellowing." "He was a shouter who always made me tremble in fear. . . and would always terrorize and frighten his subordinates." Furthermore, the nurse reported that "he even shouted at a fracture during an operation with his resident surgeon, even through the patient was only under local anesthesia. That's what they say." These statements of Hildebrandt's former nurse were most likely not exaggerated. Even the daughter of one of his colleagues, the sanitary officer, Richard Schneider (1869-1962), described Hildebrandt as "a tyrant and irascible, a man who could bellow like an exploding bomb."[20] The surgeon and Nobel Prize Winner of 1956, Professor Werner Forssmann (1904-1979),

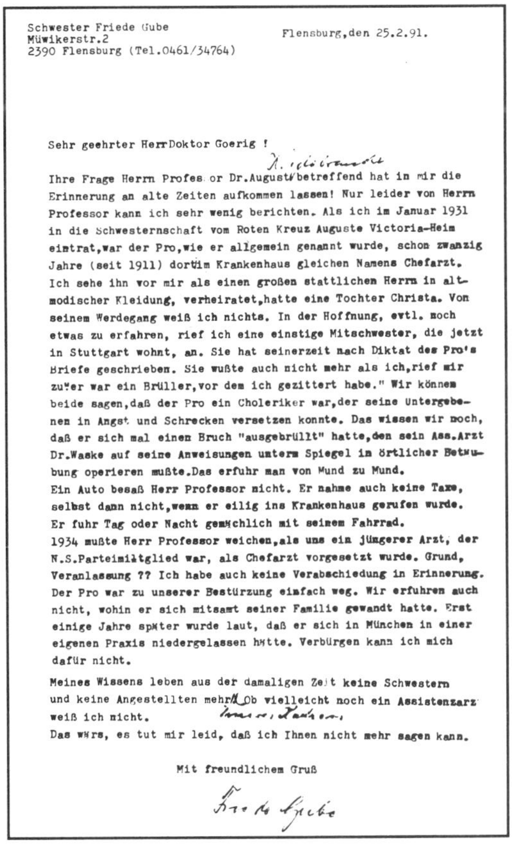

Schwester Friede Gube
Müwikerstr.2
2390 Flensburg (Tel.0461/34764)

Flensburg,den 25.2.91.

Sehr geehrter HerrDoktor Goerig !

Ihre Frage Herrn Profes or Dr.August betreffend hat in mir die Erinnerung an alte Zeiten aufkommen lassen! Nur leider von Herrn Professor kann ich sehr wenig berichten. Als ich im Januar 1931 in die Schwesternschaft vom Roten Kreuz Auguste Victoria-Heim eintrat,war der Pro,wie er allgemein genannt wurde, schon zwanzig Jahre (seit 1911) dort im Krankenhaus gleichen Namens Chefarzt. Ich sehe ihn vor mir als einen großen stattlichen Herrn in altmodischer Kleidung, verheiratet,hatte eine Tochter Christa. Von seinem Werdegang weiß ich nichts. In der Hoffnung, evtl. noch etwas zu erfahren, rief ich eine einstige Mitschwester, die jetzt in Stuttgart wohnt, an. Sie hat seinerzeit nach Diktat des Pro's Briefe geschrieben. Sie wußte auch nicht mehr als ich,rief mir zu"er war ein Brüller,vor dem ich gezittert habe." Wir können beide sagen,daß der Pro ein Choleriker war,der seine Untergebenen in Angst und Schrecken versetzen konnte. Das wissen wir noch, daß er sich mal einen Bruch "ausgebrüllt" hatte,den sein Ass.Arzt Dr.Waske auf seine Anweisungen unterm Spiegel in örtlicher Betäubung operieren mußte.Das erfuhr man von Mund zu Mund.
Ein Auto besaß Herr Professor nicht. Er nahme auch keine Taxe, selbst dann nicht,wenn er eilig ins Krankenhaus gerufen wurde. Er fuhr Tag oder Nacht gemächlich mit seinem Fahrrad.
1934 mußte Herr Professor weichen,als uns ein jüngerer Arzt, der N.S.Parteimitglied war, als Chefarzt vorgesetzt wurde. Grund, Veranlassung ?? Ich habe auch keine Verabschiedung in Erinnerung. Der Pro war zu unserer Bestürzung einfach weg. Wir erfuhren auch nicht, wohin er sich mitsamt seiner Familie gewandt hatte. Erst einige Jahre später wurde laut, daß er sich in München in einer eigenen Praxis niedergelassen hätte. Verbürgen kann ich mich dafür nicht.

Meines Wissens leben aus der damaligen Zeit keine Schwestern und keine Angestellten mehr. Ob vielleicht noch ein Assistenzarzt weiß ich nicht.
Das wärs, es tut mir leid, daß ich Ihnen nicht mehr sagen kann.

Mit freundlichem Gruß

Fig. 6. Description of Hildebrandt's character by a former nurse.[22]

wrote briefly of Hildebrandt in his autobiography, "Memories of the Self-Experimenting Surgeon": "He was an unscrupulous egotist: Hildebrandt's Villa was practically a Chinese Museum. As active military surgeon in the suppression of the Boxer Revolt, he instinctively took precious palatial and temple treasures and brought them home."[23]

When Forssmann did his research on cardiac catheterisation, he was subordinated to the already mentioned surgeon,[24,25] Schneider, who led the aseptic surgical department of the Eberswalde hospital.[20,23] Hildebrandt had become chief of the aseptic department. Although working together for a long time before 1913, a few years after Hildebrandt had become the chief of the surgical department.

Priority Claim of the Discovery of Spinal Anesthesia and the Role of Hildebrandt in this Argument

This brief sketch of his personal background sheds a bit of light on the problems which make Hildebrandt an interesting character even today: he played an important role in the priority claim for the discovery of spinal anesthesia. He was also one of the most vehement opponents in this controversy. The dispute created a commotion, not only among professionals, but also excited the general public in Germany, Europe and the United States.

At the end of April, 1901, a major German magazine of medicine and surgery published an extensive article concerning the use of spinal anesthesia. The author, Friedrich Hahn, an Austrian, had probably attended the German Surgical Congress in Berlin and had heard, not only Bier's report, but also the controversy.[26,27] Hahn wrote that Bier deserved the greater praise for the development of spinal anesthesia, without discrediting the contributions of Corning. He wrote that ". . .no one would be more surprised as Corning himself to find his method, not fully developed, to be the center of such a scientific debate." It was not until many years after these initial references that the priority claim to the discovery of spinal anesthesia would again become a major topic.

In the spring of 1905, one of a series of articles written by Dr. Philipp Bockenheimer (1875-1935) was published in the "Zeitschrift für Ärztliche Fortbildung," concerning the "Technic and Indication of Local Anesthesia."[28] Bockenheimer was a resident surgeon of the Royal Clinic in Berlin. He wrote that "Corning was the discoverer of the spinal anesthesia. . ." and ". . .after it had been forgotten Bier and Tuffier has merely rediscovered and correctly realized the use of this technic." Once again the priority claim was to become a topic of discussion.

Surprisingly, another article concerning spinal anesthesia was published a few weeks after Bockenheimer's series of articles in August, 1905. It was Hildebrandt himself who wrote the article in another reputable German surgical journal.[29] The former assistant of Bier began with, "Corning from New York is the one to be praised for the analgesia of the intestinal area and lower extremities." He further wrote that Corning, the father of spinal anesthesia, had not "by chance," but rather "slowly, tendentiously and almost with a comical wariness developed his technic; the many articles show clearly how many stages he must have gone through to fully develop his method. This important discovery is not merely an accidental one but is the discovery of the goal oriented activity of a brilliant scientist."

A few months later, in January 1906, another medical assistant from the same surgical clinic, Bruno Bosse, voiced his opinion in a lecture at the "Charité Hospital Society for Physicians."[30] The internist colleague, Paul Lazarus, had referred to Bier's spinal anesthesia and its possible analgesic indications for internal medicine.[31] Bosse, after discussing the lecture, stated that "actually it was the American Corning and not Bier who discovered the technic." Of course, his opinion fully agreed with that of his superior, by then chief surgeon Otto Hildebrand (1858-1927), who should not be mistaken with August Hildebrandt, as both worked at the same surgical department at the Charité (Fig. 7).[3] "Head surgeon Hildebrand has sent me here today to discuss the experience

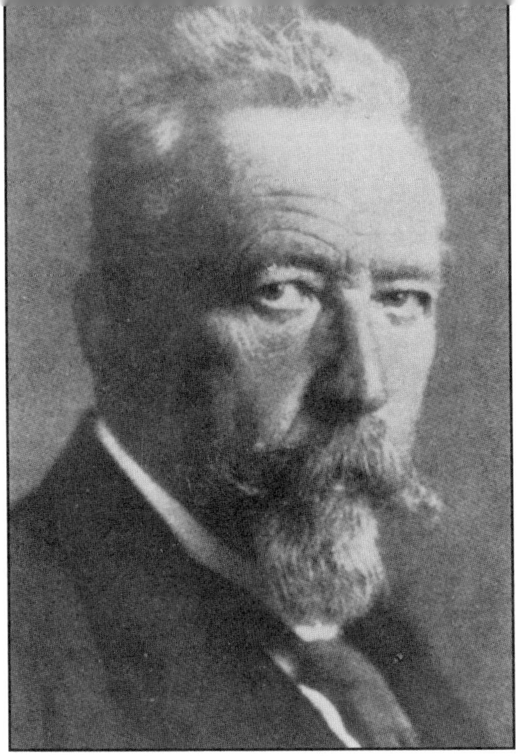

Fig. 7. Otto Hildebrand (1858-1927).[47]

gathered with use of spinal anesthesia by our surgery department."[30]

Even Bockenheimer's opinions in his published articles were in agreement with his superior, the reputed Ernst von Bergmann of the Surgical Department of Royal University in Berlin. Thus, the two leading surgeons of the two most renowned clinics of Berlin had decided in Corning's favor.[3]

A half-year later, following the publication of these three articles, Bier answered the accusations of his colleagues in an article published by a weekly medical journal.[32] This of course accentuated the debate which until then had been limited to the area of Berlin. The previous articles had been primarily published in the Berlin medical journals. Bier's article started heated discussions throughout the entire German speaking countries and created a new dimension in this debate. After all, Bier was a German and, in a time of exceptional national pride, it was practically impossible to give credit to an American named Corning for a "German discovery." Replying primarily to Hildebrandt's article, Bier mentioned "the unpleasant priority debate," which "would have been entirely unnecessary when the resident surgeons of these two university clinics would not have tried to give Dr. Corning the credit of discovering and introducing spinal anesthesia."[32] He once referred to the Congress of German Surgeons that had taken place in 1905, where he had first reported his discovery and also mentioned that great physicians like Paul Reclus (1847-1914) of France considered him as the father of this method: "C'est Bier et Bier seul qui a marqué et réalisé la méthode."[33-35]

Because Bier had attacked, not only Hildebrandt and Bosse of the Surgical Clinic of the Charité, but also the resident surgeon Bockenheimer of the Royal University Clinic, Bockenheimer later published a reply to Bier's accusations.[36] He repeated the already mentioned arguments of Hildebrandt and added that Bier had even given up the method because of the initially observed side effects. This of course did not prevent American and French surgeons from further using his method of local anesthesia by the subarachnoid route.

Even one of the neighbors of the German speaking countries, the Swiss surgeon Fritz DuMont (1854-1932), doubted Bier's claim to being the inventory of spinal anesthesia.[37] In his well-known "Textbook for General and Local Anesthesia," he expressed the following: "We have proof of the fact, that Bier was the first to popularize the method and therefore it is unnecessary to claim that he also discovered medullary anesthesia." Bockenheimer mentioned this in his reply and ended the article with a request to further develop the technique rather than continue a pointless priority claim.

Bier adamantly rejected Bockenheimer's claim that he had discontinued the method because of its side-effects and spoke of an "entirely false statement" that was merely a "figment of his imagination."[38] Again, he referred to the inherent risks of this procedure and that further experimentation would be critical and necessary. Nevertheless, he prophesied an excellent future for this type of local anesthesia. Again, he emphasized that fact that he had made the discovery entirely without the knowledge of Corning and that it was he who had introduced its practice in surgery. He then ended his repartee with, "we will allow the unbiased to decide who is right and who is wrong."

One year later, in 1907, Bruno Bosse published a monograph on "Spinal Anesthesia."[39] In his preface he claimed Corning to be the discoverer of the procedure. Furthermore, he classified the discovery as "one of the greatest of the twentieth century that all began in 1885 with a hopeful and cautious paravertebral injection. Corning knew very well that the anesthetic would be resorbed from the venous plexus and transported to the vicinity of the spinal column. Corning cautiously experimented until he, in 1894, finally had an anatomically and technically perfect intradural procedure that was proven to be of use for the operated patient."

And with that ended a debate for which the cause will perhaps forever remain unknown. Hans Killian (1892-1982), a pioneer of German anesthesiology, saw a possible cause in the misleading title of Corning's first publication.[40] The presentation of Corning's experiment had been regarded in a superficial manner. He began his experiments with small amounts of cocaine solution that he injected into the vertebral column and between the vertebrae, and only later attempted intradural injections, although without waiting for a drop of spinal fluid to appear.[11] Furthermore, Corning injected substances such as antipyrine, caffeine and strychnine, which is not exactly proof of a clear conception of developing spinal anesthesia. On the other hand, he meticulously noted his observations and made the application as a substitute for etherization in genitourinary or other branches of surgery. Most historians therefore claim August Bier to be the propagator of spinal anesthesia, even though he was not the first to call it so.[3] He was, however, the first physician to see a wide range of possibilities for the Quinckian Lumbar Puncture and, unlike Corning, was first to realize its importance of the field of surgery.

The end — an Unglorious Chapter

As fate would have it, after the death of Ernst von Bergmann in the spring of 1907, Bier was called to take his place as head of the Surgical Department of the Royal University Clinic in Berlin.[7,19] This was the final chapter of the unfortunate priority debate, ending with a common newspaper report of Bier's activities as head of the department. On May 8, 1907, on the first page of the Berliner Zeitung (BZ), the following was printed: "The New Ruler — An Insult To The Physicians Of Berlin" (Fig. 8).[41]

The first action Bier took on May 6, 1907, as head of the surgery department, was to fire a few residents.[41] This of course caused a bit of turmoil. In the BZ-article, the priority debate was mentioned, but he main topic was, "the many disagreements between the schools of Bonn and Berlin. . . . It is obvious that under these circumstances Professor Bier would have to contend with the different opinions of the former Bergmann assistants; astonishing, however, is the gruff manner with which the new chief showed his opposition. He has fired each and every resident surgeon of the Bergmann Clinic. Such an action is normally not that of newly appointed directors."[42] Bier gave his subordinate assistants the lawful six weeks notice, i.e. until the 15th of July. Dr. Bockenheimer and Dr. Coenen (1875-1963) were two of the many residents who were forced to leave. Philipp Bockenheimer had specialized in surgery at the Charité and published a reputable textbook of operative surgery.[7,43] He

Fig. 8. Public discussion about the "New Ruler" in the BZ.[40]

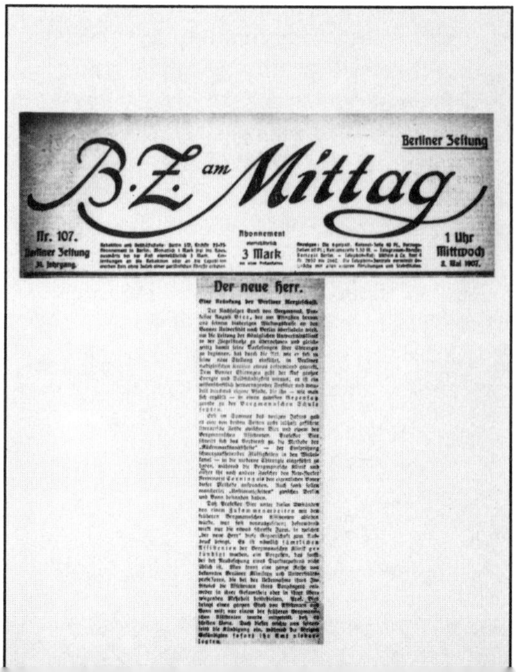
B.Z. am Mittag
Berliner Zeitung
Nr. 107.
Abonnement
3 Mark
1 Uhr
Mittwoch
Der neue Herr.

emigrated to Mexico where, according to the German Medical Calendar, he died in 1935.[44] Hermann Coenen specialized in surgery also at the University of Breslau. In 1923, he was nominated professor of the Surgical Department of the University of Münster, a position he held until his retirement in 1945.[45]

Both Bockenheimer and Coenen were known to be vehement advocates of Corning's priority to the discovery of spinal anesthesia. It was obvious that Bier had personal reasons for not wanting to have two such residents as his subordinates. The manner in which he fired his residents was an intense topic of discussion in many of the leading German newspapers: "The manner in which director Bier used his command has caused to say the least, a bit of commotion among his colleagues and is a daily topic for the physicians of Berlin. According to the little information that has filtered into the public, the professor has begun his direction with a few expulsions. . . . It is of course understandable that a new head physician will often have a difference of opinion with older medical residents, especially when discussing the future direction of their scientific work and the cooperation of a new head of the department. Nothing of the sort was a cause of his actions. . . . We believe there should have been a milder solution to the obvious problem that professor Bier had with his subordinates."[42] This was the last comment on the expulsion of the medical assistants. A few days later, on the 29th of May, the same newspaper printed the following about Professor Bier's inaugural speech: "It began with a lively trampling of feet."[43]

On the third of March, 1907, one day before Bier became director of the Surgical Department of the Royal Clinic, August Hildebrandt had held his inaugural speech as surgeon of the Charité. The title of his speech was, "The Treatment of Penetrating Stomach Wounds in Battle Field."[13,17] Whether the topic was asked for by the committee of the clinic, or whether Hildebrandt would rather have discussed the topic of Bier's new directorship, is difficult to determine.

References

1. Bier A: Versuche über Cocainisirung des Rückenmarkes. Dtsch Zschr f Chir 51:361, 1899.
2. Thorwald J: Das Weltreich der Chirurgen. Steingrüben Verlag, Stuttgart 1957.
3. Secher O: Who was Hildebrandt? The History Anaesthesia Society. Volume 8a, Proceedings of the June 1990 meeting. Huddersfield 46-49.
4. Quincke H I: Über Hydrocephalus. Verhandl Kongr Innere Med 10:322, 1891.
5. Bethe H: Heinrich Quincke 1842-1922. Sein Leben und Werk unter besonderer Berücksichtigung der Kieler Fakultätsgeschichte. Karl Wachholtz Verlag, Neumünster 1968.
6. Bier A:Weitere Mitteilung über Rückenmarksanaesthesie. Arch f klin Chir 64:236, 1901.
7. Vogeler K: August Bier, Leben und Werk. J.F. Lehmann's Verlag, Berlin - München 1942.
8. Corning JA: On the prolongation of the anaesthetic effect of the hydrochlorate of cocaine, when subcutaneously injected. An experimental study. New York Med J 41:317, 1885.
9. Corning JA: Spinal Anaesthesia and Local Medication of the Cord. New York Med J 42:483, 1885.
10. Corning JA: A further Contribution on Local Medication of the Spinal Cord, with Cases. New York Med Rec 17 March, 1888.
11. Corning JA: Pain in its neuro-pathological, diagnostic, medico-legal and neuro-therapeutics-relations. Philadelphia 1894.
12. Fink R: c/o University of Washington, personal communication concerning JL Corning, March 1991.
13. Brehmer (family of August Hildebrandt) personal communication concerning Hildebrandt, Dec 1990, Jan 1991, May 1991.
14. Küttner H: Unter dem Deutschen Roten Kreuz im Südafrikanischen Kriege. Verlag von S. Hirzel, Leipzig 1900.

15. Hildebrandt A: Briefe von der Deutschen Ambulanz des Rothen Kreuzes in Südafrika. Münch med Wochenschr 47:509, 540, 738, 1900.
16. Hildebrandt A, Graf: Die Verwundungen durch die modernen Kriegsfeuerwaffen, Ihre Prognose und Therapie im Felde. Teil I. Allgemeiner Teil, II. Spezieller Teil, Berlin 1905/1907.
17. BZ am Mittag, Ausgabe vom 5.5.1907: Hinsweis zu Dr. August Hildebrandt als neuer Privatdozent der medizinischen Fakultät.
18. Diepgen P. Der Chirurg August Hildebrandt. Deutsches Medizinisches Journal 1:39, 1957.
19. Wagner D: c/o Institute for the History of Medicine at the University of the Charité, personal communication concerning August Hildebrandt, letter March 91.
20. Schneider M: (son of Dr. Schneider) personal communication concerning Hildebrandt, February 1992.
21. Köhler: c/o Bürgermeister von Süderhasted, personal communication concerning Hildebrandt, Dec 1990.
22. Gube F: (former nurse at the hospital at Eberswalde), personal communication concerning August Hildebrandt, Feb 1991.
23. Forssmann W: Selbstversuch - Erinnerungen eines Chirurgen. Droste Verlag. Düsseldorf 1972.
24. Forssmann W: Die Sondierung des rechten Herzens. Klin Wochenschr 8:2085, 1929.
25. Forssmann W: (son of W. Forssmann) personal communication concerning Werner Forssmann, March 1991.
26. Hahn F: Ueber subarachnoidale Cokaininjektionen nach Bier. Zbl f d Grenzgebiete d Med u Chir 9:338, 1900.
27. Hahn F: Ueber subarachnoidale Cokaininjektionen nach Bier. Zbl f d Grenzgebiete der Med u Chir 8:305, 1901.
28. Bockenheimer P: Technik und Indikationen der lokalen Anaesthesie. Zschr f ärztl Fortbildung 488, 1905.
29. Hildebrandt A: Die Lumbalanaesthesie. Bln klin Wschr 34:1083, 1905.
30. Bosse B: Diskussionsbemerkung auf der Sitzung der Gesellschaft der Charité - Aerzte. Bln klin Wschr 12:367, 1906.
31. Lazarus P: Zur Lumbalanaesthesie. Bln klin Wochenschr 12:367, 1906.
32. Bier A: Zur Geschichte der Rückenmarksanästhesie. Münch med Wochenschr 1059, 1906.
33. Réclus P: De la méthode de Bier. Bulletin Médical 22, 1901.
34. Réclus P: La méthode de Bier. Bulletin Médical 38, 1901.
35. Bier A: Ueber den jetzigen Stand der Rückenmarksanästhesie, ihre Berechtigung, ihre Vortheile und Nachtheile gegenüber anderen Anästhesierungsmethoden. Arch f klin Chir 77:198, 1905.
36. Bockenheimer P: Zur Geschichte der Lumbalanaesthesie. Erwiderung an Herrn August Bier-Bonn auf seinen Artikel in der Münch med Wochenschr 1906; 22: Münch med Wochenschr 40:1669, 1906.
37. DuMont F: Handbuch der Allgemeinen und lokalen Anaesthesie. Urban & Schwarzenberg, Wien-München 1903.
38. Bier A: Erwiderung auf vorstehenden Artikel von Bickenheimer. Münch med Wochenschr 34:1669, 1906.
39. Bosse B: Die Lumbalanaesthesie. Urban & Schwarzenberg, Berlin und Wien 1907.
40. Killian H: Die Geschichte der rückenmarksnahen Anästhesien. In: Die rückenmarksnahen Anästhesien. Internationales Symposium in Minden 1972, Hrg. von Nolte-Meyer, Georg Thieme Verlag, Stuttgart 1973.
41. BZ am Mittag, Ausgabe vom 8.5. 1907: Der neue Herr. Eine Kränkung der Berliner Aerzteschaft.
42. BZ am Mittag, Ausgabe vom 9.5. 1907: Assistentenkündigungen an der Chirurgischen Klinik.
43. BZ am Mittag - Ausgabe vom 29.5. 1907 Hinweis für Biers Antrittsvorlesung als neuer Leiter der chirurgischen Klinik.
44. Reichsmedizinalkalenders für das Jahr 1935, Thieme Verlag Stuttgard 1935.
45. Toellner R: c/o Institute for the History of Medicine at the University of Münster, personal communication concerning Hermann Coenen.

WHO WAS OTTO KAPPELER?

M. GOERIG
Department of Anaesthesiology, University Hospital Hamburg, Germany

A few years following the discovery of the anesthetic properties of ether as well as chloroform, extensive monograph appeared in England and the U.S. In the German speaking countries, comprehensive textbooks concerning the indications, methods, and disadvantages of the different anesthetics were not published. So an extensive German monograph of anesthesiology did not exist until 1880. Until then, most of the analgetic methods were handled in surgical textbooks, as in the chapter on anesthesia by the surgeon Neputek Nussbaum (1829-1890) of Munich, in 1867, or by Paul von Bruns (1846-1916) of Tübingen, in 1878.[1,2]

The Swiss surgeon Otto Kappeler (1841-1909) had been the first author to publish an extensive handbook on the specialty of anesthesiology representing the full knowledge at that time (Fig. 1, Fig. 2). This handbook was considered to be a standard for the later appearing textbooks.[3] This alone is reason enough to examine the biography of Kappeler. But this was not all Kappeler had done for modern anesthesiology. A few of his experiments and inventions will be mentioned here, which is a picture of a man who believed in *In somno securitas.*

The Biography of Kappeler

Kappeler was born on March 19, 1841, in Frauenfeld, Switzerland, the son of an esteemed physician.[4,5] He studied medicine at the University of Zürich, where since 1860 the famous Theodor Billroth (1829-1894) had been working.[6] Kappeler was for a short time subordinate to Billroth and was, as he later wrote, "happy to briefly follow the path of this wonderful man."[7] He finished his dissertation in the winter of 1862, writing on the subject of Purpura.[5]

Having received a license to practice as a physician in the Canton of Thurau and Zürich, Kappeler travelled and further studied in the clinics of Vienna, Prague and Paris to learn the newest surgical achievements of Europe.[8,9] In July, at the age of 23, he was selected as chief resident of the hospital in Münsterlingen near the Konstanz lake.[10,11] At one time, he is said to have described the hospital as a monastery that resembled a medieval mortuary.[5] Kappeler was allowed to have the hospital rebuilt, which

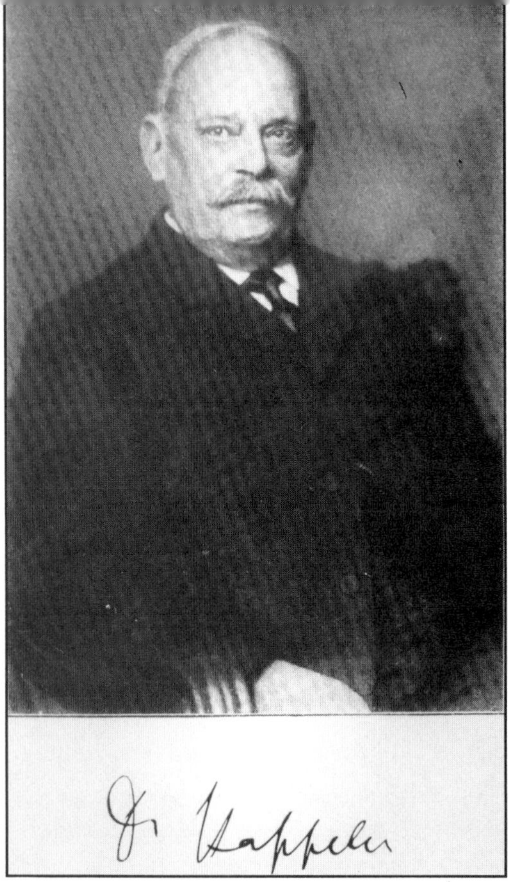

Fig. 1. Otto Kappeler (1841-1909).[6]

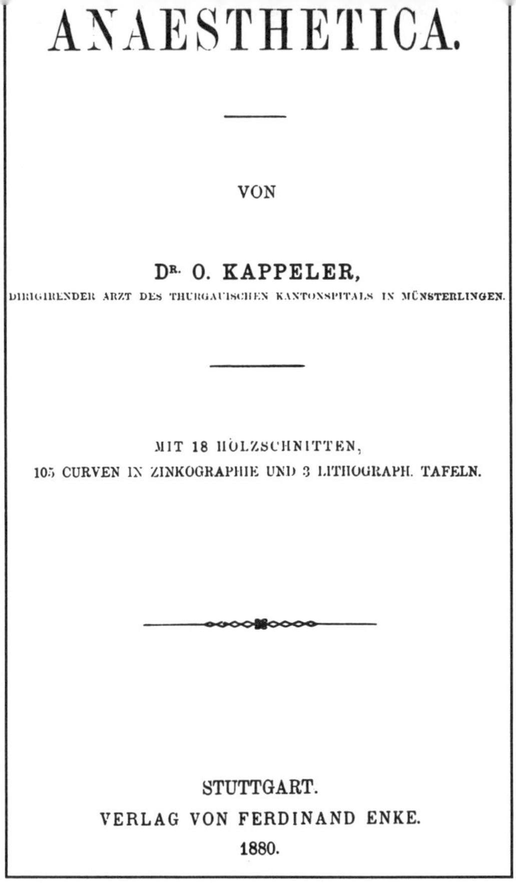

ANAESTHETICA.

VON

DR. O. KAPPELER,

DIRIGIRENDER ARZT DES THURGAUISCHEN KANTONSPITALS IN MÜNSTERLINGEN.

MIT 18 HOLZSCHNITTEN,
105 CURVEN IN ZINKOGRAPHIE UND 3 LITHOGRAPH. TAFELN.

STUTTGART.
VERLAG VON FERDINAND ENKE.
1880.

Fig. 2. Frontispiece of his textbook "Anaesthetica."[3]

bettered immensely the hygiene required for surgery, and in the following years he studied intensely the effects of different narcotics.[6]

In 1880, Billroth — who had moved in the meantime to Vienna and was the editor of the textbook series, "German Surgery" — asked Kappeler to write an extensive textbook on the subject of anesthesia.[5] Famous surgeons, such as Ernst von Bergmann (1836-1907), Friedrich Wilhelm von Esmarch (1823-1908), Theodor Kocher (1841-1917) and Friedrich von Trendelenburg (1844-1924) were also co-editors of this textbook series, each writing of his own special area in surgery.[6] Although not a professor, Kappeler's reputation among his colleagues can be seen in being allowed to publish with such famous surgeons. Billroth once said to Kappeler: "That you have done so much for medicine without being a professor means more to me than any professor who can do two times as much."[5] In February, 1896, Kappeler moved to Konstanz in Germany, where he accepted the post of head surgeon at the city hospital.[9,12]

In 1909, Kappeler had appendicitis, an illness for which he had always recommended early operation.[8] At his deathbed, the surgeon is said to have whispered: "Make my journey swift." Otto Kappeler died on May 11, 1909, and was later to be honored with the title "Father of German Anaesthesiology."[5]

Anesthesia Related Contributions of Kappeler

In his handbook, Kappeler paid special attention to safety measures from both the theoretical and the practical point of view.[3] He suggested a continuous monitoring of the patient's face, pupils, pulse and respiratory rate for each and every narcosis. He wrote detailed descriptions of the cardiovascular effects of different anesthetics, and made an extensive analysis of ether and chloroform from a collection of more than 1500 graphic curves drawn with the Marey Sphygmograph (1830-1904), which he had chosen the most suitable for didactic purposes, and with which he was able to demonstrate the principal differences

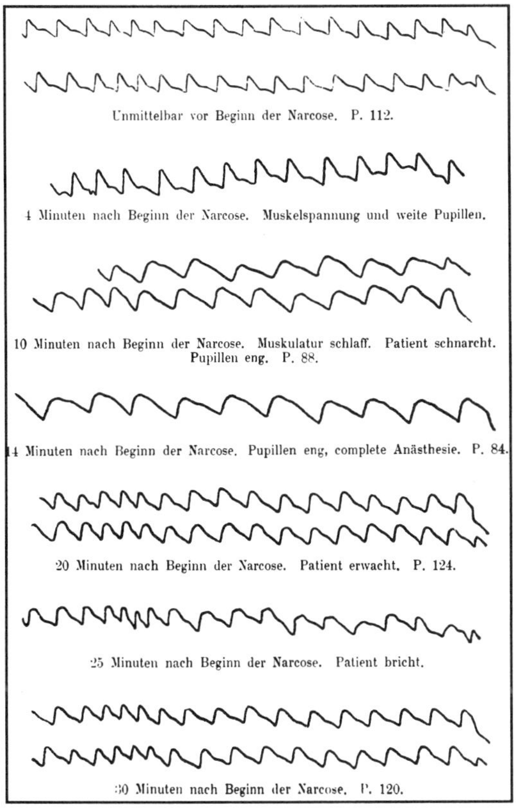

Fig. 3. Sphygmographic pulse curves under chloroform anesthesia.[3]

between these two anesthetics (Fig. 3). Kappeler recorded 10 second radial measurements with a sphygmograph designed by Brequet, serial number 35901. Kappeler was one of the first surgeons to place such an extensive sphygmographic documentation in an anesthetic textbook.[3,13,14] It was only years later that other medical authors inserted such reproductions of documentation in their textbooks.[15]

Kappeler was convinced that the most frequent dangers for a patient under general anesthesia were caused by disturbances of the circulation. For this reason, he made a detailed graphic analysis of every death caused by chloroform, gathering the information from medical reports of 1865-1876.[13] He described the necessary steps to be taken in the case of the life endangered patient: "Of utmost importance is artificial respiration since only so might the toxic gas evaporate and allow oxygenated blood

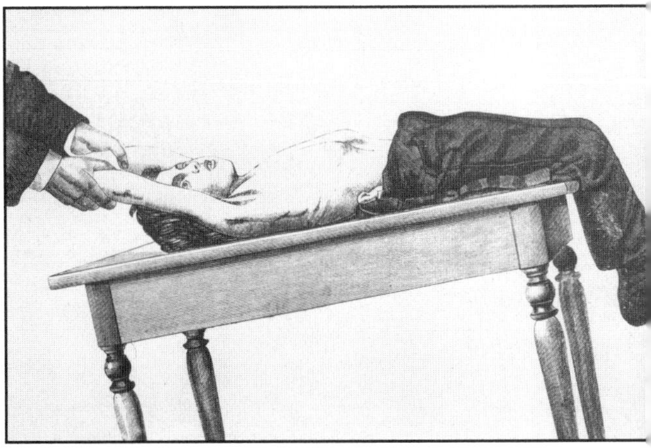

Fig. 4a. Howard's maneuver for resuscitation - inspiration.[3]

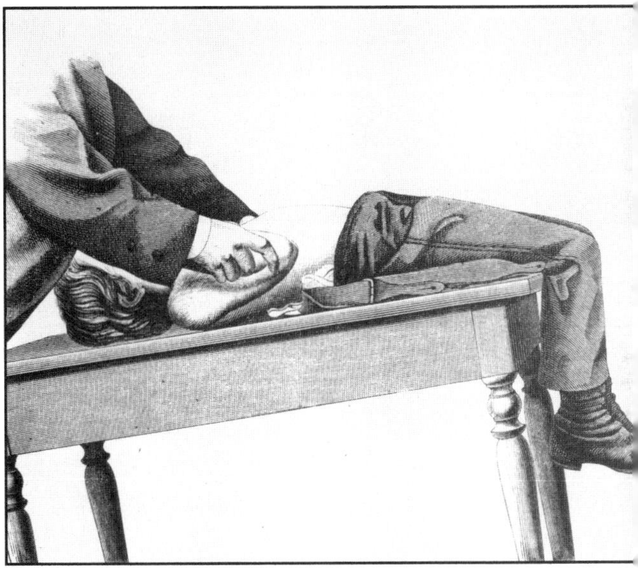

Fig. 4b. Howard's maneuver for resuscitation - exspiration.[3]

to again circulate through the body.[13] He emphatically suggested the use of the Englishman Howard's artificial respiratory and resuscitive measures (Fig. 4a, Fig. 4b). He strongly suggested keeping an open airway with the so-called Esmarch-Heiberg (1823-1908) (1843-1975) technique, and described his own technique of this procedure, the so-called Kappeler maneuver (Fig. 5). Experimenting with autopsy cadavers, he was able to prove the effectiveness of this method.

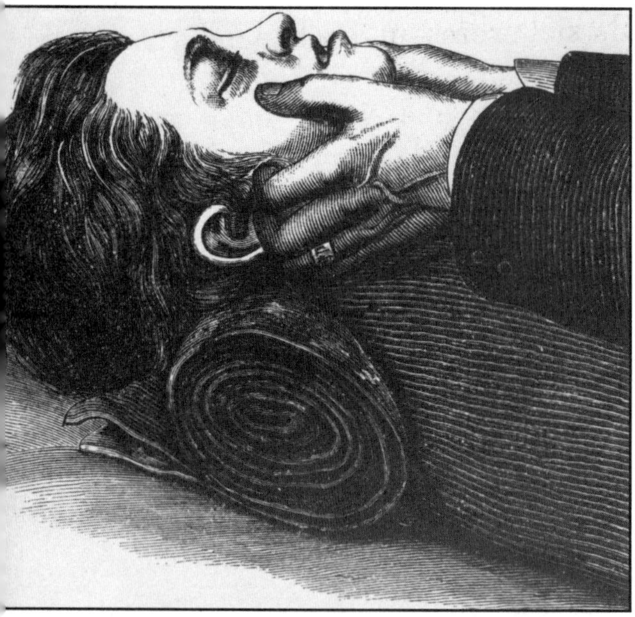

Fig. 5. The so-called Kappeler-Maneuver.[3]

Interestingly, Kappeler pointed out the advantage of blowing air through a larynx-catheter, and also the necessity of the tracheotomy with the use of Trendelenburg's tracheal tube. Although doubting the effect of electroacupuncture, he felt that the Faradisation of the phrenical nerves was a useful procedure.[3]

At the end of his book, he outlined the possible advantages of mixed anesthesia in general and morphine-chloroform narcosis. He referred to the methods of local analgesia, describing in particular the use of ether spray, a method introduced some years previously by Benjamin Ward Richardson (1828-1896).[16] He doubted the effectiveness of subcutaneously injected morphine as a local analgesic, and these doubts were proven correct in later years. With the exception of an Italian translation in 1884, Kappeler's handbook was not revised:[17] this was more than likely due to the fact that, between the years 1884-1890, many of the methods of local anesthesia were rapidly being developed and thus outdating the information contained in his handbook. A new textbook rather than a new edition was required.

Although many short monographs on anesthesia and anesthesiology appeared in the German-speaking countries between the years 1890-1910, none were as extensive as that of Kappeler.[18-20] Every medical author praised this standard textbook, and even 28 years later the obstetrician, Benno Wilhelm Müller (1872-1947), in his 800 page textbook praised Kappeler for his practice.[21,22]

After writing the handbook, Kappeler engaged himself with the technical possibilities of instruments designed to hinder the overdose of anesthetics.[6,22] He developed a simple apparatus that was easy to handle and usable in everyday practice (Fig. 6a, Fig. 6b).[6] There were, of course, already apparatuses with relatively exact dosing abilities, but these were still in the experimental phase. One exception was an instrument developed by the pharmacologist, Julius Geppert (1856-1937), designed for hospital use.[23] Although widely acclaimed, it was rarely used as it was too cumbersome for daily use in practice. Moreover, most surgeons operated in their own practice or in the home of their private patients. This was the main reason Kappeler decided to design a more manageable instrument.[6]

The Kappeler Apparatus

Kappeler developed his own apparatus for narcosis between the years 1888-1890, which he then patented at the German Patent Bureau in Berlin in 1890.[24] The model resembled the then popular model of Junker (1828-1901), which was used worldwide in many different varieties.[25-29] It is plausible that Kappeler had first seen this model used by the surgeon Edmund Rose from Berlin (1836-1914), who had been the chairman of the Surgical Department of the University in Zürich from 1867-1881.[30] The Kappeler apparatus could be described as follows:[25,29,31] The air is led through a tubular system of vaporized chloroform and into the middle of a bellows closely resembling that of Junker. The concentration of this chloroform-air-gaseous mixture depended on the temperature, the amount of air sucked into the tubular system, and the amount of chloroform present in the system. The difference between Kappeler's and Junker's

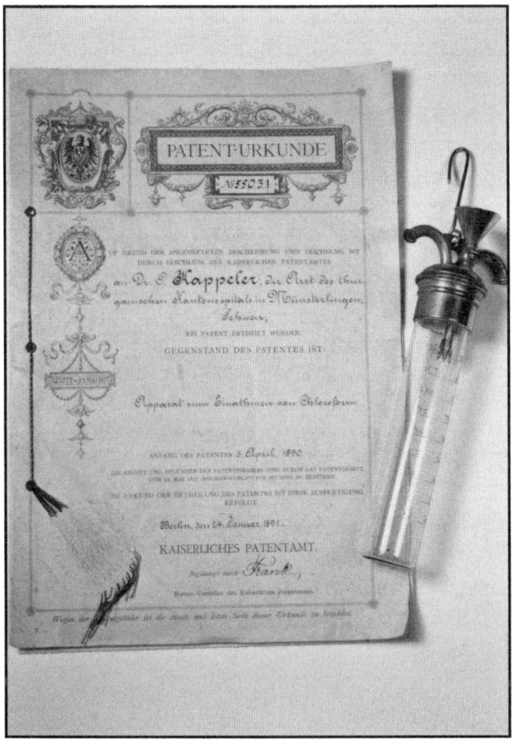

Fig. 6a. Patent-document 1891.[39]

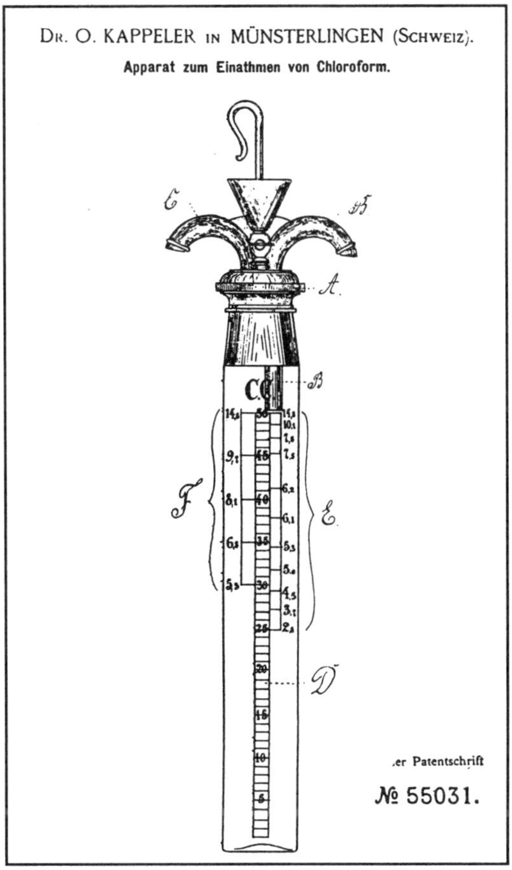

Fig. 6b. Kappeler's anesthetic apparatus.[24]

apparatus was that the air was not pumped through the liquid, but instead was led over the surface of the liquid chloroform. The bellows of the apparatus was so constructed that, with every 30 pumps, 3 liters of air could be conducted through the system. This meant that a patient with a respiratory volume of 8 liters would have to breathe the remaining 5 liters through a valve in the mask. As a result of intensive experimentation, Kappeler's apparatus could continuously show the amount of chloroform used for the anesthesia.

The apparatus had three measuring scales: the scale in the middle showed the remaining amount of chloroform, the scale on the right showed how many grams of chloroform every 100 liters of air contained, and lastly the scale to the left showed the grams of chloroform in 100 liters of air when one did not begin with a full flask. The advantages of the apparatus were described as follows:[22,26,32] 1) minimal amounts of chloroform were used. These amounts were less than those of any other available apparatus; 2) the induction of anesthesia was described by patients as pleasant, due to the dosing ability; and 3) the overall amount of anesthetic used could be estimated and controlled with fair precision.

The last point represented a not-to-be-underestimated development toward a safer anesthesia apparatus, and it was with certainty a clear alternative to the then popular drop method. Kappeler emphasized that it in no way excluded the danger of accidental death, but that it nevertheless represented a plausible solution.[32]

Unfortunately, it is difficult to determine just how many of Kappeler's apparatuses were in use. Although referred to and described in textbooks such as Müller's "Narkologie" or Max von Brunn's (1875-1924) "Allgemeine Narkose," his apparatus was not to be found in any of the leading German medical mail-order catalogues or medical instrument store catalogues.[22] Barbara Duncum mentioned Kappeler (she had falsely named him Oscar Kappeler), along with his invention, in her book which was published in 1946.[31] She stated that this variant of Junker's apparatus was rarely used in Europe.[31]

Further Contributions of Kappeler

As the conflict developed between the use of chloroform and ether throughout Europe at the end of the 19th century, it was Kappeler of the German Surgical Society who suggested that the conflict could be solved with statistical data.[6,33,34] The documentation of 240,806 chloroform and 46,233 ether anesthesia was presented before an examination board, of which the surgeon Julius Gurlt (1825-1899) was the chairman.[34] One out of every 2,907 chloroform anesthesias was the cause of an accidental death, whereas the ratio of ether was one to 14,646! This result finally forced ether into its place as the leading anesthetic for major operations and at the same time banned chloroform from further use in German-speaking countries.[34,35] A similar result was attained in England, the documentation being examined by the Royal Medical Committee of Medicine and Surgery.[36,37]

Kappeler himself made no secret of the fact that he preferred chloroform and, though not opposing ether, he did point out its specific risks, in particular its flammability near candles and gas lamps.[33] At a time when electricity was more a novelty than commonplace, the danger of the explosiveness of ether was not to be underestimated, especially when operations taking place in private practices were lighted with candles and gas lamps. He listed many cases in which operations with ether had ended in disaster. Kappeler was one of the first physicians in Germany to concern himself with safety measures to be taken during the use of anesthetics. It was not until the 1920's — after many such disasters with ether had occurred — that the solution to the problem of ether's volatibility was solved.[38]

It seems that Kappeler did not perform any extensive animal experiments in order to test the toxicity of the different anesthetics. However, he did register the circulatory effects of patients under these narcotics, constantly improving his documentation. As a result, he came to the conclusion that "all of the major anesthetics create an extreme vasodilation by blocking the vasoconstrictors."[14] This he was able to conclude through his sphygmographical documented pulse examinations. He therefore believed that a newly introduced anesthetic should be tested, not only with animal experimentation, but also with frequent pulse measurements of healthy patients before, after and while under narcosis.[14]

A presentation of Kappeler's work would not be complete without mentioning the fact that his primary concern was the patient. He suggested a morphine-chloroform anesthesia in order to alleviate preoperative fears with light sedation and thus make the operation easier for the team and patient.[3] He believed that postoperative pain should be treated with morphine and that the patient should be placed in a well-aired but heated room since he had proved the falling of body temperature after major operations.[3]

The best way to summarize Kappeler, his life philosophy and his views concerning the development of anesthesiology would be with a quote from Kappeler himself: "It is obvious for us physicians that experience with the ill or operated patient is of primary importance to medical progress."[32]

References

1. Nussbaum N: Anästhetica. In Pitha-Billroth: Handbuch der Chirurgie. Enke Verlag, Erlangen 1867.
2. Bruns V. v: Handbuch der Chirurgischen Praxis. Erster Band, Verlag der H. Laupp'schen Buchhandlung; Tübingen 1873.
3. Kappeler O: Anaesthetica. Deutsche Chirurgie, Lieferung 20. Enke Verlag, Stuttgart 1880.
4. Amman J: (c/o Kantonsspital Münsterlingen), personal information concerning O. Kappeler, Oct 1989.
5. Brunner C: Dr. Otto Kappeler. Correspondenzblatt f. Schweizer Aerzte 14:3, 1909.
6. Meisel H: (family of Dr. Kappeler, Konstanz) personal communication concerning O Kappeler, summer 1989, 1990.

7. Kappeler O: Zur Erinnerung an Theodor Billroth. Correspondenzblatt f. Schweizer Aerzte 24:161, 1894.
8. Vischer Dr. Otto Kappeler, Konstanz 1909.
9. Rode: c/o Konstanz Hospital, personal information concerning O. Kappeler, summer 1991.
10. Amman J, Studer K: 150 Jahre Kantonsspital Münsterlingen. Münsterlingen 1990.
11. Boshard R: Zur Geschichte des thurgauischen Kantonsspitals Münsterlingen und des Medizinalwesens im Kanton Thurgau bis 1895. med. Dissertation Zürich; 1936.
12. Fromm: (c/o archives of the city of Konstanz) personal communication concerning O. Kappeler, January 1992.
13. Kappeler O: Beiträge zur Lehre von den Anaestheticis. I. Ueber den Chloroformtod. Langenbeck's Arch klin Chir 35:1-30, 1888.
14. Kappeler O: Beiträge zur Lehre von den Anaestheticis. I. Ueber den Chloroformtod. Langenbeck's Arch klin Chir 35:1-30, 1888.
15. Lyman H: Artificial Anaesthesia and Anaesthetics. 1881.
16. Benjamin WR: A new method of producing local anaesthesia applicable to dental surgery. Trans Odont Soc GB 45-68, 1866.
17. Kappeler O: Anestesici. Enrico Detcen Editore, Napoli 1884.
18. Hankel E: Handbuch der Inhalations - Anaesthetica. 2., vollständig neubearbeitete und vermehrte Auflage. Verlag von Alfred Langkammer, Keipzig 1898.
19. Koblanck Die Chloroform-und die Aethernarkose in der Praxis. Verlag von J.F. Bergmann, Wiesbaden 1902.
20. DuMont F: Handbuch der Allgemeinen und Lokalen Anaesthesie. Urban & Schwarzenberg, Berlin - Wien 1903.
21. Müller WB: Narkologie. Ein Handbuch der Wissenschaft. Verlag von R. Trenkel, Berlin 1908.
22. Brunn M: v Die Allgemeinnarkose. Verlag von Ferdinand Enke, Stuttgart 1913.
23. Geppert J: Eine neue Narkosemethode. Dtsch med Wochenschr 433, 1899.
24. Deutsches Patentamt München, personal information concerning the Kappeler apparatus, summer 1989.
25. Kappeler O: Beiträge zur Lehre von den Anaestheticis. III. Ueber die Methode der Chloroformirung, insbesondere ueber Chloroformirung mit messbaren Chlorofromluftmischungen. Langenbeck's F Arch klin Chir 40:844, 1891.
26. Kappeler O: Chloroformapparat. Illustrirte Monatsschrift für ärztliche Polytechnik, März 1891.
27. Junker F: Description of a new apparatus for administration of narcotic vapours. Med Times Gaz Nov 30, 590, 1867.
28. Thomas KB: Ferdinand Edelbert Junker. Anaesthesia 28:531, 1973.
29. Thomas KB: The Development of Anaesthetic Apparatus. A History based on the Charles King Collection of the Association of Anaesthetist of Great Britain and Ireland., Blackwell Scientific Publications, London 1975.
30. Winau R, Vaubel E: Chirurgenin Berlin - 100 Portraits. Walter de Gruyter Verlag, Berlin-New York 1983.
31. Duncum BM: The development of inhalation anaesthesia. Oxford University Press, 1946.
32. Kappeler O: Weitere Erfahrungen und neue Versuche über die Narkose mit messbaren Chloroformluftmischungen. Bruns Beitr f klin Chir 24:247, 1892.
33. Kappeler O: Chloroform versus Aether. Correspondenzblatt f Schweizer Aerzte 19:282, 1889.
34. Brunn R: v Über die weitere Entwicklung der Anästhesie. Ciba Zeitschrift Nr. 60: Die Anästhesie, Wehr/Baden, 1953.
35. Julliard G: L"ether est - il préferable au chloroforme? Revue Médicale de la Suisse Romande 2:6, 1891.
36. Killian H: Narkose zu operativen Zwecken. Verlag von Julius Springer, Berlin 1934.
37. Killian H, Weese H: Die Narkose. Ein Lehr und Handbuch. Thieme Verlag, Stuttgart 1954.
38. Goerig M, Pothmann W, Pokar H: Excess gases - a historical review. The History of Anaesthesia Society. Proceedings of June 1991 Meeting-Rotterdam.

MAX TIEGEL
A Forgotten Pioneer of Anesthetic Apparatus

M. GOERIG*, K. AYISI and H. POKAR***
Department of Anaesthesiology and Department of Cardiovascular Surgery***
University Hospital Hamburg, Germany

The development of chest surgery in the last decades is closely related with the development of anesthesiology.[1] Especially, the technical development of anesthetic equipment has made numerous intrathoracic operations possible, making chest surgery the specialty it is today.[2,3] Due to serious complications such as pneumothorax and pneumonia, chest operations were often only attempted in emergency situations.[4,5]

The first step to improve the survival of patients undergoing thoracic surgery was taken by the Beeslau surgeon, Ferdinand Sauerbruch (1875-1951).[6] Sauerbruch introduced his concept of the low pressure chamber at the German Surgical Congress in Berlin in 1904.[6,7] At the same meeting, the internist, Rudolph Brauer (1865-1951) of Hamburg, promoted the use of a high pressure procedure, which he specially developed for intrathoracic operations.[8,9] Sauerbruch considered Brauer's alternative "unphysiological" and rejected the tracheal intubation technique of Franz Kuhn (1866-1929) for lung operations.[10,11] The advantages of the intubation technique, in comparison to the conventional methods, had been extensively pointed out by Kuhn.[11] Sauerbruch also questioned the usefulness of the intratracheal insufflation technique, recommended for these purposes by the American physiologists, Samuel James Meltzer (1851-1920) and his colleague John Auer (1875-1948).[12,13] Because of his authority, Sauerbruch was able to force a general acceptance of his low pressure technique, although he later acknowledged the practice and advantage of intubation.[4,10] Unfortunately, Sauerbruch was a major cause of the delayed acceptance of intubation in Europe, and in particular the German-speaking countries.[14]

Just as Kuhn was the creator and promoter of the intubation technique in anesthesia, and Meltzer and Auer were the inventors of intratracheal insufflation, Max Tiegel is considered to be the developer of positive pressure ventilation apparatus. Although Tiegel had been responsible for much of the technical advancements of anesthetic apparatus until the

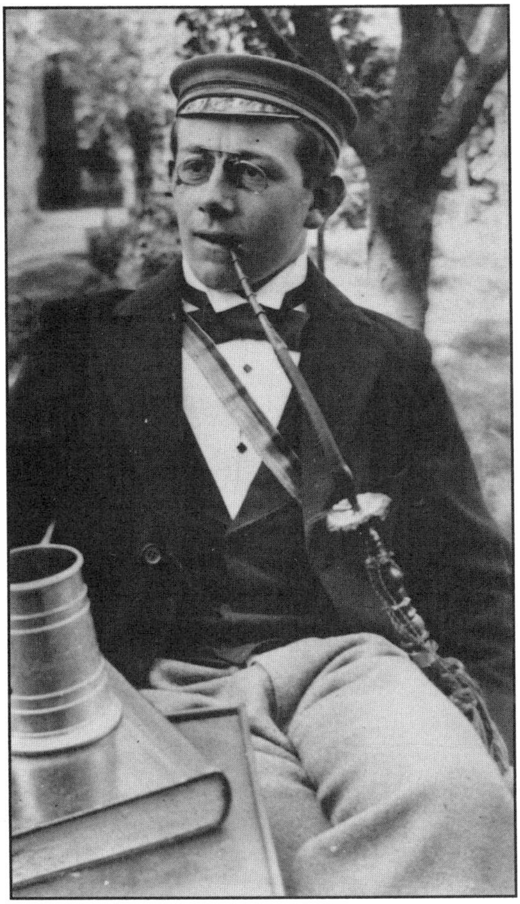

Fig. 1. Max Tiegel as a student, *circa* 1895.[24]

late 30's, his name had been more or less forgotten. Up until the 1950's, every popular German surgical and anesthesiologic textbook author had referred to his technical contribution for the development of this kind of anesthetic apparatus.[15-23] In contrast to his important contributions to our specialty, little biographic data has been available about Tiegel. That is why it is worthwhile to provide a short review of Tiegel and his anesthetic related contributions.

Biography

Max Tiegel was born on August 8, 1877, in Wansen, near Breslau, Germany, the son of a general practitioner (Fig. 1).[24] After finishing his medical studies, he began his dissertation on an obstetric topic before moving to Frankfurt and beginning his career at the Institute of Pathology. Between the years 1902-1905, he was resident surgeon of the Breslau University, where he was subordinate to the great Johannes von Miculicz-Radecky (1850-1905), whose teacher was Theodor Billroth (1829-1894). Ferdinand Sauerbruch (1875-1951) and Adolf Henlewere also working at the same institution when Tiegel attended the surgical department (Fig. 2). In the years 1905-1907, he finished his surgical studies as subordinate to the

Fig. 2. Max Tiegel* as a resident surgeon at the Department of Surgery at the Breslau University, please note Ferdinand Sauerbruch.**[24]

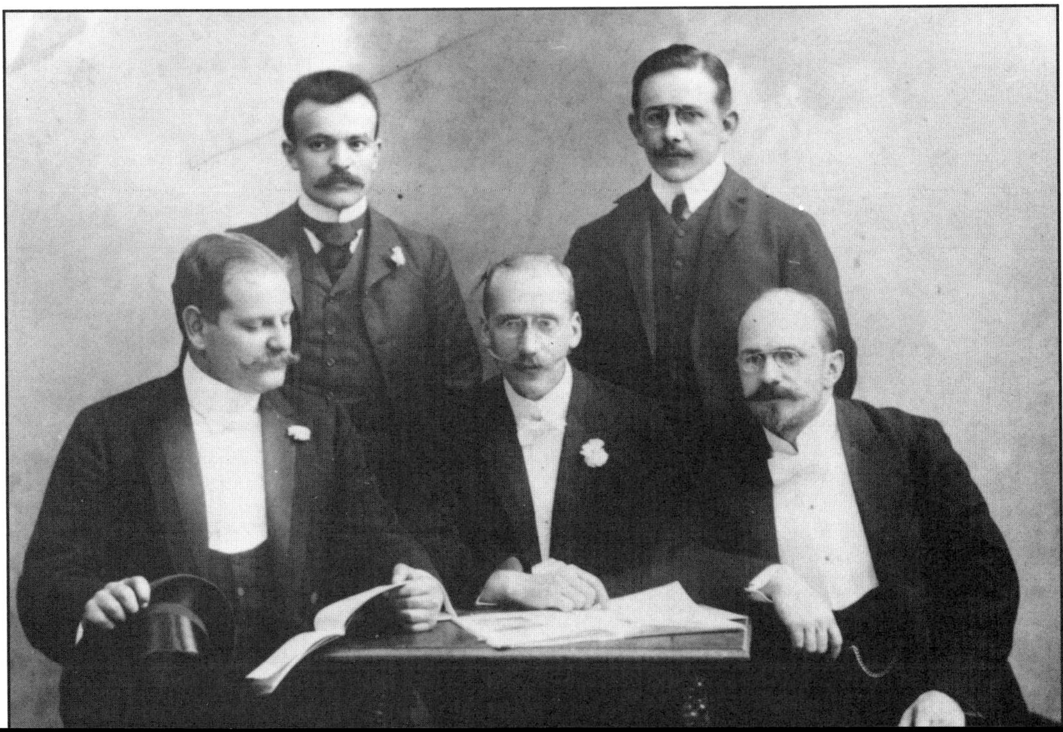

magnificent obstetrician and surgeon Hermann Johannes Pfannenstiel (1862-1929), better known as the discoverer of the neonatal hemolytic syndrome. He then moved to Dortmund, where he was a medical resident to Henle until 1919, actively participating in World War I between 1915-1918. Finally, until his early retirement in 1937, Tiegel was Chief surgeon of two different hospitals in Trier.

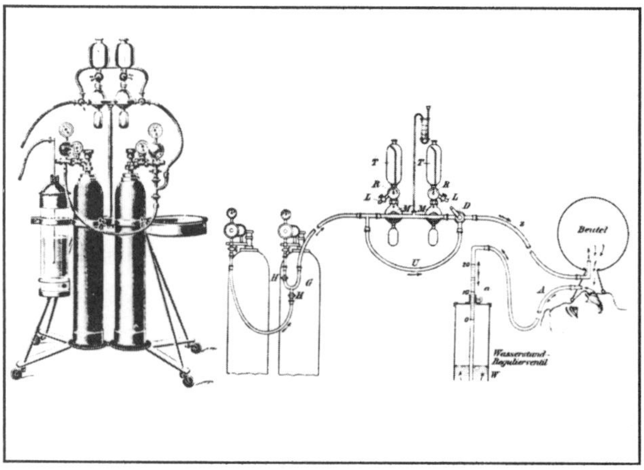

Fig. 3a. Tiegel's positive pressure anesthesia apparatus, scheme of the device.[26]

Scientific Work — the "Tiegel Apparatus"

Tiegel published his first relevant anesthetic article in 1905 during his residency in the Surgical Department of the Breslau University Clinic.[25] On the topic of intrathoracic operations, he outlined the advantages and disadvantages of both the low and high pressure techniques, which where at the time a major subject of surgical interest. Tiegel took the side of Sauerbruch and considered Brauer's high pressure technique to be absolutely unphysiological and especially dangerous for the lung and the heart of the patient.

A few years later, in 1908, he backed off from his dogmatic belief in the low pressure technique.[26] In a short notice which appeared in the most reputable German surgical journal at that time — Zentralblatt für Chirurgie — Tiegel presented his first apparatus for high pressure narcosis, describing it as "merely to be used provisionally in the case of emergencies, (a device) which nevertheless has proven its usefulness in extended intrathoracic operations and thus a great help to all those confronted with similar situations" (Fig. 3a, 3b). The central part of the described apparatus was a snugly fitting mask (resembling the so-called

Fig. 3b. Tiegel's positive pressure anesthesia apparatus, in daily surgical use.[27]

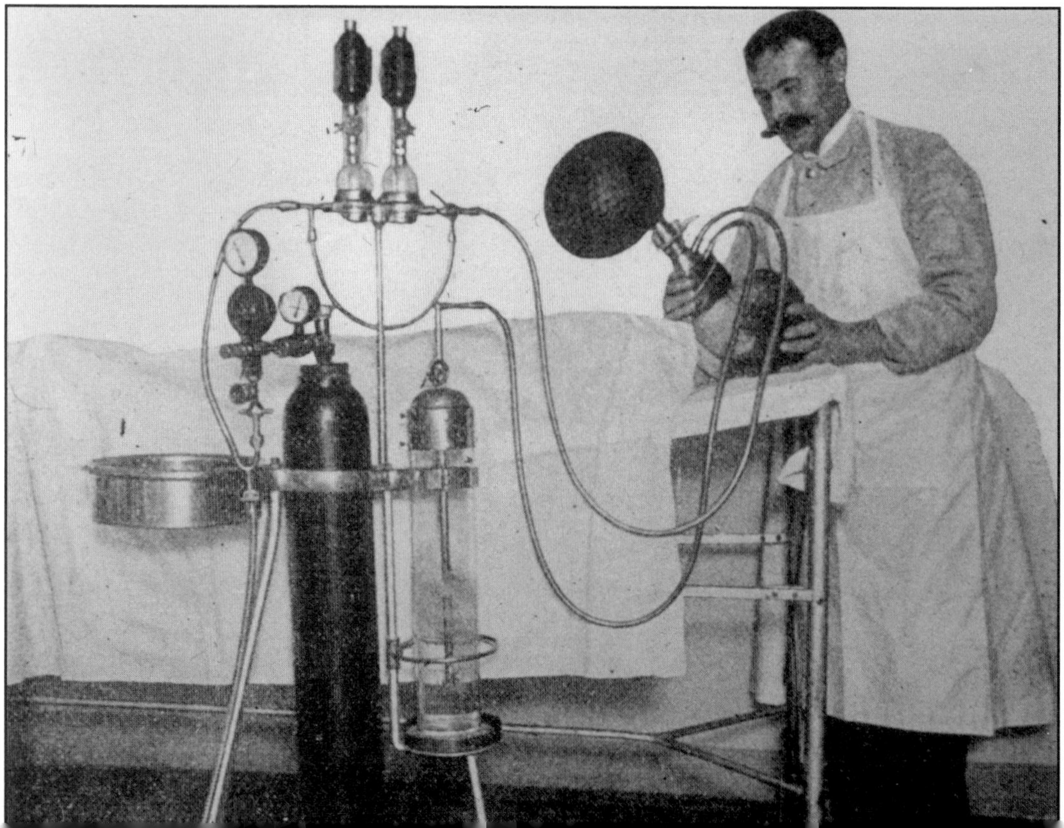

Wanscher (1846-1906) mask, Wanscher having been a Danish surgeon) which was connected to a rubber balloon with a soft rubber tube. A special protective reservoir was built into the mask in order to collect any vomit, allowing a major operation to be continued without the interruption of having to remove the mask. The balloon, which was connected to the primary source of the narcotic, served not only as a reserve for the inhaled gas, but also compensated through its elasticity for any deviation of the patient's respiration. A system of high pressure was achieved through the patient's own respiratory pressure, the exhalations being led through a one-way tube into a hydraulic tank in which the desired pressure could be regulated. Tiegel emphasized the necessity of maintaining an open airway, which was frequently closed by the patient's receding tongue. Of the many possible solutions for such instances, he suggested tying the tongue with a silk noose and then firmly replacing the mask. In the following years, Tiegel published further reviews concerning the technical improvements of the apparatus, which was developed and manufactured by the Georg Haertel Company in Breslau.[27,28] This producer was, except for the Dräger Company in Lübeck and the Lautenschläger Company in Munich, the only reputable manufacturer of anesthetic apparatus.[29]

In 1909, Tiegel not only reported the technical improvements of his apparatus, but also published an article in which he listed the various indications of his high pressure technique. Besides its advantages in intrathoracic operations, he saw its applicability in the patient with a pronounced tracheal stenosis, whether it was caused by a thyroid struma or an aneurysm of the ascending aorta.[30] The increased oxygen flow of the apparatus was exceptionally useful in the surgery of patients suffering from one- or two-sided pneumothorax or mediastinal flutter, which could be immediately observed with only slightly higher pressures. He also advocated the benefits of increasing the amount of oxygen, which was mixed with air, to enable the surgery with a collapsed lung.[31] In animal experiments, he had proved the harmlessness of a slightly increased intrabronchial pressure on the pulmonary circulation and lung tissues. Tiegel also expressed the necessity of checking the apparatus before each and every operation.[27] He had designed a special device with which he could be sure that oxygen and no other gas was contained in the flask.[32] Occasionally, a company would accidentally deliver flasks filled with carbon dioxide, and with his device such happenings could be filtered out. Tiegel had only once experienced such an accident, and fortunately he had realized the mistake before any damage could be done. His own experience had therefore been the cause of inventing such a device.

In the early 1930's, he was again much involved in the development of an ether anesthesia technique.[24] His goal was to improve the quality of anesthesia and to reduce the incidence of postoperative complications, such as vomiting and pneumonia, through the heating of ether.[33]

Many technical improvements of the last decades have been devoted to the decrease in gas temperature caused by ether vaporization. At the turn of the century, the surgeon Arthur Läwen (1876-1958) of Leipzig was unsuccessful in promoting his "Thermophor" device for drop ether narcosis.[34] In the early 1920's, Henle and Tiegel therefore designed a new apparatus for oxygen-ether-chloroform-anesthesia (Fig. 4).[35,36] An incandescent lamp within the vaporizer prevented the drastic temperature decrease of the inhaled gas mixture. As one of the more widely appearing apparatuses on the market, its advantages were advocated in all current surgery and anesthesia textbooks in Germany.[17-19]

The Dr. Tiegel-Dräger Apparatus

A further development of this device was the Tiegel-Dräger Apparatus which was introduced in the early thirties (Fig. 5).[29,37] Ether was dropped into a special vaporizing chamber, i.e. onto a silver plate which was electrically

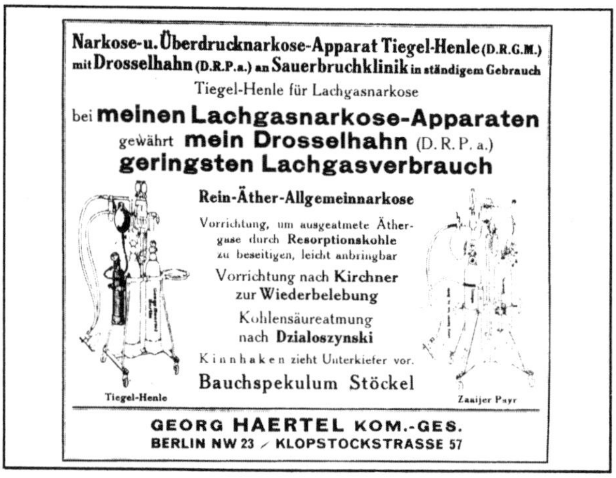

Fig. 4. Advertisement of the Tiegel-Henle Apparatus, please note the reference to the favorable use of active coal-filter (*circa* 1927).[65]

Fig. 5. Tiegel-Dräger Apparatus.

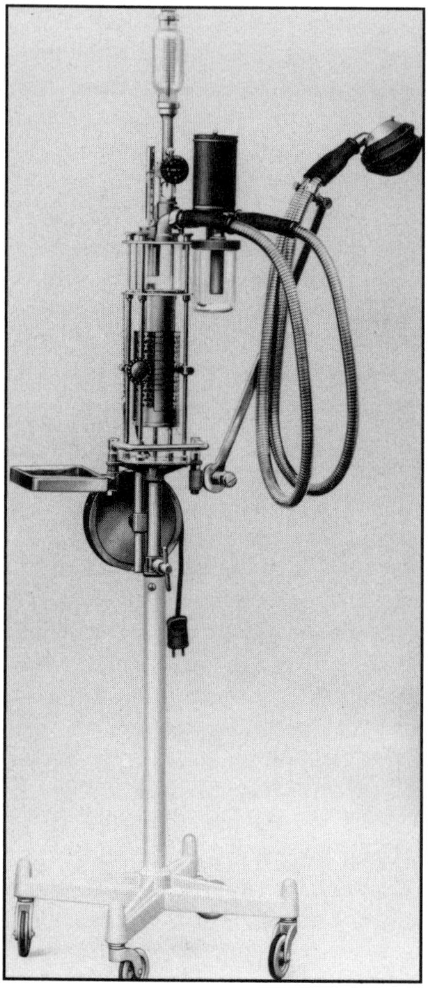

heated to a temperature of 50 degrees C in order to extend and thus rarefy the gas.[38-40] The heated and rarefied ether vapor was then combined with an air-oxygen mixture and thereafter inhaled by the patient. The anesthesia with this "High pressure mixed ether vapor" as Tiegel called it, was characterized with a minimal narcotic consumption, a negligible excitation phase, and caused little if any postoperative vomiting.[40,41] The popularity of this anesthesia technique is uncertain.[29] Only one publication concerning it could be found in the German medical literature, in which the advantages of the method were declared unproven.[42] In any case, the volatility of ether was a major concern.[43] Therefore, the development of new apparatus was indeed called for.[44] At the beginning of the twenties, the concept of recirculating the expired narcotic gas became a reality, not only in the U.S., but on the European continent as well.[44] A major reason this technique was introduced into daily practice was to reduce the cost for expensive anesthetics such as nitrous oxide and newly available vapors like narcylen.[45] Since the use of oxygen mixed with narcylen had caused deadly explosions, a new anesthetic apparatus was direly needed.[37,45,46] Furthermore, some of the new inhalation agents such as narcylen had an unpleasant pungent odour which could be removed with a filter system of active carbon placed within the narcotic circle system.[44,46,47] Because of its success, the carbon filter became an integral part of the German recirculatory devices. In the years of these technical developments, many renowned German surgeons had published articles with reports of possible dangers of chronic inhalation of gaseous narcotics.[48-50] An active coal filter was one of the various solutions. Another solution had been a specially constructed mask.[49] At the height of these discussions, Tiegel published a series of articles in which he reviewed the various problems of "Narcosis with High Pressure Ether Vapor."[38-41,43,51-53] In close collaboration with the Physics Institute of the University of Bonn, he investigated the applicability of an active coal filter in his new narcotic device and was able to prove the hypothesis.[54] He was further convinced that the active coal, when integrated into the filter system, would immensely decrease the possibility of an explosion caused by the oxygen-ether mixture.[38,54] He mentioned that such a filter would also improve the operating room conditions, which until then had been constantly "impregnated with ether."[38,43] The head engineer of the Dräger Company in Lübeck had published a monograph in which he stated to have proved the effectiveness of the integrated filter system for anesthesia apparatus.[37] He also denied the possibility of an explosion caused by a heated filter since "it could only be heated to body temperature." The active coal filter system was therefore primarily integrated as a safety measure into all narcotic devices produced in Germany and advocated for general use in every operating room.[29]

After 1934, Tiegel was in close technical contact with the Dräger Company, as he had ceased collaboration with the Georg Haertel Company in Berlin.[29,55] Thus, the new anesthesia apparatus was produced by the Dräger Company and sold as "Dr. Tiegel-Dräger-Apparat." According to the at one time head engineer of the company, Josef Haupt, the apparatus was produced until 1940, when the Second World War intervened.[29] In an advertisement of Dr. Tiegel's apparatus in 1937, the following advantages were listed: "soporification without excitation," "an expeditious awakening," "the absence of postoperative side-effects," "a precise and simple control of the anesthesia."

Tiegel then published an article in which he vehemently opposed the decision of the military medical service to use chloroform instead of his developed ether field narcosis apparatus.[56] According to the surgeon Martin Kirschner (1879-1942), a reputed surgeon of the University of Heidelberg, chloroform was the preferred anesthetic because it was not as explosive as ether; moreover, the incidence of postoperative pneumonia was said to be less in all probability.[57] In another article, Tiegel emphasized the analeptic attributes of his ether field device, which he believed should be a major consideration for surgery on wounded soldiers.[56] He was by no means the only physician who critically opposed the use of chloroform as a narcotic. Several leading German surgeons agreed with Tiegel's arguments and refused vehemently Kirschner's recommendations.[56] Following the publication of these series of articles in the leading German surgical journal, Zentralblatt für Chirurgie, Tiegel was forced to leave his post in Trier for reasons undetermined.[24]

During the war he published no other articles, and it was only afterward that he wrote some case reports concerning, "The healing of Tuberculosis and Cancer with the Inhalation of Ether vapor."[58-60] Tiegel seemed to have followed the homeopathic concept of August Bier, who was well-known for his support of a "scientific related homeopathy."[61] Already in 1937, Tiegel had written in a footnote that Bier had pointed out the therapeutic success of the use of minimal amounts of ether in the treatment of postoperative pneumonia; however, he did not describe this process in detail.[56]

After the war, Tiegel continued his collaboration with the Dräger Company in Lübeck, proposing a new version of his apparatus as an "anesthetic device for the general practitioner" (Fig. 6).[29,58] This model closely resembled his field device with heated water.[56] According to the retired chief engineer Haupt, only a few of these models were produced.[29]

Further Remarks on Max Tiegel

If one were to outline the various stages of the technical development of anesthetic apparatus, it would be obvious that Max Tiegel made major contributions in Germany to the transition from a simple narcotic technique to a complex anesthesiologic system. Nevertheless, an appraisal of his anesthetic related contributions would be incomplete without mentioning his various publications concerning the perioperative course. For example, he expressly argued for appropriate premedication, he maintained furthermore that postoperative oxygen inhalation was absolutely necessary for the thoracic patient.[24,31] He foresaw the eventual

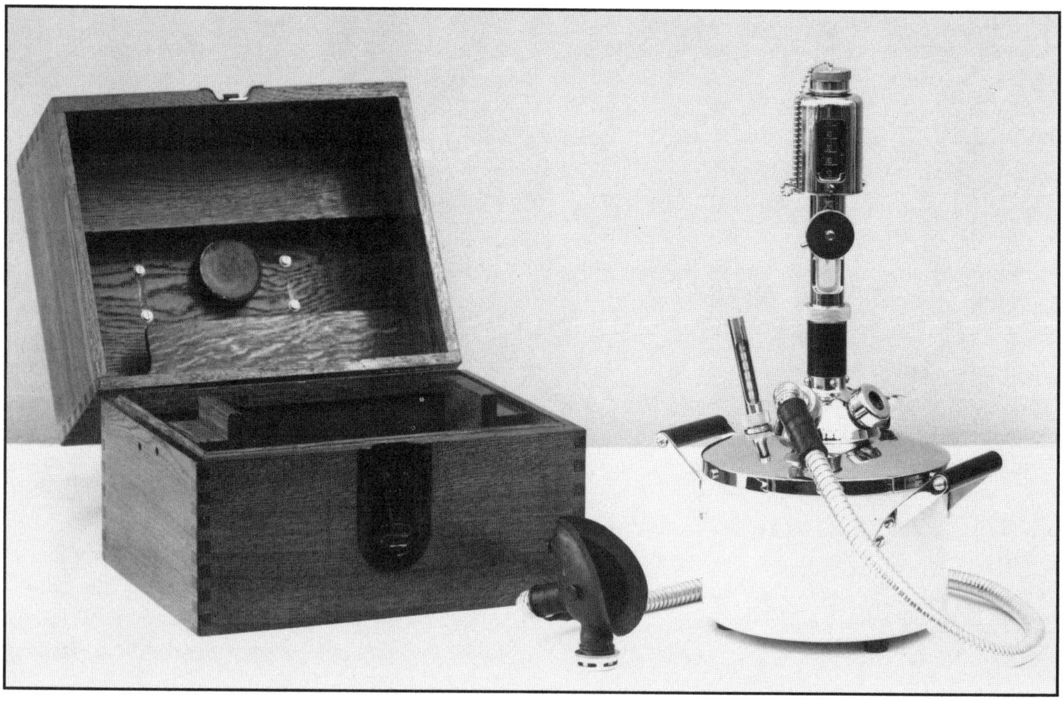

Fig. 6. Tiegel's last technical development, an "apparatus for the practitioner, using heated ether", *circa* 1951.[66]

use of insufflation, not only for the patient who had aspirated during anesthesia, but also for comatose patients.[30] Frequently, he pointed out the importance of correctly positioning the drains of patients who had undergone a chest operation so as to permit the outflow of wound secretions, thus preventing possible atelectasis or tension pneumothorax.[62] For the latter, he had designed for its relief the so-called Tiegel-Vent.[63] It is still used today in special situations, although it has been replaced to a large extent by the Heimlich-Vent, a system introduced in clinical practice in 1965.[64]

In 1912, he analyzed the advantages of the Meltzer-Auer intratracheal insufflation technique by presenting a case report: A child had accidently inhaled a bean and suffered from serious asphyxiation. After an immediate tracheotomy and a futile attempt to extract the foreign body from the trachea, the situation became so extreme that Tiegel then forced a thin Nelaton catheter (1807-1873) past the hindering body and through this catheter insufflated the lung with pure oxygen. This led to an immediate improvement of the life-threatening dyspnea after which the patient was able to cough up the foreign body. Although the procedure needed to be repeated for the next few days, the child had no further complications and survived.[30]

It is important to mention the fact that Tiegel was far from being an advocate for specialization in anesthesiology.[24] He believed that special training for such an activity was unnecessary. He did, however, believe in a standardised mechanisation of the anesthesia technique, in which he saw the simple, uniform and secure basis of a well-proven and safe ether narcosis. He was convinced that,with his high pressure gas device, anesthesia would be "no longer a skill" requiring a specialist.[39] Tiegel's lifelong denial of anesthesiology as a specialty is unimportant when compared with his numerous technical contributions to this field. Although he would have never admitted it, Max Tiegel was indeed an anesthetic-inspired surgeon (Fig. 7). (See following page).

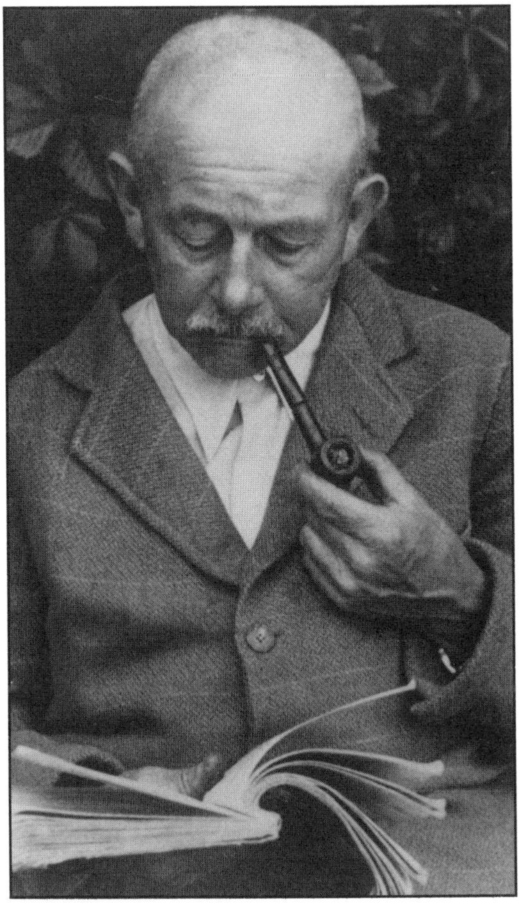

Fig. 7. Max Tiegel, *circa* 1950.[24]

References

1. Rendell-Baker L: History of thoracic surgery. In: Mushin WW, Rendell-Baker L, eds. The Principles of Thoracic Anaesthesia Past and Present. Oxford: Blackwell Scientific Publications, 1953.
2. Rendell-Baker L, Pettis JL: The development of positive pressure ventilators. In: The History of Anaesthesia. Ed. R.S. Atkinson and T.B. Bouldon: International Congress and Symposium Series Number 134 — The Parthenon Publishing Group Carnforth — New Jersey 1989.
3. Wiedemann K, Fleischer E: Zur Geschichte der Anästhesie in der Thoraxchirurgie. Pneumothoraxproblem, Intubation, Einlungenventilation. Anästh Intensivmed Notfallmed Schmerztherapie 1:3, 1992.
4. Neugebauer J: Weltruhm deutscher Chirurgie — Johann von Miculicz. Haug Verlag, Ulm/Donau 1964.
5. Nissen R: Historical Development of Pulmonary Surgery. Am J Surg 89:9, 1955.
6. Sauerbruch F: Zur Pathologie des offenen Pneumothorax und die Grundlage meines Verfahrens zu seiner Ausschaltung. Mitt Grenzgeb Med Chir 13:399, 1904.
7. Sauerbruch F: Die Chirurgie der Brustorgane. Chapter: Aus der Geschichte der Thoraxchirurgie. Springer Verlag, Berlin 1920.
8. Brauer L, Petersen: Über eine wesentliche Vereinfachung der künstlichen Atmung nach Sauerbruch. Hoppe Seyler's Zschr 41:299, 1904.
9. Brauer L: Die praktische Durchführung des Ueberdruckverfahrens. Dtsch med Wochenschr 38:1489, 1905.
10. Goerig M: Franz Kuhn (1866-1929) zum 125. Geburtstag. Anästh Intensivmed Notfallmed Schmerztherapie 8:416, 1991.
11. Kuhn Fr: Die Überdrucknarkose mittels peroraler Intubation. Zbl f Chir 42:1177, 1904.
12. Meltzer A: Dr. Samuel James Meltzer and Intratracheal Anesthesia. J Clin Anesth 2:54, 1990.
13. Meltzer SJ; The Value of Continuous Intratracheal Insufflation of Air (Meltzer) in Thoracic Surgery with Description of an Apparatus. Med Res 77:493, 1910.
14. Goerig M, Filos K, Renz D: Joseph O'Dwyer — Ein Wegbereiter der endotrachealen Intubation und Druckbeatmung. Anästh Intensivth Notfallmet 5:244, 1988.
15. Brunn M: v. Die Narkose. Enke Verlag, Stuttgart 1913.
16. Gerlach W: Überdrucknarkoseapparate. Eine kritische Besprechung nebst Mitteilung über einen neuen vereinfachten Apparat Dtsch Zschr f Chir 123:204, 1913.
17. Härtel Fr: Anleitung zur Schmerzbetäubung. Kurzes Lehrbuch der Lokalanästhesie, Allgemeinnarkose und sonstiger Anwendung der Betäubungsverfahren. Verlag von Theodor Steinkopff, Dresden-Leipzig 1936.
18. Hesse Fr,Lendle L, Schoen R: Allgemeinnarkose und örtliche Betäubung. Verlag von Johann Ambrosius Barth, Leipzig 1934.
19. Killian H: Narkose zu operativen Zwecken. Springer Verlag, Berlin 1934.
20. Kirschner M: Allgemeine und spezielle Chirurgische Operationslehre. Vol. III, Springer Verlag, Berlin 1940.

21. Pels-Leusden Fr: Chirurgische Operationslehre für Studierende und Ärzte. Urban und Schwarzenberg, Berlin-Wien 1925.
22. Semb C: Die Chirurgie der Lunge. In: Kirschner, M., Nordmann, O. Die Chirurgie. Vol V: Die Chirurgie der Brust., Urban &Schwarzenberg, Berlin und Wien 1941.
23. Kingreen O: Chirurgische Operationslehre. Urben & Schwarzenberg Verlag, München-Berlin 1952.
24. Balz D: (granddaughter of Tiegel) personal communication, November 1991, February 1992.
25. Tiegel M; Sollen die Operationen in der Brusthöhle unter Anwendung des Saugerbruch'schen Überdruck-oder Unterdruckverfahrens ausgeführt werden ? Bln Klink 209:1, 1905.
26. Tiegel M: Ein einfache Apparat zur Überdrucknarkose. Zbl f Chir 22:679, 1908.
27. Tiegel M: Ueberdrucknarkose. Bruns Beitr klin Chir 64:356, 1909.
28. Tiegel M: Weitere Mitteilungen über die Ueberdrucknarkose. Bruns Beitr klin Chir 68:584, 1909.
29. Haupt J: personal communication. January, February 1992.
30. Tiegel M: Der Wert der trachealen Insufflation für die Nachbehandlung Tracheotomierter. Zbl f Chir 40:1364, 1911.
31. Tiegel M; Die Bedeutung der Sauerstoffatmung in der Thoraxchirurgie. Zbl f Chir 47:1529, 1911.
32. Rosenthal O: Kurze Mitteilung über Gefahren der gebräuchlichen Sauerstoffanwendung. Münch med Wochenschr 48:2483, 1909.
33. Tiegel M: Verbesserung der Äthernarkose durch stärkere Erwärmung der Verdunstungstemperatur. Zbl f Chir 13:797, 1932.
34. Läwen A: Uber die Vorwärmung von Aether- und Chloroformdzämpfen für die Narkose. Münch med Wochenschr 40:2097, 1911.
35. Henle A: Bemerkungen zur Beseitigung der Narkosegase und zur Äthernarkose mit dem Überdruckapparat. Zbl f Chir 1:17, 1926.
36. Schröder H: Die technischen Hilfsmittel für die Inhalationsnarkose. Heinecke Verlag, Berlin 1938.
37. Haupt J: Der Dräger Narkoseapparat - historisch gesehen. Drägerwerk Lübeck, Medizintechnik, 1970.
38. Tiegel M: Narkose mit hochsgespanntem Ätherdampf. II. Technik der Narkose. Zbl f Chir 40:2313, 1934.
39. Tiegel M: Narkose mit hochgespanntem Ätherdampf. V. Die Mechanisierung der Narkose: ihre Steuerung und Normung. Zbl f Chir 9:485, 1935.
40. Tiegel M: Narkose mit hochgespanntem Ätherdampf. VI. Apparat für Narkose und Überdrucknarkose mit hochgespanntem Ätherdampf und für Sauerstoffdruckatmung. Zbl f Chir 8:438, 1936.
41. Tiegel M: narkose mit hochgespanntem Ätherdampf oder Äthergasnarkose. IX. Bemerkungen zur physikalischen Grundlage der Narkose. Zbl f Chir 51:3034, 1936.
42. Weisener E: Ueber Erfahrungen bei Inhalationsnarkosen mit hochgespannten Aetherdämpfen. Münch med Wochenschr 44:1789, 1936.
43. Tiegel M: Narkose mit hochgespanntem Ätherdampf. II. Die Verhütung der Explosionsgefahr. Zbl f Chir 50:2908, 1934.
44. Goerig M; Aktivkohlefilter zur Eliminierung volatiler Anaesthetika. Anaesthesist 39:637, 1990.
45. Goerig M, Pothmann W, Pokar H: Excess gases - a historical review. The History of Anaesthesia Society. Proceedings of June 1991 Meeting - Rotterdam.
46. Rimarski W: Die Narzylenbetäubung in sicherheitstechnischer Hinsicht. Münch med Wochenschr 10:386, 1925.
47. Schmidt H: Hat die Narzylenbetäubung prinzipielle Nachteile und Fehler ? Dtsch med Wochenschr 6:236, 1927.
48. Kirschner M: Zur Hygiene des Operationssaales. Zbl f Chir 39:216249, 1925.
49. Hölscher Fr: Zur Beseitigung der ausgeatmeten Narkosegase. Zbl f Cir 25, 1928.
50. Perthes G: Schutz der am Operationstisch Beschäftigten von Schädigung durch die Narkosegase. Zbl f Chir 16:852, 1925.
51. Tiegel M: Narkose mit hochgespanntem Ätherdampf. VII. Reine Äthernarkose ohne pränarkotische Vorbereitung. Zbl f Chir 10:552, 1936.
52. Tiegel M: Narkose mit hochgespanntem Ätherdampf. VIII. Rauschnarkose. Zbl f Chir 11:619, 1936.
53. Tiegel M: Narkose mit hochgespanntem Ätherdampf X. Klinische Erfahrungen (Oberflächliche Kurznarkosen bei Frauen). Zbl f Chir 20:1162, 1936.

54. Lauer F: Narkose mit hochgespanntem Ätherdampf. III. Physikalische Grundlagen der Äthernarkose mit hochgespanntem Ätherdampf. Zbl f Chir 40:2330, 1934.
55. Nitschke M: c/o Industrie-und Handelskammer zu Berlin, pers. communication concerning the Georg Haertel Company, March 1992.
56. Tiegel M: Narkose mit hochgespanntem Ätherdampf (Äthergasnarkose). XI. Feldnarkosenapparat. Zbl f Chir 16:927, 1937.
57. Kirschner M: Die Schmerzbekämpfung im Felde. Der Chirurg 8:269-76, 1936.
58. Tiegel M: Zum Kampf gegen den Krebs. Hippokrates 3:57, 1951.
59. Tiegel M: Ueberhitzte Aetherdämpfe bei Lungentuberkulose. Ars Medici 4:260, 1952.
60. Tiegel M; Inhalationen hochgespannter Aetherdämpfe. Ars Medici 2:110-4, 1952.
61. Vogeler K: August Bier, Leben und Werk. J.F. Lehmann's Verlag, Berlin - München 1942.
62. Tiegel M: Zur Frage der Thoraxdrainage. Zbl f Chir 10P:347, 1910.
63. Tiegel M: Zur Technik der Lungennaht. Münch med Wochenschr 46:2209, 1905.
64. Heimlich HJ: Heimlich flutter valve: Effective replacement for drainage bottle. Hosp Topics 43:122, 1965.

CARL-LUDWIG SCHLEICH AND THE SCANDAL DURING THE ANNUAL MEETING OF THE GERMAN SURGICAL SOCIETY IN BERLIN IN 1892

M. GOERIG, and J. SCHULTE am ESCH
Department of Anaesthesiology
University Hospital, Hamburg, Germany

Primum non nocere — derived from this premise, the surgeon Carl Ludwig Schleich reported on his own first results of a new form of local anesthetic technique which he called "infiltration anesthesia."[1] This happened exactly 100 years ago in Berlin at the annual congress of the German Surgical Society. Having presented a review about his technique, the indications and the pros and cons of his method, Schleich even went so far as to denounce any kind of chloroform anesthesia as dangerous. As a consequence, he denied the need for any general anesthesia for most surgical procedures from the humanistic and ethical point of view, as well as for legal aspects related to the state of art of his inaugurated "Infiltrationsanaesthesie" technique.[1]

With this statement at the end of his presentation, and due to his unfavorable statements, a tumult arose in the audience.[2] The chairman of the session, Heinrich Adolf von Bardeleben (1819-1895), asked the audience if there was any interest for further discussion about this topic. Furthermore, he asked the gathering if the expressed statement concerning the risks of general anesthesia reflected the opinion of the audience and was accepted as such. As nobody followed the arguments of Schleich, he had to leave the podium before any discussion could start.[3] Schleich left the congress, even though none of the congress participants knew anything about the new technique in detail.[4]

Even though the infiltration technique was later praised by the renowned German surgeon, Ernst von Bergmann (1836-1907), and that Schleich's suppression was a blot on German surgery, the general acceptance of Schleich from the established German medical world was faint.[5,6] Possibly, this led to the estrangement between Schleich and the medical world, and further to polarisation among the surgeons.[7]

August Bier (1861-1949), the forerunner of spinal anesthesia and intravenous local anesthesia, commented in 1922 on the attitude of Schleich's colleagues as follows: "Confused

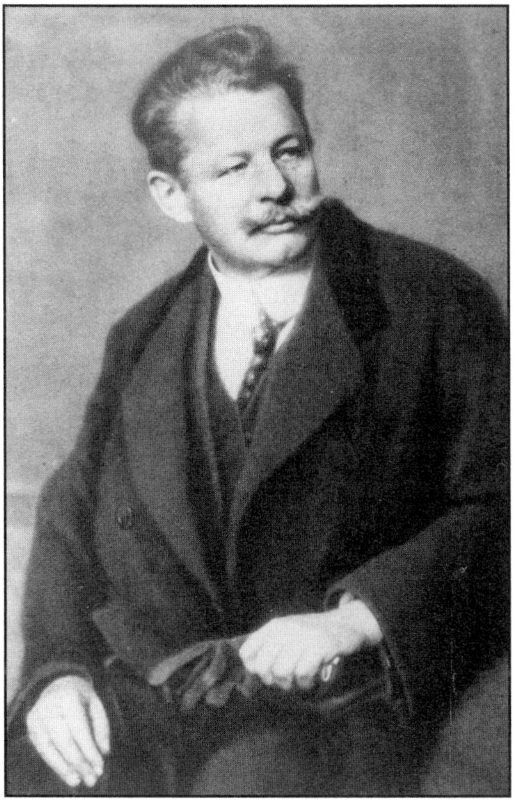

Fig. 1. Carl Ludwig Schleich (1859-1922).[4]

between hate and affection, his character swings in history" — an interpretation which is certainly valid today.[8]

Biography

Carl Ludwig Schleich was born on June 19, 1859, in Stettin, the son of a well-known ophthalmologist (Fig. 1).[2,9] In the years between 1881-1886, he studied medicine at the Universities of Zürich, Greifswald and Berlin, where he graduated in 1887 (Fig. 2, Fig. 3). As a visiting student, he worked with the surgeons Bernhard von Langenbeck (1810-1887) and Ernst von Bergmann (1844-1907), as well as with the most outstanding pathologist of that time, Rudolf Virchow (1821-1902). In 1889, he set up his private clinic for general surgery and gynecology, which became a mecca for physicians and surgeons from all over the world in subsequent years. In his clinic at the Belle-Alliance Platz in Berlin, he surgically treated several patients daily, exploiting to the maximum the infiltration technique, which evidently was the less dangerous alternative to the overall feared general anesthesia at that time.[10] In 1894, Schleich published his monograph — Painless Operations — which was controversially discussed from the

Fig. 2. No. 5693 - Carl Ludwig's signature when he enrolled as a medical student at the University of Zürich (1879).[33]

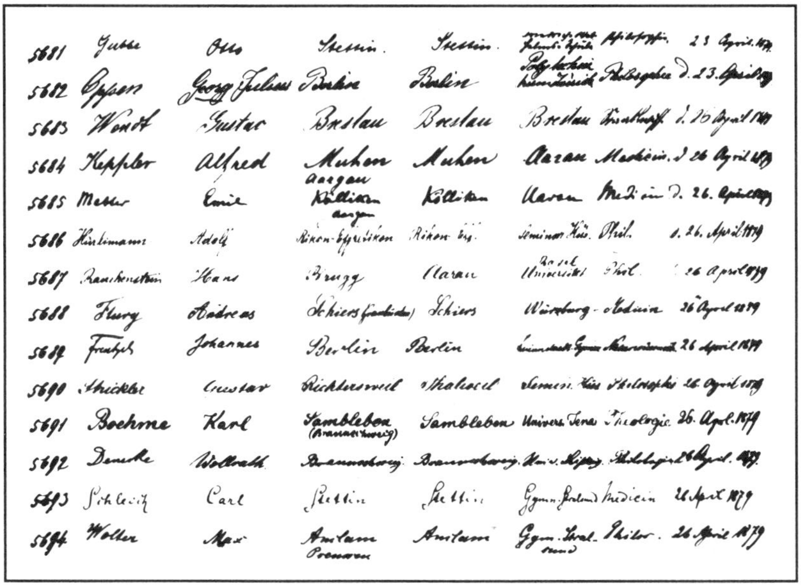

5681	[illegible]	Otto	Stettin.	Stettin.	[illegible]	Philosophie	23 April 1879
5682	[illegible]	Georg Julius	Berlin	Berlin	Polytechnicum Zürich	[illegible]	d. 23. April 1879
5683	Wendt	Gustav	Breslau	Breslau	Breslau	[illegible]	d. 26 April 1879
5684	Keppler	Alfred	Muhen Aargau	Muhen	Aarau	Medicin	d 26 April 1879
5685	[illegible]	Emil	Kölliken Aargau	Kölliken	Aarau	Medicin	d. 26. April 1879
5686	[illegible]	Adolf	Rikon-Effretikon	Rikon [illegible]	Seminar Küs.	Phil.	d. 26. April 1879
5687	Rauchenstein	Hans	Brugg	Aarau	Basel Universität	Phil.	26 April 1879
5688	Flury	Andreas	Schiers (Graubünden)	Schiers	Würzburg	Medicin	26 April 1879
5689	[illegible]	Johannes	Berlin	Berlin	[illegible]	[illegible]	26 April 1879
5690	Strickler	Gustav	Richterswil	Thalweil	Semin. Küs	Philosophie	26. April 1879
5691	Boehme	Karl	Sambleben (Braunschweig)	Sambleben	Univers. Jena	Theologie	26. April 1879
5692	Deneke	[illegible]	Braunschweig	Braunschweig	Univ. Leipzig	Philologie	26 April 1879
5693	Schleich	Carl	Stettin	Stettin	Gymn. Stralsund	Medicin	26 April 1879
5694	Wolter	Max	Anclam Pommern	Anclam	Gymn. Stralsund	Philos.	26 April 1879

Ueber einen Fall von
pulsirendem Knochensarcom
(Sarcoma aneurysmaticum)
des Oberschenkels mit Spontanfractur des Femur und des
Humerus nebst Bemerkungen über die
Aetiologie einiger Formen von Spontanfracturen.

Inaugural-Dissertation
zur
Erlangung der Doctorwürde
in der
Medicin, Chirurgie und Geburtshülfe,
welche
nebst beigefügten Thesen
mit Zustimmung der Hohen Medicinischen Facultät der Universität Greifswald
am
Montag, den 16. Mai 1887
Mittags 12 Uhr
öffentlich vertheidigen wird
Carl Schleich
aus Stettin
Assistenz-Arzt der chirurgischen Universitäts-Klinik

Opponenten:
Dr. Vierow, Assist.-Arzt d. chirurg. Klinik.
Dr. Koenig, Assist.-Arzt d. chirurg. Klinik.
Pomorski, Assist.-Arzt a. pathol.-anat. Institut.

Greifswald.
Druck von Julius Abel.
1887

Fig. 3. Frontispiece of the medical thesis of C.L. Schleich 1887.[34]

Schmerzlose Operationen.

Oertliche Betäubung mit indifferenten Flüssigkeiten.

Psychophysik
des
natürlichen und künstlichen Schlafes.

Von
Dr. C. L. Schleich.

Mit 32 Abbildungen im Text.

Berlin.
Verlag von Julius Springer.
1894.

Fig. 4. Frontispiece of his textbook "Schmerzlose Operationen," edited in 1894.[4]

beginning, but which was nevertheless published in several editions until 1904 (Fig. 4).[11]

Appointed professor in 1900, he became the surgical chief of the newly built Lichterfelde Hospital in Berlin, but he terminated this activity after a short time as he had unsurmountable disagreements with the director of the hospital.

In the following years, not medical publications but literary essays were the center of his activities. All-round talented, Schleich had formed contacts with numerous poets and artists during his years of studies.[4,6] Among these, men like Strindberg, Haupmann, v. Munich were friendly with Schleich.[2,12] As an essayist and narrative writer, he found the recognition which was refused for him for his scientific work.[9] When Schleich died on March 7, 1922, at a sanatorium near Berlin, he was said to be suffering from addiction to alcohol and morphine (Fig. 5a, Fig. 5b).[13] His reputation within established medical circles was more that of a troublemaker than of an individual who had by his impetuous actions paved the way for infiltration anesthesia.[9]

State of the Art of Local Anesthesia Before 1890

Local anesthesia did not come into being in one single moment, as Walter Artelt wrote.[14] It was not the work of a single person. Dozens of scientists contributed to the development of the local anesthesia method, either by personal exchange of experiences or independently from each other. The early period of local anesthesia is well-known, when the Austrian ophthalmologist Carl Koller (1857-1944)

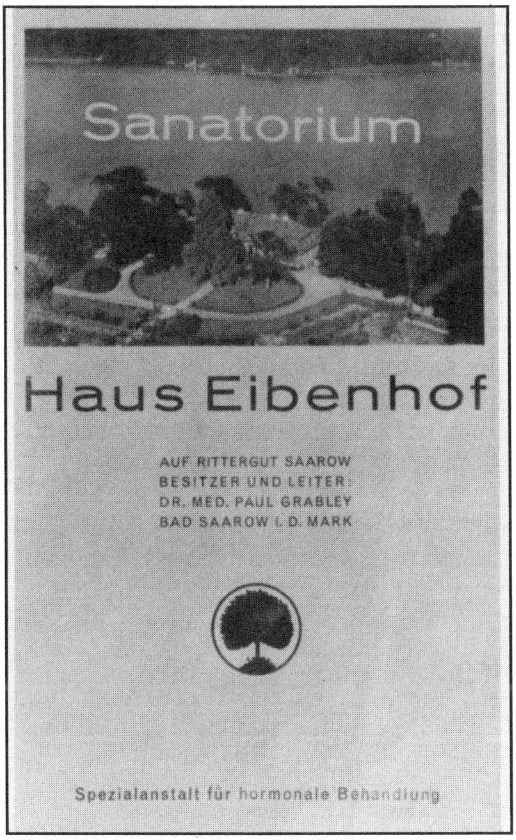

Figs. 5a, 5b. Advertisements of the sanatorium, where C.L. Schleich probably died, *circa* 1928.[13]

reported on the analgesic properties of cocaine.[15] Parallel to the widespread use of topically administered cocaine, cocaine injections were made in operative medicine.[16] In local anesthesia there was a dramatic change. Within a few years: it became possible to carry out surgical interventions without the overall feared general anesthesia.[17] While surgery had been limited essentially to the limbs and superficial tissues before, now operations opening the body cavities became possible; intracranial, thoracic and abdominal interventions became a reality.[18]

However, the initial enthusiasm about this new procedure became clouded within a few months due to frequent observations of serious and sometimes life-threatening, even lethal, complications.[19] Another problem was seen in a potential cocaine addiction, which was more and more discussed in the medical journals.[20] It seemed as if the fate of this anesthetic technique was sealed. Therefore, more and more supporters were heard proposing a return to the well-established general anesthesia. In fact, those supporting the local cocaine anesthesia had emphasized the dangers of chloroform anesthesia, characterizing cocaine as plainly

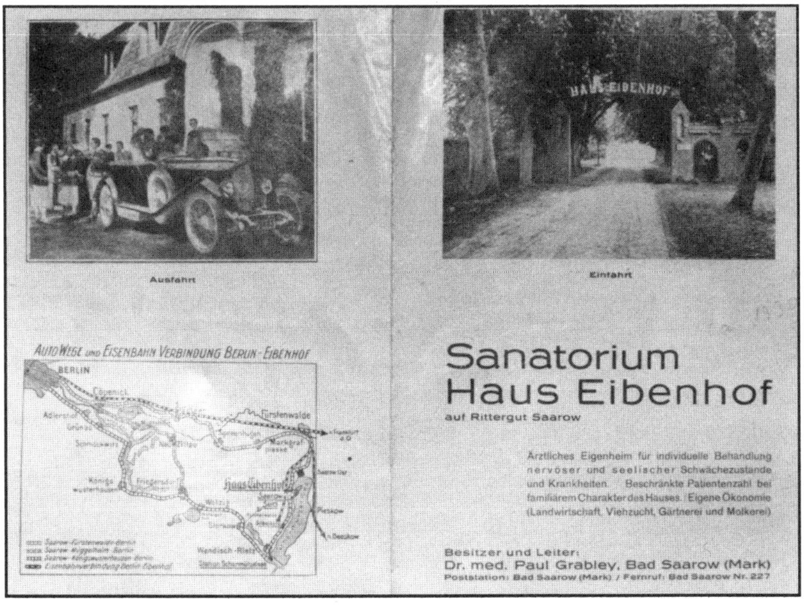

harmless. Would the chloroform, regarded as dangerous from every point of view, be replaced by cocaine, which could be even more dangerous?

In this situation of insecurity regarding cocaine use, Schleich initiated a new discussion about the advantages of his "infiltration anesthesia" technique. Moreover, he praised his alternative as absolutely safe in comparison to the dangerous chloroform technique.[1,21-23] Altogether, these interpretations could not be accepted by the attending congress surgeons, especially when he claimed that his procedure had to be used for medicolegal reasons.

When Schleich was presenting his paper, it is likely that most surgeons had already discontinued any infiltration anesthesia and preferred again using chloroform anesthesia. Most of the surgeons refused the concept of cocainization of the tissues with highly concentrated solutions. What were the main differences between the common technique of local anesthesia and the new one of the unknown surgeon who was not an attending assistant at a reputed university clinic, but did these researches at his private clinic, an institution which was dismissed as hotels with obstacles by the renowned surgeon Friedrich von Trendelenburg (1844-1924)![24]

Schleich's "Infiltration Technique"

In this private clinic, Schleich developed his procedure towards the end of the 1880's. After he had completed extensive surgical procedures in more than 400 patients, almost without any additional inhalation anesthetic like chloroform or ether, he gave a detailed report on his experiences in 1891. The method consisted in completely infiltrating the tissues with an anesthetic solution to a suitable depth in the immediate field of operation by making a series of successive overlapping injections. Schleich not only increased the safety of his method by the pharmacologic technique of diluting the cocaine solution, but he also endeavored to augment the effectiveness of his method by combining several mechanical, thermal and chemical factors.[23] Usually, the operative field was markedly cooled and the tissue infiltrated in layers, always interrupted by newly cooling with ether-spray.[17] It is worth mentioning that he never emphasized this effective additional trick, but it is quite understandable that he thus intensified the analgesic effect of the infiltrated cocaine without augmenting its toxicity. Depending on the extent of the surgical procedure, Schleich used solutions with different concentrations. For extensive operations, he recommended the weak solution of 0.01 percent of cocaine; the so-called normal solution contained 0.1 percent of cocaine and the strong preparation 0.2 percent. This last solution was preferred for infiltrations of inflamed tissue.[11] Repeatedly, he reported on his technique, which was primarily used by general practitioners, in contrast to the surgeons who often refused to use it.[26-31] From today's point of view, this development is difficult to understand, but it seems that the leading surgeons had decided to punish him with want of respect.[4,6,9] This appraisal was revised some years later when the reputed German surgeon, von Bergmann from Berlin, confessed to the false interpretation of his previous chairman, von Bardeleben, before the same audience.[5,6] Later the outstanding surgeon, Johannes von Miculicz (1950-1905), reported excellent results with the Schleich infiltration technique, but he never praised him for this development at all.[4] Another leading surgeon in Germany, Hermann Kümmell (1852-1937) from Hamburg, realized the tremendous advantages for further progress in surgery with Schleich's publication and widely used his technique.[4] It seems that a first step towards a reconciliation with the German Surgical Society was tried. Nevertheless, mainly due to the personality of Schleich or to the circumstances that he had made his first experiences with "established surgeons," there was always some discord between both parties.[9]

Further Contributions

This critical relationship between Schleich and established surgical medicine was burdened by the heavy criticism of Schleich concerning the lack of skilled persons using anesthesia techniques.[11] He analyzed and accused the general attitude towards anesthesia, which was characterized by apathy, so that administration was entrusted to students and junior house officers, many of whom came to the task without having been prepared by even the most rudimentary instruction. Furthermore, no responsibility was attached to the surgeons, either for the conduct of administration or for the results of anesthesia. He therefore called for a reformation of this system and began to agitate for a change in medical education.

He asked for skilled anesthetists and systematic teaching, and once more, with his demands in this direction, the majority of surgeons vehemently rejected rather than agreed with his proposals.[11] Once more, he had become the "enfant terrible" with the surgeons. Even decades later, another German surgeon, Friedrich Pels-Leusden (1866-1944), could write in a reputed surgical textbook, "Narcosis specialists simply do not exist and hopefully never will!"[32]

As is known in Germany anesthesia as a specialty has been accepted since 1952, when the German Society was founded. Nearly 60 years before, Schleich had called for such specialization, but until this day no one has praised the merits of Schleich in this direction. That is why Schleich was a man before his time. He realized the need for a safe local anesthetic technique as well as the need for skilled anesthetists and — the most important fact — he never stopped calling for their realization.

References

1. Schleich CL: Die Infiltrationsanästhesie (locale Anästhesie) und ihr Verhältnis zur allgemeinen Narcose (Inhalationsanästhesie). Verh Dtsch Ges f Chir 1:121, 1892.
2. Thorwald J; Das Weltreich der Chirurgen. Steingrüben Verlag, Stuttgart 1957.
3. Trendelenburg F: Die ersten 25 Jahre der Deutschen Gesellschaft für Chirurgie. Verlag von Julius Springer, Berlin 1925.
4. Schleich CL: Besonnte Vergangenheit. Vier Falken Verlag, Berlin 1920.
5. Bergmann E: Ueber die vor der Sitzung von Herrn Schleich demonstrirte Infiltrations-Änästhesie. Verh Dtsch Ges f Chir 101, 1892.
6. Silló-Seidl G: Ärzte ohne Nobelpreis. Ärzte, deren Entdeckungen Millionen geholfen haben. Ariston Verlag, Genf 1978.
7. Gottstein A: Carl Ludwig Schleich. Klin Wochenschr 18:924, 1922.
8. Bier A: Carl Ludwic Schleich. Abl f Chr 19:665, 1922.
9. Kausch W: Carl Ludwig Schleich. Klin Wochenschr 18:924, 1922.
10. Wettley A: Die wissenschaftliches Odyssee des chirurgen Carl Ludwig Schleich 1859-1922. Med Klin 29:1324, 1959.
11. Schliech CL: Schmerzlose Operationen. Oertliche Betäubung mit indifferenten Flüssigkeiten. Psychophysik des natürlichen und künstlichen Schlafes. Verlag von Julius Springer, Berlin 1894.
12. Pohl FH: Arzt, Denker und Dichter. Vor 100 Jahren (19.7.1859) wurde Professor Dr. Carl Ludwig Schleich in Stettin geboren. Ostdeutsche Monatshefte 25:598, 1959.
13. Gohrbrandt E: Carl Ludwig Schleich zum 100. Geburtstag. Zbl f Chir 28:1089, 1959.
14. Artelt W: Carl Ludwig Schleich und die Lokalanästhesie. Eine Erwiderung. Zahnärztl Mittlg 33:152, 1942.
15. Keys T: Die Geschichte der chirurgischen Anästhesie. Springer Verlag, Berlin-Heidelberg-New York 1968.
16. Killian H: Geschichte der Kokalanästhesie. In Lokalanästhesie Thieme Verlag, Stuttgart 1964.
17. Braun H: Zur Geschichte der örtlichen Betäubung. Chirurg 10:462, 1929.
18. Matas R: Local and regional anesthesia: a retrospect and prospect. Am J Surg Part I 189, Part II 362, 1934.
19. Darmstaedter E: Begründung und Ausbau der Cocain-Localanästhesie. Schmerz, Narkose, Anästhesie 10:196, 1938.
20. Rieh K: Der Anteil der Zahnheilkunde an der Ausbildung der Kolalanästhesie im 19. Jahrhundert Dtsch Zahnärtzl Wochenschr 21:187, 1939.
21. Schleich CL: Drei Laparatomien ohne Chloroformnarkose unter Anwendung der localen combinirten Aether-Cocainanästhesie, Bln klin Wochenschr 35:862, 1891.
22. Schleich CL: Ueber locale Anästhesie, mit Krankenvorstellung. Bln klin Wochenschr 51:1202, 1891.

23. Schleich CL: Local-Anästhesie und Narkose. Bln klin Wochenschr 13:269, 1900.
24. Braun H, *In* Grote LR: Die Medizin der Gegenwart in Selbstdarstellungen. Verlag von Felix Meiner, Leipzig 1925.
25. Schleich CL: Ueber locale Anästhesie. In: Leyden, E v und Klemperer, F: Die Deutsche Klinik, Urban & Schwarzenberg Berlin-Wien 1900.
26. Briegleb K: Die Schleich'sche Infiltrationsanästhesie. Therapeutische Monatshefte 12:650, 1897.
27. Briegleb K: "Für Schleich." Zschr f prakt Ärzte 9: 1897.
28. Briegleb K: Schleich und Oberst. Zschr f prak Ärzte 8:500, 1899.
29. Gehardi: Zur Infiltrations-Anaesthesie nach Schleich. Münch med Wochenschr 6:138, 1897.
30. Martin M: Die Anästhesie in der ärztlichen Praxis. J.F. Lehmanns Verlag, München 1905.
31. Schlesinger A: Die Praxis der lokalen Anästhesie. Urban & Schwarzenberg, Berlin-Wien 1902.
32. Pels-Leusden F: Chapter of pain therapy. In: Kirschner M, Schubert A. ed.: Allgemeine und spezielle chirurgische Operationslehre. Vol I Springer Verlag, Berlin 1927.

THE AVERTIN STORY

M. GOERIG
Department of Anaesthesiology, University Hospital Hamburg, Germany

In the early centuries, the rectal mucosa was frequently used to absorb various substances.[1] A few months after the anesthetic qualities of ether had been published, the rectal resorbtion of narcotic substances was also researched. In 1847, the surgeon, Ivanovich Pirogoff (1810-1881), was the first physician to achieve a deep narcosis with the use of an ether enema.[2,3] In the same year, he described the technique in his monograph, "Recherches pratiques et physiologiques sur l'ethérisation."[2] Because the enemas strongly irritated the lower intestinal mucosa, and the dosing of the narcotic was difficult to control, this anesthesia method was soon forgotten.

At the beginning of the 20th century, the lower intestinal route for narcosis was again attempted, this time with a higher rate of success, by the Swiss surgeon, Fritz DuMont (1854-1932).[4] A few years later, in 1911, another Swiss surgeon, Arndt, proposed the use of a 5 percent aqueous solution of ether in a 1 liter enema given to the patient after premedication with a combination of pantopon and scopolamine or hedonal, administered as an intravenous hypnotic drug.[5] At about the same time, the American, James Taylor Gwathmey (1863-1944), was involved with the development of this procedure.[6] His oil-ether solution was frequently reported to achieve good anesthetic results. Nevertheless, this technique did not become popular in Europe.[7,8]

The Development of E 107, Also Called Avertin

This, in brief, was the situation when the I.G. Farben Company introduced a new water soluble hypnotic. The chemical name of the drug was tribromethanol, a bromine derivative of alcohol, which had been synthetisized at the chemical laboratories in the Germany county of Bayern by Nobel prize winner, Richard Willstätter (1872-1942) (Fig. 1) and his colleague Walter Duisberg.[9-11] They reported their experiments before the German Chemical Society in 1922.[12]

This bromine-containing preparation was of special interest because of its resemblance to another narcotic called Bromoform, which had already been successfully used for the therapy of whooping-cough. Tribromethanol, better known as E 107 (E for Elberfeld, where the

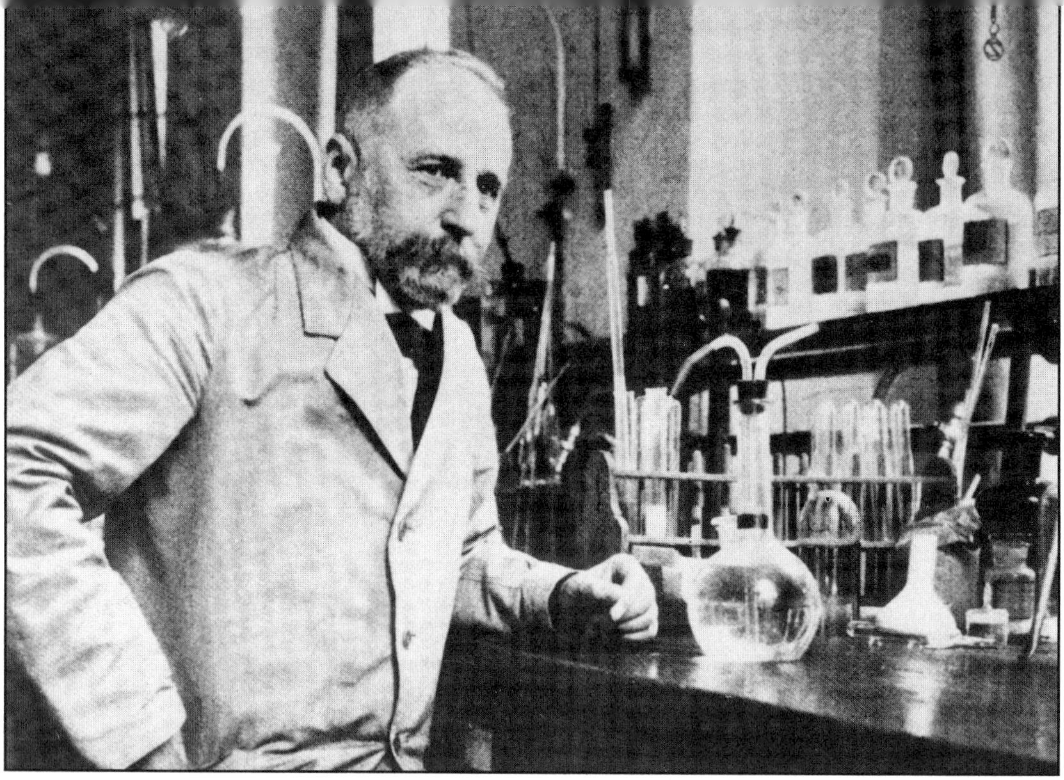

Fig. 1. Richard Willstätter in his lab (ca 1915) (1872-1942).[9]

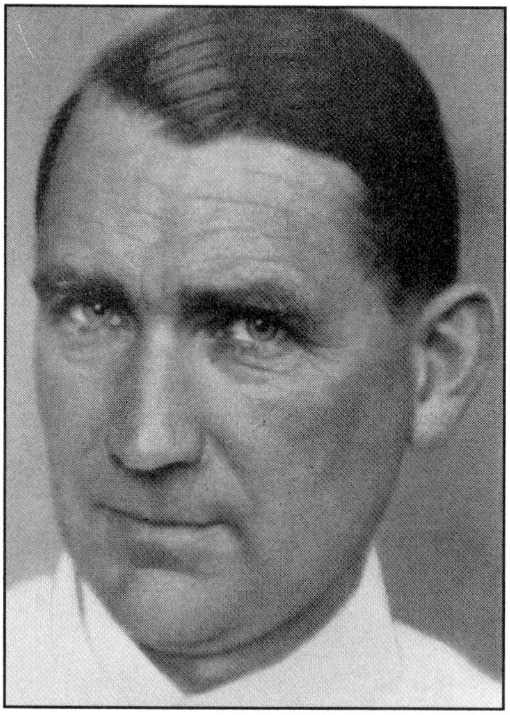

Fig. 2. Fritz Eichholtz (1889-1967).[13]

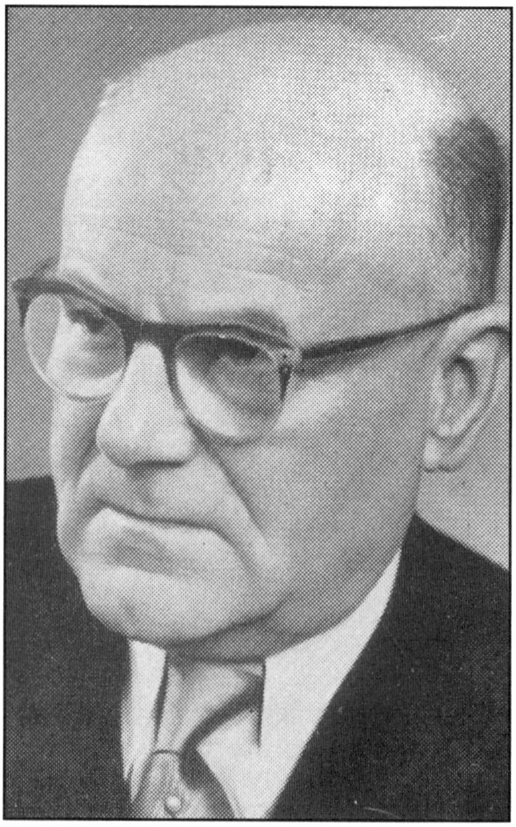

Fig. 3. Otto Butzengeiger (1885-1968).[14]

Bayer labs were situated) was first tested in the University Pediatric hospital of Düsseldorf on children suffering from whooping-cough.[12] The new leader of the pharmacology laboratory of I.G. Farben in Wuppertal Elberfeld, Fritz Eichholtz (1889-1967) (Fig. 2), had discovered the further possible use of Tribromethanol as a rectal narcotic.[13] He gave it to the surgeon, Otto Butzengeiger (1885-1968) (Fig. 3) of the Wuppertal Elberfeld Hospital, for clinical testing.[14]

First Clinical Experiences

At the 51st Congress of the German Surgical Society, the leader of the I.G. Farben pharmacologic research laboratory, Eichholtz, reported on some pharmacologic properties of the new anesthetic drug.[15] Fritz Eichholtz was born on August 15, 1889, in Lippstadt.[16] He became head of the research laboratory of I.G. Farben in Elberfeld in 1925. A short time later, he began his investigations on the application of Tribromethanol as a rectally administered narcotic. Accepting a post as professor of the Königsberg Institute of Pharmacology, he left I.G. Farben in 1928. After the world war II, he became chief of pharmacology at the University of Heidelberg, and it was here that he died in 1967.[13,16]

Chemical and Pharmacologic Qualities of E 107

Tribromethanol is an alcohol with the chemical formula CBr_3CH_20H, characterized as a white, water soluble, powdered crystal. According to the instruction leaflet of I.G. Farben, the 2 percent solution of Avertin required individual dosing, with a maximum allowable dose of 0.08-0.1 gm.17 This maximum dose was reduced in cases of cachexia, dehydration and in obese patients.[18] The rate of the resorption was often influenced by the method of application and by the position of the patient. It was also stated that the addition of sedatives increased the narcotic effects of Avertin on a basis of individual metabolism.[1] The drug was said to have been extensively tested in animals and that appropriate clinical tests had also been made. As a result of liver metabolism and kidney filtration, metabolites could be observed in urine samples 48 hours after initial use.[17] In an analysis of the absorptive qualities of Avertin, it was reported that, following use of 15 grams of a 3 percent solution, 50 percent of the narcotic would be absorbed after 10 minutes, and 75 percent after 20 minutes.[19,20] In a later investigation, it was determined that the narcotic solute had a higher rate of absorption than water solution, a major reason for the overdose complications observed in its earlier clinical testing (Fig. 4).[21] The excretion of the glucuronide metabolite was considered to be the result of liver detoxification.[18] A blood level of milligrams was required for Avertin to take effect.

The surgeon Otto Butzengeiger was the first to report on the narcotic effects of Avertin as rectally administered in a 300 patient study.[22,23] Otto Butzengeiger was born on April 4, 1885, in Arnberg, Franken. After finishing medical school and writing his doctorate, he first began a study of internal medicine before he finally chose surgery to be his specialty. At first a resident surgeon of the city hospital of Wuppertal, he later became head surgeon of the department. On July 11, 1968, he passed away in Wuppertal. Aside from his participation in testing Avertin, Butzengeiger made no other contribution to the field of anesthesiology.[14]

Butzengeiger's positive results with Avertin were due to his extreme care in application, sometimes giving only a fraction of the allowed dose. In his opinion, the maximal allowable dose was only 0.1 g/kg, because of his practice of giving patients a premedication dose of 0.5-0.75 mg of veronal the night before and 0.2 mg of Pantopon on the day of the narcosis. If the patient was not anesthetized after 10 minutes, he then administered an additional dose of 0.025 g/kg of Avertin. He considered the absolute maximal dose to be 1.5 g/kg. Most of the patients received the Avertin in their rooms instilled through a special rectal tube. They were then brought into a darkened room for 10 minutes before the operation was started. In cases of especially painful surgical procedures,

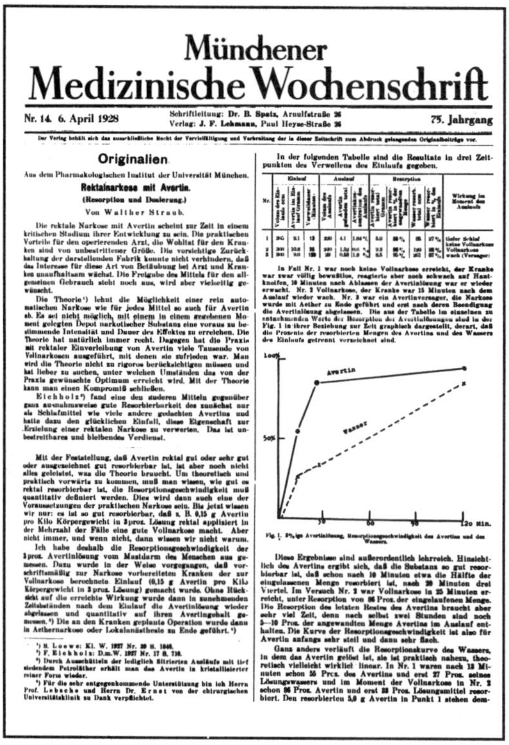
Münchener
Medizinische Wochenschrift

Nr. 14. 6. April 1928 — Schriftleitung: Dr. B. Spatz, Arnulfstraße 26 — Verlag: J. F. Lehmann, Paul Heyse-Straße 26 — 75. Jahrgang

Der Verlag behält sich das ausschließliche Recht der Vervielfältigung und Verbreitung der in dieser Zeitschrift zum Abdruck gelangenden Originalbeiträge vor.

Originalien.

Aus dem Pharmakologischen Institut der Universität München.

Rektalnarkose mit Avertin.

(Resorption und Dosierung.)

Von Walther Straub.

Fig. 4. Frontispiece of the publication series, in which the term "basal anesthesia" was first used.[19]

ether was added to the regimen. At the end of the operation, the remaining Avertin solution was sucked out of the rectum and the patient allowed to sleep off the effects of the narcotic. Butzengeiger emphatically noted that Avertin was not to be used when a deep narcosis was required. He also recommended a continual monitoring of the patient's respiratory and pulse rates. Because of these precautionary measures, unlike other clinical testers, he attained positive results.[17,24,25] Respiratory depression was a greatly feared complication of overdosage.[26,27] Severe irritation of the mucosal membrane, at times life-threatening, remained an unsolved problem. Claiming these serious side effects were typical, the celebrated surgeon, Ferdinand Sauerbruch (1875-1951) of Berlin, attacked the manufacturers of I.G. Farben for their irresponsible actions. He claimed that the complications were the major cause of an increase in the mortality rate of his clinic, further stating that the narcotic was an operational risk for every patient and refused to further test the narcotic.[28] Hans Killian (1892-1982) wrote, "E 107 had been offered in a stage when it should not have been allowed to undergo clinical examination."[29] Although other clinical investigators also reported these severe side effects, Sauerbruch's evaluation was taken seriously for he was at that time the leading surgeon in Germany. His critical comments were reported in the daily press as well. Nevertheless, all this was not enough to stop the wave of professional enthusiasm for the "intestinal narcosis."[30]

It should be noted that many physicians and patients were more apprehensive of the frequent accidental explosions caused by gaseous narcotics such as Narcylen.[31] Wealthy patients therefore demanded to have this so-called "harmless" narcosis technique. The fact that Eichholtz proclaimed that the substance would not be made available to the general public showed how seriously such criticism was taken by the manufacturers themselves.[15]

More Chemical Analysis and Pharmacological Studies

Further analysis proved that heating the solution to 40° C during its preparation and before its application created dibromacetaldehyde, a by-product responsible for Avertin's strongly corrosive side-effects.[20,25] Consequently, the manufacturer recommended that Avertin solution should only be heated to body temperature during its preparation and application. Later, the Bayer Company produced the so-called "Avertin-Fluid."[25] One milliliter of which contrasted 1 gram of the Avertin solute. Until that time, the narcotic had only been available in its crystal powder form. Avertin solutions prepared by medical personnel were to be kept in thermos flasks. They were not to be reheated after cooling, so as to avoid the formation of harmful crystallized products.[17] Moreover, before each use of the narcotics, a so-called congo red test had to be performed in

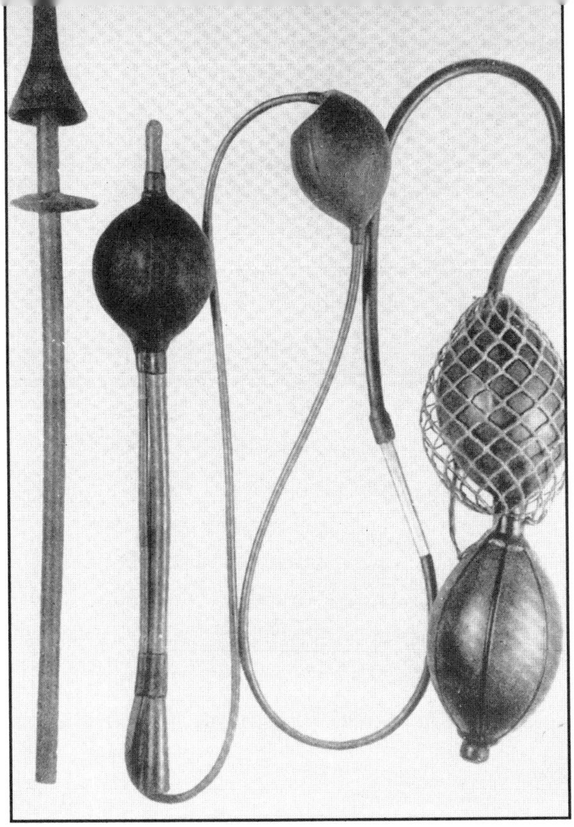

Fig. 5a. Specially designed devices for the application of Avertin, on the left side the device of Butzengeiger, on the right the device of Nordmann.[62]

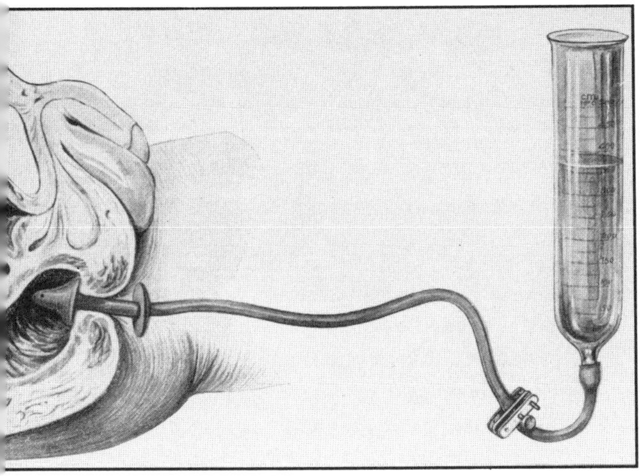

Fig. 5b. Another device "in situ."[69]

order to notice any toxic by-products. In the following years, there were no more reports of severe complications (Fig. 5a, 5b).

Process of an Avertin Narcosis

The procedure for Avertin anesthesia was as follows:[1,17,18,32] Usually the patient had a cleansing enema on the night before operation. Narcosis was attained in 5-10 minutes following application with a specially designed device and was without the accustomed excitation phase of a gaseous narcotic (Fig. 6a, 6b). A deep anesthesia suitable for an operation was attained after 30 minutes. Avertin possessed good amnestic qualities and did not cause any postoperative vomiting. Respirations became shallow and the mean blood pressure decreased about 30 mm Hg during the course of the operation. The patient woke up an average of 8 hours after the operation. Most patients were surprised to have been operated on due to the exceptional amnestic properties of the drug.

Pharmacological Interventions for Influencing the Avertin Narcosis

Various substances were tried to counteract the respiratory depression and influence the pharmacokinetics of the avertin narcosis .[32-36] Aside from thyroxin and diuretics, the use of an infusion combined with the injection of 15-20 I.U. of insulin on the night before operation was recommended in order to increase the glycogen stores of the liver. This was believed to increase the rate of glucuronisation of Avertin metabolites and expedite its renal excretion.
"Weckamine" like Lobelin, Cardiazol or Coramin was used to counteract the respiratory depression. Coramin was so effective that "no Avertin without Coramin" became a byword in every operation theater. Coramin had been proven effective, not only in animal experiments but also in clinical tests, increasing both the respiratory volume and respiratory rate of patients undergoing Avertin anesthesia. Many life-threatening situations could thus be avoided. This fact was pointed out by one of the leading anesthesiologists at that time in Germany. Hans Killian (1892-1982), when he published an historical review in the mid-sixties.[8] It is worth mentioning that the inhalation of oxygen-carbon dioxide was advocated to overcome respiratory

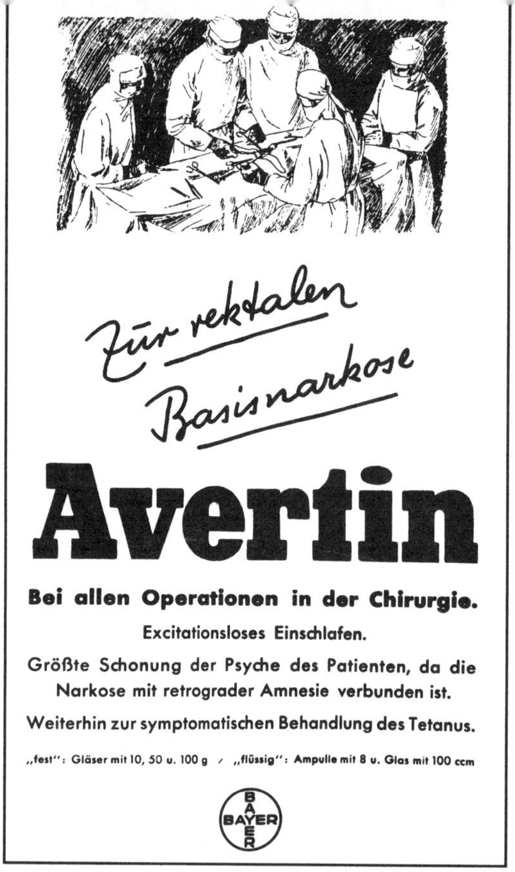

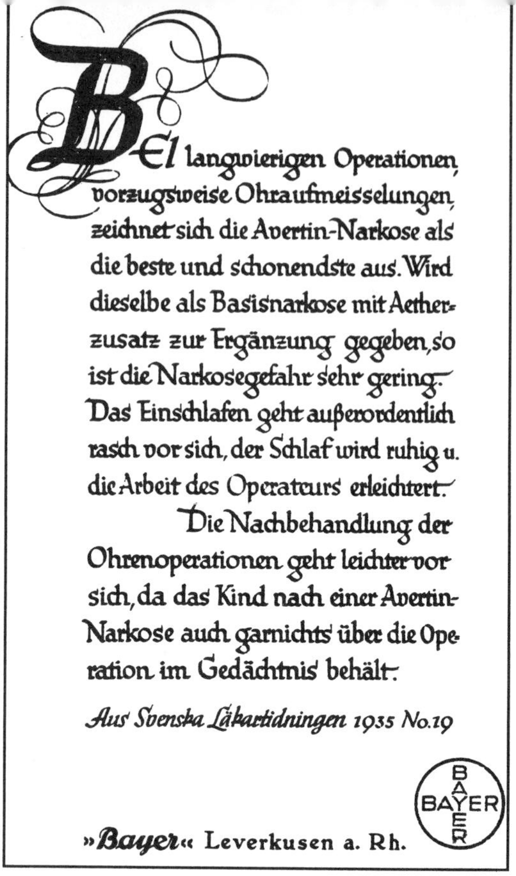

Fig. 6a,b,c. Various advertisements of Avertin, published in medical journals.[69]

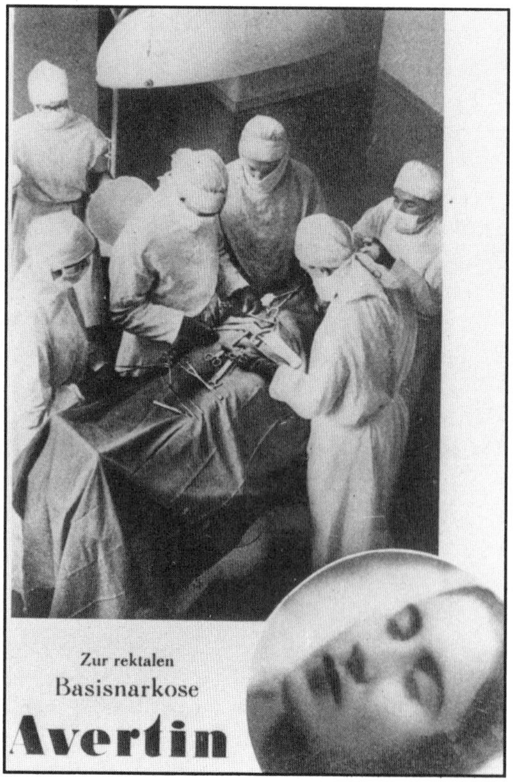

depression.[8,37] In order to prevent blood pressure decrease, ephedrin or Ephetonin was subcutaneously injected or intravenously infused before the operation was started.

Indications for the Avertin Pre-Narcosis

After the frequent occurrence of the above mentioned complications, many surgeons allowed the use of Avertin only as a basal narcotic. The pharmacologist, Walter Straub (1874-1944) of Munich, undertook an intensive investigation of the respiratory depression caused by the drug.[21] He was able to prove that the absorption rate of the anesthetic was higher than that of its water solvent, which had been the cause of the frequent complications.[20,21] It was the reason for a toxic level of Avertin in the blood, and this overdose was the cause of the respiratory depression. He recommended the use of a 3 percent solution and the use of Avertin in a dose not exceeding a maximum of 0.1 gram/kg body weight. In such low doses the narcotic could only be used as a basal narcotic, or as a supplement to ether in more painful operations. He discouraged the use of Avertin as a full narcotic with a higher dose. This opinion had also been that of Butzengeiger. As a supplementary narcotic, the drug was used for amnestic reasons during surgical procedures performed under any kind of local anesthesia.[38] Nevertheless, its application during spinal anesthesia was discouraged for fear of an additional decrease in the patient's blood pressure.[17] Morbid patients were understandably anesthetized only with a reduced dose of the drug.[39] Contraindications were seen in patients with liver and kidney diseases, septic processes, and ileus.[39,40] There was a difference in opinion as to whether or not it should be used in the presence of lung diseases.[1]

Avertin for the Symptomatic Therapy of Tetanus

In the following years, Avertin as a basal narcotic was used in a wide range of surgical fields.[1] There was practically no field of surgery where it had not been administered at one time or another. A major cause of its success was its minimal excitation at the induction of anesthesia and its excellent amnestic properties.[17] It was also a popular narcotic for pediatric, thyroid, and brain surgery.[1,32,41-45] Its well-known antiemetic qualities were an added advantage to brain operations.[41,44]

At the height of its success, the surgeon Arthur Läwen (1876-1958), at that time the chairman of the Department of Surgery at the University of Marburg, discovered yet another indication for Avertin.[46-48] He had been the first to report the symptomatic administration of Avertin for tetanus and in 1927 reported a case in which he had used a total of 154.4 grams of the drug during a therapy that lasted 13 days.[47] The patient had only survived this severe intoxication with a concomitant high dose of antitoxin. Läwen further analyzed the combined use of Avertin and curare in animal experiments.[49] He noted an increase in the effectiveness of both drugs and therefore advocated their simultaneous use in cases of tetanus.[49] As early as 1910, Läwen had already proposed the combination of artificial respiration and medical treatment with curare for these patients.[46,50]

Avertin as an Intravenous Induction Agent

Martin Kirschner (1879-1942), head surgeon of the University Clinic in Königsberg, later in Tübingen and finally in Heidelberg, had a major part in the development of Avertin.[51] Because of the complications of the rectal narcotic (primarily respiratory depression and an abrupt decrease in blood pressure), he at first discontinued its use in his clinic;[52] two years later, however, he was the first to publish an article on its possible intravenous applications.[53] He primarily used it as an induction agent and then continued the anesthesia with ether, but with time he broadened its application for minor, short lasting operations.[54] It is quite possible that he had been inspired by a speech by the surgeon, Rudolf Bumm (1899-1942) of the Charité in Berlin, concerning the intravenous application of Pernocton.[55] At the 1929 Congress of Surgery, Kirschner presented a report of his clinical experience with this new intravenous route.[56] In Avertin Kirschner had a hypnotic that could easily be controlled and one that also had amnestic properties. He considered two possible indications for the drug: one was its use as an induction narcotic followed by a gas narcotic for major operations; another was its use as an ultrashort hypnotic agent for small surgical interventions.[54] After a direct puncture of the vein, the drug was infused in a 2-3 percent NaCl solution that was body weight measured over a graduated drain tube within 45 sec. The specially designed set was developed by Kirschner himself.[56] With a careful chosen dose of 0.03 mg per Kg body weight, he claimed to have infrequently experienced cases of apnea or severe depression in blood pressure. He reported a 3 percent incidence of thrombophlebitis at the injection site and one fatally-ending pulmonary embolism. He also noted that care should be taken to avoid parainfusions or injections that could lead to unnecessary connective tissue damage.[54] Only one year later such a complication was reported which eventually necessitated the amputation of the patient's upper extremity.[57] Surprisingly, Kirschner stood by his intravenous Avertin, even after the introduction of Evipan.[58]

With the invention of his electrocoagulation

for the trigeminal ganglion, Kirschner simultaneously praised the advantages of the intravenously infused hypnotic drug, which never induced any respiratory depression during this painful maneuver.[59] He himself had experienced enough cases of respiratory paralysis when Evipan had been injected. In spite of his excellent results with intravenous Avertin, this technique never gained any popularity in Germany. A possible explanation for this was probably the introduction of the newly developed barbiturates such as Evipan.60

Evaluation Among Experts

The rectal technique of Avertin basal narcosis was described in detail in all current textbooks of surgery and anesthesiology of the 30's and 40's.[4,7,30,40,61-66] After 1945, Avertin basal anesthesia was still commonly used, even though many of the more effective intravenous narcotics already had become available. Even in the early 60's, the drug was widely used. In the U.S., Vincent J. Collins "Principles of Anesthesiology."[66]

Summary

In evaluating the almost 40 years in which Avertin was used, it can be stated that the clinical tests were correctly carried out by many of the hospitals, but the serious complications were due to the lack of care in which an erroneous overdose of the drug was used. After observing the severe intestinal irritation after the application of Avertin, Sauerbruch had probably not realized that his criticism of the manufacturer was uncalled for since the misuse of the narcotic had in truth been an iatrogenic complication.

Other complications were later also proved to be iatrogenic and were eliminated as soon as an appropriate instruction was printed. Unnoticed was the fact that, because of this severe criticism, the anesthetic was to become one of the most analyzed and investigated drugs of all time.

This is perhaps the reason why Avertin remained an important part of the anesthesiologic regimen for such a long time.

References

1. Anschütz W, Specht K, Tiemann: Die Avertinnarkose in der Chirurgie. Ergeb Chir und Orth 23:1930.
2. Pirogoff I:Recherches practiques et physiologiques sur l'éthérisation. St. Petersburg 1847.
3. Secher O; Nikolai Ivanovich Pirogoff. Anaesthesia 41:829, 1986.
4. Brunn M von: Die Allgemeinnarkose. Verlag von Ferdinand Enke Stuttgart 1913.
5. Arndt: Die Rektalnarkose mit Aetherlösungen. Arch f klin Chir XL:19, 1911.
6. Gwathmey JT: Oil-ether anesthesia. Lancet 2:1756, 1913.
7. Killian H: Narkose zu operativen Zwecken. Springer Verlag, Berlin 1933.
8. Killian H: Fünfzig Jahre Anaesthesiologie. Ein Rückblick. Anaestheist 10:315, 1963.
9. Dees de Sterio A: Der Dank des Vaterlandes - Richard Willstätter. Ärzteblatt Rheinland-Pfalz 5:408, 1981.
10. Willstätter R, Duisberg W: Zur Kenntnis des Trichlor-und Tribrom-Äthylalkohols. Ber Dtsch Chem Ges 2283, Verlag Chemie, Leipzig und Berlin 1923.
11. Stoll A: Aus meinem Leben. Verlag Chemie, Weinheim 1950.
12. Hörlein H: Zur Geschichte des Voluntals und Avertins. Die Pharmazie, Verlag Dr. Werner Saenger, Berlin 5:563, 1950.
13. Doerr W: c/o University Heidelberg, personal communication concerning Fritz Eichholtz, summer 1990.
14. Butzengeiger KH: personal communication concerning his father, Professor Otto Butzengeiger, Oct. 1990.
15. Eichholtz F: Die Rectalnarkose mit E 107. Arch f klin Chir 148:94, 1927.
16. Doerr W: Fritz Eichholtz (15.8.1889-29.12.1967). Jahrbuch der Heidelberger Akademie der Wissenschaften für das Jahr 1968.
17. Bayer Drug Company: Avertin - Drug Information. Leverkusen 1931.
18. Anschütz W: Die Darmnarkose mit Avertin. Soc. Int. de Chir, IX. Congres, Madrid 15-18 Mars 1932. Imprim. med. et scient. Bruxelles 1932.
19. Straub W: Rektalnarkose mit Avertin (Resorption und Dosierung). Münch med Wochenschr 14:593, 1928.

20. Straub W: Rektalnarkose mit Avertin (Ausscheidung und Nebenwirkung). Münch med Wochenschr 30:1279, 1928.
21. Straub W: Klinisches und Pharmakologisches zur Avertinnarkose. Klin Wochenschr 49:2346, 1928.
22. Butzengeiger O: Die Rectalnarkose mit E 107. Arch f klin Chir 148:95, 1927.
23. Butzengeiger O: Klinische Erfahrungen mit Avertin (E 107). Dtsch med Wochenschr 17:712, 1927.
24. Butzengeiger O: Zur Avertinaussprache Abl f Chir 4:204, 1929.
25. Butzengeiger O: 20 Jahre Avertinnarkose. Chirurg 5:208, 1948.
26. Nordmann O: Die Rektalnarkose mit E 107. Zbl f Chir 17:1055, 1927.
27. Roedelius E: Aussprache auf dem Deutschen Chirurgentag in Berlin 1927. In: Arch f klin Chir 148:54, 1927.
28. Sauerbruch F: Aussprache auf dem Deutschen Chirurgentag in Berlin 1927. In: Arch f klin Chir 148:99, 1927.
29. Killian H: Die bisherigen Ergebnisse mit der Avertinrectalnarkose. Narkose und Anästhesie 3:119, 1928.
30. Mühsam E: Rektalnarkose mit Avertin. Schmerz 2:106-29, 1928.
31. Rimarski W: Die Narzylenbetäubung in sicherheitstechnischer Hinsicht. Münch med Wochenschr 10:386, 1925.
32. Goldschmidt EF, Harvey SC: Rectal administration of Tribromethanol. Am J Surg 18:78, 1933.
33. Killian H: Über die Unterbrechungsmöglichkeiten der Avertinnarkose. Klin Wochenschr 10:1446, 1931.
34. Killian H: Coramin als Antagonist bei Vergiftungen durch Hypnotika und Narkotika. Klin Wochenschr 11:192, 1932.
35. Killian H: Die bisherigen Ergebnisse der Verwendung des Coramin in hohen Dosen. Klin Wochenschr 12:243, 1933.
36. Specht K: Coramin bei Avertinnarkose. Zbl f Chir 22:1345, 1932.
37. Löhr W: Schwere isolierte Atemzentrumlähmung bei Avertinnarkose mit Laudanon-Skopolaminvorbereitung und ihre Behebung durch Kohlensäureinhalation. Zbl f Chir 463, 1930.
38. Kirschner M: Die Kombinatin verschiedener Verfahren der Schmerzausschaltung. Chirurg 9:265, 1935.
39. Hesse F, Lendle L, Schoen R: Allgemeinnarkose und örtliche Betäubung. Verlag von Johann Ambrosius Barth, Leipzig 1934.
40. Härtel F: Anleitung zur Schmerzbetäubung. Kurzes Lehrbuch der Lokalanästhesie, Allgemeinnarkose und sonstiger Anwendung der Betäubungsverfahren. Verlag von Theodor Steinkopff, Dresden-Leipzig, 1936.
41. Dandy: Avertin anaesthesia in neurologic surgery. JAMA 22:18-1860, 1930.
42. Ebhardt K; Erfahrungen mit der Avertinbasisnarkose, insbesondere auch in der Kinderchirurgie und beim Krankentransport. Zbl f Chir 8:452, 1930.
43. Hornung R: Rektale Anwendung von Avertin zur Betäubung des Geburtsschmerzes. Münch med Wochenschr 14:595, 1928.
44. Olovecrona H: Allgemeine Technik der intrakraniellen Operationen. Anästhesie. Vol III. In: Die spezielle Chirurgie der Gehirnkrankheiten. Ed. H. Schum, Enke Verlag, Stuttgart 1941.
45. Sievers R: Die Avertinvollnarkose im Kindesalter. Zbl f Chir 4:194, 1928.
46. Goerig M, Schulte am Esch J: Reminiscences about Arthur Läwen - an extraordinary pioneer in anesthesia. Third Intern. Symp. on the History of Anesthesia, Atlanta 1992.
47. Läwen A: Avertin zur Behandlung des Tetanus. Zbl f Chir 238:2370, 1927.
48. Läwen A: Weitere Erfahrungen über die symptomatische Behandlung des Tetanus mit Avertin. Zbl f Chir 4:194, 1928.
49. Melzner E: Experimentelle Untersuchungen über die Behandlung des Wundstarrkrampfes mit einer Kombination von Curarin und Avertin. Dtsch Zschr f Chir 212:308, 1928.
50. Läwen A: Experimentelle Untersuchungen über die Möglichkeit den Tetanus mit Curarin zu behandeln. Mitt Grenzgeb Med u Chir 16:803, 1906.
51. Goerig M, Beck H: Martin Kirschner - an outstanding surgeon and anesthetist. Third Intern. Symp. on the History of Anesthesia, Atlanta 1992.
52. Kirschner M: Zur Theorie und Prazis der Mastdarmbetäubung mit E 107. Münch med Wochenschr 22:197, 1927.
53. Kirschner M: Eine psycheschonende und steuerbare Form der Allgemein betäubung. Chirurg 15:672, 1929.

54. Kirschner M; Ein neues Verfahren der Allgemeinbetäubung. Zbl f Chir 30:1894, 1929.
55. Bumm R: Intravenöse Narkosen mit Barbitursäurederivaten. Klin Wschr 6:725, 1927.
56. Kirschner M: Erfahrungen mit der intravenösen Avertinnarkose. Arch f klin Chir 162:361, 1930.
57. Freiensten W: Die intravenöse Avertinnarkose nach Kirschner. Klin Wochenschr 16:742, 1930.
58. Kirschner M: Intravenöse Kurz - und Rauschmarkose mit Evipan. In: 57 Tagung der Dtsch. Gesellschaft für Chirurgie. Arch f klin Chir 177:48, 1933.
59. Kirschner M; Die Punktionstechnik und Elektrokoagulation des Ganglion Gasseri. Arch f klin Chir 176:580, 1933.
60. Weese H, Scharpf, W: Evipan, ein neuartiges Einschlafmittel. Dtsch med Wochenschr 58:1205, 1932.
61. Frey R, Hügin W, Mayherhofer O: Lehrbuch der Anaesthesiologie. Springer Verlag, Berlin-Göttingen-Heidelberg 1955.
62. Gohrbrandt P: Die Allgemeine Betäubung. In: Bier-Braun-Kümmel. Chirurgische Operationslehre. ed A. Fischer, E. Gohrbrandt, F. Sauerbruch. Vol. I, Johann Ambrosius Barth, Leipzig 1952.
63. Killian H, Weese H: Die Narkose-Ein Lehr-und Handbuch. Georg Thieme Verlag, Stuttgart 1954.
64. Kingreen O: Chirurgische Operationslehre. Urban & Schwarzenberg Verlag, München-Berlin 1952.
65. Schmidt W: Allgemeine Chirurgie. Theoretische Grundlagen der operativen Medizin. Ein Lehrbuch für Studierende und Ärzte. Johann Ambrosius Barth, Leipzig 1964.
66. Collins VJ: Principles of Anesthesiology. Lea & Febinger 1966.

MARTIN KIRSCHNER
An Outstanding Surgeon and Anesthetist

M. GOERIG and H. BECK
Department of Anaesthesiology,
University Hospital Hamburg, Germany

"Cries and groans have no place in the operating room" claimed the surgeon Martin Kirschner at the end of the 1920's.[1] This statement, with which he began the chapter on pain alleviation in his textbook of general and special surgery, displays Kirschner's emphasis on the importance of adequate perioperative pain therapy. The extensive representation of various anesthetic devices and techniques is historical proof of just how much Kirschner contributed to this specialty. Many of his pain-relieving methods leave much to be desired, but this was probably due to the general non-acceptance of anesthesiology as a specialty.

A typical example of this lack of acceptance is the following statement by the reputable German surgeon, Fredrich Pels Leusden (1866-1944), concerning the surgical textbook written by Kirschner and Otto Nordmann (1878-1946): "Narcosis specialists simply do not exist and hopefully never will!"[2]

In the later editions of his textbook, his chapters on anesthesia became even more detailed.[3,4] This was for Kirschner a logical consequence of the ever continuing specialization of surgery. Many of Kirschner's contributions to anesthesiology and pain therapy, developed in the 30's, are still applicable today. In a memorial to the 50th anniversary of his death, a review of a few of his more important contributions are presented.

Biography

Martin Kirschner was born on October 28, 1879, in Breslau, belonging to a family of surgeons from his father's side (Fig. 1).[5] His grandfather had been a surgeon serving Frederick the Great in the Seven Year War, and he was probably the reason why the young Martin chose medicine as a profession.[5] He studied at the universities of Freiburg, Straßburg and Munich, writing his medical doctorate on "Syryngomyelia and Tabes Dorsalis."[5,6] After receiving his license to practice in 1904, he was a medical resident under the internist Rudolf von Renvers in Berlin.[7,8] It was at this time that Kirschner's father became mayor of the city of Berlin.[5] In 1907, deciding to see the eastern

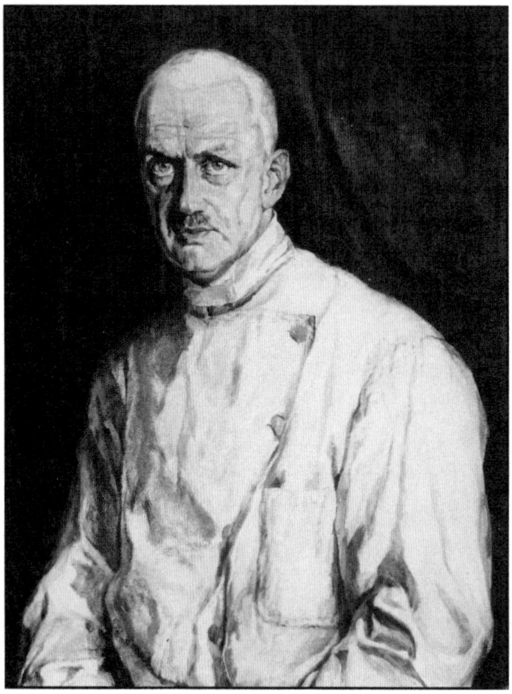

Fig. 1. Martin Kirschner (1879-1942).[5]

world, he travelled to Ceylon and India. It was during his journey that he realized the inadequacy of physicians in emergency situations. Upon his return to Germany, the 28-year-old Kirschner accepted a residency in the Surgical Department of the University of Greifswald, at Königsberg, and was appointed professor. He later accepted the post of chief of surgery at this University in 1917, when Payr left to go to the University of Leipzig as chief.[5] During the Balkan wars, Kirschner gained the recognition as a reputable surgeon. It is worth mentioning that during this time he published several reports of the war atrocities he had seen as chief of a German Red Cross Ambulatory Corps.[9,10,11,12] Kirschner led the surgical department in Königsberg until 1927, when he moved to Tübingen. Seven years later, he became head surgeon to what his predecessor and many colleagues believed to be "The Worst Surgical Clinic in Germany," the University Clinic of Heidelberg.[5] There he remained chief of surgery until his death in 1942.[5]

Kirschner was an excellent surgeon and developer of surgical techniques. Above all, his name is connected with the improvement of the wire extension for bone fractures, the first successful pulmonary embolectomy (the patient lived longer than Kirschner himself), and the introduction of a new technique in the operation for esophageal cancer.[5,13,14,15,16] He was also responsible for many of the modernisations and expansions of the surgical clinics of Königsberg, Bübingen and Heidelberg. He published more than 200 scientific articles on the topics of surgery, anesthesia and hygiene.[5] In 1927, he founded a reputable textbook of surgery and was the editor of a new surgical journal – "Der Chirurg" – in which he and others reported the latest advancements in the area of anesthesiology.[1] These numerous anesthesia related articles played a major role in the development of German Anesthesiology. The following is a brief description of a few of Kirschner's contributions to the development of anesthesia and analgesic methods.

Prophetic Concepts

Shortly after moving to Tübingen, Kirschner published a report titled, "Essential problems of Surgery," in which he discussed, not only topics of surgery, but also those of emergency medicine and anesthesiology.[18] He outlined the basic concepts of emergency medicine and the transportation of severely wounded patients. He even mentioned the possibility of the chain of patient transfer existing today. He himself considered his own ideas to be "fancies of Jules Verne that were perhaps too futuristic to be fulfilled." Nevertheless, he believed that, in a time of radios and televisions, anything could be possible. Kirschner also discussed the applicability of the aeroplane as a means of transportation, seeing not only its speed of travel, but also its lack of vibration as an advantage to the automobile. He mentioned also that the only remaining problem was that of the runway, but perhaps in the future that aeroplanes would be invented which could use a shorter runway than that which they required at the time. "Since aeroplanes are being developed that can land and take off on ever shorter runways, it would perhaps be wise to construct such runways for newly built hospitals to take advantage of the ever increasing possibility of using aeroplanes as vehicles for patient transport." Kirschner wrote this before the helicopter had been invented. He discussed another unsolved surgical problem within his article. In order to be fully cognizant of the severely wounded patient, he strongly suggested that operations should be with a "continual graphic representation of the heartbeat, pulse rate and blood pressure to observe any associated major deviations of these parameters." It was 10 years later that Vienna's surgeon, Fritz von Schürer (1896-1990?), actually recommended such a device with the invention of his Kardiotron.[19] Kirschner mentioned pain alleviating techniques, such as Avertin anesthesia and various local anesthetic methods, stressing the importance of such sedation and anxiolysis. A revolutionary idea was a conceptual solution to the problem of parenteral nutrition, in particular for the cachectic patients: "Should not we be able to develop a solution that can be parenterally tolerated and yet provide the needed nutrition for a longer duration?"[18]

The First Realizations

In the early thirties, Kirschner described the realization of some of his concepts at the newly built University of Tübingen in a series of articles published in the reputable surgical journal, "Der Chirurg."[20,21] His first action, when he moved from Königsberg to Tübingen, was to build a new hospital wing for postoperative and ill patients, following a concept created seven years earlier by the Boston neurosurgeon, William Harvey Cushing (1869-1939). Kirschner pointed out the advantages of such a department for high risk patients, stating that "the care and night round could be supervised by serious and experienced medical personnel." He also believed that "the head of such an intensive care department should have a knowledge and experience necessary for such a serious undertaking, capable of taking appropriate actions when such actions were called for."[20] This belief is a reality in the intensive care units of today.

Further Realizations

Another modern concept — probably due to his analysis of the ever increasing number of automobile and train accidents — was that of a "mobil surgical unit" (Fig. 2). In many ways, this concept resembles that of today's ambulancy: "The physician should be able to go to the wounded patient and not vice-versa."[22] These were the premises with which he propagated an idea which today is an irreplaceable part of clinical practice. It should be mentioned that Kirschner had thought not only of applying this concept to public accidents such as aeroplane, fire and theater accidents, but also had considered it necessary in the case of war. One year later, World War II broke out. In reviews concerning the treatment of wounded soldiers, he repeatedly pointed out the necessity

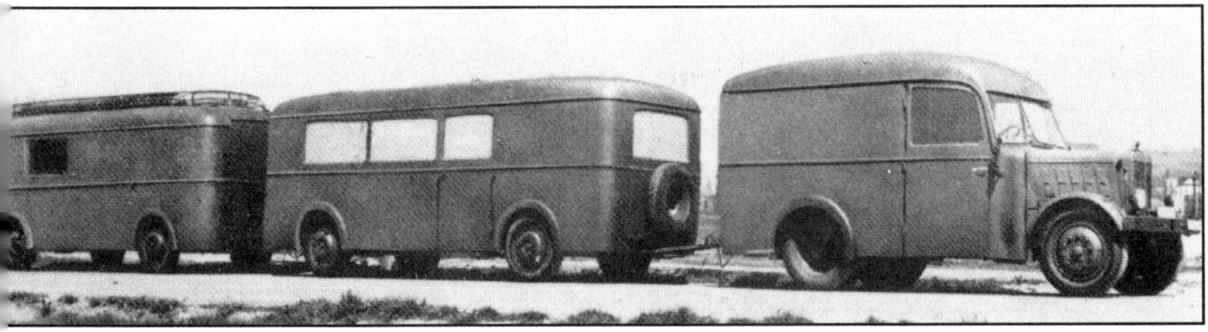

Fig. 2. Kirschner's ambulance, *circa* 1938.[22]

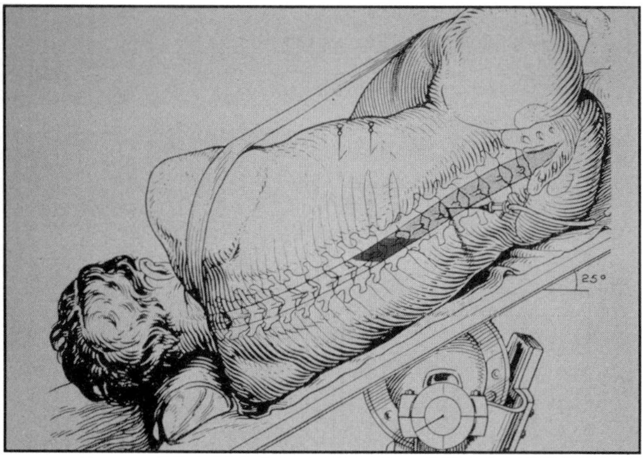

Fig. 3a. Positioning of the patient when "segmental anesthesia" is performed.[3]

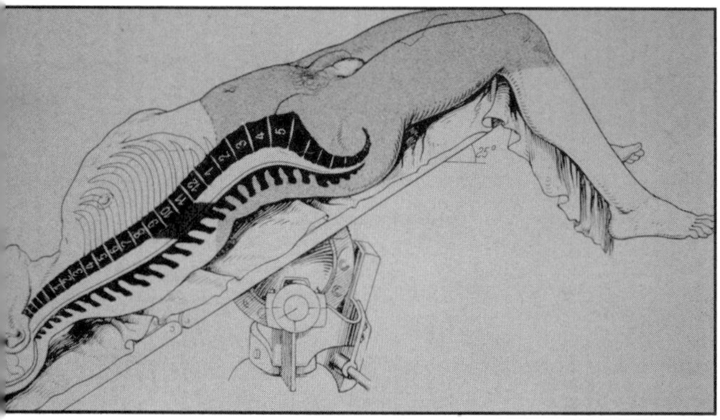

Fig. 3b. The position of the anesthetic charge and the extent of anesthetic area in low spinal anesthesia.[3]

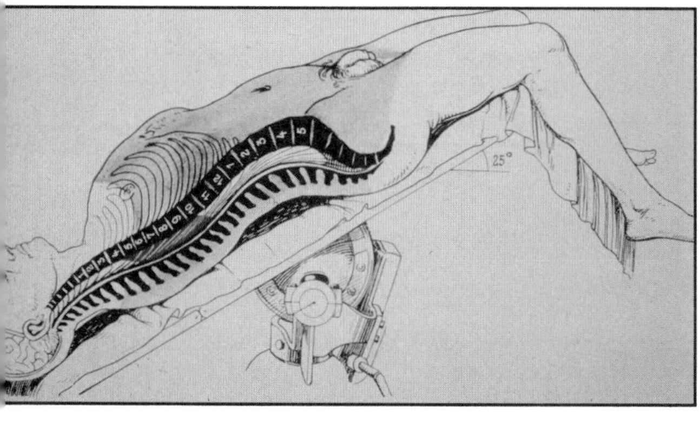

Fig. 3c. The position of the anesthetic charge and the extent of anesthetic area in high spinal anesthesia.[3]

of adequate pain therapy.[23,24] He adamantly promoted the frequent as well as liberal use of analgetics; a belief which was to slowly replace that of the common medical commandment, "nihil nocere."[24,25,26] Besides the use of regional anesthetics for spinal anesthesia, he also advocated the intravenous administration of pain alleviating drugs, such as Morphine, Eukodal, Pantopon and Scopolamine among others.[24] He had recognized the importance of Evipan in 1934 as a hypnotic to be used in all military hospitals, although he noted the difficulty of its appropriate dosing.[27,28]

Kirschner's Segmental and Lumbal Anesthesia Technique

The modified technique of spinal anesthesia and high pressure anesthesia are two of Kirschner's important contributions to the development of anesthesiology.[5] In 1919, Kirschner had already displayed his interest in spinal anesthesia, publishing an article concerning its complications: spinal headache, circulatory disturbances and respiratory arrest associated with this procedure.[29] He attributed these complications to the pharmacologic impurity of the then commonly administered tropacocain, and saw no further use of his clinic for spinal anesthesia. Years later, in 1931, he was the first to report the success of his newly conceived segmental anesthesia (Fig. 3a, 3b, 3c).[30] A major problem of the former "caudallumbar anesthesia" was the initial side-effect of the drastic decrease of blood pressure and the uncontrolled distribution of the anesthetic within the spinal fluid. The conceptional idea of a segmental anesthesia was that it would only affect the sensory nerves of a desired area, the air injected into the subarachnoid space hindering the uncontrolled distribution of the anesthetic.[30,31,32] The patient was positioned on his side in a head-down position of about 25 degrees. Then the patient's buttocks were in a higher position than the head. A spinal tap was then made with a syringe specially designed for this technique by Kirschner himself. Air was injected into the sacral end of the spine in order to prevent the uncontrolled distribution of the following hypobaric anesthetic. The fluid level of the drug could be controlled, the desired level attained by drawing out or newly injecting a predetermined amount of air into the subarachnoid area. The local anaesthetic was then fractionally injected, the needle left in place so as to allow any necessary compensatory injections. The control of the distribution was astonishingly exact when the procedure was practiced by an experienced operator. Nevertheless, the procedure was too complicated and time consuming for the patient who would have to wait for hours in the head-down position until the anesthetic lost its effect. Out of 1000 procedures performed with the described method, only three had related life-threatening complications, one of these ending with the death of the patient.[33,34] Other complications included a drastic decrease in blood pressure, which could not be alleviated with the injection of Ephetonin The incidence of post-spinal headaches was said to be less than with the conventional method. Although Kirschner repeatedly proclaimed in various articles that his segmental anesthesia was "safe and advantageous for the patient," the technique did not become popular among surgeons.[5]

In 1931, Kirschner introduced another variant of local anesthesia, the so-called "High Pressure Local Anesthesia" which, unlike the former variant, achieved more frequent use among operating physicians (Fig. 4).[35] The new method was a variant of the original Schleich infiltration procedure. Shortly after his death, a monograph written by Kirschner appeared with an exact description of, and a list of indications for, the high pressure technique. A preferred local anesthetic solution of 5 percent Novocaine was injected with specially designed needles of appropriate length. The procedure was carried out 10-20 minutes before the operation, allowing the anesthetic to take effect. Kirschner saw an advantage in the almost immediate effect of the anesthetic which, due to its facilitated tissue infiltration, required only one injection site. Each and every nerve fiber was infiltrated with anesthetic so that the distribution was more even, widely spread, and less time consuming

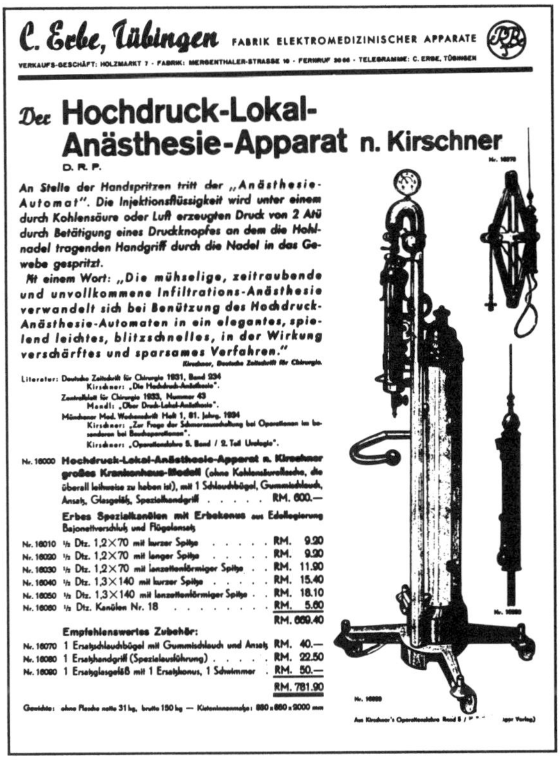

Fig. 4. Apparatus for "High-Pressure Local-Anesthesia," designed by Kirschner, *circa* 1930.[47]

than any of the former methods.[1,35]. Furthermore, an anemic state was attained through the hydrostatic pressure created in the injected tissue and the vasoconstrictive effects of the suprarenin, both of which reduced bleeding tendencies.[36] This effect had already been pointed out by the inventor and most powerful advocate of the infiltration technique, Carl Ludwig Schleich (1859-1922).[37] Kirschner often combined his high pressure technique with other methods of anesthesia, general anesthesia as well as other techniques of local anesthesia.[35] Another advantage of the method was seen by Kirschner in the lack of postoperative pain, which was of exceptional value for the patient. He did, however, expressly warn of possible block of the autonomic nerves that could pathologically affect the blood vessels and internal organs.[35] The high pressure technique was later to be "considered a milestone in the history of local anesthesia."[35] Indeed, it had been considered to be just as important as the discovery of the infiltration method by Schleich or the innovation with use of vasoconstrictive drugs, such as adrenalin, first used by Heinrich Braun (1862-1934).[36] The segmental and high pressure local anesthesia were frequently used in Kirschner's clinic.[5,33] Nevertheless, because of the difficulty and experience required to carry out such maneuvers, both methods were not commonly practiced in other surgical departments.[5]

Intravenous Avertin Anesthesia

In the middle of the twenties, Kirschner intensively researched avertin, a then usually rectally administered hypnotic developed by the company I.G. Farben.[38] Kirschner discontinued the clinical use of this preparation as toxic reactions of the rectal mucosa had been reported when administered.[38] Moreover, severe blood pressure decreases and the risk of apnea were not uncommon during the first trials of its uses. Two years after its clinical introduction for rectal use, he was the first to report its application as an intravenous narcotic.[39,40] Often, he applied it as an induction for major operations, which was then followed by any gas narcotic. Kirschner needed a hypnotic which could be controlled and one which had the amnestic abilities a hypnotic should have; he was convinced that avertin fulfilled these requirements. The avertin preparation he injected intravenously was in a solution of 3 percent sodium chloride, diluted with respect to the body weight of the patient with a device specially designed by Kirschner himself (Fig. 5). With his carefully chosen dose of 0.03 mg per kg body weight, Kirschner claimed to have infrequently had cases of apnea or severe decreases in blood pressure.[41] He reported that care should be taken to avoid parainfusion or injections that could lead to unnecessary connective tissue damage. He reported a 3 percent incidence of thrombophlebitis at the injection site and one fatal pulmonary embolisation. All in all, this anaesthesia technique did not find widespread use in German clinics, most likely because of the popularity of the intravenous barbiturates which had been introduced in 1932 and which thereafter rapidly gained general acceptance.[5,28] Kirschner believed that his surgical colleagues had not accepted avertin because it could only be used as a highly diluted solution.

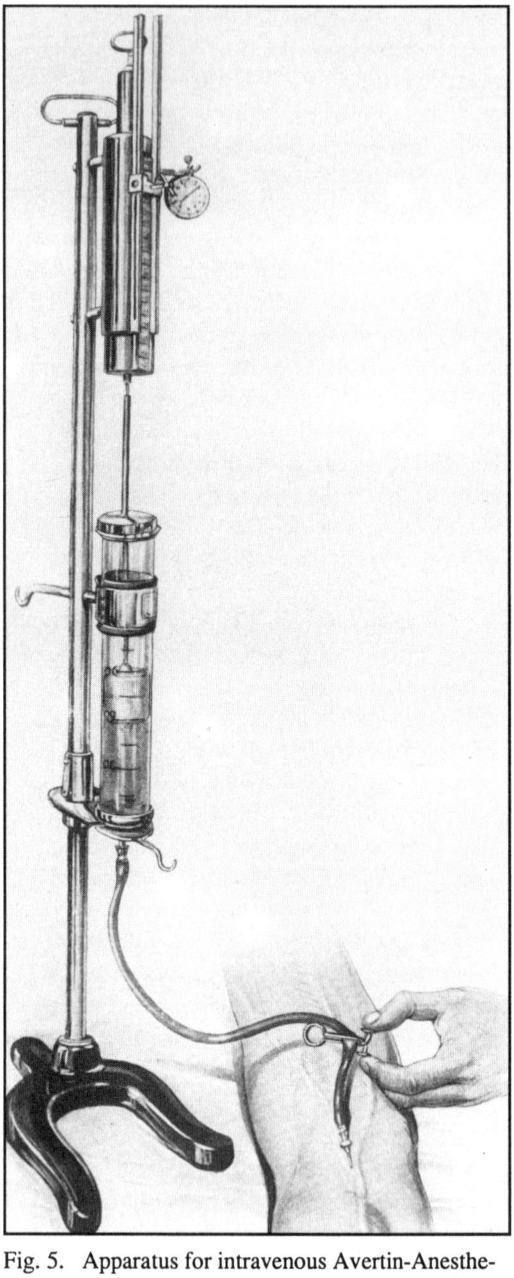

Fig. 5. Apparatus for intravenous Avertin-Anesthesia, designed by Kirschner, *circa* 1930.[41]

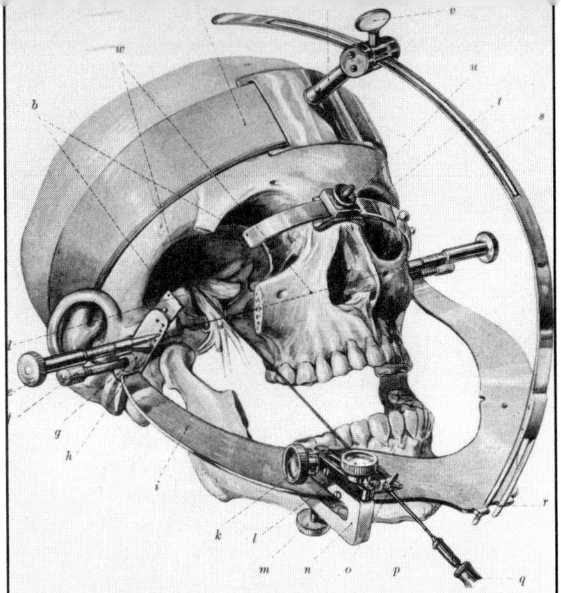

Abb. 5. *Der am Kopfskelet befestigte Zielapparat.* *a* = Säule der Feststellvorrichtung des Zielbügels; *b* = Haltebügel; *c* = Stirnband für die Befestigung der Feststellvorrichtung des Haltebügels; *d* = Mandrin des Punktionsspießes; *e* = Feststellschraube des Zielbügels; *f* = Feststellschraube des Haltebügels; *g* = Ohrzapfen des Haltebügels; *h* = Löcher des Haltebügels für die Spitze der Feststellschraube des Zielbügels; *i* = Zielbügel; *k* = Mikrometerschraube zur Horizontalverschiebung des Punktionsspießes; *l* = Mikrometerschraube zur Vertikalverschiebung des Punktionsspießes; *m* = Feststellschraube des Zielschlittens; *n* = Zielschlitten; *o* = Arretierreiter des Punktionsspießes; *p* = Trokarhülle des Punktionsspießes; *q* = Handgriff des Punktionsspießes; *r* = Einhängezapfen für den Feststellbügel des Zielbügels; *s* = Feststellbügel des Zielbügels; *t* = Nasensteg des Haltebügels; *u* = Feststellschraube des Haltebügels; *v* = Stellschraube des Feststellbügels; *w* = Verbindungslinie der Spitzen der Feststellschrauben des Zielbügels, die durch die For. ovalia geht.

Fig. 6b. The device *in situ*.[42]

Retrospectively, the intravenous route of avertin by Kirschner is considered to be one of the first successful uses of a hypnotic for the induction of anesthesia which found its daily application in surgical practice.

Pain Therapy and the Electrocoagulation of the Ganglion Gasseri

An assessment of Kirschner's anesthesiologic contributions would be incomplete without mentioning the introduction of his electrocoagulation of the Ganglion Gasseri for the purpose of alleviating the excruciating pain of trigeminal neuralgia.[42] With the help of a direction device, a specially prepared needle, which with the exception of the end had been coated with a layer of nonconducting material, was inserted through the foramen ovale of the cranium until the nerve complex was reached (Fig. 6a, 6b). The needle was directed with a milliampère sensing device which displayed the conductivity of the nerve fibers as soon as the ganglion was located. The ganglion and the surrounding tissue were then electrocoagulated until a state of nonconductivity was attained, representing the total elimination of nerve fibers primarily responsible for the neuralgia.[42,43] A similar needle had been developed by the Tübingen surgeon, Georg Perthes (1869-1927), and had been used for electrically guided localization of peripheral nerves.[44] Kirschner, who had become the successor of Perthes in Tübingen, when he died in 1927, was probably inspired by this device, thus further developing it into a electrocoagulation needle as well. After extensive experimentation, the correct size of the needle was attained and could therefore easily and precisely be directed into the trigeminal ganglion. The safety and precision of this technique was a major achievement which had been almost impossible with the "blind puncture method" popularized by the German surgeon, Fritz Härtel (1877-1940?).[45] An

Fig. 6a. Kirschner's device for the electrocoagulation of the Ganglion Gasseri.[42]

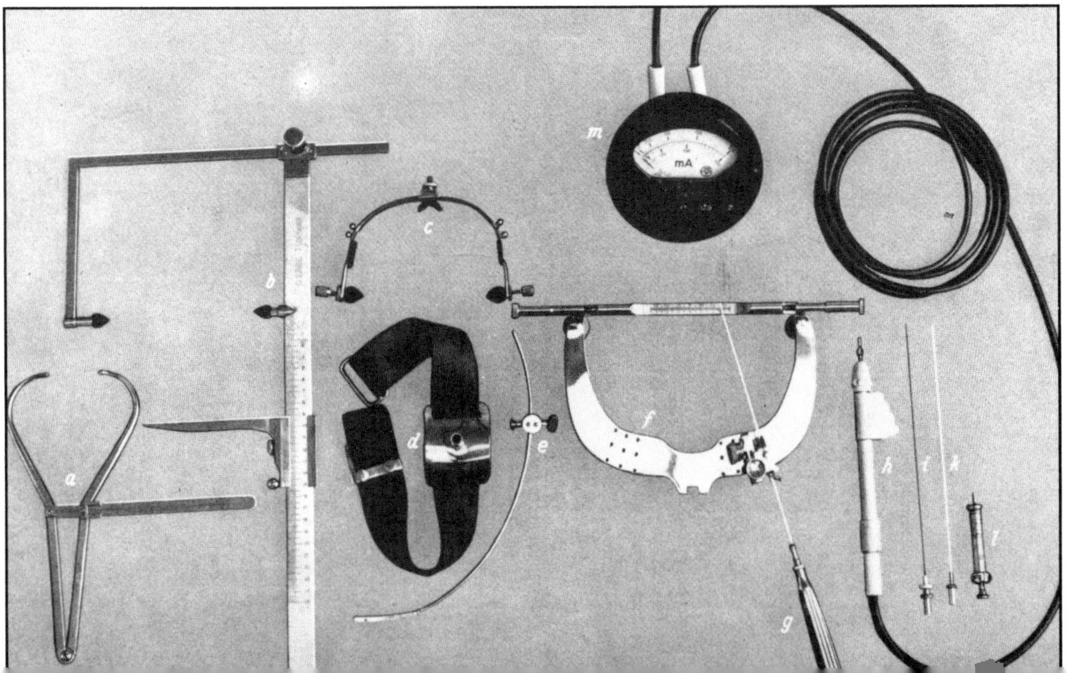

intraoperative stereoscopic X-ray control of the needle position was used in doubtful cases.[42] Kirschner routinely carried out this procedure following a rectally administered Avertin basic-narcosis.[42,43] An anesthesia either with avertin intravenously or chlorethyl was needed for the two otherwise extremely painful periods during the insertion and coagulation. The correctly positioned needle would lose its conduction abilities as soon as the ganglion was entirely destroyed since only non-conducting coagulated tissue was left. Sometimes, Kirschner also injected 0.2-0.5 ml of 70 percent alcohol into the tissue to insure its destruction.[42]

In a first review of this treatment in 73 patients, an average symptom-free period of two years had been attained. Complications, occurring especially when carried out by an inexperienced operator, were lesions of the cranial nerves lying near the ganglion.[42] Kirschner reported one entire loss of sight, an abducent paresis, and paralysis of the oculomotorius, vagus and recurrens nerve. He particularly advocated the value of such an electrocoagulation in cases of brain tumor near the trigeminus ganglion.[5,42]

He also considered chordotomy to be of great value to the patient suffering from unbearable pain. He pleaded for such a surgical intervention in selected cases, and sometimes he performed this difficult surgical procedure himself. These and other invasive pain-alleviating operations are successfully carried out today in the so-called "Pain Clinics."

The Concept of Perioperative Medication for Patients under Local Anesthesia

Kirschner believed in practicing his patient oriented concepts. He was renowned for operating on a large percentage of his patients under any local anesthetic method, in particular with his high pressure and segmental techniques. In longer operations, he tried to alleviate the stress of the patient under local anesthesia with music played into headphones (Fig. 7).[32,46] Later, he discussed the possibility of using a television set, a technique absolutely new at that time, nowadays more and more asked for by patients, rarely realized within the operating theaters!

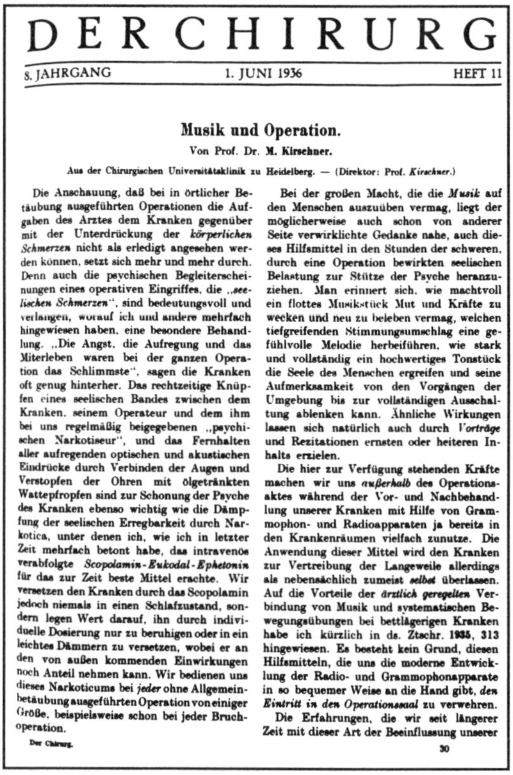
DER CHIRURG

8. JAHRGANG 1. JUNI 1936 HEFT 11

Musik und Operation.

Von Prof. Dr. **M. Kirschner.**

Aus der Chirurgischen Universitätsklinik zu Heidelberg. — (Direktor: Prof. *Kirschner*.)

Die Anschauung, daß bei in örtlicher Betäubung ausgeführten Operationen die Aufgaben des Arztes dem Kranken gegenüber mit der Unterdrückung der *körperlichen Schmerzen* nicht als erledigt angesehen werden können, setzt sich mehr und mehr durch. Denn auch die psychischen Begleiterscheinungen eines operativen Eingriffes, die „*seelischen Schmerzen*", sind bedeutungsvoll und verlangen, worauf ich und andere mehrfach hingewiesen haben, eine besondere Behandlung. „Die Angst, die Aufregung und das Miterleben waren bei der ganzen Operation das Schlimmste", sagen die Kranken oft genug hinterher. Das rechtzeitige Knüpfen eines seelischen Bandes zwischen dem Kranken, seinem Operateur und dem ihm bei uns regelmäßig beigegebenen „psychischen Narkotiseur", und das Fernhalten aller aufregenden optischen und akustischen Eindrücke durch Verbinden der Augen und Verstopfen der Ohren mit ölgetränkten Wattepfropfen sind zur Schonung der Psyche des Kranken ebenso wichtig wie die Dämpfung der seelischen Erregbarkeit durch Narkotica, unter denen ich, wie ich in letzter Zeit mehrfach betont habe, das intravenös verabfolgte *Scopolamin-Eukodal-Ephetonin* für das zur Zeit beste Mittel erachte. Wir versetzen den Kranken durch das Scopolamin jedoch niemals in einen Schlafzustand, sondern legen Wert darauf, ihn durch individuelle Dosierung nur zu beruhigen oder in ein leichtes Dämmern zu versetzen, wobei er an den von außen kommenden Einwirkungen noch Anteil nehmen kann. Wir bedienen uns dieses Narkoticums bei *jeder* ohne Allgemeinbetäubung ausgeführten Operation von einiger Größe, beispielsweise schon bei jeder Bruchoperation.

Bei der großen Macht, die die *Musik* auf den Menschen auszuüben vermag, liegt der möglicherweise auch schon von anderer Seite verwirklichte Gedanke nahe, auch dieses Hilfsmittel in den Stunden der schweren, durch eine Operation bewirkten seelischen Belastung zur Stütze der Psyche heranzuziehen. Man erinnert sich, wie machtvoll ein flottes Musikstück Mut und Kräfte zu wecken und neu zu beleben vermag, welchen tiefgreifenden Stimmungsumschlag eine gefühlvolle Melodie herbeiführen, wie stark und vollständig ein hochwertiges Tonstück die Seele des Menschen ergreifen und seine Aufmerksamkeit von den Vorgängen der Umgebung bis zur vollständigen Ausschaltung ablenken kann. Ähnliche Wirkungen lassen sich natürlich auch durch *Vorträge* und Rezitationen ernsten oder heiteren Inhalts erzielen.

Die hier zur Verfügung stehenden Kräfte machen wir uns *außerhalb* des Operationsaktes während der Vor- und Nachbehandlung unserer Kranken mit Hilfe von Grammophon- und Radioapparaten ja bereits in den Krankenräumen vielfach zunutze. Die Anwendung dieser Mittel wird den Kranken zur Vertreibung der Langeweile allerdings als nebensächlich zumeist *selbst* überlassen. Auf die Vorteile der *ärztlich geregelten* Verbindung von Musik und systematischen Bewegungsübungen bei bettlägerigen Kranken habe ich kürzlich in ds. Ztschr. 1935, 313 hingewiesen. Es besteht kein Grund, diesen Hilfsmitteln, die uns die moderne Entwicklung der Radio- und Grammophonapparate in so bequemer Weise an die Hand gibt, *den Eintritt in den Operationssaal* zu verwehren.

Die Erfahrungen, die wir seit längerer Zeit mit dieser Art der Beeinflussung unserer

Der Chirurg. 30

Fig. 7. Frontispiece of Kirschner's article "Musik und Operation."[46]

Synopsis

If one is to remember Kirschner's contributions to pain alleviation procedures, one must mention his segmental spinal anesthesia and the high pressure local anesthesia. A mention of his development of intravenous avertin anesthesia, which was originally intended as a suppository for basic anesthesia, is also necessary. Important were his concepts of perioperative anxiolytic and sedative procedures for patients under local anesthesia, whether they were attained pharmacologically or with the newest technical inventions such as the radio or television. Long-sighted were his recommendations concerning the avoidance of chronic contact with gas narcotics. As a pain therapist, he mastered the use of chordotomy to alleviate the pain of incurable cancer patients and introduced the electrocoagulation of the Ganglion Gasseri in order to temporarily cure trigeminal neuralgia. Prophetic were his suggestions with respect to intensive care units and emergency care. A modern concept which he realized was the intensive care unit which he had ordered to be built in 1930. The question as to whether Kirschner considered anesthesia a specialty or not must remain unanswered. We would not be wrong in considering him to be a passionate surgeon, but he was also a surgeon with the thoughts and actions of an anesthesiologist: "Divinum est sedare dolorem."

References

1. Kirschner M, Schubert A: Allgemeine und spezielle chirurgische Operationslehre. Vol I Springer Verlag, Berlin 1927.
2. Pels-Leusden F: Die Bekämpfung des Schmerzes in der Chirurgie. Vol. I In: Kirschner-Nordmann: Die Chirurgie, Urban & Schwarzenberg Verlag, Berlin-Wien 1926.
3. Kirschner M: Die Eingriffe am Harnapparat und an den männlichen Geschlechtsteilen. Vol. 5 II In: Allgemeine und spezielle chirurgische Operationslehre. ed.: Kirschner, M. Springer Verlag, Berlin, 1937.
4. Kirschner M: Allgemeine und spezielle chirurgische Operationslehre. Vol III, Springer Verlag 1940.
5. Kirschner H: (son of M. Kirschner) personal communication. Dec. 1991, Feb. 1992.
6. Nordmann O: Martin Kirschner. Arch f klin Chir 204:1, 1942.
7. Bauer KH: Martin Kirschner. Arch f klin Chir 69:1589, 1942.
8. Redwitz V: Martin Kirschner. Mitt. aus den Grenzgeb. Med und Chir 46:1, 1942.
9. Kirschner M: Bemerkungen über die Wirkung der regelrechten Infanteriegeschosse und der Dumdumgeschosse auf den menschlichen Körper. Münch med Wochenschr 61:2445, 1914.
10. Kirschner M: Kriegschirurgische Erfahrungen vom Balkankriegsschauplatz. Dtsch med Wochenschr 40:99, 1914.
11. Kirschner M: Berichte über die werste Hilfsexpedition nach Bulgarien. Gesamtüberblick über die Zusammensetzung, Reise, Tätigkeit und die chirurgischen Erfahrungen der Abordnung. Hrg.: Central-Komitee der Deutschen Vereine vom Roten Kreuz. Springer Verlag, Berlin, 1914.
12. Kirschner M: Die II. Hilfsexpedition nach Adrianopel. a) chirurgische und sonstige Beobachtengungen in Adrianopel. Hrg.: Central-Komitee der Deutschen Vereine vom Roten Kreuz. Springer Verlag, Berlin 1914.
13. Kirschner M: Ein durch die Trendelenburg'sche Operation geheilter Fall von Embolie der Art. Pulmonalis. Arch klin Chir 133:312, 1924.
14. Zenker R: Die Chirurgie Martin Kirschners in unserer Zeit. Münch med Wochenschr 122:318, 1980.
15. Romm S: The person behind the name: Martin Kirschner. 104, 193.
16. Schmitt W: Martin Kirschner zum 100. Geburtstag am 28.10. 1879. Zbl f Chir 21:1434, 1979.
17. Borst HG, Klinner W, Oelert H: Herzchirurgie. In: Kirschner'sche Operationslehre. Springer Verlag Berlin, Heidelberg, New York 1991.
18. Kirschner M; Wesentliche Probleme der Chirurgie. Dtsch med Wochenschr 37:1541, 1927.
19. Schürer v. F: Das Kardiotron, ein Apparat zur objektiven Messung der Harzfrequenz, des Blutdruckes und der Atmung während der Operation. Arch f klin Chir 189:388, 1937.
20. Kirschner M; Zum Neubau der Chirurgischen Universitätsklinik Tübingen. II. Der Krankenbau. Chirurg 2:54, 1929.
21. Kirschner M; Zum Neubau der Chirurgischen Universitätsklinik Tübingen. III. Der Behandlungsbau. Chirurg 3:202, 1930.
22. Kirschner M: Die fahrbare chirurgische Klinik. (Röntgen-, Operations- und Schwerverletztenabteilung). Chirurg 20:712, 1938.
23. Kirschner M: Die Schmerzbekämpfung im Felde. 8:269, 1936.
24. Kirschner M: Die operative Schmerzstillung im Kriege. Der Deutsche Militärarzt. 4:153-63, 1939.
25. Kirschner M: Lokalanästhesie. Schmerz-Narkose-Anästhesie 2:49, 1939.
26. Kirschner M: Die Wichtigsten Aufgaben des Frontchirurgen nach den Erfahrungen der letzten Kriege. Chirurg 22:768, 1939.
27. Kirschner M: Intravenöse Kurz — und Rauschmarkose mit Evipan. In: 57. Tagung der Deutschen Gesellschaft für Chirurgie. Arch f klin Chir 177:48, 1933.

28. Weese H, Scharpf W: Evipan, ein neuartiges Einschlafmittel. Dtsch med Wochenschr 58:1205, 1932.
29. Kirschner M; Häufung über Zustände der Lumbalanästhesie. Zbl f Chir 18:322, 1919.
30. Kirschner M: Eine gürtelförmige, einstellbare und individuell dosierbare Spinalbetäubung. Chirurg 5:633, 1931.
31. Kirschner M; Spinal Zone Anesthesia. Surg Gynecol Obstet 3:317, 1932.
32. Weisser C, Sprotte G: Martin Kirschner's spinal zone anesthesia. The History of Anaesthesia Society, Meeting May-June 1991, 1991; Vol 9B:68.
33. Philippides Erfahrungen mit der Kirschner'schen Spinalanästhesie. Arch f klin Chir 181:479, 1935.
34. Kirschner M; Zur Frage der Schmerzausschaltung bei Operationen im besonderen bei Bauchoperationen. Münch med Wochenschr 1:1, 1934.
35. Kirschner M: Die Hochdrucklokalanästhesie. Springer Verlag, Berlin 1944.
36. Braun Hch: Die Bedeutung des Adrenalin für die Lokalanaesthesie. Langenbecks Arch klin Chir 69:150, 1903.
37. Goerig M: Carl Ludwig Schleich and the Scandal during the Annual Meeting of the German Surgical Society. Third International Symposium on the History of Anesthesia. Atlanta 1992.
38. Kirschner M: Zur Theorie und Praxis der Mastdarmbetäubung mit E 107. Münch med Wochenschr 22:917, 1927.
39. Kirschner M: Eine psycheschonende und steuerbare Form der Allgemeinbetäubung. Chirurg 5:673, 1929.
40. Kirschner M: Ein neues Verfahren der Allgemeinbetäubung. Zbl f Chir 30:1894, 1929.
41. Kirschner M; Erfahrungenmit der intravenösen Avertinnarkose. Arch f klin Chir 162:361, 1930.
42. Kirschner M; Die Punktionstechnik und Elektrokoagulation des Ganglion Gasseri. Über "gezielte" Operationen. Arch f klin Chir 176:580, 1933.
43. Kirschner M: Die Behandlung der Trigeminusneuralgie (Nach Erfahrungen an 1113 Kranken). Münch med Wochenschr 11:235, 1942.
44. Goerig M, Schulte am Esch: J. Georg Perthes – Ein Pionier moderner Regional-anesthesie-Techniken ? Anaesthetist Regionalanesthesie 13:1, 1990.
45. Härtel Fr: Intrakranielle Leitungsanästhesie des Ganglion Gasseri. Zbl f Chir 21:705, 1912.
46. Kirschner M: Musik und Operation. Chirurg 11:429, 1936.
47. ERBE-Company, personal commuincation, September 1990.

THE STORY OF DR. JUAN MARÍN
THE FATHER OF COLOMBIAN ANESTHESIA

J.S. GRAVENSTEIN
Department of Anesthesiology
University of Florida, Gainesville, Florida, USA
and
ERNESTO ROJAS
Department of Anesthesiology
Instituto de Seguros Sociales, Bogotá, Colombia

Modern anesthesiologists complete medical school and at least three years of residency in order to acquire the information and master the skills requisite for the practice of anesthesia. We must wonder how the pioneers in anesthesia prepared themselves for their tasks; they had neither books nor mentors. Indeed, some early anesthetists were not even medically trained. We know little about these pioneers. How did they learn their craft? How did they come to formulate the concepts they needed for their practice? How did they develop instruments to help them in their daily work?

The earliest pioneers have long since vanished. Indeed, the oldest, still-living anesthetists, octogenarians and nonagenarians, started their careers around 1930, a time when textbooks on anesthesia had been published, societies had been formed, prominent teachers had been recognized, and anesthesia machines had become available. Schools for nurse anesthetists and residency training programs had been established. This was certainly true in the United States and Great Britain, but in many other countries conditions were quite different.

We had the good fortune of interviewing Dr. Juan Marín, a colleague who gave his first anesthetic in 1932, in Colombia, South America. He began his work as a chloroformist, even though he had had no formal teaching in anesthesia, no textbook on anesthesia, and no anesthesia machine. Indeed, in his country an anesthetist might be neither a nurse nor a physician. Juan Marín recalls vividly his early days of anesthesia when he had to make his own observations, draw his own conclusions, and make his own instruments. He did all of that magnificently, and now he is celebrated in his

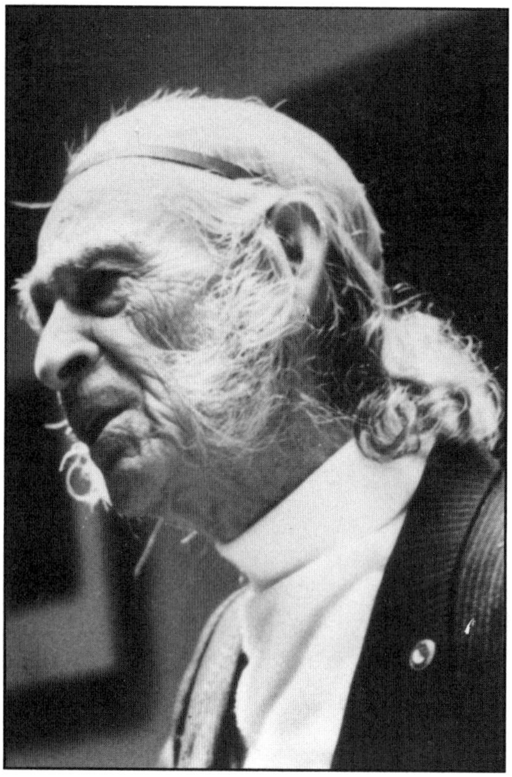

Fig. 1. Juan Marín around 1990.

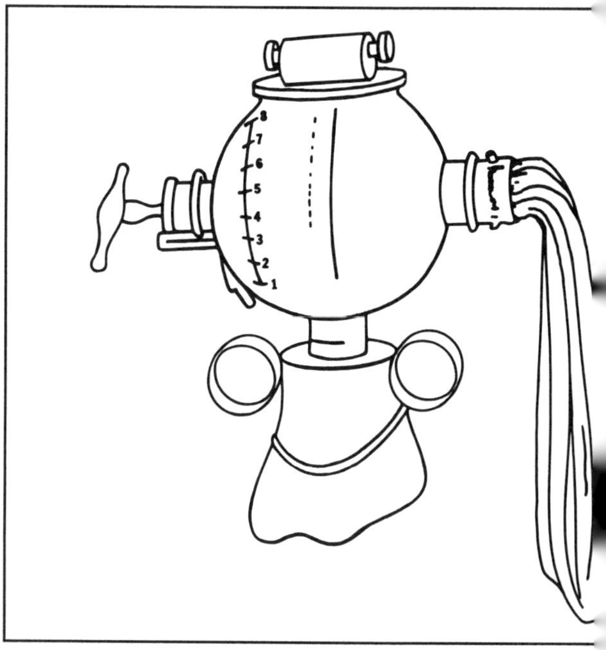

Fig. 2. The Ombrédanne mask: the metal sphere contained cotton which was soaked with ether. A pig's bladder served as breathing bag. The dial on the left could be turned to allow mor or less of the respired air to pick up ether. The apparatus, a truly closed rebreathing system, makes no provisions for the addition of oxygen or the removal of carbon dioxide and thus disarmingly ignores basic physiologic and anesthetic principles.

country as the father of Colombian anesthesia.[1,2] The story of Juan Marín is worth telling because it grants us a vivid picture of the conditions that confronted some of our forefathers; it also affords us a look at the intellectual approach that leads to inventions in general. Finally, we are allowed a glimpse at a fascinating and complex man.

Juan Marín's Career

Juan Marín Osorio was born on June 21, 1907, in rural Sonsón, in the vicinity of Medellin, in Colombia. His parents owned a little land, which enabled them, in 1928, to send their son, Juan, to the Colombian National University, in Bogotá, to study medicine. Fortunately, the tuition was only about $20 per year, an advantage because Juan Marín was not immediately successful in his studies of anatomy, which he had to repeat for 4 years. The haze that so kindly obscures the harsher truths of distant events now makes it difficult to discern whether Marín did not wish to learn what his professors taught, or whether his professors did not teach what he wished to learn. One reason for his seeking an education in medicine had been Marín's curiosity about the seat of the soul. We confidently assume that his medical school did not offer anatomical dissection exercises of the locus in which the soul was to be found.

In 1932, still enrolled in anatomy classes, he attended surgical lectures conducted by Professor Juan N. Corpas, in St. John's Hospital of Bogotá. To one surgical demonstration in an amphitheater, Marín entered late and the annoyed surgeon invited him to give the anesthetic.

"But I cannot," Marín said. "I have never given an anesthetic in my life."

"Can you count to ten?", the surgeon enquired. That he could, Marín admitted. "Well, that is all you need to know for anesthesia," Dr. Corpas states. Those two sentences should secure for Professor Corpas a place in medical history, as they distill the essence of an attitude toward anesthesia that was prevalent for many years. "Here," Dr. Corpas continued, "you take this mask, hold it over the patient's face, and when I say one, you turn the dial to one. And when I say three, you turn it to three, and so on. That is all there is to anesthesia."

Thus Marín, the persistent student of anatomy, gave his first ether anesthetic with an Ombredanne mask in front of his classmates and the professor of surgery. The patient survived, and perhaps this first success in Marín's career influenced his future. But not before another event took his life on a wild detour.

The reader may surmise that a young man who wonders about the anatomical seat of the soul might also be curious about the corporeal realization of other abstract concepts. Juan Marín, as most of his countrymen, was brought up in the Catholic faith. He had often participated in the Eucharist and had accepted the wafer, the transubstantiated body of Christ. Perhaps Juan Marín knew about the centuries old theological debates that have swirled around the eucharistic doctrine, or perhaps his inquisitiveness sprang from much simpler ideas; whatever the motive, one Sunday, before receiving the sacred wafer, he pulled out his handkerchief and dried his tongue. Then, instead of eating the host, he concealed it in the pages of his notebook and carried it home to examine it for evidence of the transubstantiation. The next day he showed it to his friends. Unfortunately, he was overheard and a witness informed the archbishop, who mobilized the police, and they arrested Juan Marín. After 5 days in jail, and barely escaping a 5-year prison sentence, Juan Marín was set free. Neither his parents nor his anatomy professor found his secular scrutiny of a religious object amusing. Juan lost his financial support from home and was barred from continuing his studies of anatomy in medical school.

With this event bad times started for Juan Marín. Bad times and good times. Bad times because he had lost all support and he often went hungry; and good times because, through the offices of a friend, he became a chloroformist at the Catholic Hospital de la Misericordia for children. Sister Maria Ermelina, a nun, taught him how to give chloroform to children, using a semi-closed or open drop technique. His efforts were not rewarded with money, lodging, or even food. A kind colleague offered him a place to sleep, and a loving cook an occasional meal.

It was more than a year before his work was rewarded with a modest stipend, and more than 8 years before he finished his medical education—without formally graduating. In 1945, he accepted the position as chief of anesthesia in St. Joseph's Hospital in Bogotá. And from then on Mr. Juan Marín's career accelerated. On September 23, 1949, he founded the Colombian Society of Anesthesiology. In 1956, without having written the usually required thesis, he was finally granted the title of Doctor of Medicine. Dr. Juan Marín, accompanied by his newly-wed wife Hilda, then left Colombia for Venezuela, where they stayed until 1973. When he returned to Bogotá, he assumed the position of Chief of Anesthesia at the Military Hospital and later the Social Security Hospital. The years were kind to him and he was able to work part-time until 1983. Dr. Juan Marín, now a widower, and his two sons live in Bogotá, Colombia.

Chloroform Anesthesia in the Mid 1930's

Even though by 1930 much had been written about the disadvantages of chloroform for anesthesia, it was still widely used.[3] In the Hospital de la Misericordia of Bogotá it was the principal anesthetic and it was only given by open methods (endotracheal anesthesia was not introduced until 1948). Preoperative visits were not conducted, examinations were not performed by anesthetists, and premedications were usually not given, even though morphine and atropine were available and their effects appreciated.

Juan first met each patient when the child was rolling into the operating room. The patient was placed on the operating room table, a strap over the knees, the arms tied to the sides of the table. Neither intravenous drip nor fluid by subcutaneous or intraperitoneal clysis was given. Nor was oxygen used. No monitors were applied. First the patient's nose was protected against the concentrated chloroform with a dab of vaseline. When this was forgotten, some patients suffered necrotic lesions on or around their noses. Sister Maria Ermelina taught Juan to prepare the anesthesia workstation by setting on a small table a glass bottle of chloroform and a gauze pad, which was to be folded into a little tent, into the point of which a cotton ball was placed which was to be soaked with chloroform and firmly placed over the patient's face.[4] Regularly, the patients passed through a stage of wild excitement before the onset of surgical anesthesia. Caffeine was injected intramuscularly when a patient's life appeared to ebb during the anesthetic.

Because the dangers of aspiration were not recognized, patients with a full stomach were accepted for anesthesia just as those who had been fasting. When a patient did vomit during induction, Juan was taught to turn the patient's head to the side and, with his fingers, wipe out the child's mouth. A very small vomiting child Juan might take by the feet and hold upside down, perhaps while clapping the patient's chest. Yet, he could recall but one patient who aspirated and died.

Tonsillectomies were common. For this the child was anesthetized while lying down and, when deep under the chloroform, was sat up on the table and the surgeon would rapidly remove one tonsil. Then the child was put down again, reanesthetized, and once again sat up for removal of the other tonsil. Bleeding was controlled by packing the tonsillar fossa. When postoperative bleeding required the ligature of the bleeders, Marín would put the patient into a head-down position and reinduce anesthesia. This time the surgeon would apply his stitches and ligatures with the patient in the head-down position.

For about 8 years, Juan gave 3 to 4 chloroform anesthetics every working day; that would perhaps be as many as 8,000 anesthetics. He can recall only one child who suffered a cardiovascular collapse following tachycardia during early surgical stimulation of the pharynx under light chloroform anesthesia. Electrocardiography was not available and there was no way of distinguishing ventricular fibrillation from cardiac standstill. The patient expired and resuscitation was not attempted. He also remembers two patients in whom jaundice developed early postoperatively. His recollections, then, resemble those published by Edward Lawrie who recalls 1 death attributed to chloroform anesthesia out of 17,300 anesthetics administered over almost 9 years.[3]

In 1941, Dr. Rafael Barberi-Zamorano, surgeon and mentor in the Hospital de la Misericordia of Bogotá, was instrumental in obtaining the first anesthesia machine for the hospital, a Heidbrink equipped with oxygen, cyclopropane, and carbon dioxide. Later, in 1945, when Juan Marín assumed responsibility for anesthesia in the St. Joseph's hospital, he became chief of 4 anesthesia-nurse-aids who had been trained by an intern to give anesthesia. His hospital had 4 Heidbrink machines with oxygen, ethylene, and cyclopropane, and one McKesson machine for nitrous oxide with which only Hans, an Austrian hospital mechanic, gave anesthesia. The nurses-aides found the machine too complex.

Of Concepts and Inventions

What happened when a young, demonstrably curious farmer's son is confronted with the phenomena of anesthesia? How does he bring order into the profusion of observations? What concepts will he formulate to overcome this difficulty or ameliorate that disadvantage? Juan Marín was impressed by many events during anesthesia and to his credit, and true to his character, he accepted nothing as given dogma.

Take the excitement phase he observed over and over again when the chloroform cap was placed on the face of his little patients. To understand why they struggled, he placed the chloroform tent on his own face and found it to be intensely unpleasant. For thousands of patients his predecessors had accepted that offense as a necessary evil. Not so with Juan Marín! He experimented with the different concentrations of chloroform and eventually he put one drop on the gauze, gave it to the patient for three breaths, took the gauze off, put two drops in, put it back on the patient for three breaths, took it off again and after adding three drops gave it to the patient for another three breaths, and so on, until anesthesia was established.

How much of the anesthetic to give was another question with which Juan had to come to grips. The nurses had taught him to watch the motion of the arms and movement of the chest, and to touch the patient's cornea with the finger to test for the absence of the reflex and thus establish the presence of surgical anesthesia. Marín had observed the gradual dilatation of the pupils as anesthesia deepened, first losing their response to light and finally becoming dilated and fixed. He called the widely dilated pupil the "open window to eternity." Later he learned of Guedel's stages of anesthesia, and he applied these stages to concepts that explained how a conscious patient can be rendered comatose and yet move, and how later motor activity ceases but heart and lungs continue to function. He offered the concept of the three aspects of life:

— *the mental life,* reflected by consciousness and awareness.
— *the life of motion,* expressed by muscular activity, but not necessarily awareness.
— *the vegetative life,* as revealed in he reaction of the pupil, and in the actions of heart and lungs.

Anesthetia had to suppress the mental life and the life of motion and it had to spare the vegetative life; indeed, the patient had to be maintained in the narrow confines of this stage. Recognizing that respiratory and cardiac functions were also under the influence of the vegetative life, he began to monitor cardiac function during anesthesia, feeling for the pulse and listening for heart sounds. During the stage of motion, he discovered that the heart rate might accelerate and, when the pupils were dilated, the heart rate slowed. Juan Marín soon appreciated that bradycardia went hand-in-hand with excessively deep anesthesia and that, at times, it was necessary not only to take away the chloroformed sponge but also to push on the chest to stimulate the heart. The advantage of listening to the heartbeat and the difficulty of doing this while administering chloroform caused him to make a stethoscope, which he built himself as he had no money to buy even the components. He use old phonograph records, which he cut and then heated so that he could roll a short cylinder which served as the chest-piece. One end he covered with a piece of tin through which he made a hole, and into which he inserted the rubber tubing that led to his earpiece, an olive-shaped object also molded from the phonograph record. The earpiece was difficult to shape and painful to wear, so he settled for a monaural stethoscope, probably the first to be used. The membrane of the chest-piece he made out of pig bladder, which he obtained from a butcher shop. This was in 1934. He did not publish a description of this invention. Later, he was given a binaural instrument so that he could hear the conversation in the operating room.

Listening to the heart sounds through his precordial stethoscope, he began to appreciate that he could also hear breath sounds; but in order to auscultate them he had to move the chest-piece of the stethoscope away from the heart. Therefore, he built a second stethoscope which he placed over the right side of the patient's chest, switching from one stethoscope to the other to listen to either breath or heart sounds. Because this was laborious, he interposed a three-way stopcock, which enabled him to listen to either heart or breath sounds by doing nothing more than switching a little stopcock. Because stridor developed in many of his patients during anesthesia, he prepared an additional stethoscope head which he placed over the patient's jugular notch. Then, with a four-way stopcock, he had the option of listening to breath sounds, laryngeal sounds, or heart sounds. This invention he called the panphonoscope.

Juan Marín's Contribution to Organized Anesthesia

A tree that blooms and distributes its seeds can start a forest. In 1936, when Juan Marín (long before he had completed medical school) gave his first lecture on the dilation of the pupil and the stages of anesthesia, he probably did not realize that he was the seed of anesthesiology in Colombia.

In 1946, as chief of anesthesia—but not yet a doctor—Juan Marín attempted to establish a first school for anesthetists. However, neither physician nor nurse applied, the reputation of anesthesia being too shallow to attract any self-respecting professional. So a year later, Juan invited the teenage daughters of hospital physicians to learn how to give anesthesia. That broke the ice and soon a dentist and three Sisters of Charity enrolled. The specialty slowly took root. In 1948, the first medical student signed up and within 12 months 8 medical students and 12 high school graduates attended Juan Marín's school of anesthesia. In 1949, Marín received an invitation to attend the First Latin American Congress of Anesthesiology in Buenos Aries. How could he attend without bringing the greetings of a Colombian Society of Anesthesia? As none existed, what was more natural than to quickly found the Colombian Society of Anesthesiologists, in whose name he then brought greetings to Buenos Aires.

Once established, anesthesiology flourished in Colombia. Juan Marín contributed papers, lectures, and more importantly than anything else, the example of a dedicated physician specialist, which was emulated by his many pupils who now hold important positions in the Americas.

The Emblem of Colombian Anesthesia

The anesthesia emblem, designed by Juan Marín in 1947, had its origin in an innocent question posed by one of the physician-daughters enrolled in his school of anesthesia, who asked about a badge that she might wear on her graduation. Marín considered different motifs and finally presented a beautiful composition that speaks to anesthesia, the state in which sleep adjoins death. In Greek mythology, the night has twin sons, Thanatos (death), and Hypnos (sleep), who carry flaming torches, pointing toward the floor, to light a path through the dark. Between the torches, the emblem shows the small flame of life which the anesthetist must guard. In the upper half, the sun of consciousness, half obscured by the dark, rises or sets. Around the emblem we read: *anaesthesia deorum ars,* or "anesthesia, the art of the Gods," which reminds us of Genesis: "and the Lord God caused a deep sleep to fall upon Adam, and he slept and He took one of his ribs and closed up the flesh instead thereof."

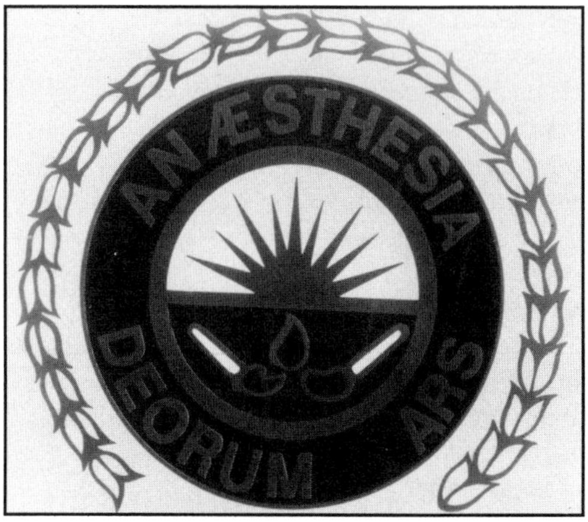

Fig. 3. Marín's emblem: *Anesthesia Deorum Ars;* the divine art that guards the small flame of life, aflicker between the torches of Hypnos (sleep) and Thanatos (death). The dark night half obscures the rising or setting sun of consciousness.

The emblem has found wide recognition. The Societies of Anesthesiologists of Colombia, Costa Rica and Guatemala, as well as the Latin-American Confederation, have adopted it as their own, and it also graces the Journal of the Colombian and Guatemalan Anesthesia Societies (letter by Solera Andara D, President of the Asociacion de Medicos Anestesiologos de Costa Rica, to Dr. Ernesto Rojas, January 20, 1992).

In 1964, Dr. F.F. Foldes suggested to Dr. Juan Marín that he further develop the emblem as a medal, measuring 8 cm in diameter and carrying the additional inscription: "WFSA – President." From 1972 until 1984, during official business, the Presidents of the World Federation of Societies of Anesthesiologists, Drs. Foldes, Mayrhofer, Gomez, Bonica and Parsloe wore the medal on a neck ribbon. Unfortunately, the medal was lost some time after 1985 (Mayrhofer O: Personal Letter to J.C. Gravenstein, March 1992; Foldes FF: Letter to J.S. Gravenstein, February 19, 1992; Samayoa R: Personal communication, 1992).

Juan Marín and Euthanasia

Early in his tenure as a chloroformist, Juan Marín had to give anesthesia to a newborn with a huge omphalocele. The surgeon attempted a repair. However, even under deep anesthesia it was impossible to close the defect and so the surgeon covered the intestines with gauze. Juan Marín anticipated that infection and dehydration would soon cause the baby to suffer a miserable death. He could not countenance that fate for the baby and, over the objections of the operating room sister, he administered an overdose of chloroform to the baby to spare its futile suffering. Marín recalls other instances where the terrible and hopeless plight of a patient had persuaded him to shorten the patient's torment.

Many years had passed when his beloved wife, mother of his two sons, fell ill with cancer of the uterus with widespread metastases and extension into the bladder and rectum, resulting in fecal fistulae. She required much morphine, became more and more debilitated and soon was no longer able to leave her bed. Juan saw her suffering and how unbearable her agony had become. He turned to God and called out: "Jehovah, Your daughter is suffering so much! Don't You hear the urgent calls of this wretched patient who loves You so much? She cries for You continuously and she prays the 23rd Psalm: 'The Lord is my Shepherd; I shall not want . . . Thy rod and Thy staff they comfort me.' On Mt. Horeb, You commanded Moses to smite the rock and when he did, water miraculously appeared from out of the rock. Please, Jehovah, do no less of a miracle for my beloved wife who is Your faithful and devoted daughter!" (Transcribed during an interview with Dr. Juan Marín in February, 1991.)

But God did not hear these desperate cries. After a week Marín repeated his plea, but again to no avail. The disease took its terrible course and after another week Juan Marín called his two sons and asked them to say good-bye to their mother. Then he sent them out of the house. Don't come back during the night because I need to be alone with your mother, he told them. At seven o'clock that evening she was awake and asked for light and water and he turned on the light and he gave her water. Fifteen minutes later she complained that her pain was very stubborn and that she needed more relief. They spoke a little and then she dozed off and he put more and more morphine into the infusion and he held her hand until the great window to eternity was opened for her. At ten o'clock she was dead. Marín said: "The two most important nights when a man and a wife should be alone together are their first night and their last night."

Juan Marín struggled with the concept of euthanasia, but rather than quietly practicing what he believed to be correct, he published a paper titled "Eutanasia."[5] In it he discusses the Karen Quinlan case and he quotes Ambrose Paré, the famous barber-surgeon who had given the following account: "In a stable where we boarded our horses, we found four dead soldiers and three others wounded and leaning against the wall. They could not see or hear, nor could they speak and their garments were still smoking as they had been engulfed by the flames of gunpowder. I contemplated their fate and was filled with pity for their misfortune. At that moment an old soldier appeared and asked me if there was a way of helping them. I answered, no, there was not. The old soldier then directed himself toward the men, drew his saber and slit their throats swiftly and without malice. I told him that he had committed a villainous act, but he answered that every day he prayed to God and asked: 'If I am ever to find myself in such a state, please let there be someone capable of doing what must be done to prevent further terrible suffering.'"

Marín comments dryly that Paré had accomplished nothing by feeling pity and contemplating the terrible fate of these soldiers. Paré had, however, kept the Hippocratic oath of never advising anyone to resort to poison and of refusing anyone who asks for such poison. In contradistinction, the old soldier, who had lived intensely through the bitter experience of war, had delivered his comrades from their pain. With that he had accepted the risks of eternal damnation and his own death, which would have been decreed by a council of war. Marín writes, "This old soldier, without any directive but with an infinite feeling of compassion and without fear of contrary rulings, resolved, before God and man, to do what neither physicians nor humanitarians nor theologians had been willing to undertake."

Marín realized that publication of his actions involving euthanasia would cause an uproar in the press, and that it might have led to his incarceration. But he held the deeply felt conviction that a good physician must act, at times against his personal wishes, to help his patients—even with euthanasia if there is no other means of alleviating unbearable suffering in the inexorable course of a fatal disease.

Conclusion

Of the pioneers in our specialty we often know only a few dates and little else. We had the rare opportunity to talk to Juan Marín, a pioneer who began to practice anesthesia without the benefit of formal teaching. He had to formulate concepts by which to accommodate his clinical observations. He had to devise his own techniques and equipment with which to improve his practice. We were privileged to have learned a little about his life and his convictions. His deeply held beliefs are those of an honorable and brave man who stands up for his profession and for what he believes to be his duty toward his patients and his family.

References and Notes

1. Santander Blanco Saladén: Los Dioses de la medicina moderna; Periodico Universal de Catagena, Colombia, 3/18/1952.
2. Juan Marín, el padre de la anesthesiologîa en Colombia. La Republica, Domingo 9 de Septiembre de 1984 (newspaper account).
3. In the third volume of his : Essays on the first Hundred Years of Anaesthesia (Wood Library-Museum, sponsored by the American Society of Anesthesiologists, 515 Busse Highway, park Ridge, Ill 60068) W. Stanley Sykes cites some 30 references on delayed chloroform poisoning in children—dating back to the late 1890s—and he provides probably the best discussion of the worries expressed by some and the success with chloroform experienced by others.
4. While this description is reminiscent of the "Hyderabad chloroform cap, as advocated by Lawrie E: Chloroform: a manual for students and practitioners, London: Churchill, 1901, Juan Marín does not recall ever having seen this book or heard of Lawrie during his years as a chloroformist.
5. Marín J: Eutanasia: *Revista Colombiana De Anestesiologia,* 207-15, 1977.

THE FOUNDATION OF THE DEPARTMENT OF ANESTHESIA AT UCSF

WILLIAM K. HAMILTON
Professor Emeritus, Department of Anesthesia

The establishment and development of academic anesthesia departments in the United States is a relatively recent event. The vast majority of such units appeared on the scene after World War II. It is of interest that, in some medical schools, departments seem to have developed readily, while others were characterized by lack of interest or repeated unsuccessful attempts.

This review will deal with anesthesia at the University of California in San Francisco (UCSF). This department eventually achieved at least a modicum of success which has persisted to the present time. However, until more than a decade after the end of World War II, UCSF had nothing resembling a program of creditable teaching or research. Why was academic anesthesia slow to develop at the University of California in San Francisco? Why did this failure occur in a university which was a recognized leader in education, while very successful departments developed in situations which seemed less favorable? This review, covering a period from the 1920's to 1960, is presented not as a model, but as a series of events which suggestions provide toward answers to the above questions. In addition, the review uncovers some interesting anecdotes which bear on questions facing the specialty of anesthesiology today.

In the late 1920's and 1930's, the University of California in San Francisco had an anesthesia unit which provided operating room anesthesia service and some teaching to medical students on the surgical service. The unit appears to have been almost entirely hospital based, with little if any reference to the School of Medicine. The chief was Dr. Mary Botsford, a graduate of the University of California, class of 1896. She had taken another physician, Dr. Dotty Wood, under her tutelage, and with some other physicians anesthetized patients for the Department of Surgery, of which anesthesia was a division. There was no residency training program, no research, and the physician staff practiced privately in the city of San Francisco in addition to University Hospital duties.

There is evidence that this group did very well in areas of clinical anesthesia. A report published in 1932 reviews experience in 551 brain operations from the period of 1921 to 1930[1]. The patients ranged in age from 3 days to 79 years and were anesthetized in a variety of positions, including the now dreaded sitting position. The electrocautery was used in all procedures. The operations included 18 tumors, many of which were located in the posterior fossa. There were 54 Gasserian ganglionectomies and 13 transsphenodial hypopysectomies. All patients were anesthetized by open drop ether and in *none* was endotracheal intubation used. Nitrous oxide was avoided because it increased intracranial pressure, and no narcotics were given. Fluid was administered largely by clysis and only 16 units of blood were administered. Intraoperative mortality is not mentioned and only three postoperative deaths related to anesthesia are listed. One of these was from pneumonia, one from lung abscess and one from cardiac dilation. There were no explosions. This very satisfactory outcome was accomplished without many adjuvant drugs and procedures considered so important and perhaps essential in the 1990's. Such success under those conditions must make us think seriously about today's dogma concerning narcotics in intracranial surgery, the dangers of explosive anesthetics, the very essential nature of endotracheal tubes and the frightening consequences of posterior fossa surgery in the sitting position. How many of the "facts" we teach with vigor in any era cycle to nearly opposite opinions in another day?

In 1935, Dr. Botsford succumbed to mandatory retirement policies. She was replaced by her pupil, Dotty Wood, a graduate of the neighboring Stanford University School of Medicine, whose training had been entirely by preceptorship with Dr. Botsford. Dr. Wood was apparently an extremely skilled clinician and may be the first documented neurosurgical anesthesiologist. She established quite a reputation for her ability to get cases underway rapidly. She was reputed to have any patient ready for surgery in less than five minutes. She is also reputed to have been approximately five feet tall and remarkably obese. Anecdotes relate that she spent entire cases under the neurosurgical drapes administering ether by open drop and insufflation. Further anecdotes tell of lunch being brought to her for consumption without emerging from these drapes.

At that time there were four other physicians in the anesthesia unit, all of whom were women. In this day of affirmative action and equal opportunity, the preponderance of women in UCSF Anesthesia might reflect a progressive appearance of the women's movement, but more likely is an example of the lesser status simultaneously given to women and to this new "specialty." Dr. Phyllis Harroun, one of the women physicians, has stated she was ill for many years following graduation from medical school and took up anesthesia because it was a place where she could obtain work.

In the mid-thirties, anesthesia in the state of California received a boost when Stanford University imported Dr. William Neff from Canada and Dr. Arthur Guedel came from Indiana to far away Los Angeles. Stanford actually began residency training at this time but there were still no residents and no formal teaching program in the University of California.

The names of three persons who were not anesthesiologists appear repeatedly in this history. The first of these was Dr. Chauncey Leake, a very well known pharmacologist, teacher and philosopher. He was an early believer in structure-activity relationships of drugs and he developed divinyl ether (Vinethene) as a result of his observations on the actions of ethylene and ethyl ether. While Vinethene achieved some popularity throughout the United States, it was essentially never used in Dr. Leake's own institution. Dr. Wood stated that she tried it once and didn't like it and the chief of surgery is rumored to have prohibited its use. The reasons for this prohibition are unknown. Dr. Leake's interest in anesthesia and its research is further documented by his tales of frequent meetings with Dr. Guedel and his active role in the recruitment of Dr. Neff to Stanford. In spite of his interest and activity in anesthesia, the personnel for the anesthesia unit at the University of California admit to little contact with Leake or his activities. This gives a stark message about the academic and intellectual environment at that time.

The second name is that of Dr. Howard Nafzigger, a neurosurgeon and chief of the Department of Surgery. He was a very influential and powerful man and is still a legend in the institution. It is not known with certainty what his thoughts were about anesthesia, but rumor has it he did not favor establishment of the new specialty as an independent, academic unit. Many will think this was the most important factor delaying development of anesthesia.

The third name is that of Mr. Drury, the hospital director. He controlled everything financially related to anesthesia. Under him, the hospital did all of the billing and kept the income of the physicians at a very low level. He is alleged to have had a tight rein on the actions of the anesthesiologists and was critical of any activities not strictly related to service.

In 1940 a decision was made that real professional anesthesia was desirable for the University of California. The factors basic to this decision are unknown, but it is not unreasonable to assume that the anesthesia movement was becoming prevalent throughout the United States and had produced a teaching unit at Stanford University — a close neighbor of the University of California. This activity resulted in the recruitment of Dr. H.R. Hathaway who apparently promised a residency program and an academic department. Dr. Carl Fischer, a medical student at the time, relates that Hathaway was enthusiastically received by surgeons and students. However, he was advised to "settle in" for a time before beginning the residency training program. The entrance of the United States into World War II interfered with many of the plans and physician training followed the irregular patterns consistent with the fluctuating availability of physician manpower. Dr. Fischer's promised residency training was put on hold until his return from military service in 1945. Some physicians who preceded him in discharge from the service received training under Hathaway, but Fischer appears to have been the first formal fully trained UCSF resident.

Misfortune best describes Hathaway's career in San Francisco. In addition to the manpower problems, rumors of substance abuse and associated deterioration were widespread, and his career ended in tragedy at about the time World War II ended. The son of a prominent faculty physician died on the operating table during an appendectomy, the anesthesia for which was being administered by Dr. Hathaway who was found asleep at the head of the table. Hathaway was relieved of his duties. The specter of substance abuse in our specialty did not suddenly appear in the 1970's and 1980's.

A bright side of the history accompanies that sad tale. The name of Phyllis Harroun must be highlighted as the savior of anesthesia at UCSF at that time. During the war it was Dr. Harroun who really ran things. She worked with medical students, did clinical and animal research, and provided excellent clinical anesthesia.

Much of her research involved the then new drug curare. She is believed to have been a pioneer in the development of apneic techniques and to be among the first to note that a pregnant dog could be paralyzed by this agent without apparent effect on the intrauterine fetuses[2,3,4.] Later, Dr. Harroun became quite interested in the molecular mechanisms of anesthesia. Her activities at UCSF demonstrated that teaching and research could in fact be done by the proper person. She dealt with heavy workloads and oppressive administrations and accomplished much in spite of these obstacles. Certainly her contributions to the development of this department and the specialty have not been adequately recognized. Much of this history is found in a taped conversation of Drs. Harroun and Fischer.

Dr. Harroun has related an interesting story about the place of endotracheal intubation in anesthesia during this period of time. She relates that she had been in the department for five years without ever having passed an endotracheal tube. At this time, while anesthetizing a patient for gynecologic surgery which lasted quite a long time, she increased the depth of anesthesia and rather secretively performed laryngoscopy. She then placed a woven wax endotracheal tube in the trachea and was quite excited to feel the respiratory gasses passing through this tube. She thought it unwise to leave the tube in place, however, and removed it to continue anesthesia with an oropharyngeal airway in place.

The departure of Hathaway was followed by the recruitment of Dr. Frank Murphy. There was no formal search as we know the process today. Dr. Murphy had served with one of the UCSF senior surgeons during World War II and this appears to have been his only qualification. Not much can be said for Dr. Murphy's contributions. He is not remembered as a good teacher and did little if any research. He is reputed to have spent a great deal of time in his office in conversation with a variety of people while allowing others to perform the daily tasks in the operating room. The fledgling residency program did continue although records of training are scarce. Murphy can be credited with one accomplishment and that was wresting from the hospital administration freedom in managing the economic affairs of the unit. He was able to institute professional fee billing which he apparently accomplished very effectively. Murphy's tenure is described by some who worked with him as one of great financial success for Dr. Murphy and lack of proper development in the department. The attending faculty was characterized by rapid turnover because of the unfavorable financial situation for junior faculty. Teaching was limited to the operating room, with the exception of four or five lectures per year given by faculty members from outside the specialty. Pre- and post-operative patient contact by anesthesia personnel did not occur. Obstetrical anesthesia service was given minimal attention and the closely affiliated San Francisco General Hospital was totally ignored by the University anesthesia personnel. It was alleged that the failure to cover the General Hospital was based on the lack of private fees therefrom. This so antagonized the chairman of the Department of Surgery that he set about to improve the situation in his Division of Anesthesia. His efforts were aided and abetted by the decision of the Residency Review Committee for anesthesia which failed to accredit the program in 1955. An adverse report of the Residency Review Committee was rendered following a site visit by Dr. Lucien Morris. The anesthesia residents apparently refuted Murphy's claims of multiple classes and seminars.

This then represented two failed attempts to institute an academic program in anesthesia. It is not difficult to recognize ample cause for these failures. The directorship had never been in the hands of stable and accomplished leaders. The hospital and the school, and perhaps the Department of Surgery, may have failed to yield control or least failed to encourage development. Nevertheless, it must be recognized that research had been recognized and rewarded in many units of the school, including the Department of Surgery. There is no evidence that requests for more research resources were denied — or even made. The lack of properly aggressive leadership is evident and must assume a great share of the blame.

Dr. Murphy resigned and moved from San Francisco. After his departure, Dr. Neri Guadagni, whose memory has supplied a portion of this story, was named as acting chair of the unit — still within the Department of Surgery. At this time a formal widespread, national search was undertaken. This search ended with the appointment of Dr. Stuart C. Cullen, who had just completed 20 years of leadership at the University of Iowa. There he had developed a successful unit widely recognized for its teaching and its research in addition to the excellent clinical service.

At the time of Cullen's appointment, there were concomitant changes of significance to the entire medical school. Dr. Julius Comroe had moved to San Francisco from the University of Pennsylvania and had established a large and active Cardiovascular Research Institute. Dr. Comroe's work with Dr. Robert Dripps in Philadelphia had convinced him of the potential contributions to research by academic anesthesiologists. Dr. Comroe had also become acquainted with Dr. John Severinghaus while at Penn. Dr. Severinghaus had taken part of his residency with Cullen at Iowa and all of this meshed to lure Cullen to this previously undistinguished anesthesia position. Additionally, a colleague at the University of Iowa, Dr. Robert Featherstone, had assumed the position of chair of the Department of Pharmacology in San Francisco. He, too, was influential in Cullen's decision. The cooperative attitude of basic scientists Comroe and Featherstone had a tremendous influence on the research potential and the research development for this new department. It is probably also of great significance that the chair of the Department of Surgery, the director of the hospital and the dean of the medical school somewhat reluctantly agreed to Cullen's demand for departmental status. A new hospital had just been built and space for growth and development was quite readily available.

It is also worth recalling that this was a time of explosive growth of the National Institutes of Health with generous support of research in all academic disciplines.

This remarkable coincidence of so many factors resulted in the very rapid development of a larger and very successful Department of Anesthesia in 1958 which has continued to grow and develop to the present time.

The record reveals a dramatic and abrupt change from repeated failure to outstanding achievement. Obviously there is not one single reason, but rather the confluence of a proven effective leader placed in a newly receptive atmosphere with what today seems to be unbelievable resources in terms of dollars and space. We have no way of knowing whether the leadership of Cullen applied in 1940 or 45 would have succeeded where Hathaway and Murphy failed. It seems unlikely that either of the latter would have succeeded even with the improved environment which accompanied Cullen's arrival on the scene. Good leaders probably beget better resources and rather certainly can improve attitudes. Thus, they have potential to succeed in modest environments. On the other hand, leaders who have proven to possess only limited capabilities have had some success in favorable environments. The sharp contrast in this story effectively demonstrates the extremes of poor leadership combined with unfavorable environment, immediately followed by creative leadership added to a receptive, resource-rich environment.

References

1. Wood DA: Survey of anesthesia given in 550 brain operations in the years 1921 to 1930. Anesth Analg; 11:201-5, 1932.
2. Harroun P, Hathaway, HR: Use of curare in anesthesia for thoracic surgery; Preliminary Report. Surg Gynecol Obstet; 82:229-31, 1946.
3. Harroun P, Beckert FE, Hathaway, HR: Curare and nitrous oxide anesthesia for lengthy operations. Anesthesiology; 7:24-28, 1946.
4. Harroun P, Beckert FE, Fischer, CW: Physiologic effects of curare and its use as adjunct to anesthesia. Surg Gynecol and Obstet; 84:491-8, 1947.

THE MEDICAL EDUCATION OF CRAWFORD W. LONG, M.D.

WILLIAM D. HAMMONDS
Emory University, School of Medicine
Atlanta, Georgia, USA

Much has been said and written about Crawford W. Long and his discovery of anesthesia. At times debate about that discovery obscures facts about the man who made the discovery. What is known is often presented in poorly documented form, such as the 1954 TV dramatization that presented Long as a rustic backwoods physician.[1] This paper presents information about Crawford W. Long, the man, and about his education.

The facts of Dr. Long's medical education make a fascinating story and give a new perspective to the man, his life, and his discovery of anesthesia. During his medical education, far reaching changes occurred that continue to influence medical education to this day.

His undergraduate years were spent at Franklin Academy (later to become the University of Georgia) in Athens, Georgia. He roomed with Alexander Stephens, who was to become Vice-President of the Confederate States. They lived in a building constructed between 1800 and 1804, now known as "Old College." Their second storey room is marked by a brass plaque. He was a good student and graduated second in his class in 1835 with an A.M. degree.

In that era, most medical students entered medical school without a college education. One study of the medical students of the 1830's found that between 4 and 7 percent were college graduates.[2] Another 10 percent had some college education, but had not graduated.

After completion of his college education, Long returned to Danielsville, Georgia, to teach in the Danielsville Academy, a school that his father had founded. He wished to begin the study of medicine immediately, but he was only 19 years old, and his father did not want him to begin at so young an age and preferred that he teach for a year. After completing one term as a teacher, he entered a medical apprenticeship with Dr. George R. Grant of Jefferson, Georgia, in 1836.

The apprentice system education in the United States had its origins in the guild system of the crafts of medieval Europe. In this country, the apprentice system was used in preparation for careers in medicine, law and the ministry.

Over 90 percent of American physicians were educated in this system between 1620 and 1820. Formal medical school education began to be more widely appreciated in the 1830's. Waite,[3] in a survey of Ohio physicians in 1835, found that only 20 percent had academic medical degrees, although many others had attended some medical school classes. By 1843, one survey showed that nearly half of all practicing doctors in the United States had an academic medical degree, the remainder having been educated entirely in the apprentice system.[4] The term of apprenticeship was usually three years and did not terminate until the apprentice was 21 years of age. During the term of study, the apprentice helped the doctor with his patients and was allowed to read the preceptor's books. There was no formal curriculum. The standard fee in Crawford W. Long's day was $100.00 per year. Having students was both a way for doctors to supplement their income and an indication that the doctor was held in high regard. The apprenticeship contracts were legally binding until age 21, but by the late 1830's were easily dissolved by mutual agreement between preceptor and student. Crawford W. Long completed only one year of his apprenticeship with Dr. Grant. By that time he was 21 years old and certainly had his preceptor's blessing to leave, because they remained friends afterwards. He left to pursue a university medical education leading to the M.D. degree.

In 1837, Crawford Long made the long and dangerous horseback trip to Lexington, Kentucky, to enter the Medical Department of Transylvania University. This school was established in 1799 and was the first in what was then the American West. Transylvania University had a distinguished medical faculty and was said to have the finest medical library in the United States. The library was one of the greatest attractions of the school and was started in 1821 when Charles Caldwell used $11,000.00 from the City and State to purchase books in Europe. The medical department closed in 1859, but the library still exists intact. It is from this library that Crawford W. Long may have first learned about the use of ether in medicine.

Among the books there is *A Manual of Materia Medica and Pharmacy* by Edwards and Vavasseur and printed in 1829. The book listed ether as an "antispasmodic" which was used to calm, and it was also described as producing "a sort of intoxication, not so lasting as that of alcohol." It was a major component of Hoffmann's anodyne used for many different kinds of pain. The idea that ether could be used to treat pain was not a foreign concept at the time of Crawford W. Long's medical education It is known that Crawford W. Long used Hoffmann's anodyne from a description of his treatment of spider bite written in his own hand in the 1840's.

Advantages of the medical education at Transylvania were said to include less expense by avoiding the long journey to the east, but also that Lexington offered "less danger from dissipation, folly, and extravagance."[5] Crawford W. Long's sponsor continued to be Dr. George Grant, his former preceptor.

In 1838, after a single year, Crawford W. Long left Transylvania University. His departure might have been due to the political unrest then present at that institution. The turbulence started in 1836, when a member of the medical faculty proposed that the Medical Department be moved to Louisville, Kentucky. Lousiville was a rapidly growing town located on the Ohio River, and thus had much better transportation than landlocked Lexington. Since the income of the medical faculty was directly related to the number of students recruited and the number of tickets to their lecture series sold, some members of the medical faculty favored a move to the more populous and better located Louisville. The trustees of Transylvania were outraged at the thought of the Medical Department moving away from the parent institution, a practice that was to become common in later decades with the proliferation of medical schools, many of which were chartered by geographically distant universities. The trustees investigated the charges in 1837 and responded by firing all six members of the Medical Department. Crawford W. Long was not the only student to leave; enrollment dropped by 15 students that year.

In a way, this upheaval marked the end of

an era when there were few medical schools and payment for teaching in them was relatively poor, and the beginning of the proliferation of schools run for profit, an era that did not end until 1910 with the publication of the Flexner report.

Crawford W. Long chose to complete his medical education at the University of Pennsylvania medical school. It was the first in the United States, organized in 1769. It was one of the most respected of the existing 35 medical schools at the time Crawford Long entered.

He spent six months at the University of Pennsylvania, from October 1838 to March 1839. Requirements for graduation from the 1839 catalogue included:

> 1. the student must have attained the age of 21 years; 2. the student was required to take the same course of lectures twice. Because there were no laboratories for teaching and few demonstrations, the lecture was the only teaching method in widespread use at that time. Medical educators felt that the student should attend the same course of lectures twice to master the large amount of information presented; 3. the student was required to have one course of clinical instruction. Practical clinical experience was a serious shortcoming of all medical schools of the early 1800's. The University of Pennsylvania had tried to meet that need by encouraging students to attend classes at the Almshouse, later called Blockley and still later Philadelphia General Hospital. In 1815, the medical students petitioned trustees to allow them to do their clinical studies at the Almshouse or Pennsylvania Hospital. During CWL's attendance there, the University of Pennsylvania permitted the clinical studies to be done at either hospital. Although not adequate, the opportunity for clinical study was better than at most medical schools of the day; 4. the student was required to take one course of lectures if "ad eundem." Because he had attended one course of lectures at another "approved" university, Transylvania, he was admitted in an "Ad eundem grandum" status, meaning that he had an equivalent first year at another school; 5. the student was required to write a thesis on a medical topic; 6. the student had to pay the $40.00 graduation fee; and 7. the student had to attend the public commencement.

Figure 1. shows the ledger book for 1839. In it are recorded the date, number, name of graduate, state of residence, if the student was an "ad eundem" graduate. . . the school they transferred from, and their local address. On the facing page of the ledger book, (Fig. 2), was listed the title of their thesis, the professor who sponsored them, and whether or not the fee had been paid.

Crawford W. Long's thesis was titled, "Functional Amaurosis," and was written under the sponsorship of William Gibson, M.D.,

Fig. 1. The ledger book in 1839 showing the date and number of graduate Crawford W. Long.

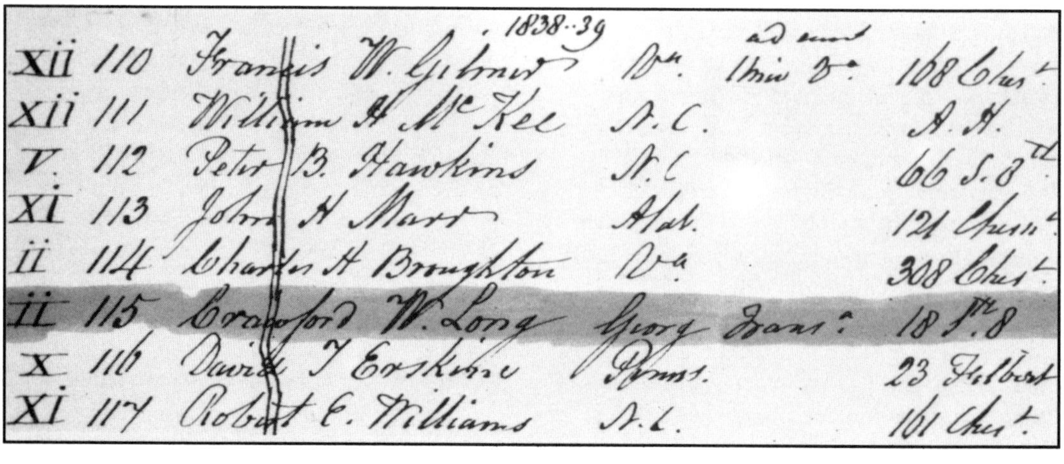
1838-39

				ad eund	
xii	110	Francis W. Gilmer	Va.	Univ. Va.	108 Chest.
xii	111	William H. McKee	N.C.		A. H.
V	112	Peter B. Hawkins	N.C		66 S. 8th
XI	113	John H Marr	Ala.		121 Chesn.
ii	114	Charles H Broughton	Va		308 Chest.
ii	115	Crawford W. Long	Georg	Trans:	18 S. 8
X	116	David J Erskine	Penns.		23 Filbert
XI	117	Robert E. Williams	N.C.		161 Chest.

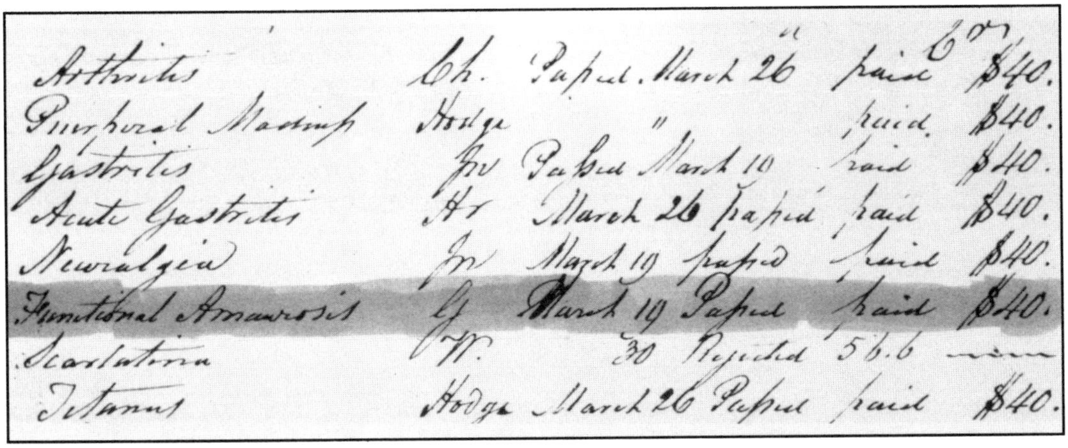

Arthritis	Ch.	Passed. March 26	paid	$40.
Puerperal Madness	Hodge	"	paid	$40.
Gastritis	Jn	Passed March 10	paid	$40.
Acute Gastritis	Hr	March 26 passed	paid	$40.
Neuralgia	Jn	March 19 passed	paid	$40.
Functional Amaurosis	Gj	March 19 Passed	paid	$40.
Scarlatina	W.	30 Rejected	56.6	—
Tetanus	Hodge	March 26 Passed	paid	$40.

Fig. 2. The facing page of the ledger.

Professor Surgery. Gibson was an Edinburgh graduate and was noted as being the first surgeon to ligate the common iliac artery. Later in his career, he had the then unique experience of doing two successful Cesarean sections on the same woman. He was said to be a close friend of Lord Byron.

Following his graduation from the University of Pennsylvania in 1839, Long went to New York to further his medical training. He spent the next 18 months "walking the hospitals" gaining experience in surgery. Frances Long Taylor[6] said in her biography of her father that he witnessed enormous suffering of patients undergoing surgery while in New York, and that this experience first fixed his attention on devising a way to prevent the pain of surgery.

Hudson's[7] study of eminent physicians, listed in the 1928 edition of American Medical Biography, found that only 10 percent of physicians educated before 1850 had hospital or "residency" training. The postgraduate training in surgery brought to a close Long's formal education. He entered his profession with the best medical education available in North America in 1840. The universities and hospitals in which he studied were at the forefront of medical education. By all indications, he continued his education by the standards of the day during his medical practice. He was an avid reader. His daughter reports that he read to the family almost every evening. She reported that his reading ranged from the classics to authors of the day, such as Wilkie Collins and Charles Dickens. He apparently read the medical literature also, and at one time was offered the position of Editor of the Southern Medical and Surgical Journal. He also demonstrated his interest in scholarship by teaching, and frequently had medical apprentices who considered him to be an excellent teacher.

While he did not write about his use of ether in a timely manner, Dr. Long did eventually report his use of ether in the *Southern Medical and Surgical Journal*[8] and wrote occasional editorials in the Athens newspaper on social and political topics. His writing gives evidence to his scholarly bent and to the quality of his education.

The picture that has emerged is that of a physician who had the best medical education available in the early 1800's, who continued to use the tools of scholarship in his professional and private life.

References

1. Branch H: *Bless the Man.* Frank Wisbar Productions, 1954.
2. Rothstein WG: *American Medical Schools and the Practice of Medicine*: A History. New York: Oxford University Press, 1987:50.
3. Waite FC: The Professional Education of Pioneer Ohio Physicians. *Ohio State Arch Hist Qt*; 48:190, 1939.

4. Rothstein WG: *American Medical Schools and the Practice of Medicine:* A History. New York: Oxford University Press, 1987.
5. Jennings WW: *Transylvania: Pioneer University of the West.* New York; 1955:209.
6. Taylor FL: *Crawford W. Long & The Discovery of Ether Anesthesia.* New York: Paul B. Hoeker, Inc. MCMXXVIII.
7. Hudson RP: *Patterns of Medical Education in Nineteenth Century America.* Baltimore, MD: Johns Hopkins University; 1966. Masters degree essay.
8. Long CW: Account of First Use of Sulfuric Ether by Inhalation. *South Med Surg J*; 38:1849.

THE LIFE AND TIMES OF ENID (JOHNSON) MACLEOD, MD, LLD

INTERVIEW by CHARLES HOPE
Dalhousie University, Halifax, Nova Scotia, Canada

On 23rd January, 1942, Enid Johnson gave the anaesthetic when Harold Griffith first administered curare for a surgical operation. She was, at the time, Anaesthetic Resident at the Homoeopathic Hospital, now called the Queen Elizabeth Hospital in Montreal. On completing her training she married Innes MacLeod, a lawyer, and accompanied him to Sydney, Nova Scotia. She established an anaesthetic practice and acted as medical officer for the Red Cross Blood Transfusion Service.

Later she returned to Dalhousie Medical School in Halifax, where she joined the Department of Physiology. She retired in 1976, was named Professor Emeritus in 1978 and received an honorary LLD degree from Dalhousie in 1985. Her story is told in an interview with Dr. Charles Hope, Professor and Chairman, Department of Anaesthesia, Dalhousie University.

THE INTRODUCTION OF CURARE FOR THE TREATMENT OF TETANUS IN ENGLAND

JEAN M. HORTON
Emeritus Consultant Anaesthetist
Addenbrooke's Hospital, Cambridge, England, United Kingdom

Tetanus, "lockjaw," occurs from contamination of wounds by the spores of the Clostridium tetani, which produces a powerful endotoxin causing intense muscle spasms. The clinical manifestations were described by Hippocrates. Until the 19th century, physicians relied upon opium and a variety of bizarre remedies such as brandy, ardent spirits, aconite, alcohol, belladonna, ether and chloroform to control these spasms. The first suggestion of a sensible therapeutic approach was made by the famous English physiologist and surgeon, Sir Benjamin Brodie (1783-1862), who reported in London in 1811[1] and 1812[2] to the Society for Promoting the Knowledge of Animal Chemistry, and through them to the Royal Society, that he had found that, by applying curare (woorara) powder, which had been given to him by Dr. E.N. Bancroft, to wounds in animals, he could preserve life by artificial respiration. He suggested that the paralyzing powers of curare might be used in the treatment of tetanus. His experiments were confirmed shortly afterwards by Professor Sewell of the Royal Veterinary College and Mr. Morgan of Guy's Hospital in London.

It should be noted that in these and subsequent reports about the use of curare that the spelling of the name of this drug varied, probably because of the attempt to spell phonetically the Indian word. Claude Bernard (1813-1878), the French physiologist, stated that there were at least thirteen different versions, ranging from urari and curari, to woorara and woorari.

In 1856 George Harley, a lecturer in Physiology from University College, London, demonstrated the antagonistic action of curare and strychnine, the practical implication being that strychnine poisoning gives rise to severe spasms similar to those of tetanus.[3] In 1857 Harley tried the effects of curare on a horse with tetanus.

The next reports on curare and tetanus started to appear from 1857. Vulpian published an article in 1857 in L'Union Medicale on "The use of curare as an antidote to strychnine and a treatment of tetanus.[4]

Claude Bernard had been reporting in his classical experiments on the site of action of curare from 1850,[5] and in 1859 presented to the Academy of Sciences in Paris a communication from M.L. Vella, who was a surgeon working at the French Military Hospital in Turin, Italy, during the French-Italian War. The report concerned the use of curare in the treatment of tetanus in a wounded soldier.[6] The curare was diluted in water and applied as a compress to the wound. Vella claimed that his use of curare had been prompted by the knowledge of the antagonism between strychnine and curare, which had already been reported by Harley. The report of this meeting and subsequent discussions prompted Sir Benjamin Brodie to write a letter to Pierre Jean-Marie Flourens (1794-1867), a French comparative anatomist, and the Secretary of the Academy of Sciences, pointing out that he had suggested the use of curare for the treatment of tetanus fifty years before.

Also in 1859 two communications on the same subject came from Paris. Manec[7] used large doses of curare as a compress and also as subcutaneous injections. Chassaignac[8] used local compresses of curare as well as giving an oral mixture diluted in julep. In all, in 1859, thirteen communications on this subject were published in French language journals, four in English language journals, and four in German. Sayres and Burall[9] in New York applied curare to a wound in a case of tetanus in 1859, but without success.

In England in 1859, the English surgeon and obstetrician, Sir Thomas Spencer Wells (1818-1897), read a paper to the Royal Medical and Chirurgical Society on, "Three cases of tetanus in which woorara was used in the treatment."[10] This was the first report in England where curare had been used to treat humans with tetanus, and concerned patients who contracted tetanus following ovariotomy, an operation of which Spencer Wells was a pioneer. Of special interest was that he used both local applications and hypodermic injections of curare.

From 1860 onwards, little or no progress was made with the use of curare because the preparations were crude and toxic, and means of long-term artificial respiration were not available.

Interest in the use of curare in the management of tetanus was renewed in 1934 by the Cambridge physician, Leslie Cole, who at that time was the foremost British authority, or indeed World authority, on the treatment of tetanus. Cole had found that cases of tetanus were frequent in East Anglia, and he was all too often confronted with patients in severe distress and danger whose treatment remained uncertain. He was aware of the work of West,[11] who had used curare in cases of muscular rigidity, and had mentioned the possibility of its use in tetanus. Cole obtained a sample of curare of the "gourd" variety, and in 1934 he reported in the Lancet[12] two cases of tetanus in which he had used subcutaneous injections of curare, but did not at that time persist with its use because the preparations were impure and he was reasonably satisfied with using the sedative action of Avertin (bromethol). Also in 1934, Florey, Harding and Fildes from Sheffield reported in the Lancet[13] on the use of curare to control tetanus spasms in rabbits. In their article they make "Suggestions for the More Adequate Treatment of Tetanus." One interesting suggestion was that cases of tetanus should be sent to suitably-equipped centers where there were specially trained staff. An early concept for intensive care units and the idea came from the department of Pathology! They also advocated the use of curare to control spasms, were aware of the risk of respiratory depression, and suggested that its administration required constant watchfulness and a team trained to use it.

It was not until the isolation in 1935 by King[14] of a pure curare alkaloid, the introduction of the first commercial preparation Intocostrin by ER Squibb and Sons, and its introduction into anaesthetic practice in 1942,[15] along with the experience of the Danish poliomyelitis epidemic in 1952, that further progress was made in the use of curare in the management of tetanus. Anaesthetists were becoming involved in the management of patients requiring artificial ventilation, and in 1958 Crampton Smith[16] from Oxford reported to the Royal Society of Medicine on his experience, together with the neurologists Ritchie Russell and Spalding, on the "Treatment of severe tetanus by total paralysis with curare and intermittent positive pressure respiration."

Meanwhile, in spite of the spread of prophylactic immunization, cases of tetanus continued to appear in the agricultural areas of East Anglia. It was suggested to Cole by the Cambridge anaesthetist, Harold Youngman, that he should try the use of curare again in the light of the availability of trained anaesthetists and ventilators. Cole at that time was reluctant to take advice from an anaesthetist. However, in 1959 a severe case of tetanus was given intravenous curare and successfully managed with controlled ventilation by the Cambridge anaesthetists.

As with many scientific discoveries, it took 150 years from a suggestion by a brilliant young surgeon who became President of the Royal College of Surgeons, President of the Royal Society and the first President of the General Medical Council, to the satisfactory use of curare to manage the spasms of tetanus.

References

1. Brodie BC: Experiments and observations on the different modes in which death is produced by certain vegetable poisons. *Phil Trans R Soc*; 101:178-95, 1811.
2. Brodie BC: Further experiments and observations on the action of poisons on the animal system. *Phil Trans R Soc*; 102:205-9, 1812.
3. Harley G: Antagonism of wourali and strychnine. *Lancet*; 619, 1856.
4. Vulpian EF: De l'emploi du curare comme antidote de la strychnine et comme traitement du tétanos. *L'Union Médicale*; XI: 25-6, 1857.
5. Bernard C: Études physiologiques sur quelques poisons américains. Le curare. *Revue de Deux Mondes*; 53:164-90, 1864.
6. Vella ML: Emploi du curare dans le traitement du tétanos. *Comptes Rendus Hebdomadaires des Séances de l'Académie des Sciences. Paris*; 330-71, 1859.
7. Manec M: Observation de tétanos traumatique; emploi du curare sans effet sensible; mort trente heures après l'invasion de la maladie; *Comptes Rendus Hebdomadaires des séances de l'Academie des Sciences. Paris*; 405-8, 1859.
8. *Lancet*, ii; 487, 1859, Woorara in tetanus.
9. Sayres LA, Burall FA: Two cases of traumatic tetanus, *NYJ Med*; 4:250-3, 1858.
10. Wells TS: Three cases of tetanus in which 'woorara' was used. *Proc Roy Soc Med Chirurg Soc, London*; 3:142, 1859.
11. West R: Curare in man. *Proc Roy Soc Med*; XXV:1107, 1932.
12. Cole L: Tetanus treated with curare. *Lancet*; ii: 4757, 1934.
13. Florey HW, Harding HE, Fildes P: The treatment of tetanus. *Lancet*; ii: 1036-41, 1934.
14. King H: Curare alkaloids. 1. Tubocurarine. *J Chem Soc*; 1381-9, 1935.
15. Griffith HR, Johnson GE: The use of curare in general anaesthesia. *Anesthesiology*; 3:418-20, 1942.
16. Smith AC: The Treatment of Severe Tetanus by Paralysing Drugs and intermittent Pressure Respiration. *Proc Roy Soc Med*; 51: 1006-8, 1958.

DENIS BROWNE'S TOP HAT

JEAN M. HORTON
Emeritus Consultant Anaesthetist
Addenbrooke's Hospital
Cambridge, England, United Kingdom

Denis Browne's Top Hat was the name given by successive generations of anaesthetists at the Hospital for Sick Children. Great Ormond Street (GOS), London, to the ether inhaler devised by the paediatric surgeon Sir Denis Browne.

Denis John Wolko Browne, K.C.V.O., M.B. B.S. (Sydney), F.R.C.S., Hon F.R.A.C.S., 1892-1967, was a pioneer of paediatric surgery who spent his working life at the Hospital for Sick Children, Great Ormond Street (GOS), London. He was the first surgeon in England to devote all his time to children and was affectionately known to all who worked with him as DB. A great original thinker and innovator, he developed many ingenious instruments for techniques specifically suited to children. Of interest to the anaesthetist are an ether inhaler (the Denis Browne Top Hat),[1] a mouth tube for delivering anaesthetic gases, a mouth gag for edentulous children, an endotracheal tube, a blood transfusion apparatus for children (modified from that described in 1927 by R.R. Macintosh)[2] and a cruciform support for use when operating on infants.[3]

Biography[4,5]

Denis Browne was born in Melbourne, Australia, in 1892, the son of an Australian pioneer in mining and sheep farming, and was educated at King's School, Paramatta, and the University of Sydney. Both at school and University he was very much an individualist and as well as being academically able, excelled at tennis, shooting, athletics and billiards.

He graduated in 1914 and immediately joined the 13th Light Horse Regiment of the Australian Imperial Force (AIF) as a medical Officer. He served at Gallipoli and in France with the ANZACS. After demobilization he elected to live, train, succeed and then die in England. After training in Liverpool and London, and taking the F.R.C.S. in 1922, he became casualty officer, then Resident Medical Superintendent at GOS, was appointed to the consultant staff in 1928, and served the hospital until 1957 when he was elected emeritus surgeon. He was appointed K.C.V.O. in 1961.

He was also interested in history, and in 1960 gave a paper at the Royal Society of Medicine on Byron's lameness, based on a careful study of the leg appliance that the poet wore.[6]

Denis Browne's Ether Inhaler (Top Hat)

When DB was casualty officer and then Resident medical Superintendent at GOS,[7] one of his duties was to deal with the enormous tonsil and adenoid waiting list which the Hospital (GOS) had acquired as a legacy of the work of the ENT surgeon George Waugh, who had propounded the need for the operation to be done by careful dissection, rather than by the generally accepted guillotine method. DB was a demon for work and organized an operation session of 25 tonsils and adenoids a day and 10 on Saturdays. On Sundays, according to James Crooks, his ENT surgeon colleague at GOS, DB would think about tonsils and adenoids. He described a tortuous vein lying between the tonsil and posterior pillar of the fauces (thought to be the cause of the bleeding tonsil), developed suitable surgical instruments for the operation, and for the anaesthesia an ether inhaler and a mouth gag for delivering the anaesthetic gases and ether. These instruments were to be found in all the major anaesthetic catalogues of the day. He attached his name to all the instruments he devised, so using one of the few advertising channels open to the medical profession.

In a letter[1] to the British Medical Journal of 6 October, 1928, DB commented on an article[8] in the British Medical Journal of 28 July, 1928, by a Mr. Sandiford (an ENT surgeon) and a Dr. Clayton (an anaesthetist) from Queen Mary's Hospital, Stratford, London, who had described the use of ethyl chloride and the guillotine for tonsillectomy. DB's letter points out that the operation for tonsillectomy should be unhurried and that the best anaesthetic was ether, and proceeded to describe his own inhaler which he said had been used in many thousands of cases. His description of his ether inhaler shows that he was familiar with and understood the workings of other ether inhalers available at that time, and their disadvantages.

In DB's own words, "The main difficulty in giving ether is to vary the concentration of the vapour from the very weak at the start to very strong when deep anaesthesia is needed. With the open method a high concentration can only be obtained by muffling the mask with towels, etc. — a crude wasteful and inexact proceeding. Also the ordinary Schimmelbusch mask has the fatal defect for ether that as soon as the fluid is poured onto the convex gauze pad it runs down into its borders, leaving a dry patch through which the patient breathes.

"The Clover inhaler, well used, gives a most excellent anaesthetic, but it is expensive, fragile, and difficult to clean, while its proper handling is a very rare accomplishment. Silk's inhaler has the sound principle of retaining the heavy ether vapour where it must be breathed by the patient, by means of a cylinder fitting below, closely to the face. The sponge, however, when soaked with ether, is almost impermeable to air, and tends to drip from its lower surface.

"My own pattern (made by Allen and Hanbury) is an aluminum 'cylinder,' 7-inches in height, and shaped to fit the face, with a Sorbo spongy rubber pad at the lower end.

"The ether is held by an oval gauze pad, seven inches by five, and at least eight layers thick, preferably hemmed so that it can be washed and used again. This is placed on top of the cylinder, and thrust down into it, on to the bars across the lower end, by a smaller cylinder mounted on a handle.

"This gives a flat gauze surface, down to which all ether poured into the inhaler runs, so that the patient's breath must pass through it; while owing to its flatness, there is no tendency to dripping."

DB considered that his inhaler had the following advantages:

"1. It will give a very high concentration of ether with a percentage of CO_2 much as in the Clover inhaler;

"2. It is very economical, its consumption of ether being only a third of that of the open method. In one department alone at Great Ormond Street this difference meant a saving of £50 a year;

"3. It is simple, cheap, easily cleaned between anaesthetics, and has that priceless quality for hospital equipment of surviving being dropped on a stone floor; and

"4. It does not cover the eyes, thus avoiding what I think to be one of the main causes of panic in children."

DB then described his main points on how to use the inhaler:

"1. Start the induction with a single drop of ether in the inhaler. Anyone who thinks this too little is recommended to experiment on himself.

"2. Keep the mask closely on the face, and as soon as the patient is breathing one strength of ether easily, increase it. A fairly wide experience of inducing all types of cases with ether has convinced me that the main causes of failure are starting with too strong a vapour, and taking the mask off for no particular reason except to see if the patient is still underneath it.

"3. As soon as the patient is deeply anaesthetized, with dilated pupils and easy breathing, hang a weighted hooked mouthpiece on the top of the inhaler and pump ether vapour through it. If this provokes no coughing, gag the mouth open and hang the tube in it to continue the anaesthetic, again carefully avoiding giving one breath of etherless air."

DB then commented that he found this method quicker and better than inducing with ethyl chloride and changing to ether, as it avoided the "no man's land" when the patient is coming out of deep ethyl chloride into shallow ether, and an expert surgeon and anaesthetist team could do about eight cases an hour. In Allen and Hanbury's Catalogue of Surgical Instruments for 1930, the ether inhaler was priced at one pound two shillings and sixpence. and the double weighted mouth tube at eight shillings and sixpence.

Working With DB and the "Top Hat"

DB was an outstanding figure of a man, well over six foot, having inherited from his forefathers strong qualities of physical statue, adventure, leadership, courage and scholarship. "Wolko," his third name, in aboriginal language means "Big Man," appropriate to this man who probably contributed more to paediatric surgery and over a wider range of conditions than any other surgeon. He was an intellectual adventurer, a rebel and a cynic who took nothing at its face value. Altogether a formidable character.

I was a senior house officer in anaesthetics at GOS from 1951-1952, and privileged to have given anaesthetics for DB, who taught me how to use his "Top Hat." In those days a senior house officer would give anaesthetics for him without any senior or consultant supervision, and I went once a week to the country branch of GOS at Tadworth Court in Surrey to give anaesthetics for an operation list for DB. Providing that one did what he asked and used his techniques, or ones of which he approved, he was very kind and tolerant with a junior and inexperienced anaesthetist. If one spent too long over an induction, he would offer to help, saying that he knew a thing or two about anaesthesia and tracheal intubation.

There is no longer a need for the "Top Hat" in paediatric anaesthesia, but it was one of Denis Browne's ingenious and useful gadgets and he ranks among those famous surgeons who have contributed to the development of anaesthesia.

References

1. Browne DB: Anaesthesia for tonsillectomy and removal of adenoids. British Medical Journal 2:632, 1928.
2. Macintosh RR: A simple method of blood transfusion. Lancet ii:22, 1927.
3. Browne DB: An aid to operations on infants. British Medical Journal 1:548, 1930.
4. Obituary. Sir Denis Browne. British Medical Journal 1:178, 1967.
5. Stephens D: Obituary. Sir Denis Browne. British Medical Journal 1:508, 1967.
6. Browne DB: The problem of Byron's lameness. Proceedings of the Royal Society of Medicine 53:440-2, 1960.
7. Crooks J: Denis Browne: Colleague. In: Nixon HH, Waterston D and Wink CAS. eds. Selected writings of Sir Denis Browne. London. Trustees of Sir Denis Browne Memorial Fund 1-2, 1983.
8. Sandiford CR, Clayton JC: The guillotine and ethyl chloride. British Medical Journal 2:149-52, 1928.

FROM SALT-FREE INTRAOPERATIVE FLUIDS TO BALANCED SALT SOLUTIONS
An Odyssey Led by Carl A. Moyer, M.D.

M. T. PEPPER JENKINS
University of Texas Southwestern Medical Center
Dallas, Texas, USA

In the past 150 years that anesthesiology, its drugs, its techniques, and its practitioners have been developing, a very few individuals could be considered as giants in their spheres of interest. In the nineteenth century a giant in physiology was Claude Bernard who, in 1879, brought us the concept of the milieu intérieur — that bit of primeval sea within us, the true atmosphere in which we live, so isolated from our surroundings that external storms cannot alter it or penetrate beyond it.[1] Our understanding of the extracellular fluid (ECF) as a large mobile body derives from our knowledge of the milieu internus.

In this century I nominate Carl A. Moyer, M.D., (1908-1970) as a giant among physiologists for his knowledge of the ECF, his application of that knowledge to the practices of surgery and anesthesiology, and his inherent gift of inspiring others to investigate his teachings and to expand his horizons further.

Carl Moyer was born in the upper peninsula of Michigan, in Baraga, in 1908. After his undergraduate degree from Northern Michigan University he entered the University of Michigan Medical School in 1930, but because of energetic digressions into organized pharmacology and experiments in physiology, he received his Master of Science degree in 1934 and did not achieve the MD degree until 1937. After four years of surgical training, still at the University of Michigan, he spent a productive clinical and research year with Henry K. Beecher, M.D., Dorr Professor of Anesthesiology, at the Massachusetts General Hospital. Among other publications resulting from this collaboration were three reports, the first definitive studies of the effects of the thiobarbiturates on respiratory control mechanisms.[2-4] Another significant achievement this year by Dr. Moyer was a profound respect for and an enjoyment of the clinical practise of anesthesiology.

Returning to the University of Michigan,

Dr. Moyer became involved in the extensive clinical research in fluid balance conducted by the Department of Surgery. A thesis developed early and continually reiterated was that there is a renal intolerance for salt solutions administered during anesthesia and operation. Expressed another way, the kidney was credited with an inability to excrete salt loads administered to the anesthetized patient. Several publications repeated this theme.[5-8] By the end of World War II, the proscription of salt solutions to the anesthetized patient was firmly fixed in the psyche and practises of surgeons and anesthesiologists in the United States and was not questioned by internists.

It was six years later, when Dr. Moyer had become Chairman of the Department of Surgery at the Southwestern Medical School in Dallas, Texas, that he questioned his earlier experimental protocols and changed his beliefs about intraoperative fluid replacement. It happened this way. In a short time during the summer of 1950, nine trauma patients in hypovolemic shock bypassed the emergency department and were brought directly to the operating rooms because of unchecked hemorrhage. Whole blood under pressure was administered via multiple veins to each patient who received no other fluids except 5 percent dextrose in distilled water. The individuals administering the anesthetic, primarily endotracheal 100 percent oxygen, became aware of the increasing loss of pulmonary compliance, plus persistent ashen-grey cyanosis, in each of these patients. At autopsy the lungs were described grossly as liver-lungs. Microscopic examination revealed many alveoli filled with red blood cells translocated from the circulation, alveolar cells still intact, and pulmonary capillaries greatly distended. Our subsequent publication described this as congestive atelectasis.[9]

In the laboratory, using anesthetized dogs bled into states of shock but without trauma, this same picture of congestive atelectasis was reproduced by the pressure re-infusion of shed blood. Further laboratory studies using radioiosotope-tagged red blood cells and tagged albumin revealed an absolute increase in pulmonary red cell mass and decrease in pulmonary plasma volume.

Therapy in laboratory studies included the administration of balanced salt solutions (BSS), fluids whose milliequivalent values for salts closely approximated those of extracellular fluid. The number of animal survivors was significant, and then under Dr. Moyer's direction we began using BSS, usually lactated Ringer's solution, for patients during anesthesia and operation.

What a courageous act of integrity it was for this man, Dr. Carl Moyer, to declare years of his previous work and publications to be invalid because of a flawed basic research protocol!

Now, what was that flawed investigative protocol? As appended to reference 5 it entailed a very sophisticated clinical study of urinary sodium excretion by a series of patients undergoing the same operation, combined abdominoperineal excision of the rectum for carcinoma (The Miles' operation, devised by British surgeon William E. Miles, 1869-1947). These patients were prepared for operation by the Miles' regiment of purging with magnesium sulfate followed by cleaning soap suds enemas. Then they received 125 ml 0.9 percent sodium chloride per hour for four hours during the anesthesia and operation. In studying urinary output no sodium was found.

Conclusions then were that, under circumstances of anesthesia and operation, there was either a renal intolerance to salt or a renal inability to excrete salt during an operation. Conclusions today would be that an adult patient prepared by the Miles' regimen would have the extracellular fluid volume diminished by two to four liters, which would be significantly further reduced by translocation accompanying the necessary trauma of such an extensive surgical procedure. Consequently, today the absence of sodium in the urine would be interpreted as the normal action of the kidney in protecting a reduced extracellular fluid volume.

Fellow workers in Dallas with Dr. Moyer included Drs. G. Thomas Shires, Ben J. Wilson,

Morris J. Fogelman, and M. T. Jenkins, all of whom continued to follow Dr. Moyer's expanding vistas of fluid balance.[10] In later years Dr. Moyer stated before an audience at a symposium on fluids at the National Research Council that he had achieved the ultimate as a teacher: one of his students, Dr. Shires, had surpassed his teacher in research into fluid balance and into the practical day-to-day application of lessons learned from his research. (We might wonder whether Dr. Coller at the University of Michigan was as generous when his trainee, Dr. Moyer, discredited the clinical rule followed by the surgery department of giving the postoperative patient 0.5 g of salt for each 100 mg percent the plasma chloride was reported below 560 mg percent.) Notably, among other important precepts, Dr. Shires had measured and defined the extracellular fluid as a large mobile mass normally entering into the dynamics of the circulation and responding to trauma and to significant blood loss by a translocation from the circulation.[11-14]

Dr. Moyer burst upon the medical scene in Dallas, Texas, in 1946, and he was recognized instantly as a dazzling medical personality who had much to offer everyone in medicine. Many of us had recently come from years of sterile medical experience during active military service, and we were entranced with his virtuosity in teaching. I, for one, initially had troubles with the concept of millequivalents per liter because of my background in milligrams percent. Dr. Moyer simplified the transition for me. "Milligrams percent," he said, using an automotive comparison, "is the number of cylinders. Milliequivalents per liter is the horsepower." Ah, instant appreciation and a glimmer of light about me!

This is a capsule description of Dr. Moyer's odyssey from advocating no intraoperative salt solutions to prescribing plenty of intraoperative salt solutions. This is only a meager description of his professional life. To capsulize his career further, it should be noted, and be a source of pride to anesthesiology, that while he was professor and chairman of surgery at Southwestern Medical School he was sorely tempted to take up the post of chairman of anesthesiology at Washington University in St. Louis. Dr. Evarts Graham, noted surgeon at Washington University, made the offer repeatedly. Was it poetic justice that, after he became Dean at Southwestern Medical School and effectuated its incorporation into the University of Texas System, Dr. Moyer left Dallas to succeed Dr. Graham as chairman of surgery at Washington University where he continued to espouse the importance of anesthesiology in the care of the surgical patient.

Because of my early work with Dr. Moyer and my continued association with the research team which remained after his departure, our intraoperative fluid regimen developed and has been previously published as follows:[15,16]

> No single regimen for fluid administration will apply to patients with varying physical status and disease processes and scheduled for a variety of operations. We acknowledge the obvious fact that throughout the world, differing routines for intraoperative fluids are followed. These routines may range from no fluids at all, to blood only, and some may include albumin or mannitol on a definitely timed basis. Under any regimen, it seems that a majority of patients survive, some because of fluid administration and others despite it.
>
> As a central theme of our precepts we feel that homeostatic mechanisms in the anesthetized patient are best maintained if fluid administration helps to preserve normal renal function while replacing ECF translocated from the dynamic pool. Our regimen, therefore, is strongly influenced by recent developments in the history of sequestered edema.
>
> A. We begin with 5 percent dextrose in water (D5W) up to 500 ml, and continue with 5 percent dextrose in balanced salt solutions (D5BS) in the following procedures:
>   1. *Intraabdominal and hip operations*: 12 to 15 ml per kg body weight during the first hour, and 6 to 10 ml per kg per hour for the next two hours, varied as indicated by the

degree of surgical manipulation (trauma), arterial pressure, pulse, urine output and, in certain cases, central venous pressure or pulmonary wedge pressure. For operations beyond three hours, we continue with a balanced salt solution without glucose at a rate to assure urinary output of 50 to 100 ml per hour.

   2. *Intrathoracic (noncardiac) operations:* 6 to 10 ml per kg per hour.
   3. *Extremities and major superficial operations:* 6 to 10 ml per kg per hour varied after the first hour as indicated by degree of operative manipulation (trauma), arterial pressure, and pulse.

B. We begin and continue with D5BS in these operations:
   1. *Intracranial procedures:* Balanced salt solutions are administered only in volumes sufficient to keep the venous channel (IV) open until the surgeon begins the closure; then begin replacement with balanced salt solutions as indicated by urine output.
   2. *Transurethral prostatic surgery:* 3 to 6 ml per kg per hour while watching closely for sudden expansion of intravascular volume by operative "washwater" absorbed through the prostatic bed.

C. We begin and continue with D5W in volumes sufficient to keep the IV open (i.e., minimal fluids where operative trauma is limited) in these procedures:
   1. *Microsurgery of the ear and larynx.*
   2. *Most ophthalmic operations.*

D. We limit the total dextrose administered to a maximum of 125g.

E. We transfuse with whole blood or its equivalent in blood component therapy when blood loss exceeds 20 percent of estimated blood volume.

F. We monitor urine output on all major trauma operations and all predicted to be lengthy procedures."

Now, nearly four centuries since Harvey's epochal publication on the circulation of the blood and four decades after Dr. Moyer's determination that the anesthesiologist should administer salt solutions during operations, balanced salt solutions are given freely, and the results have been for the betterment of the surgical patient.

References

Italicized comments followed by an* are excerpted from reference 16.

1. Bernard C: Leçons sur les phénomènes de la vie communs aux animaux et aux végétaux. Ballière, Paris, 1879.
   (Possibly this was one of the three publications in the remote past of importance to the development of intravenous fluid therapy. Harvey's description of the circulation of the blood in 1628, and Lister's proposal of the germ theory in 1875, are the other two important events.)
2. Beecher HK, Moyer CA: Mechanisms of respiratory failure under barbiturate anesthesia (evipal, pentothal). *J Clin Invest*; 20:549, 1941.
3. Moyer CA: Major changes in the fundamental relationships of the respiratory drive mechanisms during evipal and pentothal anesthesia, with special consideration of possible applications to transpleural surgery. *J Thoracic Surg*; 11:131, 1941.
4. Moyer CA, Beecher HK: Effects of barbiturate anesthesia (evipal and pentothal sodium) upon the integration of respiratory control mechanisms. A study directed toward improvement of methods for the preclinical evaluation of anesthetic agents. *J Clin Invest*; 21:429, 1942.
5. Coller FA, Moyer CA et al: Postoperative salt intolerance. *Ann Surg*; 119:533, 1944.
   *("There is a high incidence of 'salt intolerance' following general anesthesia; . . . give no isotonic saline or Ringer's solution on operative day and following two days;. . . treat fluid deficiency states on responses to test doses rather than on measured electrolytes." In the recent past this was perhaps the most significant article in influencing fluid administration during anesthesia and operation, proscribing the use of salt solutions.)**

6. Coller FA, Moyer CA et al: Translocation of fluid produced by the intravenous administration of isotonic salt solutions in man postoperatively. *Ann Surg*; 122:663, 1945.
*(Postoperative injection of 09 percent sodium chloride results in its being retained, more than 50 percent. Hypotonic solutions are retained also, although extra free water is provided for elimination by skin and lungs. Translocations, if any, are not explained.)**
7. Moyer CA et al: Some effects of an operation, anesthesia and composition of parenteral fluids upon the excretion of water and salt. *South Surg*; 15:218, 1949.
*(Volatile general anesthetic agents depress renal excretion. Further, there is depressed excretion of water, sodium, and chloride given in postoperative period. "Pre-renal deviation of fluid into injured area can scarcely be responsible.")**
8. Moyer CA: Acute temporary changes in renal function associated with major surgical procedures. *Surgery*; 27:198, 1950.
*(Salt solution is avidly retained during and after operation [combined A-P resection]. "Fundamental causes for changes in renal function during operations are still unknown." Secretion of ECF into injured areas might change renal function. There may be some distributional shift.)**
9. Jenkins MT, Moyer CA et al: Congestive atelectasis — a complication of the intravenous infusion of fluids. *Ann Surg*; 132:3, 1950.
*(In congestive atelectasis red cell mass in lungs is increased and plasma volume in lungs is decreased. This was the turning point in authors' attitudes leading to advocacy of infusing salt solutions intraoperatively. Author's intraoperative fluid regimen, 1950-59: Lactated Ringer's solution, alternating with 5 percent dextrose in L/R, 10 ml per kg body weight per hour; plus L/R equivalent to 2 X blood loss, tempered with reason as influenced by urine output. After 1959 the regimen changed as indicated in references 15 and 126.)**
10. Moyer CA: Fluid Balance: A Clinical Manual. Year Book Publishers, Chicago, 1952.
(Written before clinical electrolyte determinations became easily and rapidly obtainable, this little volume was and is a goldmine of clinical signs. Particularly well described are disturbances in body fluid equilibrium: in volume, in electrolytic osmolar concentration, in composition, in distribution, and, less well described, in rate of internal exchange.)*
11. Shires GT, Williams J, Brown F: Changing concept of salt water and surgery. *Texas J Med*; 55:1, 1959
*(This explains sequestration of ECF during operations ["third-space shift"] and the consequent reduced functional extracellular fluid and diminished renal sodium excretion. This article introduced the modern concept of fluid translocation due to trauma and/or shock.)**
12. Shires GT et al: Distributional changes in extracellular fluid during acute hemorrhagic shock. *Surg Forum*; 11:115, 1960.
(The triple isotope technic for simultaneous measurement of red blood cell mass [51-Cr], plasma volume [131-iodine tagged serum albumin], ECF volume [35-S labeled Na_2SO_4*] is described, as is the demonstrated loss of functional ECF after hemorrhage.)**
13. Shires GT, Carrico CJ, Coln D: The role of the extracellular fluid in shock. *Int Anesth Clin*; 2:435, 1964
*(Blood loss alone if sufficiently large also results in losses of ECF from the dynamics of the circulation.)**
14. Shires GT et al: Fluid therapy in hemorrhagic shock. *Arch Surg*; 88:688, 1964.
*(As described here the ECF is a very mobile huge pool of water, electrolytes, and metabolic components. Measurements here show disparate reductions of functional ECF in hemorrhagic shock, prescribing intraoperative administration of balanced salt solutions as an adjunct to blood replacement.)**
15. Jenkins MT, Giesecke AH, Johnson ER: The postoperative patient and his fluid and electrolyte requirements. *Brit J Anaesth*; 47:143, 1975.
(This report offers reasons for the administration of glucose to the anesthetized patient. The fasting patient has approximately 900 m-osmoles [45g] of non-volatile solute to the excreted in the urine daily, representing breakdown of 160g of fat and 75g of muscle protein. Intravenous glucose, up to 100g, will reduce the non-volatile solute to 200-400 m-osmoles [10-20g], which represents a small load even for the kidney having a limited concentrating ability.)
16. Jenkins MT: History of sequestered edema associated with surgical operations and trauma: In Brown BR (Ed): Fluid and blood therapy in anesthesia. *F.A.Davis Co., Philadelphia*, 1982, pp 1-31.

THE BEGINNING OF ETHER ANESTHESIA IN SPAIN
Contributions of an American Dentist

JOAQUIN C. LAIÑO, A. FRANCO GRANDE, A. CARREGAL, L. VAZQUEZ, M. VIDAL and P. PICATTO
Department of Anesthesiology
Hospital General de Galicia
Santiago de Comportela, Spain

Some years ago, our research group was able to determine the exact date of the first surgical operation performed in Spain using sulphuric ether as an anesthetic.[1] On January 13, 1847, Prof. Diego Argumosa-Obregón tested the effects of this substance in an operation on a parotid abscess in which, as in the further four trials he carried out that same month,[2] the anesthetic was administered with the Harapath inhaler that had been used by Lansdown at the end of the previous month in Bristol, England.

News of the discovery of ether anesthesia had arrived in Spain by two independent routes at the beginning of 1847. Argumosa-Obregón learned of it from a Sr. Barron (possibly an Englishman resident in Madrid), whose source was a letter sent from London by his friend Dr. Forbes, the Editor of the *British and Foreign Medical Review*.[2] Forbes had personally witnessed many of the trials of ether carried out in London hospitals. The other route was via the London press, specifically the *Times* and the *Daily News* of January 4, the *Illustrated London News* of the 9th and the *Morning Chronicle* of the 11th. It was through these media that many other Spanish surgeons first came to know of the anesthetic effects of ether.

The first Spanish news item on the discovery of ether anesthesia appeared on January 14, 1847, in *La Opinión*, a primarily political newspaper published in Madrid.[3] It read more or less as follows:

> *Surgical experiments. If we are to give credit to the English newspapers, then in spite of the claims of its supporters, it is not only magnetism that, when applied in surgical operations produces a sleep*

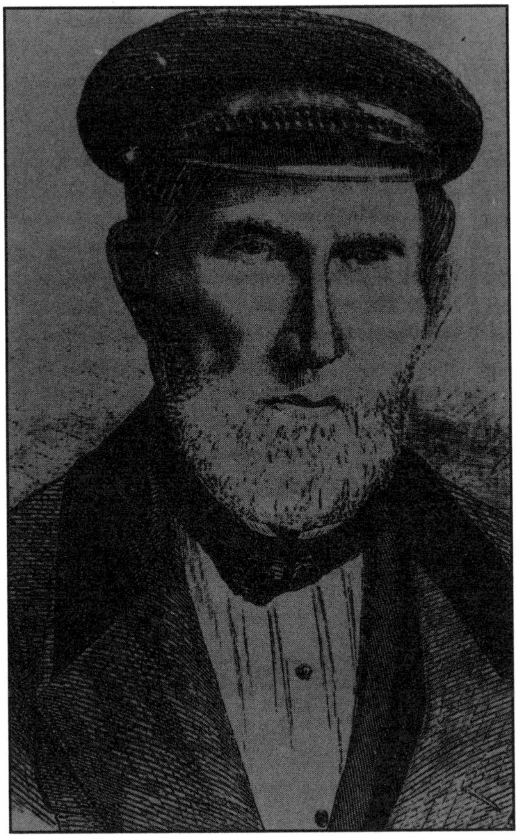

Fig. 1. Prof. Diego Argumosa Obregón.

during which the patient undergoes the operation without any pain. According to these sources, in University College Hospital Dr. Liston has performed two dangerous operations without causing the least pain, for which purpose he use ether vapour, a medium he has employed in a number of American localities (sic).

La Opinión was followed on January 23 by *El Observador*, which under the headline, "Unconsciousness of patients in surgical operations produced by inhalation of ether," reproduced the information contained in the *Morning Chronicle's* item of January 11.[4] The following day, January 24, this report was also published by *La Opinión*.[5]

January 24 also saw the first recognition of an ether anesthetic by the Spanish scientific press. In Madrid, the journal *Anales de Cirugía*, published a note headed, "A Most Important Discovery,"[6] and informed of Prof. Argumosa-Obregón's first three trials. A few days later, on January 28, *La Facultad*, another scientific journal, published two articles on the use of ether as an aesthetic, and likewise reported on Argumosa-Obergón's first trials.[7] These experiments of Argumosa-Obregón's were also publicized by the daily papers: the January 29 issue of *El Popular*,[8] and the January 30 numbers of *El Imparcial*[9] and *La Carta*,[10] all ran the following story:

> *Dr. Diego de Argumosa y Obregón, Professor of Clinical Surgery in the Medicine Faculty of Madrid, has performed a number of experiments to remove pain during operations. One has had indifferent success, for the patient did not feel a thread being passed through the nape of his neck. (sic)*

Our research has uncovered conclusive documentary proof that the second to use ether as surgical anesthetic in Spain was an American dentist called Oliver Machechan, who temporarily set up practice in Madrid. By January 28, 1847, Machechan had used ether for a number of tooth extractions, as was widely reported in the daily and political press of Madrid during the final days of that month (specifically, in *El Tiempo* on Thursday 28[11] and Friday 29,[12] in the *Eco del Comercio* on Friday 29[13] and Saturday 30[14] and in *La Opinión*[15] and *El Espectador*[16] on Sunday 31). All these reports lay great emphasis on Machechan's skill and experience, and on his high reputation on either side of the Atlantic. Machechan also used the Bristol Harapath inhaler to administer the anesthetic, and apparently achieved totally satisfactory results.[17]

Our attempts to find out more about Machechan have so far met with little success. He appears to have arrived in Madrid during the first few days of 1847 and to have stayed there only until mid-February, 1848. In that short time he seems nevertheless to have become extremely popular, having attended the cream of Madrid society — including Queen Isabel II and other members of the Royal Family. It may even be possible that members of the Royal Family were among those receiving anesthetics for extractions,[18] for on February 14, 1848, the newspaper *El Siglo* reported that the well-known dentist Dr. Rotondo was called to the Royal Palace to extract one of the Infanta Amalia's molars (Machechan may already have left town), and that the operation was performed successfully with no fuss on the illustrious patient's part and without any need for the fashionable anesthetic chloroform.[19]

It is in relation to chloroform that, in February 1848, Machechan again appeared in the Madrid press, several dental operations he performed with the help of the new anesthetic being commented on by *El Siglo* on February 9[20] and by *El Siglo*,[21] the *Gaceta de Madrid*[22] and *El Espectador*[23] on Thursday the 10th (on this latter date *El Siglo* refers to him literally as "Mr. Oliver P. Makeemkan," presumably due to an error).[21] We have been unable to uncover any further information concerning Machechan or the important role he appears to have played in the introduction of surgical anesthesia in Spain, an advance that occurred earlier in Spain than in any other European country except the United Kingdom and France.

References

1. Franco A. et all: Primeros aparatos para la anestesia etérea. Rev Esp Anestesiol Reanim; 25:445-62, 1978.
2. Fernández U: Sobre la inhalación etérea. Gaceta Médica; 76:25-27, 1847.
3. Anonymous: La Opinión. Madrid, January 14, 1847; 105:4.
4. Anonymous. El Espectador. Madrid, January 23, 1847; 135:3.
5. Anonymous: La Opinión. Madrid, January 24, 1847; 114:3.
6. Anonymous: Descubrimiento importantísimo. Anales de Cirugía; 56-7, 1847.
7. Anonymous: Del éter sulfúrico para adormecer á los que han de ser operados. La Facultad; 259:3, 1847.
8. Anonymous: El Popular. Madrid, January 29, 1847; 196:4.
9. Anonymous: El Imparcial. Madrid, January 30, 1847; 259:3.
10. Anonymous: La Carta. Madrid, January 30, 1847; 18:3.
11. Anonymous. El Tiempo. Madrid, January 28, 1847; 873:4.
12. Anonymous. El Tiempo. Madrid, January 29, 1847; 874:4.
13. Anonymous. Eco del Comercio. Madrid, January 29, 1847; 1326:4.
14. Anonymous: Eco del Comercio. Madrid, January 30, 1847; 1327:4.
15. Anonymous: La Opinión. Madrid, January 31, 1847; 120:4.
16. Anonymous: El Espectador. Madrid, January 31, 1847; 142:4.
17. Franco A, Baños G, Carregal A, Carceller J: Historia de la introdicción de la anestesia etérea en España. Una nueva contribución a su estudio. Rev Esp Anestesiol Readnim; 38:102-8, 1991.
18. Anonymous: El Faro. Madrid, February 10, 1848; 36:4.
19. Anonymous: El Observadór. Madrid, February 14, 1848; 18:3.
20. Anonymous: El Siglo. Madrid, February 9, 1848; 35:4.
21. Anonymous: El Siglo. Madrid, February 10, 1848; 36:4.
22. Anonymous: Gaceta de Madrid. Madrid, February 10, 1848; 4897:4.
23. Anonymous: El Espectador. Madrid, February 10, 1848; 441:4.

TWENTY-FIVE YEARS OF LIVING HISTORY

JOHN J. LEAHY
Philadelphia, Pennsylvania, USA

The Living History of Anesthesia Series of the Wood Library-Museum (WLM) was begun in 1966 as a private non-funded project of Drs. J. W. Pender of Palo Alto, California, and John Leahy, then of Washington, D.C., later of Chicago and presently of Philadelphia.

The project was inspired by the reading of the Faulconer and Keys Book, "*Foundations of Anesthesiology,*" published in 1965, and the realization that many of the pioneers of the specialty were still alive and available for first-hand recounting of their roles in the development of anesthesiology. This was further augmented by the publication in JAMA (Feb. 1966) of "*Videotaped Autobiographical Interviews - An adjunct to Medical Education*" by David Segal, MD of Columbia University.

The early efforts were made on 16mm color/sound film and, although cumbersome, complicated and very expensive, nevertheless preserved for us the voice, impressions and personality of many of the "greats" in our specialty who did not live until the videotape era.

The early interviews were primitive by present standards, both from the audio/video and interviewer standpoints. But they were a beginning. . . a first step. . . and we have learned much from them. Of course, the introduction of practical videotape in the late seventies was a great impetus to our project. But the most important advance was the development of a trained interviewer who would take time to thoroughly research the subject and, together with the interviewee, prepare the interview in advance. For this we are indebted to Dr. Elliott Miller of Boston who in 1980 first taped interviews of Roy Vandam, Urban Eversole and Dave Little at a TV station in Boston.

With this progression we moved from doing interviews in hotel rooms, at meetings and, on occasion, at the interviewee's home, to the professional TV/Recording studio, both commercial and University Medical-Center based. When the Living History Series began, very few Medical Centers had sophisticated TV recording facilities.

The funding of a project such as this is a most important consideration. In the early years there was none! The originators of the project tried unsuccessfully to enlist support from various sources, including pharmaceutical firms, the National Library of Medicine and the ASA. A period of nearly ten years intervened during which nothing new was added to our collection for lack of funds. We had spent much more of our own resources than could be reasonably expected and without any interest from outside sources.

Finally, during the presidency of Dr. James Eckenhoff at the Wood Library-Museum (WLM) and, succeeding him, Dr. Charles Tandy and Garth Huston, the Living History Series was adopted as an ongoing project of the WLM. New interviews are being added at the rate of up to 5 or 6 per year. The number of tapes in our collection now numbers more than one hundred, of which all are available for loan or purchase in various formats from the WLM. Arrangements have been made to exchange tapes with societies and libraries in other countries, notably Great Britain, New Zealand and Australia, as well as South America.

In this presentation we will show, briefly, some of the original films (later transferred to tape) as well as some of the most recent additions. One of our early hopes was to interview individuals at least twice. . . at the peak of their careers and again after their retirement. We illustrate this with excerpts from interviews of Dr. James Eckenhoff. Some obstacles appeared from time to time: some individuals who had made outstanding contributions to Anesthesiology refused to be interviewed. Both Scott Smith of Salt Lake City and Margo Deming of Philadelphia were in this group. Also, there were some who died prematurely such as Bob Dripps, Harry Beecher, Curtis Hickcox, Ralph Tovell, Lloyd Larrick, Henry Ruth, Digby Leigh and Ed Tuohy. In an effort to get as close as we could to these persons, we have attempted to gather panels of some of their contemporaries to discuss them. Here, for example, we show such an approach to the memory of Bob Dripps.

In addition to those mentioned above, we have included brief excerpts from interviews of Drs. Dave Little, Emmanuel Papper, "Pepper" Jenkins, John Steinhaus, Henrik Bendixen, Richard Kitz, John Severinghaus, Ted Eger, John Michenfelder and Henning Pontoppidan. (Showing time of this tape: 20 minutes)

NORMAN REYNOLDS JAMES
Australian Pioneer

PATRICIA MACKAY
The Royal Melbourne Hospital
Victoria, Australia

The second of March, 1948, saw the beginning of the modern era in anesthetics at the Royal Melbourne Hospital with the formation of the first Anaesthetic Department in Victoria and the appointment of Dr. Norman James as the foundation Director of Anaesthetics.

Norman Reynolds James was an Australian who had lived for a number of years in the United Kingdom, having worked in Wolverhamptom, the West Middlesex County Hospital, and in the Department of Anaesthetics in the University of Oxford. He had associated with the illustrious anesthetists of the time—Ivan Magill, Sir Robert Macintosh, M.D. Nosworthy and Langton Hewer. Thus, he was well qualified to develop and transform a faltering anesthetic service into a properly organized Department and to commence training candidates for the newly instituted Diploma of Anaesthetics in the University of Melbourne—the first 2 part postgraduate qualification in Anesthetics in Australia.

The hospital gave Norman James a clear brief—to provide a clinical service, establish a teaching program and to develop research. Unfortunately, proper support was not provided—either by the hospital or the surgeons of the time. It became necessary for the new director to raise funds from external sources in order to provide essential equipment for the blossoming Department. This he did with a vigor and enthusiasm which did not always meet with approval from the medical establishment, who believed that such advertisement was unacceptable. However, by 1951 the Department had become the showplace of Australia for its modern equipment and emphasis on safety—suction was provided in all anesthetic rooms; new anesthetic machines, complete with laryngoscopes and bronchoscopes, were available in every theater and a cardiac emergency trolley was introduced.

Norman James was an enthusiastic and flamboyant teacher whose message was seldom forgotten. For the first time junior resident staff received regular tuition, and certification was necessary before interns could administer anesthetics without supervision. Structured undergraduate and postgraduate programs were introduced, resulting in strong recruitment of Melbourne University graduates into anesthesia. A fulltime anesthetist resident was appointed in 1949, but the hospital did not concede the need for an increase in trainee staff until 1953, when the first anesthetic registrars were appointed.

The senior staff consisted of honorary sessional anesthetists, with the Director as the only fulltime member. This changed in 1954 when the first Deputy Director was appointed, followed by a halftime thoracic anesthetist. I was fortunate to be that Deputy and to be a disciple of Norman James. Despite preoccupation with the development of the Department, Norman also was enormously productive in the development of new equipment—always concentrating on his theme of safety. In 1950 he produced the R.M. (Royal Melbourne) Resuscitator and attempted to provide what he called "an asphyxia service" in the Emergency Department of the hospital and in the wards.

Of course he knew well that such a service was also essential in the field, where iron lungs were still being transported to the site of drowning and electrocution, and Norman lobbied hard to get his respirator installed in the ambulance service. The R.M. Resuscitator was only recently discarded in the wards of the hospital; it would be safe to predict that such equipment designed today would not be in service 26 years hence.

In 1952, the Harrington-James respirator was developed in conjunction with the Department of Physiology—this simple and quiet machine with its ability to provide negative pressure facilitated major advances in neurosurgical anesthetis and in neurosurgical techniques. This was the first respirator to be developed in Australia and presented an enormous advance on the iron tank lung respirators, still in use at the infectious diseases hospital. Thus, at the Royal Melbourne Hospital in 1955 we were able to institute prolonged ventilation and intensive care principles of management in medical conditions such as tetanus, polyneuritis and myasthenia gravis.

The theme of the Department under Norman James was safety—safety in the operating room by the training and employment of specialists in anesthesia and by the provision of adequate equipment. He was also most concerned about the considerable morbidity and mortality associated with recovery from anesthesia in the wards. Strong persuasion to outside sources enabled him to raise sufficient money to open what I believe was the first modern Recovery Room in Australia on December 18, 1953. The inaugural ceremony, well publicized in the local press, was performed by the then senior surgeon, Sir Albert Coates, who opened the postanesthetic facility with the words, "Melbourne Surgery is top class!" Just two years later a liquid oxygen system was installed and oxygen piped to all the wards.

Thus, within five years of his appointment Norman James had made the Department a showplace in Australia and there were many visitors, as Melbourne in the early fifties was the mecca for anesthetists.

Norman James displayed enormous energy and resourcefulness, had considerable management skills that he imparted to all his assistants, and had a clear vision of the widening horizons of anesthetis. Sadly, he had a long battle for recognition in the hospital—partly because he belonged to a "Cinderella" specialty and partly because his was a salaried position. Thus, in spite of all his contributions and the development of a flourishing Department, he was not granted membership of the Senior Medical Staff until 1957, and even then it was suggested that he should not have voting rights!

In the early 1960's, Norman felt that he should meet new challenges and he believed these lay in the United States, to which he emigrated in 1964. He spent the rest of his professional life at the Southwestern Medical School in Dallas with Professor M.T. Jenkins. Here he was very highly regarded for his ability as a gifted educator, and he also maintained his resourceful development of equipment and designed three ventilator models. He remained in the USA after retirement until his death in 1989, but always retained his Australian citizenship.

In the 16 years of his leadership in the Department of Anaesthetics at the Royal Melbourne Hospital, Norman Reynolds James—the first Director, provided a critical link in the chain and was a true pioneer of modern anesthesia in Australia.

NURSE ANESTHETISTS:
Establishing their Right to Practice in the United States

SANDRA M. MAREE* and IRA P. GUNN**
Winston-Salem, North Carolina; El Paso, Texas**, USA*

The elation and optimism concerning painless surgery that accompanied the discovery of the anesthetic properties of diethyl ether, chloroform and nitrous oxide in the 1840's were slowly replaced by the reality of infection and anesthesia mishaps as serious impediments to surgical practice. It took the work of a combination of Nightingale, Semmelweiss, Koch, Lister and others to demonstrate that infections could be contained. But it was the anesthesia outcomes of a large number of nurses and a few physicians specializing in the practice that demonstrated anesthesia's safety in the United States.

By 1876, many surgeons were turning first to Catholic hospital sisters, and then nurses educated in the Nightingale tradition, to administer their anesthesia. They believed that the key to anesthesia safety lay in its provision by experienced personnel. Indeed, the work of Alice McGaw, nurse anesthetist for Drs. Charles and William Mayo, and other nurse anesthetists proved their case.

It should be remembered that nurse utilization in the provision of anesthesia services coincided in time with the passage of state medical practice acts, which were shortly followed by nurse practice acts. Medicine chose to claim the whole of health care as its domain, and ever since other health professionals have been carving out their scopes of practice. It is therefore not surprising that some legal challenges to nurse anesthetist practice by physician anesthetists occurred as the success of their practice became known. Had nurse anesthesia proved a failure, no challenge would have been necessary.

The early formalization of educational programs for nurse anesthetists, prior to 1912, gave evidence that the nursing specialty was taking root. Shortly thereafter, two challenges to nurse anesthetist practice resulted in favorable legal precedents. The first occurred in Ohio.

In 1912, Dr. George Crile and the Lakeside Hospital were challenged for using nurses to provide anesthesia services. One such nurse was

Agatha Hodgins, the founder of the American Association of Nurse Anesthetists. Dr. Crile received a letter from the secretary of the Ohio State Medical Board informing him of its position that no one other than a registered physician could administer an anesthetic. The board also noted that the Attorney General concurred in his opinion.[1] In 1916, the Interstate Association of Anesthetists petitioned the Ohio State Medical Board to take action against Lakeside Hospital as the chief source in the use of nurse anesthetists. To prevent denial of recognition of its nursing school, Lakeside Hospital discontinued the anesthesia school. Dr. Crile continued to argue in favor of nurse anesthesia, however. This challenge led to an exemption being enacted in the Ohio Medical Practice Act in 1919 excluding nurse anesthetists from charges of practicing medicine when qualified by education and supervised by a physician. The Lakeside school reopened in 1917.

The second legal action resulted from a restrictive ethical code passed by the Kentucky Medical Society. The resolution called for an end to the use of non-physician anesthetists and recommended that physicians not employ anyone other than physicians as anesthetists, except in emergencies. Further, the resolution urged physicians not to refer cases to hospitals where nurses were allowed to give anesthetics. Any doctor "violating" the terms of the resolution would no longer be considered a member in good standing of the Association. In *Frank v. South,* Dr. Louis Frank, a surgeon, and Margaret Hatfield, his nurse anesthetist, sued the State Board of Health so the question could be definitely answered.

In deciding the case in favor of Ms. Hatfield and Dr. Frank, Judge Hart ruled that Ms. Hatfield was not practicing medicine within the meaning of Kentucky law. It states, "these laws have not been enacted for the peculiar benefit of the members of such professions, further, than they are members of the general community, but they have been enacted for the benefit of the people . . . While the practice of medicine is one of the most noble and learned professions, it is apparent that such a construction ought not to be given to the statute which regulates the profession, that the effect of it would be to invade the province of the professions of pharmacy, dentistry or trained nursing, all of which are professions, which relate to the alleviation of the human family of sickness and bodily afflictions, and to make duties belonging to those professions also the practice of medicine within the meaning of the statute." The decision enunciated clearly the purpose of state practice acts. They are designed to protect the public, not professions. It further reminded physicians that the legislature was the sole body for defining the exclusive legal privileges for professionals. Anesthesia was one of them.[2]

In the 1930's, during the great depression, the final major legal challenge to nurse anesthetists was mounted by a group of California physician anesthetists. Dr. Verne Hunt, a surgeon from Mayo Clinic, moved to St. Vincent's Hospital in Los Angeles. He invited Dagmar Nelson to come from Minnesota to California to work at the hospital as an anesthetist. His interest in bringing Ms. Nelson to California was due to the death from asphyxiation of one of his patients, a 23-year-old undergoing minor surgery. The anesthetic had been given by a young man with little experience in anesthesia.[3]

The California physician anesthetists first sought an injunction to restrain permanently Dagmar Nelson from administering anesthetics. On July 12, 1934, in the Superior Court of Los Angeles, Dagmar Nelson went on trial for violating the California Medical Practice Act: practicing medicine without a license. The physician anesthetist argument was the practice of medicine for the following reasons: 1) the surgeon, being separated from the anesthetist by a screen, could in no way supervise the actual administration of an anesthetic; 2) an anesthetic is a drug, and in so administering the drug the anesthetist used judgment as to amount; and 3) in observing the signs of anesthetia and acting as those signs indicated, the anesthetist is making a diagnosis of the patient's condition.[4] The defense argument was: 1) the giving of drugs upon direct or understood instruction of a physician was a recognized practice and within the limits of the definition of nursing; 2) the recognition and the reporting of changes in a patient's condition and acting accordingly under the direct or understood supervision of a physician was within the practice of medicine; 3) nursing education as accepted by law gave instruction in the administration of anesthetics and the recognition of the signs and stages of anesthesia; and 4) it is an established practice within the law for registered nurses to give anesthetics as a nursing duty.[5] The twelve-day trial ended July 27, 1934. The decision rendered by the California Supreme Court confirmed that nurses were commonly used as anesthetists by surgeons and hospitals, and as practiced Dagmar Nelson was practicing nursing and not medicine. In an address to the Midsouth Postgraduate Nurse Anesthetists' Assembly in Memphis in February, 1941, Dr. Hunt stated, "I believe that as I may have had something to do with maintaining and enhancing the status of nurse anesthetists, they have likewise had much to do with rearing me surgically for which I continue to be grateful."[6]

The Dagmar Nelson court challenge coincided with the formation of a national association of nurse anesthetists. There are over 24,000 Certified Registered Nurse Anesthetists (CRNA's) today who administer more than 65 percent of the 26 million anesthetics given annually in the United States. The demand for CRNA's is great. The US Department of Health and Human Services study on CRNA manpower needs documents a current shortage of approximately 7,000 CRNA's and projects a need for 35,433 by the year 2010. In order to meet this need, the number of students graduating from nurse anesthesia must triple.

Nurse Anesthesia in the United States is the oldest of nursing specialties. Education and experience required to become a CRNA include: 1) Bachelor of Science in Nursing (BSN) or other appropriate degree; 2) graduation from an accredited school of nurse anesthesia education of at least 2 years in length; 80 percent of these programs are within a graduate university framework; and 3) passing a national certification examination following graduation and completing a continuing education and recertification program every two years thereafter.[8]

On June 9-10, 1989, The International Federation of Nurse Anesthetists (IFNA) was founded in Teufen, Switzerland. In addition to the United States, other charter members included Austria, the Federal Republic of Germany, Finland, France, Iceland, Norway, South Korea, Sweden, Switzerland and Yugoslavia.[9] Known non-member countries in which nurse anesthetists practice include: Algeria, Australia, Botswana, Bulgaria, China, Congo, Denmark, Ethiopia, Ghana, Hungary, Israel, Kenya, Luxembourg, Malaysia, The Netherlands, Poland, Rwanda, Saudi Arabia, Spain, Thailand, Tunisia, Vietnam an Zimbabwe.[10]

Despite continuing periodic challenges concerning practice modalities, nurse anesthetists remain a vital anesthesia resource in the United States in all types of practice settings. While there remains a critical shortage of this provider, nurse anesthetists have established their practice rights. Additionally, they have strengthened and acquired the political acumen which, when combined with quality services, have made these professionals long-term survivors.

References

1. Thatcher V: *History of Anesthesia With Emphasis on the Nurse Specialist,* Philadelphia, 111, 1953.
2. Bankert M: *Watchful Care: A History of America's Nurse Anesthetist,* New York, 62-63, 1989.
3. Ibid 90.
4. Ibid 91.
5. Ibid 92.
6. Ibid 94.
7. Gray S, McFadden P: Nurse anesthetist spotlight. *RN,* 56:103-7, 1992.
8. Gray S: Nurse anesthetists. *Graduating Nurse,* 24-26, 1992.
9. Caulk R, Maree S: A new beginning: The International Federation of Nurse Anesthetists. *AANAJ,* 58:158-64, 1990.
10. Caulk R: The International Federation of Nurse Anesthetists (IFNA). *CRNA Forum,* 8:3-19, 1992.

THE INTRODUCTION OF NITROUS OXIDE INTO OBSTETRIC ANESTHESIA

GERTIE F. MARX and TATYANA KATSNELSON
Department of Anesthesiology
Albert Einstein College of Medicine
Bronx, New York, USA

Nitrous oxide was introduced into obstetric anesthesia in 1880 by Stanislav Casimirovicz Klikovicz (1853-1910), a young physician working at the St. Petersburg Clinic for Internal Diseases under the guidance of the well-known internist, Professor Botkin. Born in the Russian-occupied part of Poland, Klikovicz had his medical education at the Academy of Medicine and Surgery in St. Petersburg.[1] Besides being fluent in Polish, Russian and German, he had sufficient knowledge of English and French to correctly quote Horace Wells, Paul Bert and many other previous nitrous oxide investigators.

Requested by Professor Botkin to test the therapeutic importance of nitrous oxide in his department, Klikovicz began his "experiments" late in 1879. His first report on the subject was published in the St. Petersburg Medical Journal in April, 1880.[2] Using 4 parts of N_2O and 1 part of O_2 in patients with angina pectoris, he noted marked improvement after 5 to 10 inhalations of the gas mixture. In June of the same year, a second paper appeared in the same journal discussing the benefit of N_2O-O_2 in abolishing reflex-induced nausea and vomiting in patients, as well as in dogs.[3] Based on these findings, he tested his gas mixture for the treatment of hyperemesis gravidarum. He then began to study the effect of N_2O-O_2 in the *one* situation in which severe pain of short duration develops with regularity, i.e., the birth process. Starting the inhalation at the onset of the uterine contraction and continuing it for the duration, he noted that each of the five women so treated ceased to cry. Consciousness was maintained, permitting use of the auxiliary forces of labor. Maternal and fetal heart rates changed minimally, and the infants were born without any signs of asphyxia.

These two preliminary reports were soon followed by two detailed descriptions of his experiences with a larger number of parturients. The first paper, in Russian, appeared late in 1880 in a collection of essays by physicians of the Institute of the Imperial Medical-Surgical Academy of St. Petersburg (Latest Research in Various Branches of the Medical Sciences), and included 20 parturients.[4] The second paper, in German, was published early in 1881 in the Archives for Gynecology; by then 25 women had been studied. The contents of the two papers are similar, with the exception that the second report contains the results of tocodynamometry in three cases.[5]

Klikovicz manufactured the nitrous oxide himself in a rather complicated process. Suffice it to say, he heated ammonium nitrate to 240° C in a glass retort, purified the evolved gas by passage through two Wolff bottles, and stored the pure gas in a zinc plated gasometer. He then added oxygen to produce a mixture containing 80 percent N_2O and 20 percent O_2. Because of difficulty in placing the gasometer next to the labor bed, he transported the gas mixture in gutta-percha cushions, which he connected via India-rubber tubes with a water-containing, "double-necked" bottle standing next to the parturient's pillow. A second tube, fitted with a wooden or hardrubber mouthpiece, was attached in such a way that the inhaled mixture traversed the water in the bottle. Thus, the gas not only contained oxygen but also was saturated with water vapor, preventing dryness in the throat.[4,5]

Klikovicz wrote that he felt obliged to use this gas mixture on himself to better understand its action. Based on the results, he concluded that, while not totally ideal, there were two undeniable advantages: rapid effect and harmlessness, which should not be denied patients in pain.[4,5]

In both the Russian and the German versions, Klikovicz described his routine in obstetric pain relief as follows: with watch in hand, one must first teach the inhalation of nitrous oxide from the mouthpiece during a painfree interval. One should coach the woman to exhale deeply and then inhale as much gas as possible, because the effect appears faster when the gas remains in the lungs for a longer period of time. One should begin the first anesthesia early in order to attain good pain relief; a late start will prevent the deep inhalation and thus render the effect incomplete. One should also warn the parturient of the possibility of a short-lasting feeling of intoxication. Thereafter, the inhalation is begun at one-half to one minute prior to the anticipated next contraction. Two to five breaths of the gas mixture usually suffice to produce the desired effect. There is no need to use the gas between contractions. Encouraged by the successful pain relief, the parturient will rapidly learn to take deep breaths and to manage the mouthpiece on her own as soon as she feels the impending contraction.[4,5]

Klikovicz also studied the effect of nitrous oxide on the strength, frequency and duration of the uterine contractions. In most women, he accomplished this by manual palpation through the abdominal wall. He soon observed that, in contrast to chloroform, this gas mixture did not alter uterine activity.[4,5] To confirm this finding, he borrowed a tocodynamometer which he employed in three parturients. The longest duration of labor in the three women undergoing tocodynamometry was 2 1/2 hours and, during the entire period, the character of the contractions remained comparable with or without nitrous oxide inhalation.[5]

Concluding, Klikovicz inferred that his 25 cases may not comprise a sufficiently large number to make definitive recommendations. However, there remained no doubt that relief of labor pain was desirable as long as it did not interfere with the birth process, and that the advantages of nitrous oxide-oxygen in obstetrics far outweighed its disadvantages.

He listed the following advantages: 1) it is totally harmless for mother and fetus and does not slow the progress of labor; 2) it undoubtedly relieves the pain in all stages of labor; 3) it causes no loss of consciousness, permitting use of the auxiliary forces of labor; 4) it does not induce nausea, vomiting, headache or excitement; 5) it can be administered throughout labor without cumulative effect consequent to recovery in the intervals between contractions; and 6) it does not require the presence of a physician.

The main disadvantages are its relatively high cost and its lack of portability.[4,5]

References

1. Richards W, Parbrook GD, Wilson J: Stanislav Klikovich (1853-1910). Pioneer of nitrous oxide and oxygen analgesia. Anaesthesia 31:933-40, 1976.
2. Klikowitsch S: Ueber die therapeutische Wirkung des Stickoxyduls bei einigen Krankheiten. St. Petersburger Medizinische Wochenschrift 15:117-8, 1880.
3. Klikowitsch S: Weitere Untersuchungen über die therapeutische Wirkung des Stickoxyduls. St. Petersburger medizinische Wochenschrift 15:249, 1880.
4. Klikovich SK: The use of nitrous oxide for pain control in labor. Latest Research in various Branches of the Medical Sciences (Collection of Essays by Doctors of the Imperial Medical-Surgical Academy). St. Petersburg, XVIL:361-83, 1880. (Translated from Russian)
5. Klikowitsch S: Ueber das Stickoxydul als Anaestheticum bei Geburten. Archiv f. Gynäkologie XVIII:81-108, 1881.

The authors thank the St. Petersburg Public Library and the Library of the New York Academy of Medicine for providing copies of the original articles.

DR. OTOJIRO KITAGAWA, A JAPANESE PIONEER IN THE CLINICAL USE OF INTRATHECAL MORPHINE

AKITOMO MATSUKI
Department of Anesthesiology
University of Hirosaki School of Medicine
Hirosaki, 036 Japan

Introduction

John J. Bonica[1] quotes John Milton's words in his famous book "The Management of Pain," "Pain is perfect miserie, the worst of evils, and excessive, overturns all patience."

These words mean that physicians' true duty and mission are to do their best to attenuate or relieve pain in their patients, not only in the operating theaters, but also in outpatient clinics and surgical wards. Professor James Young Simpson of Edinburgh, the discoverer of chloroform anesthesia, once described human suffering or pain as follows:[2] "I most conscientiously believe that the proud mission of the physician is distinctly two-fold, namely, to alleviate human suffering, as well as preserve human life."

It has been widely accepted that the new era of pain control began when Yaksh et al[3] reported the analgesic effect of intrathecal narcotics in experimental animals in 1976 and when Wang et al[4] applied this method in 1979 to treat eight patients suffering from intractable pain in the back and legs caused by metastatic cancer. However, little is known, even to Japanese medical historians, about a Japanese surgeon who succeeded in producing prolonged pain relief by intrathecal narcotics in his patients about 75 years earlier than Wang et al did.

2. A brief biography of Dr. Otojiro Kitagawa

Otojiro Kitagawa (Fig. 1) was born as the third son of Yadayu Kitagawa in Shiga prefecture of Japan (Fig. 2) on June 17, 1864. In 1881, he went to Tokyo to enter the German language school. At that time, German was the most important foreign language to learn for a physician. Three years later he entered the Faculty of Medicine of Tokyo Imperial University. He studied hard at the University, but he left the faculty in 1887 to go to Germany

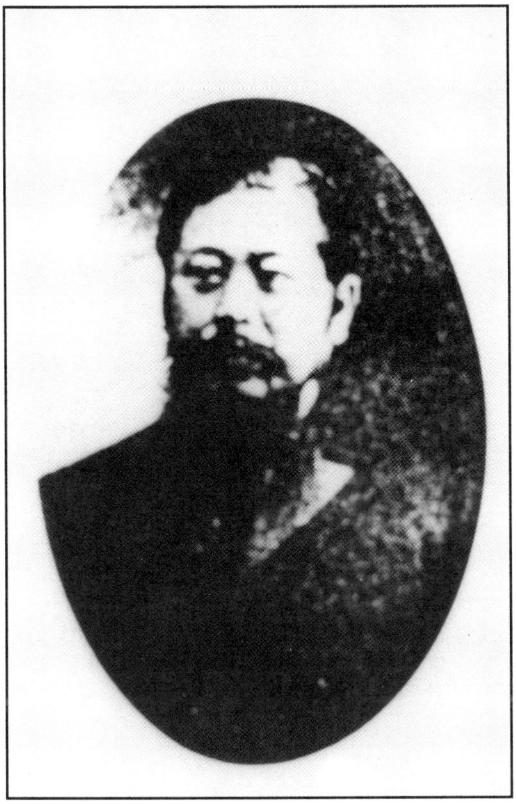

Fig. 1. Portrait of Dr. Kitagawa.

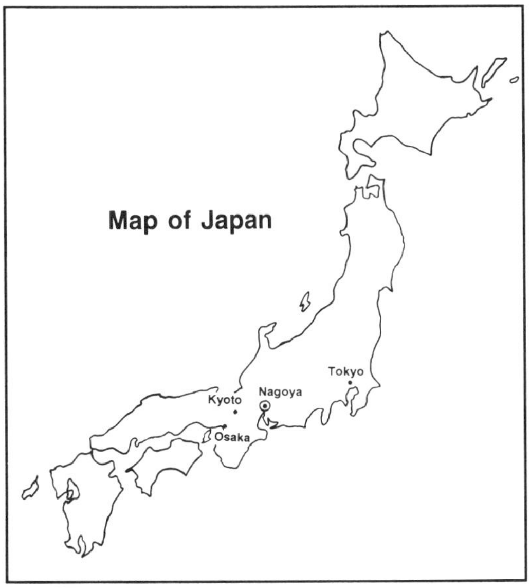

Fig. 1a. Map of Japan.

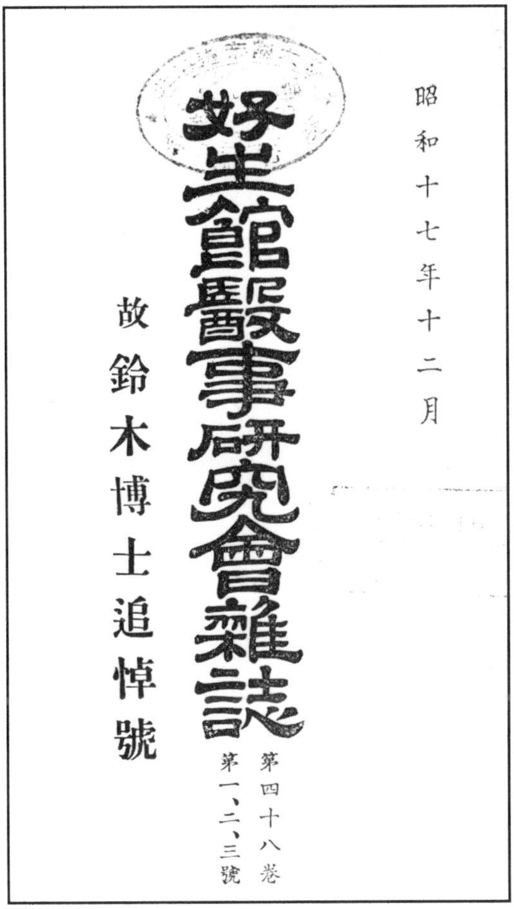

Fig. 2. The last volume of Ko-Sei-Kan Medical Journal.

to study German medicine in depth. He entered the University of Berlin and later the University of Würzburg, where he studied surgery and pathology. Dr. Kitagawa and Dr. Ishiguro, later a Viscount, and the Surgeon-General, stayed in the same apartment house in Berlin. Dr. Ishiguro stayed in Berlin to study the German system of military medicine by order of the War Minister.

Dr. Kitagawa came back to Japan in December, 1899, suffering from a pleuritis. Dr. Ishiguro recommended that he go back to Japan. After six months of recuperation, Dr. Kitagawa was asked by Dr. Ishiguro to take over the directorship of Wakayama Prefectural Hospital in Wakayama City. He worked for the hospital for only one year. He then moved to Nagoya

City to become the director of Nagoya Ko-sei-kan Hospital, replacing Dr. Nobuyuki Yokoi, the director of the hospital and Kitagawa's father-in-law, who had died suddenly in 1891.

He was very active and worked hard as a director, surgeon and clinical investigator, as well as being the administrator of the medical association of both Nagoya City and Aichi prefecture. He was the first in Japan to perform a Gasserian ganglionectomy to relieve trigeminal neuralgia.[5]

In 1895, he founded the Ko-sei-kan medical journal club in his hospital, and also began to publish a Journal, "Ko-sei-kan Journal of Medical Meeting," which included the papers presented at the journal club. The journals were published even after his death in 1922, and the final 48th volume was issued in 1942. He also founded a Pathology Institute in the hospital. He was productive in writing 118 medical papers in his lifetime, most of them concerning surgery an pathology. Dr. Kitagawa was an excellent administrator as well as a surgeon. He was the president of the Medical Association of Nagoya City for 14 years, from 1907 through 1921, and also was the President of the Medical Association of Aichi prefecture for several years from 1909. He died from uremia on Oct. 19, 1922, and was buried at Yakoto cemetery in Nagoya City. The gravestone of his family is located in this cemetery (Fig. 3).

3. Intrathecal morphine for pain relief

Dr. Kitagawa was the first in the world to administer intrathecal morphine successfully in man, as well as the first to perform spinal anesthesia in Japan. In 1899, August Bier[6] of Germany reported the administration of spinal anesthesia with cocaine, and this information was conveyed to Japan four or five months later. As foreign medical journals were brought to Japan by ship at that time, Dr. Kitagawa must have read Bier's paper in the last month of 1900 or in the early months of 1901. As a surgeon, he was much interested in Bier's work and decided to give spinal anesthesia to his patients sometime in 1900 (the exact date is not known to us). He presented the results of his clinical

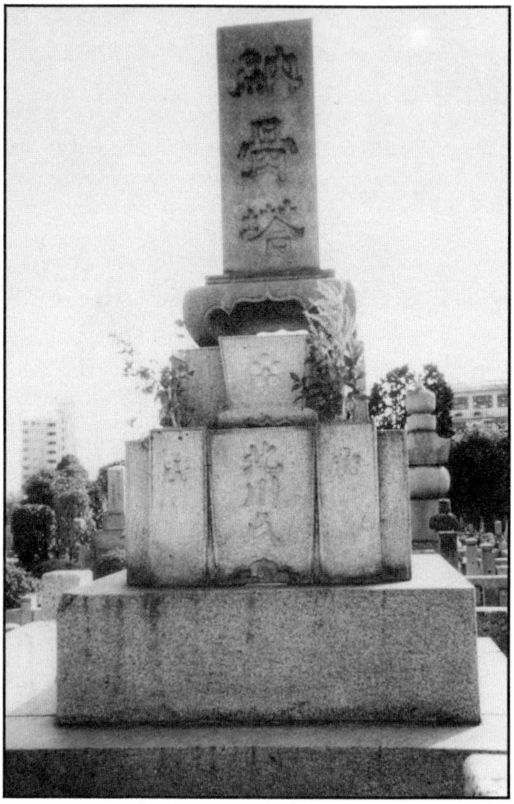

Fig. 3. The gravestone of Dr. Kitigawa in Yakoto Cemetery.

observations at the 3rd annual meeting of the Japanese Society of Surgery on April 2, 1901. His presentation was immediately published in the April 13 issue of the Tokyo Medical Journal, No. 1200, 1901[7]

In the paper, Kitagawa presented a short history of spinal anesthesia in European countries and then referred to six patients he had treated. Their profiles of age, sex, diagnosis, performed operation, local anesthetics used, effect and duration of analgesia were noted. Patients 1, 2, 5 and 6 received spinal anesthesia with either 10-15 mg of cocaine or 20 mg of eucaine for surgical operation. The duration of anesthesia was 30 to 40 minutes for patient 1 and 2, but not known for patient 5 and 6.

Patient 3 was a 33 year-old male suffering from painful lumbar spondylitis. He was given 10 mg of intrathecal morphine in a combination with eucaine 20 mg (the concentration is not known). The effect of analgesia was remarkable and the patient was completely relieved of severe pain for two days. Patient 4 was a 43 year-old female also complaining of low back pain caused by lumbar spondylitis. Kitagawa gave her subarachnoid morphine 10 mg in combination with eucaine 20 mg. Her pain was completely relieved for several days. The spinal was given to these two patients, not for producing surgical anesthesia, but for the definite purpose of pain relief only. Each 10 mg of morphine would have been enough to

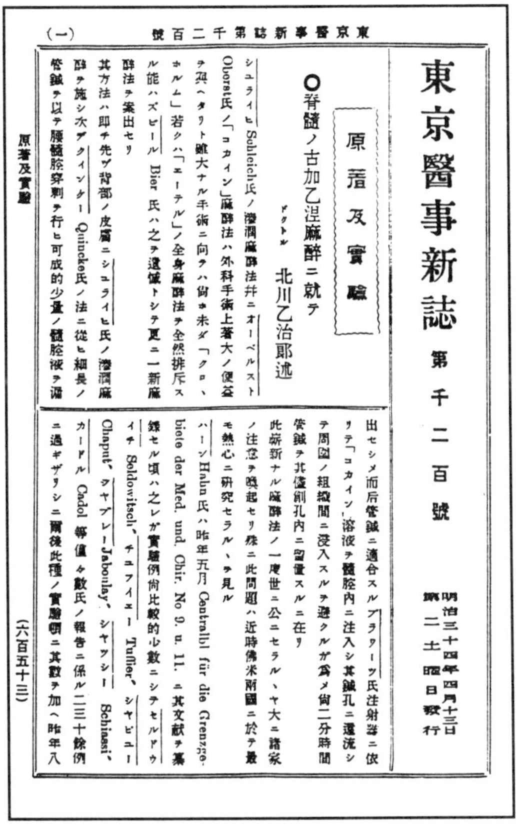

(一)　東京醫事新誌第千二百號

東京醫事新誌　第千二百號

明治三十四年四月十三日　土曜日發行

原著及實驗

○脊髓ノ古加乙涅麻醉ニ就テ

ドクトル　北川乙治郎述

シュライヒSchleich氏ノ浸潤麻醉法幷ニオーベルストOberst氏ノ「コカイン」麻醉法ハ外科手術上著大ノ便益ヲ與ヘタリト雖大ナル手術ニ向テハ尚ホ未ダ「クロヽホルム」若クハ「エーテル」ノ全身麻醉法ヲ全然排斥スル能ハズビールBier氏ハ之ヲ遺憾トシテ更ニ一新麻醉法ヲ案出セリ

其方法ハ即チ先ヅ背部ノ皮膚ニシュライヒ氏ノ浸潤麻醉ヲ施シ次ヅクインケーQuincke氏ノ法ニ從ヒ細長ノ管鍼ヲ以テ腰髓腔穿刺ヲ行ヒ可成的少量ノ髓腔液ヲ漏出セシメ而后管鍼ニ適合スルプラワーツ氏注射器ニ依リテ「コカイン」溶液ヲ髓腔内ニ注入シ其鍼孔ニ還流シテ周圍ノ組織間ニ浸入スルヲ避クルガ爲メ尚二分時間管鍼ヲ其儘鍼孔内ニ留置スルニ在リ

此嶄新ナル麻醉法ノ一度世ニ公ニセラルヽヤ大ニ諸家ノ注意ヲ喚起セリ殊ニ此問題ハ近時佛米兩國ニ於テ最モ熱心ニ研究セラルヽヲ見ル

ハーンHahn氏ハ昨年五月Centralbl für die Grenzgebiete der Med. und Chir. No 9. u. 11. ニ其文獻ヲ纂錄セル頃ハ之レガ實驗例尚比較的少數ニシテセルドウイチSoldowitsch、チュフイエーTuffier、シャピユーChaput、ヂャブレーJaboulay、シャアシーSchiassi、カードルCadol等僅々數氏ノ報告ニ係ル二三十餘例ニ過ギザリシニ爾後此種ノ實驗例ニ其數ヲ加ヘ昨年八

原著及實驗　(六百五十三)

Fig. 4. Dr. Kitagawa's original paper.

produce profound respiratory depression in the above two patients, but they did not develop any respiratory depression. A possible reason for this was that, because a large sized spinal needle was used, there was leakage of the cerebrospinal fluid containing morphine from the subarachnoid space to the epidural space and the neighboring tissues.

The author believes that Dr. Kitagawa must have known that intrathecal morphine was effective for pain attenuation and not for surgical anesthesia. This belief was clearly substantiated by Kitagawa's comment[8] on Dr. Omi's paper[9] on spinal anesthesia which was presented at the 5th annual meeting of the Japanese Society of Surgery. He says as follows: "As I have seen many complications following spinal anesthesia, we should be more careful in giving it. But this method is very effective for pain relief in patients with ishias."

As he had experienced many complications, such as headache, following spinal anesthesia, he gave it up. Before 1901, he had experience with several thousand general anesthetics with ether or chloroform without any severe and fatal complications. He had an impression that general anesthesia was far better than spinal anesthesia.

In 1911, Dr. Ueno[10] presented a review article on spinal anesthesia at the 12th annual meeting of the Japanese Society of Surgery, and he concluded that spinal anesthesia should be limited only to surgical operations of the lower half of the body.

About 30 years passed without any important advance in spinal anesthesia in Japan until Dr. Makoto Saito (1889-1950), professor of surgery, University of Nagoya, and his disciple, Dr. Park, proposed using a hyperbaric solution and controlling the level of anesthesia by tilting the operating table. He made the hyperbaric solution with 10 percent glucose. Dr. Park presented their method at the 41st annual meeting of the Japanese Society of Surgery on April 8, 1940. Saito's method with dibucaine in 10 percent glucose has been widely accepted all over the country.[11]

Japanese anesthesiology was far behind that of the United States at the end of World War II in 1945. In July, 1950, Dr. Saklad of Rhode Island Hospital came to Japan as a member of the medical mission of the Unitarian Service and introduced endotracheal anesthesia, closed and semi-closed systems using soda lime, and continuous spinal anesthesia.[12] All these techniques were new to Japanese physicians. However, so far as hyperbaric spinal anesthesia was concerned, there was not a big gap between the two countries.

4. Conclusion

A brief biography of a Japanese surgeon, Otojiro Kitagawa, is described. He was the first physician to give intrathecal morphine to attenuate severe pain in man in the world, and he was also the first to perform spinal anesthesia in Japan.

It was fortunate for him that he gave up intrathecal morphine soon after his trial in two patients because he had no effective measure to overcome respira-tory depression, which might have occurred after 10 mg of intrathecal morphine.

References

1. Bonica JJ: The Management of Pain. (second edition) Philadelphia, Lea and Febiger, p 203, 1990.
2. Simpson JY: On a new anaesthetic agent, more efficient than sulphuric ether. *Lancet* II:549-50, 1847.
3. Yaksch TL, Ruty TA: Studies on the direct spinal action of narcotics in the production of analgesia in the rat. *J. Pharmacol Exp Therap* 202:411-28, 1976.
4. Wang JK, Nauss LA, Thomas JE: Pain relief by intrathecal applied morphine in man. *Anesthesiology* 50:149-51, 1979.
5. Kitagawa O: A case report of Gasserian ganglionectomy for severe trigeminal neuralgia. *Tokyo Med J* 1123:1745-51, 1899.
6. Bier A: Versuche über Cocainisirung des Rückenmarkes. Deutsche Zeitschrift für Chirurgie 51:361-9, 1899.
7. Kitagawa O: On spinal anesthesia with cocaine. *J Jap Soc Surg* 3:185-91, 1901.
8. Kitagawa O: Comment on Dr. Omi's paper of spinal anesthesia. J Jap Soc Surg 5:303-4, 1904.
9. Omi K: On spinal anesthesia. *J Jap Soc Surg* 5:284-305, 1904.
10. Ueno S: Local anesthesia. *J Jap Soc Surg* 12:129-69, 1911.
11. Matsuki A (ed): Monograph of Japanese History of Anesthesiology. Vol. 4, History of spinal and epidural anesthesia. Tokyo, Kokuseido, 1990.
12. Fujita T, Matsuki A (eds): Monograph of Japanese History of Anesthesiology. Vol 3, Dr. Saklad and Japanese Anesthesiology, Tokyo, Kokuseido, 1989.

THE DEVELOPMENT OF ANAESTHESIA IN ZIMBABWE

A. G. McKENZIE
Division of Anaesthetics,
Parirenyatwa Hospital, Harare, Zimbabwe

Early Days

Thomas Morgan Thomas, one of the first missionaries to settle in Zimbabwe (in 1859), recorded that the indigenous African people knew of the medicinal qualities of local herbs and trees. They brewed beer from indigenous corn, millet or maize, and some smoked Isangu (wild hemp, dagga), becoming "stupefied or intoxicated by the narcotic fumes."[1] Cupping (blood letting)[2] and extraction of teeth[3] were performed, but I have found no records of intoxicants being administered to relieve the pain of such surgery. A measure of local anesthesia seems to have been available in the form of powdered roots for relief of toothache.[4] (See Table I).[5] Probably the first general anesthetic on Zimbabwean soil was administered by one of the early missionaries: they had undergone a six month course of basic medical practice before leaving England.[3] The wife of the Rev. C.D. Helm, who went to Hope Fountain Mission in 1875, is recorded to have administered chloroform to a patient,[6] though the date is unstated.

Under the British South Africa Company: 1890-1923

The bulk of the Pioneer Column set off from Macloutsie (in Botswana) on 27 June, 1890, and arrived at "Fort Salisbury" on 11 September. Medical men were included by Rhodes and in surgery they had learned the use of anesthesia.[3] There was a "well-fitted ambulance" wagon drawn by oxen,[3] but I have been unable to find details of the medical stores carried. Fortunately, the health of the Pioneers during the journey was excellent[7] and there is no record of any requirement for anesthesia along the way.

Two men were documented users of anesthesia in 1891, namely, Dr. Richard Frank Rand and John Strachan. On 15 May Dr. Rand used chloroform to anesthetize John Cooper-Chadwick, whose badly injured hands had to be amputated. The operation, which lasted three and a half fours, was performed under candlelight at the recently founded Salisbury Hospital.[9] Dr. Rand,[3,10] (Fig. 1.) from Essex, England, came to South Africa in 1889. On the invitation of Rhodes he became Surgeon

TABLE I

MEDICAL PLANTS USED TOPICALLY FOR TOOTHACHE

INDIGENOUS NAMES	ENGLISH NAME	BOTANICAL NAME	FAMILY	ACTIVE PRINCIPLE
MAPFUTA MUPFUTA	CASTOR OIL PLANT	RICINUS COMMUNIS	EUPHORBIACEAE	?
MUPFENJE MUFENJE	CABBAGE TREE	CUSSONIA ARBOREA	ARALIACEAE	?
METETI MUTITI	LUCKY BEAN TREE	ERYTHRINA LIVINGSTONIANA ERUTHRINA ABYSSINICUM	LEGUMINOSAE (FABACEAE)	?
NHUNDURWA MUNHUNDURWA	APPLE OF SODOM	SOLANUM DELAGOENSE S. INCANUM S. PANDURIFORME	SOLANACEAE	SOLANINE MAY CONTAIN SMALL AMOUNTS OF OTHER ATROPINE-LIKE SUBSTANCES*

* Atropine (d 1- hyoscyamine) has local anesthetic activity, about half that of procaine.

Captain to the B.S.A. Co.'s Police and accompanied the Pioneer Column to Fort Salisbury. There he took charge of the (only) hospital and remained Police Surgeon until he resigned in 1892, when he entered private practice.

John Strachan,[4] a Scot, used nitrous oxide for painless extraction of teeth. He qualified as a Chemist and Druggist in 1878 and also trained in dentistry at Guy's Dental Hospital. Early 1891 he left Johannesburg, South Africa, for Salisbury (now Harare). Very heavy rains were in full force at the time, and his journey was delayed by swollen rivers.[11] He passed through posts of the B.S.A. Co.'s Police en route and was consulted 'on the road' by a number of patients needing teeth extracted. He had with him some bottles of compressed nitrous oxide gas.[3] Strachan's wagon, stocked with drugs and chemists' requirements, arrived in Salisbury at the end of July, 1891.[3] He set up practice in a

Fig. 1. Dr. R.F. Rand MB, CM FRCS (Eng.), MD (Edin). *Reproduced from "Tropical Victory" (M. Gelfand) by kind permission of Mrs. E. Gelfand.*

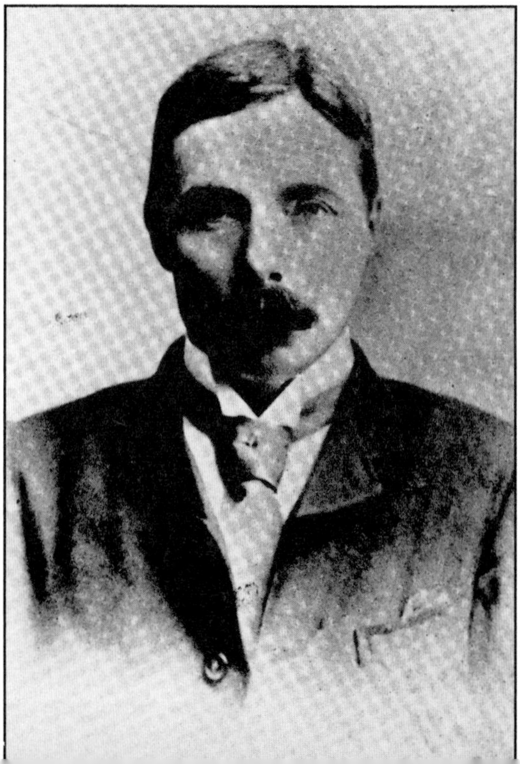

pole and dagga hut, the "Lion Dispensary," (Fig. 2), which displayed his chemist and dentist sign. His advertisement in the Mashonaland Herald of 15 August, 1891, read, "painless extractions by means of nitrous oxide (or laughing gas)."

In 1904 an American dentist, Dr. Westcott Byron-Moore, came to practice in Southern Rhodesia. He used nitrous oxide which he made on his own premises. He also tried local anesthesia using cocaine tablets — injecting the drug around a tooth to be extracted. Unfortunately this technique often resulted in sore gums and sloughing in the sockets. The use of nitrous oxide alone was far from ideal: with the methods of administration available at the time, it afforded only about one minute of good anesthesia. In 1910 Byron-Moore visited America and brought back information on improved techniques. Firstly, he learned how to prolong the duration of general anesthesia (up to three to five minutes) by passing the nitrous oxide gas through three wash bottles, the last of which contained an ounce of each chloroform and alcohol. The final gas mixture of nitrous oxide plus chloroform was called vitalized air. Secondly, he started to use procaine for "conductive anesthesia," preparing his own injections by dissolving procaine tablets in water.[4]

One of the earliest medical practitioners to devote a considerable amount of time to anesthesia was Dr. N.S. MacNaughton, who was registered in Southern Rhodesia in 1912.[12] He later became expert in the use of the Shipway apparatus.[13] He was joined in 1919 by Dr. J.E. Hurworth in what was known as the Huggins medical partnership.[14]

Southern Rhodesia ("Responsible Government"): 1923-1953

In 1926, Dr. Hurworth was appointed as Anaesthetist at the Salisbury Hospital, this probably being the first such post in the country.[15] In the 1930's, Dr. Hurworth gave the majority of anesthetics in Salisbury (Fig. 3.), though he continued his general practice.[13] Some interesting observations on anesthesia in the 1930's and 40's are to be found in the late Professor Gelfand's book, "A Service to the Sick" (1976, Mambo Press).[16] Mr. Barton Gilbert related his impression of the anesthetic room at the Salisbury African Hospital in 1943. There was a Boyle's machine, Clover's bag anesthetic apparatus, and bottles of chloroform and ether. He recalled that the "rag and bottle" method of anesthesia was commonly used at that time. He also recorded a case of cardiac arrest following induction of anesthesia with chloroform. Ether was difficult to use in the warm climate, because it evaporated rapidly and ice tended to form all over the mask. Most Government Medical Officers serving in the

Fig. 2 Strachan's chemist shop and dental practice: *circa* 1891.
Strachan's Photo Pharmacy (Pvt.) Ltd.

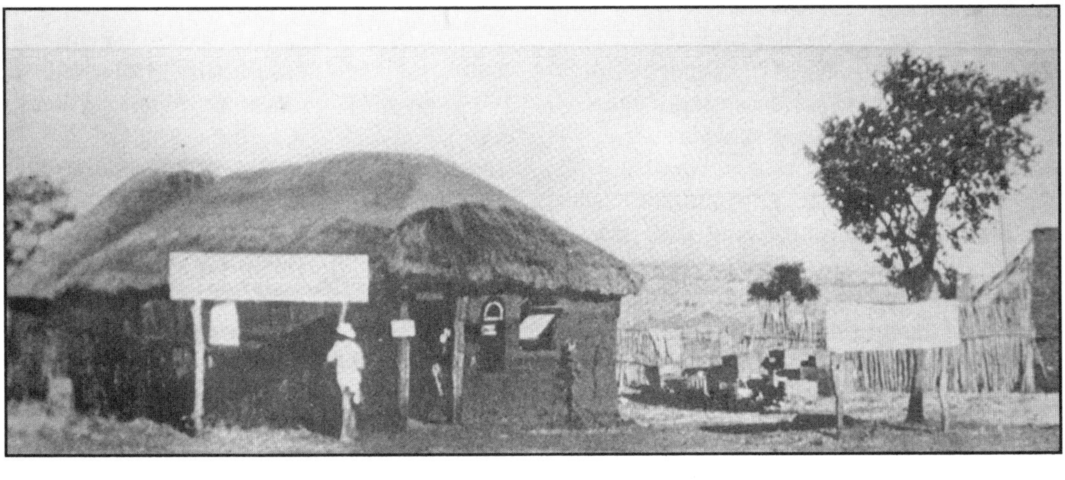

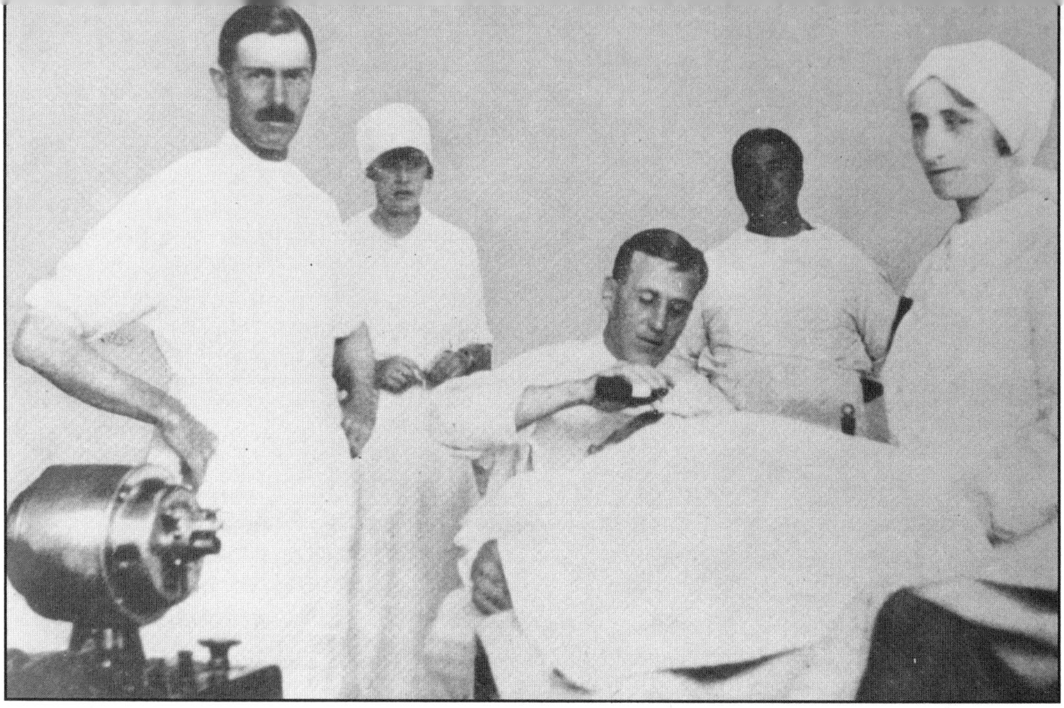

Fig. 3 The operating theatre of the Salisbury Hospital in 1924. While the surgeon, Dr. Huggins looks on, the anaesthetist, Dr. Hurworth, is administering a volatile anaesthetic, probably chloroform. This he is most likely dripping onto a Schimmelbusch mask (not visible) — the "rag and bottle" method. *Reproduced from "Tropical Victory" (M. Gelfand) by kind permission of Mrs. E. Gelfand.*

1930's and 40's gave anesthetics from time to time. In some rural areas in the 1930's, relatives or friends of patients had to be enrolled to act as anesthetists. As time passed Nursing Assistants and Medical Assistants were taught to give anesthetics.[16]

It is pertinent to look at the health services present in the country at that time.

In 1950 Dr. G.V.S. Wright (D.A. Eng.) arrived and was the first man in Souther Rhodesia to devote himself full time to anesthetics.[17] He recalls that when he arrived the standard of anesthetics was mediocre (though it improved to a high standard a decade later). He was horrified to find patients being strapped to the operating table with a wide band of webbing prior to induction. The usual anesthetic technique in 1950 was intravenous induction with thiopental and maintenance with nitrous oxide-oxygen-ether or cyclopropane. The cylinders of anesthetic gases came by rail from Johannesburg, South Africa, often getting lost in transit. Thus there were often shortages of oxygen and/or nitrous oxide and/or cyclopropane. On one occasion there was only one cylinder of oxygen in Salisbury. Consequently, the anesthetists often resorted to "rag and bottle." A fair number of spinal anesthetics were also given at that time. Muscle relaxants had just been introduced. The anesthetists used to collect blood for operations and did the blood grouping and cross-matching themselves.

Federation of Rhodesia and Nyasaland: 1953-1963

In 1958 halothane was introduced into anesthetic practice in Southern Rhodesia, since when it has remained the most commonly used volatile anesthetic in the country. Dr. G.V.S. Wright was probably the first to use it.[18] He also instigated (in the same year) the formation of the Association of Anaesthetists of Rhodesia.[19]

In 1959 local manufacture of oxygen was commenced (OXYCO: personal communication). Also Dr. Wright introduced the technique of hypothermia for "open heart surgery,"[20] having acquired the know-how on a visit to Denver. In 1962 he visited Boston and brought back a Foregger machine with which extra-corporeal work was commenced[17] (but continued for only a few years).

The country's first Medical School was opened in 1963.

Southern Rhodesia/Rhodesia: 1964-1979

Intensive care had its beginnings in 1966 when Dr. R.A. Cahi (Government Specialist Anesthetist at Harare Central Hospital) decided to ventilate a child with tetanus. The child was kept in a side-room adjoining the operating theaters (personal communication). Following this episode Intensive Care Units were established.

The commercial manufacture of nitrous oxide in Rhodesia began in 1971 (OXYCO: personal communication).

In 1975 a Chair and Department of Anesthetics were created within the University Faculty of Medicine: Dr. A.K. Duthie was appointed the first Professor.[21] Taking cognizance of the shortage of anesthetists, the Ministry of Health launched a Nurse Anesthetist Diploma Course in July, 1978. The Course Director from the beginning until this day has been Mrs. M. Bagorro, Sister Tutor (personal communication).

Zimbabwe: 1980-1990 — A Decade of Majority Rule

From the anesthesia viewpoint, the most significant events in this period occurred in the University Department of Anesthetics. In 1985, Professor E.M. Chinyanga was appointed to the Chair, and the following year he launched a one-year course for registered medical practitioners leading to a Zimbabwean D.A. Besides providing tangible evidence of competence in safe anesthetic practice, this D.A. provided a basis for selection of candidates for a Zimbabwean M. Med. (Anaesth.) Course. The latter, a three-year course in two parts, commenced in 1988,[22] and five candidates were accepted at the inception of the Course. Out of these, two presented at the final examination in November, 1990, and both were successful.

In 1989, an open-heart surgery program was restarted,[23] this having been dormant for some 25 years. (In the previous year, the feasibility of such a program had been demonstrated by a team from Loma Linda University.)[24] The anesthetic demands have been well met by the University Department in Harare. Paradoxically, while there is this level of expertise in the capital city, anesthetics at some rural hospitals are still given by staff with no formal training in anesthesia. (Table II.).

TABLE II

Anesthetic Drugs Commonly Used in Zimbabwe (1991)

VOLATILE ANESTHETICS;	
	Halothane
	Trichlorethylene
INTRAVENOUS ANESTHETICS	
	Thiopental
	Ketamine
	Etomidate
MUSCLE RELAXANTS:	
	Suxamenthonium
	Alcuronium
	Tubocurarine
ANALAGESICS:	
	MEPERIDINE
	MORPHINE
	PARACETAMOL
LOCAL ANESTHETICS;	
	Lignocaine
	Bupivacaine

References

1. Thomas TM: Eleven Years in Central South Africa. Bulawayo: Books of Zimbabwe (Reprint); 87, 178-80, 300, 1970.
2. Varian HF: Some African Milestones. Bulawayo: Books of Zimbabwe (Reprint); 192, 1973.
3. Gelfand K: Tropical Victory. Cape Town: Juta; 7, 11, 14, 26-27, 33, 40-41, 1953.
4. Gelfand M: Early Rhodesian Dentists. Central African Journal of Medicine; 7:363-71, 1961.
5. Gelfand M, Mavi S, Drummond RB, Ndemera B: The Traditional Medical Practitioner in Zimbabwe. Gweru: Mambo Press; 322-24, 1985.
6. Lovemore JC (Mrs, nee Helm) in First Steps in Civilizing Rhodesia: by Jeannie M. Boggie. Bulaway: Philpott & Collins; 87, 1953.
7. Johnson F: Great Days. Bulawayo: Books of Zimbabwe (Reprint); 160, 333, 336, 1972.
8. Leonard AG: How We Made Rhodesia. Bulawayo: Books of Zimbabwe (Reprint); 31, 1973.

9. Cooper-Chadwick J: Three Years with Lobengula. London: Cassell; 152, 1894.
10. Rande RF: Reminiscences of Salisbury. National Archives of Zimbabwe: Historical Manuscripts Collection: SA 12/1/14.
11. Brown WH: On the South African Frontier. London: Sampson Low, Marston & Co.; 162, 1899.
12. National Archives of Zimbabwe: Public Health Department: 1891-1923: H5/2/3: Registers: Medical Practitioners.
13. Martin AP: Anaesthetics in Salisbury. (Letter to the Editor). Central African Journal of Medicine; 1:195-6, 1955.
14. Obituary: Dr. J.E. Hurworth. Rhodesia Herald. 19 April 1938; page 8, column 4.
15. National Archives of Zimbabwe: Ministry of Health, Correspondence, General, 1908-39:S1173/167: Salisbury Hospital, July 1925-December 1926.
16. Gelfand M: A Service to the Sick. Gweru: Mambo Press; 60, 85-88, 131, 134, 136, 138, 141, 143, 159, 1976.
17. Wright GVS: in The Nuffield Department of Anaesthetics, Oxford: 1937-1962: Jubilee Subscription Volume: compiled and edited by R. Bryce-Smith, J.V. Mitchell and J. Parkhouse. Oxford: University Press: 108-9, 1963.
18. Wright GVS: Halothane, A New Anaesthetic Agent. Central African Journal of Medicine; 4:233-5, 1958.
19. Editorial: The Association of Anaesthetists of Mashonaland. Central African Journal of Medicine; 4:135, 1958.
20. Micklem NJ, Wright GVS: Hypothermia for Pulmonary Valvotomy. Central African Journal of Medicine; 5:4667, 1959.
21. University of Zimbabwe: Records of the Secretary to the School of Medicine (with permission).
22. Chinyanga HM, Haisma H, Clark N: Progress in Postgraduate Training in Anaesthetics for Doctors in Zimbabwe. Central African Journal of Medicine; 35:420-1, 1989.
23. Marks C: Essentials of Open Heart Surgery. Central African Journal of Medicine; 36:76-83, 1990.
24. Abson P: Obituary: The Late Dr. Baldachin. Central African Journal of Medicine; 34:278, 1988.

HENRY KNOWLES BEECHER
A Man of Controversy

ELLIOTT V. MILLER
Massachusetts General Hospital
Harvard Medical School
Boston, Massachusetts, USA

Henry Knowles Beecher spent nearly all of his professional life as Anesthetist-in-Chief at Massachusetts General Hospital. He was a man of controversy. Another, and very apt, title he received is that of "Whistleblower" in the book, Strangers at the Bedside, published in 1991 by David J. Rothman.[1] As an example of controversy, many of you present here knew him and a few will probably disagree with some of the things I will say about him. I extend my great thanks to many of you who have provided me with specific information and some personal reminiscences about him.

Beecher, as a man of controversy, seemed to enjoy a serious and good fray, and the issues he chose to do battle over were almost always important. In science and in politics he was a great street fighter. In social gatherings, he was gracious and charming. Myron Laver, a colleague at MGH and later Professor at Basel, helped write a Memorial Minute and put it similarly: "In Science he was a Cyclops; in social life, a Bacchus."

Beecher was born in 1904 in Kansas under another name. I will leave it to you to hypothesize why he changed his name and whether his natural name loomed greater and more true than his adopted name. Beecher did all of his undergraduate work and graduate education in Kansas until he entered Harvard Medical School in the class of 1932. His classmates readily recall him. He then entered the surgical training program at the Massachusetts General Hospital (MGH) on the renowned West Service. Edward D. Churchill was Surgeon-in-Chief and a mentor to Beecher through most of his career. After two years of surgical training, he became a Moseley Travelling Fellow and spent a year with Professor August Krogh in Copenhagen. He returned to MGH for a final year in Surgery.

Churchill needed a Chief of Anesthesia. Several candidates were considered, including

Ralph Waters of Wisconsin. Beecher got the job, even though he was not trained in anesthesia. Julia Arrowood was a department member at the time and undoubtedly helped him. He was mostly self-taught and this dogged him through his career. He had a heavy hand when it came to pouring ether, which caused discomfort to the staff and residents who relieved him as he moved quickly from case to case administering anesthesia to important persons. But his charm and heavy ether delighted the ladies from Beacon Hill, who had a long sleep and little pain or recall. To them he was a wonderful anesthetist.

His first major text, "Physiology of Anesthesia," appeared in 1938.[2] He observed respiratory acidosis in patients breathing spontaneously during thoracotomies.[3] World War II came and Beecher became a Lieutenant-Colonel in the European Theater. Here he made other important observations, such as the morphine poisoning that occurred after adequate circulation was restored in wounded soldiers.[4] His observations on the psychologic components of pain were monumental.[5] At the Anzio Beachhead, he noted the wounded soldiers had no pain or needed little morphine.[6] Beecher quickly reasoned that the wounded soldiers knew they were alive and that their injuries were a ticket away from the war.

In the 1950's, he continued his work on pain and analgesics. He demonstrated repeatedly that placebos were "active" compounds.[7] A placebo would relieve pain as would morphine, but was markedly different. Beecher then encouraged the inclusion of a placebo in many new drug trials. This was not a uniform practice for many other workers, He was so taken with this concept that he wrote an article on some operations that seemed to have only a placebo effect, such as internal mammary artery ligation for the treatment of angina pectoris.[8] Beecher, our man of controversy, did little to endear himself to many surgeons as he wrote of the placebo effect of some surgical procedures.

His work in narcotics carried him into other interesting areas. Along with many others, he investigated narcotics antagonists as analgesics.

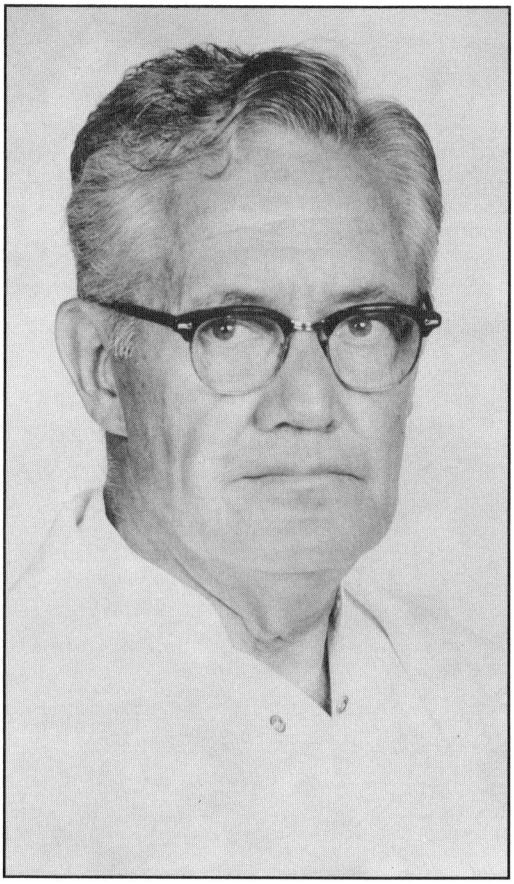

Fig. 1. Henry Knowles Beecher, (1904-1976).

He reasoned that this was a fruitful avenue since respiratory depression and addiction would probably be less of a problem. A major thesis was that narcotic analgesics did not remove postoperative pain, but rather changed the persons response to the pain.

In July of 1954, he published the now famous Beecher-Todd Report titled, "A Study of the Deaths Associated with Anesthesia and Surgery."[9] It was widely read and raised the issue that "death from anesthesia is of sufficient magnitude to constitute a public health problem."

He especially warned about the use of muscle relaxants. His colleagues in anesthesia were highly annoyed when they learned from their surgeon friends that Beecher had the gall to first publish it in Annals of Surgery rather than in an anesthesia journal. Sixteen well-known anesthesiologists wrote a 7-page critique in an attempt to refute many of his arguments. They were successful in one particular point, as is obvious in the particular statement Beecher made, "All of this adds up to the possibility that the real problem here is inherent toxicity of the muscle relaxants studied."

In 1953 and 1954, Beecher helped found the Association of University Anesthetists (now Anesthesiologists), mainly in association with Emmanuel Papper and Robert Dripps. The AUA continues to be strong, active and growing. Curiously, this also was controversial to many leading officers of the American Society of Anesthesiologists, wherein the only acceptable form of practice was fee for service. Beecher had his department on salaries.

Beecher published an article in 1966 which changed the world of human biologic research. He published "Ethics and Clinical Research" in the June 16 issue of the New England Journal of Medicine.[10] He mentioned 22 research papers (unidentified in his paper) wherein serious ethical errors in consent of the research subjects occurred. All were by prominent researchers and in prominent journals, no less than six were from the New England Journal of Medicine itself. His main thesis was that informed consent had not been obtained and that the procedures were not done for the possible benefit of the individuals. This paper caused a firestorm of wrath in the United States. But all of you here know that this condition is not tolerated today. In fact, Beecher was thereby the father of the Institutional Review Board for new research projects. Informed consent must be obtained in human research today.

This firestorm had not subsided before Beecher was again working on a controversial area. He chaired a Harvard Medical School ad hoc Committee and published this report, "A Definition of Irreversible Coma," in the JAMA, August, 1968.[11] Many groups favored care of indefinite duration, even in the presence of a persistent vegetative state. Now Beecher had stirred many legal and religious figures to oppose him. Surely, turning off the ventilator would be considered murder. Nevertheless, Beecher led the charge into this fray.

His last great adventure has a year of prologue and a very clear beginning. In May of 1972, a mass related to his distal ileum was found, which brought a close to the final life chapter four years later. He faced it all directly and courageously. He was willing to let his illness be open to public scrutiny and, one can read about it in great detail in the Case Records of Massachusetts General Hospital in the New England Journal of Medicine, August 23, 1973, wherein he is the subject of the Clinical Pathologic Conference.[12]

The honorary degrees and awards bestowed on Beecher are too many to detail here. They come to him from all over the world. I will mention that he was an Honorary Fellow in the Royal Society of Medicine (limited to 100) and Chevalier of the Legion of Honor. He was a citizen of the world, beloved by many and a thorn in the flesh of a few. He inspired either strong loyalty or animosity, loved power politics, and changed the world for us all. But, back to an early thread in our story. What was the family name to which Henry Knowles Beecher was born? It was Unangst, which if there were such a regular word in German, would mean "without fear." He lived a fearless life as a physician and scientist. He seemed fearless as he faced death. He was larger than life in many ways that were not appreciated by even those who saw him frequently.

(See References on next page).

References

1. Rothman DJ: Strangers at The Bedside, A History of How Bioethics Transformed Medical Decision Making. Basic Books, 1991.
2. Beecher HK: Physiology of Anesthesia. New York: Oxford University Press, 1938.
3. Beecher HK, Murphy AJ: Acidosis during thoracic surgery. J Thorac Surg 19: 50-70, 1950.
4. Beecher, HK: Delayed morphine poisoning in battle casualties. JAMA 124: 1193-4, 1944.
5. Beecher HK: Measurement of subjective responses. Quantitative effects of drugs. New York. Oxford University Press, 1959.
6. Beecher HK: Pain in men wounded in battle. Ann Surg 123:96-105, 1946.
7. Beecher HK: The powerful placebo. JAMA 159: 1602-6, 1955.
8. Beecher HK: Surgery as placebo. A quantitative study of bias. JAMA 176: 1102-7, 1961.
9. Beecher HK, Todd DP: A study of deaths associated with anesthesia and surgery. Ann Surg 140: 2-34, 1954.
10. Beecher HK: Ethics and clinical research. NEJM 274: 1354-60, 1966.
11. Beecher HK, et al: A Definition of Irreversible Coma. Report of the Ad Hoc Committee of the Harvard Medical School to Examine the Definition of Brain Death. JAMA 205:337-40, 1968.
12. Case records of the Massachusetts General Hospital. NEJM 289:419-24, 1973.

BASIC SCIENCE ROOTS OF CLINICAL ANESTHESIOLOGY

LUCIEN E. MORRIS
Bainbridge Island, Washington, USA

There is a tendency to feel that progress to the present status, if cause and effect are recognized at all, has been on the basis solely of anesthesiologists' own effort and struggle. Not so — we are in debt to many "assists" along the way from interested, sympathetic and politically helpful colleagues including:

a. Administrators — for example: I think of Gus H. Frankel, the founding Dean of the Medical School at Flinders University in South Australia, and Charles Bardeen, original Dean at the University of Wisconsin, who each facilitated remarkable developments in anesthesia.
b. Among the surgeons, good examples of those who helped the progress of anesthesiology are Ravdin at University of Pennsylvania and Schmidt at University of Wisconsin.
c. Numerous physicians from neurology, cardiology and pulmonary medicine have been helpful.
d. Basic scientists— especially evident are those from Pharmacology and Physiology.

It is my purpose to call attention to events and factors less appreciated, and especially to people, some of whom are today relatively unknown or mostly forgotten, who contributed in important ways to the development of the clinical specialities, and particularly to the establishment of anesthesiology as a respected clinical entity. Indeed, I believe that it was largely individuals from the basic medical sciences who recognized the need for development of academic anesthesia, attended its birthing process, and have also repeatedly extended a helping hand during the maturation years.

Sixty to one hundred years ago anesthesia was generally viewed as a merely technical exercise. Despite the relatively high incidence of apparently inevitable complications and death, few medical leaders in the United States felt the subject worthy of the attention and special interest of a physician. Even in the British medical spheres, although there anesthetics were administered by physicians, the concerns of anesthetic practice were largely technical, as revealed in the textbooks and journals of that time. Anesthetics was not in the medical curriculum despite cogent pleas for its inclusion by F.W. Silk in 1892 and Dudley Buxton in 1900.

It was in 1927 that Ralph Milton Waters joined the new clinical faculty of the University of Wisconsin Medical School in Madison. Waters had arrived at Madison with an innovative spirit and a deep curiosity about questions which had arisen in his more than ten years of previous clinical practice as a specialist anesthetist. One of his motivations to move from an established comfortable practice in Kansas City was the exciting prospect of potential collaboration with the physiologists, pharmacologists and others in the university environment at Wisconsin.

It was Dr. Waters' stated objective to teach doctors, who would go forth to teach other doctors the scientific basis for the safe practice of clinical anesthesia. That this first truly academic postgraduate anesthesia program had a tremendous impact on the growth and development of clinical anesthesiology in North America is well established. Indeed, the academic department at Wisconsin quickly became a model for both undergraduate and resident teaching, which was emulated ultimately by others and was thereby a stimulus to the development of anesthesiology throughout the world. This includes the well-known Oxford University Department, which, as I saw it during WWII, clearly reflected both flavor and organization traits adapted from Wisconsin as a result of R.R. Macintosh's visits to both Madison and NYU Bellevue Hospital, where Emery Rovenstine, Waters' eminent disciple, held forth.

Visitors flooded upon the anesthesia center at Madison. Among the earliest of these in 1930 was Geoffrey Kaye of Melbourne who had been stimulated and guided in his anesthesia interests by Francis McMechan when they met at the time of the 1929 BMA meeting in Australia. Other prominent visitors to Madison in the 1930's included Gilbert Brown, Gillert Troup, and Stuart Marshall of Australia. Ivan Magill, Edgar Pask, Stanley Sykes and Michael Nosworthy were among the prominent guests from England. Ultimately, visitors and students came from many other areas of the world as well.

Waters' tremendous impact on the development of anesthesiology was due largely to his insistence on exploration of the scientific principles basic to clinical practice questions, as well as the undoubted force of his personal dynamics. He sought and obtained supportive cooperation *from* and correlated investigative activity *with* several senior faculty from the basic science disciplines, to the benefit of participating clinical trainees at a time 20 to 40 years before it became a popular mode to include basic science research experience in residency training. The collaborative effort of Wisconsin workers added significantly to the knowledge base for the study and practice of anesthesia. Waters was encouraged and facilitated in this approach by forward looking individuals of the Wisconsin faculty, including Leake, Loevenhart and Seevers of Pharmacology, Meek in Physiology, and the Dean of Faculty, the eminent anatomist Charles Bardeen who, fortunately for all of us, had been acquainted with a prominent anesthetist, Dr. John J. Beuttner, from upper New York state. Beuttner was an invited guest at the 1930 meeting of the Anesthetists Travel Club held in Madison. Especially important was Erwin Schmidt, kindly Professor of Surgery at Wisconsin, always supportive of physician anesthesia, who also recognized and stressed the need for further knowledge and application of basic sciences during postgraduate education in all clinical specialties. Dr. Schmidt was also helpful politically in the process of establishing the American Board of Anesthesiology.

But why did it happen? How was it that Ralph M. Waters recognized the need and opportunity and was stimulated to develop a P-G educational program, the like of which had not existed for anesthesia? Part of the answer lies in the climate of thought and circumstances of the earliest decades of this century. There had been in the AMA for the fifty years of its existence a ferment of growing concern about the variability of medical school standards, which in many of the then existing proprietary schools were deplorably poor. In the early 1900's, the AMA Council on Medical

Education, having identified the needs and determined minimum standards for a proper medical curriculum, to include basic sciences, clinical experience and internship, set out to review and evaluate the programs of 160 existing U.S. medical schools. In order to assure a semblance of an independent, impartial and objective report, they coopted participation of the Carnegie Foundation for Advancement of Teaching.

Beginning in January, 1909, Mr. Abraham Flexner, of the Carnegie Foundation, and Dr. N.P. Colwell, Secretary of the AMA Council, visited and surveyed the policies, programs and qualifications of every medical school in the country. Their findings, published in 1910, commonly known as "The Flexner Report," severely criticized the limited scope of education in the proprietary schools and called for implementation of minimum standards, including medical students' exposure to basic science teaching by a full time faculty, as well as the need for a teaching hospital for introduction of clinical subjects through student participation in its clinics and bedside instruction. Widespread dissemination of this report in newspapers, and discussion of its implications through the J.A.M.A., resulted during the ensuing decade in a systematic restructuring of the viable schools, while unworthy ones, or those with lesser resources, were phased out of existence. The imposition of standards for curriculum and facilities, and the elimination of substandard medical schools, was an amazing accomplishment since neither the Council nor the Carnegie Foundation had legal powers, but had to depend on persuasion.

Fresh from the success of significant improvement of undergraduate medical education, the AMA Council on Medical Education then began, in 1920, to focus on education beyond medical school. In due course, standards referable to qualifications of trainees, of supervisor's and of facilities were promulgated for training in postgraduate specialties (but not including anesthesia at that time). The original statement (1923) is of interest because it included three recommendations:

> *First:* Review courses in anatomy, pathology and other preclinical sciences as applied to the respective specialities.
>
> *Second:* Opportunities to participate in the care of patients in both clinic and hospital environment, with a graded responsibility according to individual experience and competence.
>
> *Third:* Opportunity should be provided also for guided research experience relating to both the fundamental sciences and the clinical field.

These are still the core of sound graduate education programs in medicine. Few of us now would dispute the importance of supervised, graded responsibility, and the application of scientific method, careful observation and experimental design to the progress of every aspect of medical and surgical practice.

So the wonder is not why Waters set and attained his goals for academic anesthesia, but rather why others did not also rise to the obvious challenge. I believe the difference was the receptive environment of the new school at Wisconsin and the cooperation of that basic science faculty with the physicians in anesthesia, as is evidenced in the record of joint authorship of research papers from Wisconsin in that era.

In other centers there was a phenomenon which John Bunker has called, "the Reluctant Universities." This reluctance to recognize anesthesiology as worthy of full academic collegial membership in the university has existed to varying degree and duration throughout the world, even to the present time.

There has apparently always been a bond of interests between anesthetists and pharmacologists or physiologists. A selected few examples will emphasize the point. First, there was the association and mutual respect between John Snow and the early pharmacologist, Benjamin Richardson. In Melbourne, C.J. Martin and W.A. Osbourne provided facilities, encouragement and support for the classic research of Edward Embley. Robert Dripps at the University of Pennsylvania had scientific guidance, stimulation and early laboratory training from Richards, Lambertson, Comroe and Carl Schmidt, as well as local political support from them and their surgical colleague Ravdin, who like Erwin Schmidt viewed improvements in anesthesia and its status as a needed step toward better and more challenging surgery.

Let me return again to earlier events. In 1911, the anesthetists had been refused in their request to be allowed formation of a section in the AMA. This rejection resulted in the sequential founding of several regional societies of anesthetists, which eventually evolved into the larger ones of today.

Much of the animal research interest in basic sciences involved or required the use of anesthetics *and* a consideration of its effects. It is noteworthy also that, in the early decades of this century, aside from anatomy and pathology, the other basic sciences were struggling for their own identity and for space in the medical curriculum. So the basic scientists recognized, not only a community of interest and the importance of anesthesia, but also the urgent clinical need to *apply* some of the new information about it.

Then there were the beginnings of collation of papers, reports and writings of anesthetic interest: — the yearbooks, the quarterly anesthesia supplement to the American Journal of Surgery, and ultimately a Society Journal. All of these early efforts were edited by the indomitable Frank McMechan, who in spite of (or because of) his disabling arthritis was for 20 years the driving force behind the organization of anesthesia societies, meetings and publications. He kept on lighting and rekindling flames of activity and bringing together people with a mutual interest in anesthetics all over the western world.

The records of transactions of those early anesthesia societies in North America, and in particular the early issues of the "Yellow Journal," Current Researches in Anesthesia and Analgesia, reveal an impressive collection of basic scientist names involved in the programs and activities. On the masthead of that new journal in 1922 and '23, about half of the names are those of basic scientists. It was a time in which well-known physiologists and pharmacologists were reporting on investigative topics of fundamental importance to anesthesiology. They were not merely bystanders, but actually played a major role in the launching (birth, parenting, bringing to maturity) of anesthesiology as an academic branch of clinical medicine. Dennis Jackson, Ph.D., M.D., prominent Professor of Pharmacology at the University of Cincinnati, who had pointed the way toward use of the closed system for carbon dioxide absorption, was for a time a prime mover in the affairs of the National Anesthesia Research Society. He organized in 1923 a one week practical workshop attended by clinical anesthetists from many parts of the country. Jackson also served as President of an Annual Congress of the International Anesthesia Research Society and received a Scroll of Recognition from that Society in appreciation of his efforts. Jackson's efforts *were* outstanding, but there were many other notables as well. Subsequent Scrolls of Recognition were awarded to physiologists Howard Haggard and Yandell Henderson,and also to chemist Allan Winter Rowe and pharmacologist Walter L. Mendenhall.

The dependence of progress in anesthesiology on acquisition of knowledge from basic science research is surely undoubted. As Howard Haggard pointed out over 50 years ago, good clinical anesthesia is the application of that knowledge. We enjoy the privilege of being able to practice as applied pharmacologists and applied physiologists in so far as we acquire and use the available knowledge base. Today, an increasing proportion of those individuals seriously motivated toward academic anesthesiology have taken time for additional graduate training in a basic science. Conversely, a number of individuals have been attracted from one or another of the basic sciences into the clinical area of anesthesiology because of the evident opportunities to apply their knowledge, with consequent satisfaction of accomplishing good clinical care.

In 1945-46, The National Research Council made a brief effort to support fundamental research fellowship opportunities for academically motivated anesthetists. Simpson S. Burke at Wisconsin received one of these fellowships. Merel Harmel was also a recipient for work at Johns Hopkins under the guidance of Austin Lamont.

The process still goes on. Julius Comroe, after his move to the Cardiovascular Research Institute in San Francisco, provided research guidance and inspiration to a number of the now prominent individuals in our field. In 1958, after persuasive requests by some of us, the NIH initiated Training Grants in Anesthesia Research at four centers in the United States (U. of Washington, Columbia U., U. of California at San Francisco and U. of Pennsylvania), providing support for fellowships, many of which were served in basic science departments. From these and the Center grants which followed, there has been a steady flow of individuals into academic anesthesiology, but never enough to meet the increasing demands for faculty in the ever enlarging departments. As a corollary, those who have had the opportunity of directed exposure in basic sciences have continued those interests through membership in national and international societies, especially pharmacology and physiology.

And so it goes that, through the years, not only have we learned much that is pertinent to our specialty from the investigative efforts *of,* and sometimes collaborative efforts *with,* our colleagues in basic sciences, but have also benefited by their very real initial and continuing support of the academic aspects of our specialty.

Still today this specialty flourishes best in an environment where there is real cooperative effort between basic scientists and anesthesiologists. Those imbued with Waters' spirit and mission who went to supportive environments succeeded, while others less well received (in a less supportive environment) were less successful; partly because of the lack of "assists," partly because of the distraction of "road blocks."

We stand tall today, being lifted on the shoulders of those basic science colleagues in our medical schools, whose vision foretold the importance of academic anesthesia to the development of a clinical specialty that touches on almost all other branches of medicine.

THE EARLY HISTORY OF LOW-FLOW ANESTHESIA

JOSEPH L. ONISHCHUK
Assistant Professor of Anesthesiology
Temple University Hospital
Department of Anesthesiology
Philadelphia, Pennsylvania, USA

Introduction

"Rebreathing" has been around almost as long as inhalation anesthesia. It has been known by many names; (carbon dioxide) absorption technique, closed-system, closed circuit-anesthesia, and low-flow anesthesia (LFA). It has represented a wide spectrum of techniques, some involving hypercapnia. Many anesthesiologists are not aware of the developments that made rebreathing practical and safe, nor are they familiar with many of the people who have made contributions to the technique.

I wish to trace the early development of rebreathing and examine the motivations of its early proponents. I will also attempt to explain why rebreathing decreased in popularity during the 1950's and 1960's.

The Pioneer Era, 1850-1941

Early work on LFA was motivated by two factors, cost and safety. Gases were expensive. There were no scavenging systems. All excess (expired) gases remained in the air in the operating room. Ether and cyclopropane, both popular during this period, were explosive. Without scavenging systems, explosive gases were released into the air of the operating room. Even at this early date, anesthesiologists realized that the gases from the cylinders were cold and dry, and that this contributed to the loss of heat and humidity from the patient. They realized that rebreathing could conserve these rare commodities.

John Snow is often credited with the first use of rebreathing in anesthesia. In 1850 he created an experimental closed circuit device using potassium hydroxide to absorb carbon dioxide during chloroform anesthesia.[1] Willis Gatch recommended rebreathing as a measure of economy in the use of gas and oxygen as early as 1910. Rebreathing in a closed system with ether had been popular in the 19th century.

There were deaths associated with this technique, however, due to lack of oxygen and the high concentrations of ether that developed in the closed system. Gatch felt that the "open" method of administration was harmful because it resulted in hypocapnia, which caused "surgical shock." His closed system had no method of carbon dioxide absorption. He felt that hypercapnia was beneficial because it stimulated respiration. He did recommend, however, that rebreathing should not be done for extended periods of time.

E.I. McKesson held similar beliefs. He introduced the principle of fractional rebreathing in 1910.[2] "He developed and manufactured an apparatus (McKesson Rebreather) which provided conveniences not previously available with earlier machines for gas administration."[3] The machine automatically saved a portion of the expired tidal volume, and assisted the patient in rebreathing expired gases. This device also had no provision for carbon dioxide absorption. The controls consisted of: tidal volume pointer, rebreathing pointer, rebreathing pressure dial, mixing valve (nitrous oxide-oxygen), fine oxygen adjustment (0-50% oxygen), pressure dial. (Note that when using a nitrous oxide-oxygen mixture with this system, there was no way to determine the concentration of oxygen in the inspired gas.)

Rebreathing, as we know it now, was the result of the work of two people, Dennis Jackson and Ralph Waters. In 1915 Jackson[4] designed and built the first machine that delivered an anesthetic using a closed system with carbon dioxide absorption. Aqueous sodium or potassium hydroxide was used to change carbon dioxide to carbonate in an alkali solution.[5] What motivated Jackson to develop a rebreathing system? The high cost of nitrous oxide, oxygen and later cyclopropane figured prominently in his writings. Jackson calculated the cost of nitrous oxide anesthesia using his closed system (on a purely theoretic basis) at $0.32 per hour. He later commented:

> When I first started to work the cost (of anesthesia) was $3.00 or more per hour, mostly for asphyxia. (No oxygen was used.) Cyclopropane or ethylene, of course, could not have been used in the old way (open circuit with high FGF).

In November of 1915 Jackson presented his device to the St. Louis Medical Society and received a less than enthusiastic reception. He stated: "The profession was just not yet ready for the closed system with carbon dioxide absorption. . ." Jackson's machines were later (1915-1918) used clinically for operations at the Washington University Medical School in St. Louis.[6] On 29 September, 1920, Waters wrote to Jackson and initiated a long correspondence on carbon dioxide absorption. Jackson's work influenced Waters to introduce a simpler device, known as the "to-and-fro" rebreather. Research on CO_2 absorption for submarines and gas masks during World War I led to the development of granular forms of gas absorbents, including Wilson's "Soda Lime." This new material allowed Waters to develop a closed system of ventilation using a canister of solid carbon dioxide absorbent placed in the circuit adjacent to the mask. Waters presented a number of papers and published several articles on the "carbon dioxide absorption technique" and its advantages. In 1924, he enumerated the practical benefits:[7] 1) economy of gases, 2) convenience—"Disagreeable odors of drugs such as ether and ethylene can be kept away from the surgical teams. . .", and 3) patient welfare—"Body heat and moisture are not lost." Waters referred to his method as "complete rebreathing,"[8] as compared to McKesson's technique of "fractional rebreathing." He used complete rebreathing and filtration of carbon dioxide for 200 anesthetics and found the technique to be superior to fractional rebreathing.

> The use of filters has changed my attitude toward rebreathing. The principle of fractional rebreathing as held by McKesson, causing the patient to rebreathe approximately his excess tidal air over waking conditions seems sound if one accepts Henderson's work on carbon dioxid. I believe now, however, that this benefit was not due to retained carbon dioxid, but to retained heat and moisture.

Waters estimated that his new canister would reduce his costs for gases and soda lime to less than $.50 per hour. The apparatus was very portable. He even carried a machine and small tanks of oxygen and nitrous oxide in his car. These could be taken into a patient's home and would provide several hours of anesthesia.

Richard Foregger wrote about "closed circuit respiration" in 1929.[9] He stated:

> Closed circle respiration has been exploited for a number of years in mine rescue helmets and gas masks but to my knowledge in this country (U.S.) not for anesthetic purposes. . . . It seems that all German anesthetic apparatus have provision for closed circle respiration. . . .

In 1930, Sword and Foregger developed the circle system. They designed the system with several improvements over the to-and-fro inhaler. The carbon dioxide absorber (which was big and clumsy) was moved away from the patient's face and surgical field.[10]

Philip Woodbridge[11] summarized his experience with the carbon dioxide absorption in 1933:

> The carbon dioxid absorption technique has been used at the Lahey Clinic for over two years and has proved its great superiority. Not only has there been a marked savings in the amount of gas used, but—a matter of greater importance—the character of gas anesthesia has been greatly improved. Breathing is usually delightfully quiet, offering a marked contrast to the deep, vigorous respirations frequently seen with the common method of giving gas. Without the removal of carbon dioxid, breathing frequently resembles the panting of one who has run up a flight or two of stairs. To subject a seriously sick patient to prolonged stimulation so powerful that it calls forth this energetic, often labored, response can hardly be beneficial and might occasionally add a severe burden. The quiet breathing which results when carbon dioxid is removed bespeaks a marked saving of the patient's energy. . . . Moreover, the resultant quieting of the movements of the abdominal wall and contents is a boon to the surgeon when working within the abdomen.
>
> . . . The Expense of gas anesthesia is very greatly reduced and the danger of explosion is lessened. The patient's body heat and moisture are conserved, and his breathing is made quiet and effortless. . . The method appears to represent so distinct an advance in gas anesthesia as to deserve universal adoption.

In 1933, Waters introduced a new anesthetic agent, cyclopropane, which was explosive. Rebreathing with a closed circuit was particularly suited for use with cyclopropane. Adriani[12] wrote in 1946:

> Like many other advances in medicine, the rebreathing technique of anesthesia was slow to gain popularity. For at least ten years following it introduction, few anesthetists accepted the method. The introduction of the relatively expensive agent, cyclopropane (1933), and the increased interest in recent years in the practice of anesthesia by physicians have increased the popularity of the carbon dioxide absorption method. Today the rebreathing technique is recognized as superior to all others.

In his original article on carbon dioxide absorption in 1924, Waters remarked on one of the limitations of his technique:

> Requiring as it does, an air tight connection with the air passages, all mouth and nose work precludes the possibility of the use of the filter to full advantage.

He and Guedel overcame this difficulty in 1928 when they introduced the cuffed endotracheal tube. They reported on their technique in 1931.[13] They stated that their purposes were: 1) to prevent aspiration of operative debris into the lungs; and 2) to provide a clear field of work for the surgeon. The technique, however, also provided a sealed airway that made the closed system much more effective.

Clearly, the early anesthesiologists recognized the benefits of "rebreathing" and tried to incorporate it into their practice of the administration of general anesthesia. They designed and built their own anesthesia equipment to take advantage of LFA. In 1946, Waters presented an historical article on carbon dioxide absorption at the Ether Centennial.[14] He concluded:

> The absorption of carbon dioxide from anesthetic atmospheres is a common technic in almost every modern operating room throughout the world. It is universally abused as well as used. Many physiologic sins are committed in its name. Its advantages sometimes mask these abuses.

The Era of "Safety First," 1945-1969

After World War II, many factors contributed to the decline in the popularity of LFA. Cyclopropane had been used for rapid sequence inductions because of its swift onset. There were problems with explosions, however, even with closed techniques. When intravenous drugs such as sodium thiopental (1934) and succinylcholine (1950) became popular, they replaced cyclopropane for rapid induction and intubation. Another desirable property of cyclopropane and ether was potent muscle relaxation. When curare came into clinical use (1942), satisfactory surgical conditions could be obtained with nitrous oxide, morphine and curare, thereby eliminating the risk of explosion. Conway[15] stated, "The popularity of cyclopropane and closed systems fell in the late 1940s when safe and potent muscle relaxants became available. . . ."

The danger of hypoxia were recognized and publicized. Anesthesiologists realized that they could deliver a hypoxic mixture inadvertently when using LFA, and they did not have the technology to prevent it. Barach and Rovenstine (1945) severely criticized the deliberate use of anoxia in anesthesia and remarked on unintentional delivery of hypoxic mixtures.[16]

> Unfortunately, there is at the moment no device other than that of a (fixed) mixture (in a tank) of nitrous oxide and oxygen which will ensure the provision of 20 percent oxygen. Even among the better anesthetic appliances on the market today, the accuracy of flow meters may vary as much as 5 per cent, and anesthetists are constantly exposed to the temptation to decrease oxygen to aid the induction or to produce more profound anesthesia.

Halothane and the "new" vaporizers

In the 1950's, two developments made LFA difficult and perhaps even dangerous. Anesthesiologists didn't fully understand the properties of halothane (introduced into clinical use in 1956) or the new vaporizers (Copper Kettle, Fluotec) when they were first introduced. These vaporizers were often inaccurate and lacked several important features that were necessary to perform LFA safely.[17] Halothane was often used in in-circuit vaporizers designed for ether. Finally, the properties of the vaporizers and the anesthesia circuit changed radically when changing from spontaneous respiration to intermittent positive pressure breathing (IPPB).

Calibrated vaporizers had been in use prior to the introduction of halothane. The Copper Kettle had been developed by Lucien Morris in 1952 to deliver specific concentrations of chloroform. It was calibrated in ml/min of oxygen flow through the vaporizer, not volume percent of agent delivered. The anesthetist manually calculated the concentration of anesthetic agent delivered. When using the Copper Kettle with halothane, it was easy to remember that if one used a total FGF of 5 L/min and directed 100 ml/min of oxygen through the Copper Kettle, the delivered concentration of halothane was 1 percent. Multiples of 100 ml/min yielded predictable concentrations. Anesthesia could be delivered with a minimum of mathematics, provided these high gas flows were used. Using a Copper Kettle with low FGF, however, it was possible to deliver "lethal concentrations equalling ten to twenty times the concentration required for maintenance of anesthesia."[18]

In Britain, the TECOTA (TEmperature COmpensated Trichloroethylene Air) vaporizer had been developed so that midwives could provide safe obstetric analgesia in the home. This vaporizer was adapted for use with halothane and the "Fluotec" series of vaporizers was introduced.[19] Hill and Lowe (1962) demonstrated that the Mark II Fluotec vaporizer set at 0.5 percent halothane could deliver up to 3 percent with FGF of 500 ml and intermittent positive pressures of 20 cm in circle system.[20] "The fact that the concentrations are high at the 1/2 percent and 1 percent settings when the Fluotec feeds into a closed circle system is due to the back pressure exerted on the vaporizer by the ventilator." They reported that the Fluotec calibrations for free flow were substantially different from those obtained in a closed circle employing controlled or assisted respiration. Furthermore, reducing the dial setting failed to decrease the delivered concentration until the vaporizer was actually turned off. Eger and Epstein reported that the combination of a Mark II Fluotec vaporizer and intermittent positive pressure breathing (IPPB) could lead to "an unstable anesthetic system with positive feedback."

Hamilton[21] commented on these "new" vaporizers:

> This (the use of LFA) changed when halothane was introduced, because there were some problems associated with the use of "breathe-through" vaporizers. High flow rates facilitated delivery of a known concentration of anesthetic agent with "bubble-through" vaporizers. High flows also facilitated the use of nitrous oxide in a period when oxygen analyzers were not widely available.

Using one of the vaporizers with high flows and spontaneous ventilation might be safe. However, the combined effects of low FGF and IPPB provided a pumping effect and positive feedback that could yield a delivered concentration of halothane far in excess of the intended concentration. In 1968, a back-pressure check valve was incorporated into the Copper Kettle by the manufacturer. Its purpose was to prevent back-pressure from causing an increase in the delivered concentration of volatile agent.

In the 1960's there was an increase in the activity on monitoring anesthetic gases, especially the F_iO_2. This led to investigation into predicting the F_iO_2 during LFA/CCA. One group of anesthesiologists felt that LFA was undesirable because it required monitoring the F_iO_2. (They must have felt confident in their anesthesia delivery systems.) In 1965, Smith began investigation into the continuous measurement of carbon dioxide (infra-red) and oxygen. In his article, Nitrous Oxide and Low Inflow Circle Systems, he concluded that, in a low-flow system, one must monitor the concentration of oxygen. "Below FGF of 600 ml/min, it was necessary to deliver from 40-70 percent oxygen to maintain 20 percent in the mixed expired gas."[22]

In 1978, Gorsky reviewed the origins of the belief that CCA was dangerous.[23]

> . . .young anesthesiologists have had little experience with closed system technics (sic), since their teachers often consider the closed system dangerous.
>
> . . .several deaths resulted from the use of halothane in a closed system. One of these was reported by Foster, who administered halothane from an in-circle vaporizer in unknown concentrations. . .

He concluded:

> The complex problems of uptake and distribution, in addition to reports of anesthetic deaths with halothane in the closed system at a time when pollution by waste anesthetic gases was ignored, led to the demise of closed system techniques.

The post-war era witnessed increased emphasis on equipment safety and the avoidance of hypoxic mixtures. The introduction of halothane, (an extremely potent and non-flammable agent), new out-of-circuit vaporizers and IPPB resulted in many changes in the delivery of gas anesthesia. As a result, many anesthesiologists may have felt that LFA was dangerous and abandoned it for safer techniques.

References

1. Conway CM: Low flow and closed breathing systems. Clinics in Anaesthesiology 1:275-90, 1983.
2. McKesson EI: Some physical factors in the administration of gaseous anaesthetics. Br Med J 11:1117, 1926.
3. Barach AL, Rovenstine EA: The hazard of anoxia during nitrous oxide anesthesia. Anesthesiology 6:451, 1945.
4. Jackson DE: A new method for the production of general analgesia and anæsthesia with a description of the apparatus used.
5. Jackson DE: Anesthesia equipment from 1914 to 1954 and experiments leading to its development. Anesthesiology 16:953-69, 1955.
6. Thomason H, Jackson DE: The carbon dioxid filtration method for general analgesia and anesthesia. Anesth Analg 6:181-2, 1927.
7. Waters RM: Clinical scope and utility of carbon dioxid filtration in inhalation anesthesia. Anesth Analg 3:20-2, 1924.
8. Waters, 1924.
9. Foregger R: The position of the breathing bag. Anesth Analg 8:34-9, 1929.
10. Sword BD: The closed circle method of administration of gas anesthesia. Anesth Analg 9:198-202, 1930.
11. Woodbridge PD: Better gas anesthesia at less cost: The carbon dioxid absorption method. Anesth Analg 12:161-73, 1933.
12. Adriani J: The Chemistry of Anesthesia. Springfield, IL, Charles C Thomas, 1946.
13. Guedel AE, Waters RM: Endotracheal anesthesia: a new technique. Ann Otol Rhinol Laryngol 11:1139-45, 1931.
14. Waters RM: Absorption of carbon dioxide from anesthetic atmospheres: Historical aspects. Anesthesiology 8:330-47, 1947.
15. Conway
16. Barach AL, Rovenstine EA: The hazard of anoxia during nitrous oxide anesthesia. Anesthesiology 6:449-61, 1945.
17. Robson JG: Fluothane (halothane) in closed circuit anesthesia. Anesthesiology 20:251-60, 1959.
18. Feldman SA, Morris LE: Vaporization of halothane and ether in the Copper Kettle. Anesthesiology 19:650-5, 1958.
19. Calverley
20. Hill DW, Lowe HJ: Comparison of concentration of halothane in closed and semiclosed circuits during controlled ventilation. Anesthesiology 23:291-8, 1962.
21. Hamilton WK: Low-flow systems without calculus (or even algebra). ASA Refresher Courses in Anesthesiology 8:79-86, 1980.
22. Smith TC: Nitrous oxide and low inflow circle systems. Anesthesiology 27:266-72, 1966.
23. Gorsky BH, Hall RL, Redford JE: A compromise for closed system anesthesia. Anesth Analg 57:18-24, 1978.

THE SELLICK MANEUVER, a Historical Perspective

N.A. PACE
and
A.H. GIESECKE
Department of Anesthesiology, University of Texas Southwestern Medical Center Dallas, Texas, USA

To many anesthesiologists involved in Critical Care Medicine, the X-ray shown in Fig. 1 must be familiar. It shows an intubated young female patient with patchy infiltration and consolidation throughout both lung fields, illustrating the typical picture of aspiration pneumonitis, otherwise known as Mendelson's Syndrome (1946).

Mendelson first described the syndrome in 1945 at a presentation to the New York Obstetrical Society and subsequently published his report in 1946. Since then, the clinico-pathologic picture of aspiration of stomach contents, especially in obstetric practice, has come to bear his name. However, five years before Mendelson first described his findings, Hall (1940) had already described the syndrome. In an article in the Journal of the American Medical Association titled, "Aspiration of stomach contents, an obstetric hazard," he described 15 patients, 14 of whom were in labor, who had aspirated during anesthesia; 5 subsequently died. He recognized that the condition was not rare and carried a significant morbidity and mortality. He differentiated clinically between two types of cases: those in which the material aspirated was solid particles and those in which it was fluid. He wondered whether aspiration pneumonitis was primarily an obstetric complication, and also whether the type or amount of premedication or the analgesia used during labor had any effect on the condition. Mendelson, however, was the first to associate the clinical syndrome with the presence of acid in gastric fluid.

In an effort to avoid this complication, anesthesiologists have tried various techniques.

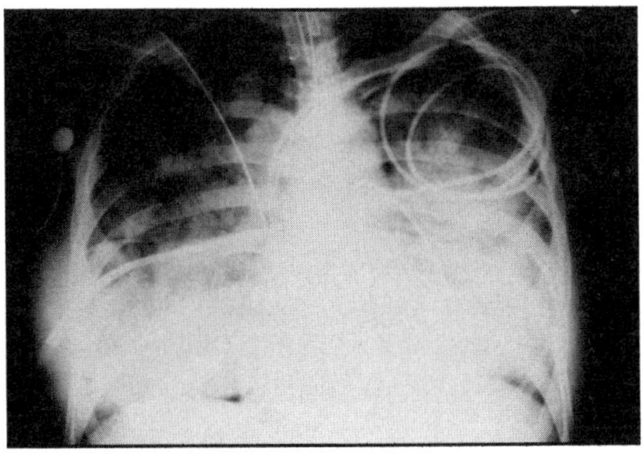

Fig. 1. X-ray showing patchy infiltration and consolidation throughout both lung fields.

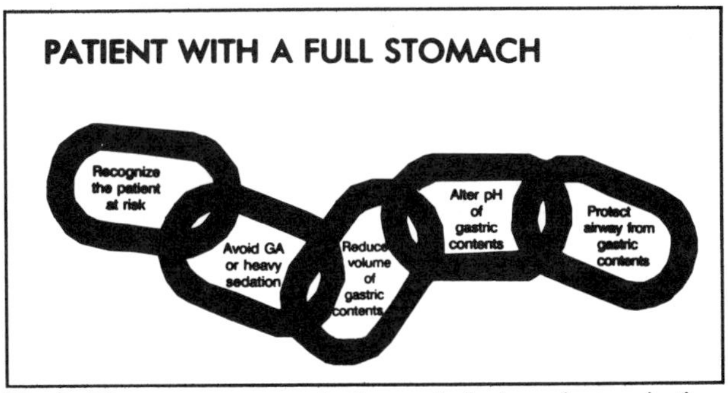

Fig. 2. The necessary steps in the prophylaxis against aspiration pneumonitis can be compared to a chain that is only as strong as its weakest link.

These measures can be compared to a chain that is only as strong as its weakest link (Hilley and Giesecke 1990) (Fig. 2). We recognize that we must consider each link, but for this lecture we concentrate on the last link; the prevention of soilage of the airway with gastric contents. One of the first methods was the induction of the patient in the semi-sitting position. The basis for this method arises from the findings of O'Mullane (1954), suggesting that the maximum expected intragastric pressure in adult patients was 18 cm H_2O. Hence, if the patient is placed in a 40-degree head-up tilt, the larynx will lie 19 cm above the gastro-esophageal junction, and therefore any regurgitated gastric contents would not reach the larynx.

Of all the precautions, the universally accepted method to protect the airway is endotracheal intubation, preceded by the application of cricoid pressure (or cricoesophageal compression) as described by Sellick (1961). He writes:

> The manoeuvre consists in temporary occlusion of the upper end of the oesophagus by backward pressure of the cricoid cartilage against the bodies of the cervical vertebrae. . . . Before induction the cricoid is palpated and lightly held between the thumb and second finger; as anesthesia begins, pressure is exerted on the cricoid cartilage mainly by the index finger . . . as soon as consciousness is lost, firm pressure can be applied without obstruction of the patient's airway. Pressure is maintained until intubation and inflation of the cuff of the endotracheal tube is completed.

Since this description, the technique has been universally called "Sellick's maneuver." However, the technique had been described almost two hundred years previously. In 1776, Mr. John Hunter, writing in Philosophical Transactions about the recovery of people apparently drowned, suggested that:

> If during (blowing air into the lungs) the larynx be gently pressed against the oesophagus and spine, it will prevent the stomach and intestines being too much distended by the air, and leave room for the application of more effectual stimuli to those parts. This pressure, however, must be conducted with judgment and caution, so that the trachea and the aperture into the larynx may both be left perfectly free.

However, the technique appears to have been used even before this. In a letter dated August 8, 1774, but published in 1776, Dr. William Cullen, professor at Glasgow and Edinburgh Universities, wrote to Lord Cathcart, the noted diplomate, in which he described the technique used by his colleague Dr. Monro.

> Whether the blowing is done by a person's mouth, or by bellows, Dr. Monro observes, that the air is ready to pass by the gullet into the stomach; but that this may be prevented, by pressing the lower part of the larynx backwards upon the gullet. To persons of a little knowledge in anatomy, it is to be observed, that the pressure should be only on the cricoid cartilage, by which the gullet may be straitened, while the passage through the larynx is not interrupted.

The same technique was reported at around the same time, and the possibility of a connection therefor arises. Dr. Monro was a colleague of Cullen's. Dr. W. Hunter was a direct pupil of Dr. Cullen. Dr. John Hunter was William's younger brother. It would not be too far-fetched, therefore, to speculate that Monro, Cullen and the two Hunters knew each other academically, if not socially. Hence they may have discussed the management of "persons apparently drowned" before the publication of the articles. It should be pointed out, however, that Cullen described cricoid pressure, whereas Hunter described gentle pressure on the larynx. An advert by Drager for the "Pulmotor" in 1921 clearly suggests that cricoid pressure was already well in use in those days. Sellick's undeniable contribution was to recommend that the maneuver could prevent regurgitation of gastric contents into the pharynx, whereas his predecessors were preoccupied with the use of the maneuver to prevent entry of air into the stomach.

Myths

A number of misconceptions appear to have arisen regarding the application of cricoesophageal compression. In his article, Sellick (1961) writes: "By tripping the sphincters at the upper and lower end of the oesophagus, a (gastric) tube increases the risk of regurgitation, and it also interferes with compression of the upper oesophagus." Such thinking is not uncommon. In an audit of current practice at our institution, 40 percent of doctors stated they would remove a nasogastric tube prior to induction because they believed the tube would interfere with crico-esophageal compression. However, such fears appear to be unfounded following an article by Salem et al (1985), clearly showing that cricoid compression was effective in obliterating the esophageal lumen in the presence of a nasogastric tube.

In an editorial in Anaesthesia, Rosen (1981) claims that only one record of failure of cricoid pressure could be found in the literature. This is the publication by Whittington et al in the Lancet (1979). However, careful examination of the two cases reported reveal that the techniques of application of cricoid pressure were inadequate. In case one the patient vomited when cricoid pressure was being applied during induction, but after the start of the injection of the induction agent. Furthermore, the patient vomited several liters of coffee colored fluid upon extubation when no cricoid pressure was being applied. Hence one cannot attribute the aspiration to failure of cricoid pressure. In the second case described, cricoid pressure appears to have been applied after thriopental and succinylcholine had been administered. Both Sellick (1961) and Crawford (1878) state that cricoid pressure must be applied before the start of induction. We do not therefor accept that these two cases represent a failure of cricoid pressure to prevent aspiration of stomach contents, but rather the failure of its correct application.

A further question regards the possibility of esophageal rupture. Sellick (1961) writes: "(Cricoid pressure) should not be used to control active vomiting because the oesophagus might be damaged by vomit under high pressure." Cricoid pressure appears to have been prematurely released in case one mentioned previously (Whittington et al 1979) because of a fear of esophageal rupture. In a letter in the *Lancet* in 1979, Rosen suggests that rupture of the esophagus, to his knowledge, had not been recorded in a young fit patient. However, in a recent case report, Ralph and Wareham (1991) describe a case of rupture of the esophagus during circoid pressure in an elderly female who suffered from a bleeding pyloric ulcer, hiatus hernia, and severe rheumatoid arthritis. Rupture of the esophagus is therefore an extremely rare complication and the benefits of its application far outweigh its risks.

Two-Handed Technique

In his original description, Sellick (1961) states that the head and neck must be fully extended during the application of cricoid pressure. This extension serves to increase the anterior convexity of the cervical spine, stretching the esophagus and preventing its lateral displacement. We believe that proper cricoesophageal compression is facilitated by using two hands. This entails placing one hand under the neck to lift the neck and head into a good sniffing position and the other on the cricoid cartilage to compress the esophagus between the broad, flat posterior aspect of the cricoid and the body of the sixth cervical vertebra (Hilley and Giesecke 1990). The use of two hands balances pressure, facilitates a good "sniffing" position, and is therefore beneficial to laryngoscopy and tracheal intubation. In certain situations, single handed cricoid pressure may be virtually ineffective because no counter pressure can be generated. One would also predict that, in certain situations, the force generated by cricoid pressure may be less than anticipated. Such situations include patients with suspected cervical trauma, and hence in a collar, and in patients who have fixed flexion deformities of the cervical spine. In such situations anesthesiologists should take extra care to avoid what we believe is now an avoidable situation, that is, aspiration pneumonitis.

In summary, the technique of cricoesophageal compression was described many years before Sellick's article in the Lancet in 1961. Despite this, Sellick deserves credit for recognizing that the technique could be usefully applied to prevent aspiration of stomach contents.

References

1. Crawford JS: Principles and practice of obstetric anaesthesia, 4th ed. Oxford: Blackwell Scientific Publications, 275, 1978.
2. Cullen W: A letter to Lord Cathcart concerning the recovery of persons drowned and seemingly dead. London, printed for J Murray, Fleet Street, No. 32, 1776.
3. Hall CC: Aspiration pneumonitis, an obstetric hazard. JAMA 114:728-33, 1940.
4. Hilley MD, Giesecke AH: The patient with a full stomach. Seminars in Anesthesia 9:204-10, 1990.
5. Hunter J: Of persons apparently drowned. Philosoph Trans 66:412-25, 1776.
6. Mendelson CL: The aspiration of stomach contents into the lungs during obstetric anesthesia. Am J Obstet Gynecol 52:191-204, 1946.
7. O'Mullane EJ: Vomiting and regurgitation during anaesthesia. Lancet 1:1209-12, 1954.
8. Ralph SJ, Wareham CA: Rupture of the oesophagus during cricoid pressure. Anaesthesia 46:40-1, 1991.
9. Rosen M: Antacids and cricoid pressure in the prevention of fatal aspiration syndrome. Lancet 353, 1979.
10. Rosen M: Editorial. Anaesthesia 36:145-6, 1981.
11. Salem MR, Joseph NJ, Heyman HJ, Belani B, Paulissian R, Ferrara TP: Cricoid compression is effective in obliterating the esophageal lumen in the presence of a nasogastric tube. Anesthesiology 63:443-6, 1985.
12. Sellick BA: Cricoid pressure to control regurgitation of stomach contents during induction of anaesthesia. Lancet 2:404-6, 1961.
13. Whittington RM, Robinson JS, Thompson JM: Fatal aspiration (Mendelson's) syndrome despite antacids and cricoid pressure. Lancet 2:228-30, 1979.

CRAWFORD W. LONG
The Influence of the Spirit of the Age of Romanticism on the Discovery of Anesthesia

E. M. PAPPER
Department of Anesthesiology
University of Miami School of Medicine, Miami, Florida, USA

Among historians of medicine it is common to be inundated by the conflicts and the quarrels among the principal participants that attended the "discovery" or invention of anesthesia. Much of the writing in the past has been devoted to attempting to assess the priority of discovery to one or another of the various principal personalties engaged in the early story of the practical usage of substances for the prevention of pain and suffering due to deliberate surgical intervention designed for the care of patients.

Among the important personalities in the early 19th century who had a major claim to the discovery of anesthesia is the native son of Georgia, the southern physician and surgeon, Dr. Crawford W. Long. Generally speaking, it is not unusual for anesthesiologists and others who have not had the opportunity nor the interest in delving deeper in to the understanding of Dr. Long's role in the establishment of anesthetic care for surgical procedures, to think that his role was either accidental or derived in whole or in large part from his social experiences with ether or nitrous oxide. The inhalation of ether or nitrous oxide for social purposes to produce alterations of emotion and mentality for the production of party related fun was commonplace. However, insufficient attention, in the present observer's view, has been paid to Long's background and his opportunities for more important participation in the discovery process than merely one of using a game to develop a major medical gift to humanity.

It seems appropriate, therefore, to re-examine the recent work of connecting medical and literary evidence in the Age of the Romantics to understand the role of Crawford Long as a major player or protagonist in the tale of the discovery of anesthesia. The cultural forces of his Age were powerful and undoubtedly had an impact upon him and his work. The almost total concentration, or perhaps even obsession, with the issue of the priority of discovery is neither the crucial nor the fascinating part of Long's work. Its importance lies in making the connection that pain prevention is not only possible, but desirable in surgery. How he came to this view is the main theme of this paper.

In one of the streams of new information which deals with the forces that had an important influence in finding ways to prevent pain and suffering, including those inflicted for useful purposes like surgical intervention, was the role of the important new development (at the time) of a different way of looking at philosophy, intellectual activities and sociological behavior. These winds of change occurred with the advent of the Romantic Period, beginning with the French Revolution in 1789 and extending at least as far as the Revolution of 1848 in Britain as well as in continental Europe. The influence of these new attitudes was also forcefully present in the then young United States. These matters and the marked changes in the culture of the West following the thinking and behavior patterns of the Augustan Age or the Century of Enlightenment are dealt with in a number of studies. One of them which relates to the influence of this new habit of thought of the Romantics is dealt with more completely than can take place in this essay in a recent study.[1]

In that essay, it is shown that a marked change in attitude toward pain and suffering takes place in the Romantic Period with the advent of the French Revolution. The change is an outgrowth of a totally new concept in Western civilization, i.e., the idea of the sanctity and importance of the individual and the value of subjectivity. In this point of view, the idea is developed that, for the first time, there is value in the idea of respect for the self. The various democratic forces that sanctify the rights and privileges of the individual, as well as the opportunity of the individual to seek the "pursuit of happiness" on the same basis as any other human being, characterize a remarkable new feature in the outlook of Western thought and emotion. Intellectuality is improved by the addition of passion.

One of the fascinating consequences of this new way of viewing experience and earthbound satisfactions and happiness is the rejection of the previously held idea that pain and suffering are inevitable and that they are the lot of all mankind.

There is ample evidence that the two major streams of influence upon modern Western civilization, i.e., the Old and New Testaments on the religious side and Greek and Roman civilization in the secular area, were designed to sanctify the presence of pain in what many viewed as the "vale of tears" in which suffering was to be expected. Sin, suffering and pain were, until the end of the 18th century or early 19th century, viewed as punishment for sin by a vengeful God. The early fathers of the Christian church added the importance of martyrdom as a secure access to everlasting life, love, and contentment in the form of heavenly immortality as a reward for suffering earthly pain in the service of God.

The secular area provided little that would lead to the diminution of the role of pain and suffering in the human condition. Much of the classical period and its writings ignore the common man or woman. The vaunted democracy of the ancient Greeks was preserved and designed only for a modest number of male citizens who were slave holders (as was Crawford Long!) and whose democracy can hardly be said to have been one of concern for comfort and freedom from pain and suffering. Only a few select freemen, who were by and large aristocrats, had the benefits of Greek Democracy. The great Greek tragedies are powered by fate and other cosmic forces. In any event, they deal only with heroes or gods of demigods. There is, therefore, nothing in the philosophical roots of the Western world as we know it today, and as it continued until the time of the major cataclysm of the French Revolution, that suggested that a world in which humans would be free of pain and suffering was desirable and worth achieving.

It was in this sort of environment that the major upheaval of the human condition, which was the French Revolution, occurred. For the first time, the message was rendered loud and clear in the Western world that each and every person had a right to certain basic freedoms and had the right to live in dignity on this earth. Happiness was not to be deferred to some afterworld as a reward for devotion to a God who is otherwise insensitive to the needs of mankind on earth.

In the world before the Romantic liberations took place there could be no interest in thinking that the relief of suffering or the prevention of pain had social or human worth. Even where the knowledge clearly existed, the connection was not made for application toward human welfare and benefit in this earthly life. Dr. Norman Bergman points out, by way of illustration, that the future Sir Humphry Davy *knew* that nitrous oxide could provide analgesia and pain relief. Davy clearly stated in one of his reports when he worked in Beddoes' Pneumatic Institute that it might even be used in surgical anesthesia — yet he himself, when injured in a painful way, proceeded to treat his own wound without the analgesic benefits of the inhalation of nitrous oxide which he clearly knew all about. Even Davy, the putative discoverer of anesthesia in the minds of some, was unprepared to see its application because the *Spirit of the Age* was not yet ready for the advent of measures designed deliberately and carefully to produce an environment in which the prevention of pain induced by surgical treatment could be obtained and was desirable to achieve.[2]

The importance of societal readiness and interest in the prevention of pain associated with surgical operations cannot be sufficiently appreciated without considering the major impact it had upon the practice of clinical medicine. The prevailing methods of taking care of sick people were sharply conditioned by the underlying and prevailing habit of thought that pain and disease were often inflicted as punishment for sin and therefore, it would be contrary to divine purposes to interfere with the condition of such patients. Whether for religious purposes or other reasons, there is clear evidence that there was no interest on the part of physicians, scientists or prospective patients who might be benefited by the use of materials which could provide a condition which came to be appreciated as surgical anesthesia. For instance, at least two of the really effective agents for the production of anesthesia — nitrous oxide and diethyl ether — were well known long before they came into actual clinical use. Their properties were well known, but the connection was not made between these properties of inducing hypnosis and analgesia that there was a role to play in clinical medicine. For example, nitrous oxide was first described and manufactured by Joseph Preistly in 1772.[3] The actual anesthetic capabilities of nitrous oxide were, as suggested above, fully described and clearly appreciated by Humphry Davy in 1800. The oft quoted passage by Davy which describes the situation reads, "As nitrous oxide in its extensive operation appears capable of destroying physical pain, it may properly be used with advantage in surgical operations in which no great effusion of blood takes place."[4] The issue with nitrous oxide is so clear as to defy any other interpretation but the fact is that a substance known to produce anesthesia well documented in its usage was actually not put into practice until society's time was ready.

The story of the other important agent first used was that of diethyl ether. It was known since 1540, having been synthesized by a Prussian botanist called Valerius Cordus. Evidently it was also synthesized by others for different purposes, including the distinguished chemist Boyle in 1680, and the great scientist of the age, Sir Isaac Newton, also synthesized ether in 1717.[3] Nothing was done with ether for clinical medical purposes, but the mind altering substances were actually used for amusement and for social occasions. From time immemorial, mind altering substances in all cultures seem to have been used for religious purposes, self-oriented pleasures or a form of social hilarity. Whatever the reasons the substances, well known to produce pain relief and the prevention of pain did not find their way into clinical usage until the brilliant connection made by Crawford Long that the analgesia and amnesia discovered after injury during thc social inhalation of ether could and should be used for beneficial clinical purposes to prevent the pain of surgical operation. It is not unreasonable to inquire why Crawford Long should be so singularly blessed with insight to make these connections between social use of drugs and clinical applications to induce surgical anesthesia. His mind was prepared by his knowledge of the changes produced by Romanticism.

One of the important handicaps which had to be overcome in thinking about the work of Dr. Long is the stereotyped image that has been handed down from generation to generation alleging that Crawford Long was a simple country doctor, implying that his knowledge and experience were not compatible with the greatness of the discovery of anesthesia. These preconceived notions are at best inadequate and at worst simply false. Crawford Long was not a simple country doctor and it is now necessary to examine some of his background and to suggest that the Spirit of the Age with all of the important new forces unleashed by the great Romantic thinkers and poets after that gains of the French Revolution made a major impression upon him which consciously or unconsciously led to making the important connection between the action of a drug and its *desirability* for *clinical* usage.

Long is the figure upon whom one can attach part of the answer to the historical puzzle as to why there was such a long delay of the entrance of surgical anesthesia into medical therapeutics. The most reasonable explanation of a change in societal readiness for anesthesia comes with the total change in Western thought and emotions powered by the Romantic poets, philosophers, artists, politicians and economists and eventually, also the medical practitioners. The spirit of secularism which was also anti-religious was no small factor in eliminating the idea that pain and suffering were punishments for sin or were the consequences of an immovable fate, or that pain and suffering were to be accepted as normal and unchanging. The marked changes in thinking of the Romantics made it not only possible but desirable to cherish each individual human being as a valuable person in the social order. The prevention of pain and suffering became conceptually desirable in such a society. The medical practitioner can, with increasing ease and while accepting these views of humanity, therefore think that the prevention of pain due to surgical intervention or to disease is an important part of his clinical mission. The linkage thus established between life science and medicine on one side and philosophy and poetry on the other comes to fruition in this fascinating age of the Romantics. It is now necessary to see where Crawford Long's experience fits into the Romantic tradition and how he may have been influenced by it.

Fortunately much of the story of Dr. Long's life, work and education has been preserved by a loving biography of him by one of his daughters, Frances Long Taylor.[5]

According to his daughter, Crawford Long as a young man was well-to-do and his parents were of "good stock," and provided him with advantages unusual even for that day. Crawford Long's father, Mr. James Long, inherited both money and slaves. According to Frances Long, her grandfather "by his industry and energy, had accumulated a fortune."[5a] Among his other activities, Dr. Long's father was active in political affairs. He was the Postmaster of the town in which they lived. He was a leader in business in many new enterprises and he became one of the larger stockholders of the new Georgia Railroad Company which was one of the first railroads to be built in the South. It became very valuable in due time. Dr. Long's father also established an academy for secondary school studies. One gets the picture that James Long was a very wealthy, highly influential citizen and a pillar of the Presbyterian Church. The elder Mr. Long was very fond of reading and in his library his granddaughter, Mrs. Taylor, describes the presence of books by Shakespeare and articles from the Tatler, the Spectator, and the extraordinary presence of a book to become famous in later years, Burton's Anatomy of Melancholy, and also novels by Maria Edgeworth (Thomas Beddoes Sr.'s sister-in-law). In those days, female writers were few in number. These works were the sign of an intellectually inclined individual with a strong leaning toward what might then have been viewed as avant-garde literature not ordinarily read in the households of establishment families. Mrs. Taylor describes her paternal ancestors as "men of position; quiet, reserved gentlemen but of forceful character and intellect, industrious and thrifty. They were interested in public affairs, founding churches and endowing schools."[5b]

On Dr. Long's maternal side were the ancestors of Dr. Long's mother, Elizabeth Ware. The Wares were participants on the side of the colonists in the Revolutionary War. Dr. Long's mother was a beautiful woman and was thought to be rather worldly since she was a member of the Episcopal Church rather than of the Presbyterian. The family was very wealthy by any of the standards of the time and Mrs. Taylor describes her childhood environment as: "we were considered a prodigal, extravagant people."[5c]

Crawford Long spent his childhood in this environment of wealth, good behavior, and the considerate treatment of slaves which was said by Mrs. Taylor to be a characteristic of many southern aristocrats. Crawford Long's education was begun early at home in reading and when he was fourteen he went to Franklin College, now the University of Georgia. Crawford Long's friendship with Alexander Stephens, with whom he shares Georgia's representation in Statuary Hall at the capitol's building in Washington, began when they were students at Franklin College. Long's biographer makes the point that he opposed secession when the Civil War came later, but was loyal to Georgia and eventually took Georgia's side to join the Confederacy.

After graduation from Franklin College, young Crawford Long spent some time teaching and also as a medical apprentice to a Dr. Grant in Jefferson, Georgia. He subsequently attended the Medical Department of Transylvania University in Lexington, Kentucky. It was a long and courageous trip by horseback from his hometown in Georgia through territory that was still inhabited to some degree by hostile Indians. The people of that part of Kentucky, according to Frances Taylor, had "the purest Anglo-Saxon blood in America."[5d] Crawford Long in that environment heard old English commonly spoken in Shakespeare's time transported to the New World. After his experience in Kentucky, Dr. Long's father decided that he should have the best possible medical education to be obtained in the United States. Accordingly, in 1838 he went to Philadelphia where he entered the Medical Department of the University of Pennsylvania. In the eyes of many, the University of Pennsylvania had the most outstanding School of Medicine in the United States at the time. It was also a large institution in one of America's oldest cities. The faculty at the University of Pennsylvania were among America's outstanding scholars in medicine.

Among them were Dr. Philip Syng Physick who was a student of the famous John Hunter in London and in turn, was one of the founders of American surgery.

At the time that Long entered Pennsylvania the professor of surgery was the very well recognized and respected William Gibson who succeeded Dr. Physick. Gibson had studied with the renowned Sir Charles Bell in Britain. Among his other interesting and very important qualifications exerting influence upon the young student Crawford Long was the fact that Gibson had been a spectator at the battle of Waterloo and was wounded by a stray bullet. Most important of all, perhaps, is that Gibson was a friend and correspondent of Lord Byron who had many interests and connections in the United States and whose works were very well received in this country immediately upon their publication. Certainly, Long was familiar with Byron's great poetry and his exquisitely told stories of resisting oppression.

Another distinguished member of the faculty was George B. Wood who taught materia medica. He was a major influence in the ethics of clinical practice both at Pennsylvania and in the country. Mrs. Taylor is lavish in her praise of Dr. Wood in stating: "no man who has held a chair in the University ever brought greater reputation to it."[5e]

After this extraordinary education in Philadelphia at the University of Pennsylvania, Crawford Long had received the best medical education that could be obtained in this country. He also did what other students had done who were contemporaneous with him in Philadelphia. They participated in the inhalation of nitrous oxide or ether vapor for the purposes of producing exhilaration, excitement for themselves and fun for the onlookers. Ether and nitrous oxide were known to Crawford Long in this particular social setting while he was still a medical student. He brought these social customs with him upon his eventual return to his native Georgia in 1841.

However, before his return home to Georgia at his father's request, Crawford Long participated in one of two experiences open only to the select few who chose to improve their medical education after graduation from Medical School. After he finished at the University of Pennsylvania, Long went to New York City to perfect himself further rather than going to Europe which was the other option. He, according to his biographer, "went to New York to perfect himself further and spent 18 months "walking the hospitals," specializing in surgery and witnessing much suffering."[5f] While in New York City exactly what he did was not quite clear form either his biographer or from papers that were left. However, it is known that he studied or at least heard lectures and made rounds with Valentine Mott and Willard Parker among others. He therefore had exposure to at least two of the outstanding physicians in New York. Valentine Mott, the first professor surgery at the College of Physicians and Surgeons, soon to be united with Columbia, was important in his many influences upon the young Georgian.

It is necessary at this point to digress some in the story of Crawford Long to establish the possible importance of Long's association with Valentine Mott during the year and a half that he spent in New York City. Valentine Mott was not only a distinguished surgeon of his period and a major force in American Surgery, but he was very highly cherished by Mr. Astley Cooper, the premier surgeon of England, with whom he studied as a young man at Guy's and St. Thomas' Hospitals in London. Mott also returned for a visit of self renewal in his later life when his teacher, now Sir Astley Cooper, was the reigning force in British surgery. It is through Sir Astley that Professor Mott met such distinguished surgeons as Barron Larrey, Napoleon's chief surgeon, and many others of similar stature.

An interesting and tantalizing fact is that Valentine Mott was a student with Astley Cooper approximately a decade before Sir Astley had the unusual experience of having as a student in surgery the then very young and future great Romantic poet, John Keats. There is no evidence that Mott and Keats knew each other, but there is evidence that the humanism expressed in vastly different ways by the great poet and the equally great surgeon was influenced by the teachings of Sir Astley, obviously in different ways, but most important to human welfare. It is tempting to think that these influences also extended to Crawford Long from Cooper through Mott to Long. Certainly, the exposure to Romantic literature is clear in the library that Long maintained for himself in which he used important literature of the Romantics as well as older classics. The undoubted crucial influence of Gibson on Long and the impact he brought of Byron's Romantic and humanistic ideas cannot be evaluated exactly, but must have been of great importance on the development of the young Crawford Long. Long was interested in literature and new ideas. In addition to the British Romantics, he was very fond of the writings of Washington Irving and Longfellow who were among the Americans who were affected positively by the British Romantics' interests in the common man and the beauties of Nature.

According to Frances Long Taylor her father enjoyed "The world . . . full of ferment, investigation, speculation and novel ideas. These they pondered over, accepting this, dismissing that, interested in all."[5g]

There is further collateral and important evidence of the impact of the thinking and poetry of the Romantic Age in the recollections of Dr. Joseph Jacobs who worked for and with Crawford Long in his drug dispensing business. In an article preserved in the archives in the University of Pennsylvania, Jacobs wrote of Dr. Long's involvement with and his interest in literature. Jacobs says that Long's "chief delight found expression, . . .in books selected from the classics of standard English literature." He says further "They have told me that his father had a wonderful collection of old books, so he was reared in a literary atmosphere. He never tired of Shakespeare plays and frequently quoted from them . . . he was fond of Burns, Byron, Coleridge, Shelley and Keats as poets."[6] There is, therefore, strong evidence that Crawford Long was not only a highly cultivated individual but specifically his interests ran to a delight in the almost contemporary great Romantic poets of his time. He therefore could not help but be influenced by their writings and their conveying of the strong Romantic concepts so well described in their work.

Further support for the influence of the Romantics upon Crawford Long is found in the 70th anniversary celebration of the first administration of ether by Crawford Long in which academic activities of an important nature were presented at the University of Pennsylvania as a memorial to their distinguished alumnus Crawford W. Long on March 30, 1912. In those ceremonies Dr. J. William White, the President of the University of Pennsylvania, pointed out the important nature of societal readiness as well as the great insight that Crawford Long had in making the connection between the characteristics of a drug or foreign substance and its usage in connection with a medical activity. Dr. White says, "but there is something else than 'facts' needed before the discovery comes. Ether may stand — as it did stand — for 300 years on the chemists' shelves while the tortures and agonies of injury, disease, even of physiological processes like parturition, go on unalleviated . . . the facts are there; the men are there. But the currents of thought, the connecting medium, are absent. By the time the 'atmosphere' has formed when the world is as it were, ready for a discovery, there have been almost invariably (perhaps under our unconscious, telepathic influences of which we as yet know nothing), several minds turning or groping in the same direction."[7] Dr. White further in his address makes the statement that it is important to understand the value of the advanced and magnificent education Long received at Pennsylvania by describing it as, "it may certainly fairly be said that when Crawford Long came here at the age of 23, he found as he could have found no where else in America, the scientific traditions, the intellectual stimulus to original thoughts and deeds, the atmosphere, in other words that was favorable, probably essential, to his later achievement."[7]

All things considered, there is clear and unmistakable evidence that Crawford Long was a child of his age and was very familiar with the best education both in medicine and in literature of the time. His living habits and his behaviors had complexities which need to be understood better. There appears to be some conflict in the fact that a wealthy slave holder would be greatly influenced by the language of the common man and its pursuits in defending natural human rights so clearly enunciated by the great Romantic poets. However, Long was a child of his time and a wealthy Georgian would be an anomaly indeed if he left his native Georgia to which he was so attached or freed his slaves. Even Jefferson was like Long with respect to slavery. Long, therefore, was a mind very well prepared and fashioned to be able to make the apparently unrelated connections between the social experiences of the inhalation of nitrous oxide or ether for fun, for mind alteration, and for pure sport to an important medical therapy. To his great credit must go the realization of the connection between injury sustained during the influence of ether inhalation and its subsequent analgesia with the crucial clinical use of employing it to prevent the pain of deliberate and planned surgery. The time had to be right. The societal readiness had to be there and the forces of human intellect had to be competent enough to make the connection between a desired and acceptable new practice in medicine i.e., the prevention and the alleviation of pain and suffering with the possibility to do so.

References

1. Papper EM: The influence of romantic literature on the medical understanding of pain and suffering — The stimulus to the discovery of anesthesia. Perspectives in Biology and Medicine; 35:3, 401-15, Spring 1992.
2. Bergman NA: Humphry Davy's Contribution to the Introduction of Anesthesia: A New Perspective. Perspectives in Biology and Medicine; 34:4, 534-41, Summer 1991.
3. Nuland SB: Doctors: The Biography of Medicine. New York, Knopf, 1988.
4. Davy H: Researches, Chemical and Philosophical, Chiefly Concerning Nitrous Oxide or Dephlogisticated Nitrous Air and Its Respiration. London: J. Johnson, 1800.
5. Taylor Frances Long: Crawford Williamson Long, Annals of Medical History; VII: 267-424, 1925.

5a. Ibid, pg. 268

5b. Ibid, pg. 270.

5c. Ibid, pg. 271.

5d. Ibid, pg. 273.

5e. Ibid, pg. 274.

5f. Ibid, pg. 273.

5g. Ibid, pg. 277.

6. Jacobs J: Some Personal Recollections and Private Correspondence of Crawford Williamson Long. Privately Printed — in Archives of the University of Pennsylvania (Atlanta, Ga. 1919).
7. White JW: Memorial to Dr. Crawford W. Long: An Account of the Ceremonies. Special Bulletin, The University of Pennsylvania, Philadelphia, April 1912.

1880'S MEDICAL POLITICS AND SPINAL ANESTHESIA

R. W. PATTERSON
Los Angeles, California, USA

Reports in American medical journals of 1900 enthusiastically acclaimed the latest European surgical advancement; analgesia accomplished by subarachnoid injection of cocaine.[1,2] Fifteen year earlier, in 1885, the report[3] by an American neurologist, Dr. James Leonard Corning, describing the extent of neural blockade resulting from the identical technique and suggesting that such a procedure would be useful during surgical procedures, was completely ignored.

Corning was 30 years old when the spinal paper was published in 1885. He was in the midst of building up a private practice of neurology in New York City, a process that depended on referrals and consultations and demanded congenial accommodation with the powerful cliques controlling hospital appointments, as well as with the general practitioners. General practitioners of the 1870's and 1880's resisted specialism as a challenge both to their conception of medicine as a unitary field and to their relative social and economic status. "Most threatening to the general practitioners were the specialists who claimed as their domain not the most difficult cases of a particular type, but all cases pertaining to a class of people."[4] Though immersed in these practical problems, Corning was already evincing a predilection for clinical investigation. He was one of numerous investigators who had been stimulated by Koller's 1884 report on the use of topical cocaine. In 1885 he published the results of his experimental studies, "On the prolongation of the anesthetic effects of the hydrochlorate of cocaine when subcutaneously injected," and a book on the subject of "Local Anesthesia."

Preceding these events and preliminary to pursuing his special interests in diseases of the nervous system, he had worked with the renowned surgeon, J. Marion Sims, and been directly exposed to situations of pain and to the problems of general anesthesia; both topics which would continue to fascinate and involve him the remainder of his life. For reasons which will be subsequently reviewed, it is apparent that American surgeons would have been reluctant to try the newly suggested procedure even had he attracted their attention with a title more appropriate to their speciality such as, "Painless Sounding of the Bladder;" or if his experiment had not involved a medical patient, "a man who had long been a sufferer from spinal weakness and seminal incontinence, and who for many years had been addicted to masturbation and other forms of sexual abuse.[3] However, at this time the selection was not inappropriate; masturbation was classified as a somatic disease[5] with a distinct cause and pathology.[6] An authority on this disease was Austin Flint, an influential New York physician and powerful political leader in the fields of medicine and neurology. Hospitals reported death from masturbation, and autopsy findings substantiated the effects of self-abuse on the spinal cord,[6] from which it followed that proper treatment would be a matter of scientific concern and not an occasion for moral condemnation or cynical dismissal. Then, as now, the medical facts being dealt with were not timeless truths, but data given through the distorting biases of our history and culture. "Medical reality exists within the embrace of society's expectation."[7]

Corning had also worked with Dr. Edward Seguin, the first Professor of Neurology at the College of Physicians and Surgeons, the President of the New York Neurological Society, and a founding member of the American Neurological Society. Through such association Corning became familiar with the turbulent strife of the expanding, embattled specialty of neurology; the politics of which formed a background and a restraint to his work on medication of the central nervous system. Extending the field of interest far beyond organic disease of the nervous system by asserting that "the mind itself was to be understood as a physical phenomenon, a function or product of the brain and perhaps even of the spinal cord," spokesmen for Neurology had precipitated a schism within their own ranks.[8] The eminent neurologist, George Beard, asserted that insanity was as much a physical ailment as smallpox or a broken leg. The clinical neurologist, with his scientific knowledge of physiology and pathology, considered himself the most competent person to treat the insane patient. In 1878 an active group of neurologists attacked the Superintendents of the Asylum Association, the members of which had the monopoly on the professional care and treatment of the insane, accusing them of being essentially committed only to custodial care — combining the tradition of "moral treatment" with a "medical response" to a social problem (the hospitalization of the destitute, aged, or "the difficult). The acrimonious controversy broke into the public sphere including, as reported in the New York Times, the Superintendent's stark rebuttal that treatment advocated by the upstart neurologists, "Direct medicament of the brain and nervous system is malpractice. . . ."[9]

Further unwelcome public observance of the professions "disarray" soon occurred as the nation's press focused on the legal proceedings following the "God-inspired" assassination of President Garfield in 1881.[10] Criminal responsibility was the trial issue. There was a public fear that vengeance might be cheated if the assassin was declared legally insane. Expert testimony reflected with clarity the personal, social and professional antagonisms that split the institutional structure of Medicine. The Superintendents, whose institutional and public role made them conscious of the expressed will of common men and the mundane strategems of politicians, were solidly behind the prosecution; "Insanity developed as a result of processes, often flawed religious education, taking place during life."[10] For the defense, the scientific cadre of Neurology proposed an intellectual argument emphasizing the hereditary causation of mental illness and criminality. Such advanced medical views were viewed with general suspicion, "as being tainted with European sensualism and materialism, atheistic, and inimical to the welfare and stability of society."[10] The will of the people prevailed; for Guiteau, death; for medicine, a persistent suspicion of professional irresponsibility and dereliction of moral duty. Many Americans in the 1880's already considered physicians a generally impious, mercenary, and cynical lot. The bitterness and near unanimity of respectable opposition to the defense experts' arguments imputed a somewhat defensive tone to medical writings generally. The striking discordance in the testimony of the opposing sides publicly proclaimed that medical science was clearly unable to settle disagreements within its own camp. Beset by pervasive flawed public image, clearly it behooved all of Medicine, and in particular those associated with the specialty of neurology, to keep a low profile and avoid the limelight.

As noted by George Beard in 1882, "The Anglo-Saxon peoples have in modern days a genius for nonexpertness in science. . . . Were we not constantly nursed at the breast of Germany, both England and America would long since have starved scientifically."[11] Unlike many of his American medical colleagues who in the late 19th century felt obliged to add a continental cachet with a year of touring European medical clinics and surgical theaters, Corning from age 14 had been schooled in Germany. He received his medical degree from Wurzburg in 1878. His dissertation was directed by the anatomist Rindfleisch in the department of Pathology. In this milieu exposure to knowledge of the spinal cord and cerebrospinal fluid was unavoidable.

By the end of the 1870's, the membranes and cavities of the brain and spinal canal had been extensively investigated and described in Germany by Magendie, Luschka, Retzius and Axel Key. In 1872 Heinrich Iraneus Quincke (1842-1922) published an informative description of the subarachnoid space, drawing attention to the fact that this was but a potential space in the dead animal. His studies, based on needle injections of dye into the subarachnoid space of living animals, demonstrated that the entire arachnoid of both cord and brain form a continuous sac.[12] Rindfleisch, the mentor of Corning, was known as an intensive investigator of the vascularity and hyperemia of the brain and spinal cord.

In 1881, using the format of the Croonian Lectures, Moxon discussed the gross and microscopic aspects of the membranes, ventricles, and spinal canal supply to the cord, Moxon tried to explain why only the legs and lower part of the spinal cord were involved in the "bends." Later named caisson disease, the problem was well described by A. Jaminet, the physician associated with building the Eades Bridge in St. Louis in 1871. Out of 352 workers, 30 were seriously affected with paraplegia,[12] or fatally. Autopsies noted copious collections of subarachnoid fluid with effusions.[13]

Corning, referring to his own studies conducted prior to 1888, describes a lumbar puncture rationale and technique that is the very model of explicitness. "I became impressed with the desirability of introducing remedies directly into the spinal canal, with a view to producing still more powerful impressions upon the cord, and more especially upon its lower segment. When a needle is thrust down between the spinous processes of the third and fourth lumbar vertebrae, . . .the point of such a needle, after penetrating the dura mater, will find itself directly in contact with the filaments of the cauda equina, which from this point downward occupies the space of the spinal canal." He further points out that "medicinal fluid now injected through the needle will thoroughly impregnate the cerebrospinal fluid bathing the filaments of the caudia, thus powerfully affecting the functions of the lower segments of the cord."[14]

Nevertheless, at a time when general anesthesia posed significant problems and disadvantages, Corning's efforts to persuade surgeons to try this simpler approach were in vain. He was sympathetic to their fears of wounding the cord, "Nor ought we to judge them harshly for this; for at that time penetration of the meninges of the cord seemed as venturesome an undertaking as did mutilation of the peritoneum at a more remote epoch."[14] In spite of Weir Mitchell's view that "the passage of a needle into the nerve of an animal causes usually a little bleeding which passes away without grave result,"[14] Corning experimented with techniques designed to lessen such possibilities and encourage clinical use. He devised a small trocar to be thrust through the skin, through which a long, fine needle could be passed till the spinal canal was entered. This technique was reinvented by Sise in 1928. Other recommendations included the use of a markedly shortened beveled needle point; needle length measurements related to the vertebra to extend confidence as to the intra- or extrathecal position of the tip; also, the planned deliberate extradural or epidural deposition of anesthetic drug. Additionally, he devised a nonpenetrating bulbous-ended outer sheath-needle combination used to apply drug to the cord by iontophoresis without instrumentally invading the subarachnoid space.

These efforts did not evoke the bold surgical trailblazing he anticipated. Their apathy continued even though, because of his 1885 paper on extending the duration of subcutaneous cocaine, he was frequently called into consultation by surgeons confronted with patients difficult to conventionally anesthetize with inhalation methods. This reminded him of times "while I was serving my medical apprenticeship with Dr. J. Marion Sims my attention was often attracted by the great difficulty often experienced in etherizing individuals of large and robust constitution and I had many a discussion on the subject with my illustrious preceptor."[15] This prompted his "endeavors to abbreviate the time necessary to place a patient under the influence of an anesthetic." His observations on the influence of the circulating blood volume to the speed of induction of general anesthesia became the subject of several communications.[15,16] The principle involved was stated in his 1882 monograph on Carotid Compression, wherein is described an external device to occlude the carotid arteries: the technique was reinvented in Germany in 1923 to circumvent the excitation phase of inhalation anesthesia.[17] Corning's prescient 1894 book, Pain, discussed the subject of pain management, a discipline that would remain dormant for the next 75 years. In one section of the book he details therapeutic irrigation of the subdural space. One of the cases treated in this manner was a patient with caisson disease; a subject he had reported on earlier in 1890.

During the 1890's there were numerous investigators tentatively employing lumbar puncture clinically: none of the American experience met with enthusiastic acceptance. In addition to the prudent cautions imposed by strife within the medical community, there was also a pervading hostility toward the profession in the public sector that mandated a measure of circumspection and reticence relating to novel observations and treatment, particularly where an "aura of experiment" was concerned. There is no more apt illustration of this chilling atmosphere than the stark pillorying of Dr. Arthur H. Wentworth in the cause of public relations.

At the end of the 19th century, cerebrospinal meningitis was one of the deadliest diseases. In 1895 Wentworth, a professor pediatrics at Harvard Medical School, faced with the diagnostic dilemma of differentiating cerebrospinal meningitis from other diseases of the spinal cord and brain, performed lumbar puncture to obtain cerebrospinal fluid for bacteriologic examination. Accounts of 27 children formed the basis of his 1895 and 1896 publications on the diagnostic value of lumbar puncture. When he presented his research to the American Pediatric Society in 1896, commentators were emphatic in support of his investigations and had no doubts as to the diagnostic value of the procedure. However, a hostile societal group was set to intervene! Previously, Professor H. Newell Martin at Johns Hopkins (whose isolated mammalian heart preparation has been claimed to be the greatest single 19th century contribution made by an American physiological laboratory), had been subjected to a vigorous and sustained attack by the antivivisectionists; a disruptive movement active throughout the 1880's and 1890's. Within a year of his presentation, in an article titled, "Human Vivisection," published by The Philadelphia Polyclinic Medical Journal, Wentworth was castigated for conducting what were seen as experimental operations on children.

In 1896 antivivisectionists proposed a bill to the Massachusetts legislature restricting animal experimentation in medical schools.

Hearings on the bill captured and held the attention of Bostonians in an extraordinary way. Not since a campus murder 50 years earlier was so much public attention, curiosity, and concern exhibited by the general public about the activities of the scientific and medical establishment. The scientists and practitioners of Boston stressed that the antivivisectionists' attacks were directed against medical science and endangered the freedom to acquire knowledge. To the President of Harvard the proposed legislation represented an attack on academic freedom and the entire educational process. The bill was not passed. But the attack was continued in 1900 with the rallying cry, "animal experimentation ultimately leads to human experimentation," and the centerpiece was to be Wentworth's experimental operations on children, i.e., lumbar puncture.[18]

Nathaniel Bowditch (Dean of the Harvard Medical School, and one of the founders of the American Physiological Society, as well as its first president) and members of the Boston Society Medical Science Defense Committee deliberately decided to mount no defense. They felt that a vigorous public debate on the issue might interfere with their efforts to raise funds for the new medical school buildings.[18] In an effort to avoid controversy during the hearings, Bowditch prepared a public apology to defuse the issue. "Dr. Wentworth's experiments on lumbar puncture have been universally and emphatically condemned by the medical profession. . . . Dr. Wentworth now entirely agrees with the opinion here expressed and regrets extremely that his enthusiasm for the advancement of medicine led him to forget his duty to his patient."[18] Wentworth himself had no input to the deliberations, nor to the statement. He had not agreed. He had no regrets for his work. He did not sign the statement. He resigned from Harvard. No one at the medical school spoke in his defense, or in defense of lumbar puncture, not event his chief Dr. T.M. Rotch, who had co-authored Wentworth's first paper in the Boston Medical and Surgical Journal.

Such an occurrence clearly emphasizes the attitudinal differences between European and American scientific developments and assimilation. In Europe, discipline was internal to the profession, scientific data and laboratory techniques were the basis of medical practice; achievement was measured in terms defined by the world of academic science. Whereas in American medical institutions, political and financial considerations were major factors in professional success, and in medical practice external social attributes determined distribution of status and influence. America lacked an organized disciplined institution capable of sustaining an authoritative and stimulating atmosphere where an audience of fellow workers could fruitfully shape their partially developed thoughts. By the early decades of the 19th century it was plain that popular politics in the United States would not support either the guidance of a "national aristocracy of talent," as envisioned by Jefferson, or the building up of scientific institutions that would bring America among the leaders of world science, as John Quincy Adams proposed.[19] Later in the 1800's, Dr. William Alexander Hammond, neurologist and organizational gadfly, had plans for a "National Institute of Letters, Arts, and Science" to function like the Royal Society of England, or the National Academy of France. An "Academy of Medical Sciences" was actually organized as a division of the fledgling National Institute, with Austin Flint Sr. as President and Hammond, Vice-President. The National Institute never materialized: the nation's intellectuals were left "to be a company of Nomads or Bedouins, each one of whom is to go his own way."[20]

During the years that the American publications of Corning (1885, 1890, 1894), Browning (1894), Jacoby (1895), Caille (1894) and Goldscheider (1895) were pointedly overlooked, similar European studies of Quincke (1887, 91), von Ziemssen (1893), Sicard (1898), Bier (1899) and Tuffier (1899) were openly proclaimed and discussed at international meetings.

After the International Medical Congress, August 1900, Tuffier's surgical clinic was visited by American surgeons. Impressed, they returned to their hospitals, satisfactorily duplicated this new form of surgical anesthesia, and published a plethora of enthused reports. Now under the protection of "authoritative" European approval, no longer having to distance themselves from possible accusations of human experiment, and with the further competitive impetus of mastering the latest surgical advance, suddenly the American surgeons could fearlessly copy a procedure that they could have pioneered.

As a Chicago Professor of Surgery, John B. Murphy, pointed out, "It is to be regretted that the Americans were so long in appreciating the great original work of Corning, and it is only another illustration that original work by Americans is many times not adopted by their countrymen until it is returned to this country with European sanction."[2]

References

1. Phelps AM: Subarachnoid injections of cocaine as a substitute for general anesthesia. The Philadelphia Med J; 6:868-9, 1900.
2. Murphy JB: Subarachnoidean injections of cocaine as a substitute for general anesthesia in all operations below the diaphragm. The Chicago Clinic; 13:427-38, 1900.
3. Corning JL: Spinal anesthesia and local medication of the cord. NY Med J; 42:483-5, 1885.
4. Blustein BE: New York neurologists and the specialization of American medicine. Bull Hist Med; 53:170-83, 1979.
5. Russell J: Cases illustrating the influence of the spinal cord in inducing paraplegia. Medical Times and Gazette, London; 2:456, 1863.
6. Engelhardt HT Jr: The disease of masturbation: Values and concept of disease. Bull Hist Med; 48:234-48, 1974.
7. Engelhardt HT Jr: The Foundations of Bioethics. New York: Oxford University Press, Chapter 5, 1986.
8. Blustein BE: A hollow square of psychological science. In : Madhouses, Mad Doctors and Madmen. A. Scull, ed. Philadelphia: University of Pennsylvania Press, 1981, 241-70.
9. New York Times: Treatment of the insane. 1879, 14 Nov., p 3, col 1.
10. Rosenberg CE: The Trail of the Assassin Guiteau. Chicago: University of Chicago Press, 1968.
11. Rosenberg CE: The place of George M. Beard in nineteenth-century psychiatry. Bull Hist Med; 36:245-59, 1962.
12. Quincke H: Zur Physiologie der Cerebrospinalflussigkeit. Arch f Anat Physiol (Leipzig); 153-77, 1872.
13. Jaminet A: Physical effects of compressed air and of the cause of pathological symptoms produced on man, by increased atmospheric pressure employed for the sinking of piers, in the construction of the Illinois and St. Louis Bridge over the Mississippi River at St. Louis, Missouri. St. Louis: R&TA Ennis, 1871.
14. Corning JL: Pain. Philadelphia: J B Lippincott Co, 1894.
15. Corning JL: On the effective, rapid, and safe induction of general anesthesia. NY Med J; 46:466, 1877.
16. Patterson RW: 1887 Manipulation of uptake and distribution. The Circular; 5:10-12, 1988.
17. Ritter C: Anämisierung des Gehirns zum schnelleren Eintritt der Narkose. Zentralblatt f Chirurgie; 36:1390, 1923.
18. Benison S, Barger AC, Wolfe EL: Walter Cannon. Boston: Harvard University Press, 1987.
19. Price DK: The Scientific Estate. Cambridge Mass.: Harvard University Press, Chapter 4, 1965.
20. Blustein BE: A New York Medical Man: William Alexander Hammond, M.D., Neurologist. Ph D diss, University of Pennsylvania; 1979.

REACTIONARY SOCIETY AND THE INTRODUCTION OF ANESTHESIA

R. W. PATTERSON
Los Angeles, California, USA

Commentators suggest that by the early 19th century the development of anesthesia as a goal-in-itself was imminently inevitable in Britain, Europe, or even in America. Pain relief as a worthy goal became an integral part of Romantic and Humanitarian idealism; a concept favorable for anesthesia was "in the air;" the idea was "ripe for the time."[1,2,3] Such considerations, though permissive of the means of amelioration of pain, were obviously not sufficient to create an understanding of the means. For more than fifty years (1795-1845), the prescient suggestions and sporadic attempts of almost a dozen eminent investigators (Pearson, Mitchill, Davy, Stockman, Hickman, Guthrie, Glover, Long, Wells, Ellsworth) faltered. Later, when priority of discovery was questioned, some guidelines were formulated that stressed as important requisites publicity and practical application. "A party can be entitled to no consideration, whose efforts have gone little beyond speculation and who has not developed the leading idea, by application or use, or when the application has been of so imperfect a character as to indicate that he had formed no just conception of its practical bearing and value. . . ."[4]

In a review of a century of progress from the vantage point of 1876, the Professor of Medicine at Harvard proudly proclaimed, "The progress in medicine has kept abreast of the other natural sciences of politics and of theology and has made equal conquests over authority, error and tradition. Crystallized by the American Revolution and the faith of Christendom, such has been the progress . . . and achievements of medial science . . . to justify the enthusiastic regard in which physicians hold their profession and to deserve the gratitude of mankind."[5] This accolade indicates nothing of the determinate conditions. Initiation in 1846 of the self-sustaining chain reaction of clinical anesthesia depended on basic short-term societal drives; individualism, economics, utilitarianism, vanity. A pragmatic American society established their desires and demands; the medical profession followed rather than led. Fifteen years earlier (1831), when chloroform was discovered by the American physician Samuel Guthrie, its usefulness as an anesthetic went unrecognized because of the theory of medicine being practiced at the time.[6] Based on the Brunonian system, all diseases had been reduced to two categories, sthenic and asthenic. The cure of the latter was to increase the amount of a theoretical body property, excitability, through the use of a group of substances known as diffusible stimuli. Included in this group were opium, nitrous oxide and ether: all were recommended for resuscitation from suffocation, narcotic overdose, and drowning. Guthrie was actually trying to produce such a stimulant when he formed the new compound, chloroform. Samples sent to the Professor of Materia Medica at Yale, Eli Ives, were confirmed to be a drug useful only as a diffusible stimulant. Collectively, orthodox physicians and dentists ignored the postulated idealistic permissive considerations mentioned above, and they were neither instigators of the discovery nor, afterwards, promoters of its use. From many examples, two illustrations of this negative attitude are: the outstanding onslaught by Dr. J.F. Flagg, who together with his brother and an infamous "committee of 7" from around the country, brought forth a malicious manifesto to suppress the growing evil;[8] and the proscription of the use of ether during the Mexican War by the Military Field Surgeon, John B. Porter. Porter contended, "It poisons the blood and depresses the nervous system; in consequence, hemorrhage is much more apt to occur, and union by adhesion is prevented."[4] Further, he pontificated, "Manly heroism, tempered in the fire of military life and honed by the excitement of battle, make soldiers insensitive to the pain of almost any operation."[9] Throughout the remainder of the century, as Pernick emphasized in "The Calculus of Suffering,"[9] surgical pain itself was not sufficient to compel anesthetization.

This stifling, authoritarian, and paternalistic attitude, based on dogma rather than substance, characterized the first 50 years of U.S. Medicine and was the source of an ever widening gulf between the professional practice of medicine and what the majority of people felt they needed, or at the very least would accept. The foremost medical educator in the new republic was Benjamin Rush. For Rush a multiplicity of treatments to fit the individual case was not just a mistake, but a form of quackery. His explicit Enlightenment faith in the simplicity, predictability, and rationality of the universe, and his Jeffersonian conviction that in real and important ways all men had been created equal, were reflected in his advocacy of reducing the concept of "Medicine" to one mankind, one disease, one therapeutic regime. Routine therapeutic measures were Calomel given till toxicity occurred; bleeding for childhood fevers; and the application of pain to drive disease out of the body. Revolted by this institutionalized triad of heroic poisoning, bloody butchery, and therapeutic pain, patients began to abandon orthodox medicine in favor of the various "irregular" sects whose practices were less productive of iatrogenic disease and suffering.[10] Thomsonianism was the most prominent and influential medical sect in the late 1830's.[11]

Thomsonian botanical therapy was designed to complement and assist the body's "healing power of nature" (an idea that was an anathema to Rush who had declared, "Gentlemen, we can have no reliance on Nature, we must turn her out of doors in our practice and substitute for her efficient art.")[12] Botanical therapy was in accord with the popular prejudice against the orthodox armamentarium of unnatural mineral remedies and human contrivances in treating disease. Equally important, in stark contrast to the corporate body of regular physicians, Thomsonianism responded sensitively to the social and intellectual needs of the populace. The sect appealed to the working man, had an affinity to the perfectionist teachings of the liberal clergy, and was in the forefront of the feminist movement that from 1830 on promoted women's rights societies, which in turn organized protests and crusades to further their concerns with political issues such as peace, abolition, and temperance. The success of Thomsonians was due in no small part to their sincere identification with radical causes.

Politically, they saw their movement as "wresting medicine from the doctors and completing the great revolution which, beginning with the Reformation, freed government from the lawyers and despots, and religion from the priests."[11] They would have every man be his own physician. Later, when this was seen to be too radical and their influence waned, the teachings of Hahnemann took over. Unlike Thomsonians, Homeopaths never had any doubts about the need for medical schools and medical societies. A sect that scorned medical learning had been supplanted by one which emphasized that its physicians were more learned in the sciences of the day than regular physicians, and that they alone could bring to bear on medicine all the newly discovered wonders of vitality, force and electricity. Increased patronage of the "irregulars," reflecting their popularity, was an economic disaster for orthodox practitioners who, through their local and state medical societies, fought to maintain their position by legal proscriptions. By 1830, thirteen states had passed licensing legislation that sought to protect fees and monopolize medical practice for trained "regular" physicians who constituted only a small fraction of the total number of medical advisors to the populace.[10]

Concurrently, in the economic realm, the vast expansion of the transportation system of canals, turnpikes, and (in the 1840's), railroads created a means of obtaining raw materials in one part of the country, assembling units in a manufacturing center, and redistributing the finished product back into the hinterland. This transition to a full-scale factory system, mass-producing goods for broad distribution, spelled the end of the era of independent handcraft and domestic production, and incidentally of a democratic homogeneous middle class, and in its stead spawned a "social revolution in which sovereignty in economic affairs passed from the community as a whole into the keeping of a special class;"[13] middlemen dealing in loans and credit. America became "blessed or cursed with financiers, security flotations, stock markets, and all the other appurtenances of industrial capitalism;[13] all were privileged institutions protected by state and federal laws.

The old-style Federalists held that voting was a privilege and not a right, and that the chief functions of government were the protection of property and of individual freedom, not the forcing of the majority will on a reluctant minority. These views were expressed in conservative state constitutions that not only restricted suffrage by property qualifications, but further removed government from the people by providing for Councils of Appointment to fill state offices and for Councils of Revision having the right to veto popular legislation. During the 1820's, popular feeling which long favored reforms to change the undemocratic aspects of the outmoded constitutions was too strong for politicians to ignore. By 1828 political reforms prevailed, all restrictions on white manhood suffrage were removed; many, for the first time voting directly for the presidential electors, expressed their democratic spirit and newly-won political might by overwhelmingly electing Jackson. By the 1830's, in most states, persons had triumphed over property.

A monopoly over medical practice was out of harmony with the spirit of the Jacksonian age which sought "to emancipate talent, enterprise, and industry from corporate restrictions; to leave the mind free to exercise its energies and allow the public freedom to encourage what it approves."[11] Organized medicine, banks, and other chartered corporations were similarly opposed as monopolies whose "all exclusive privileges, or powers, or facilities, for the accumulation of wealth, or the exclusive use and enjoyment of the bounties of Providence secured to individuals or combinations of men by legislative enactments, the free and uninterrupted enjoyment of which are denied by laws to other members of the same community."[13] By the mid-1840's popular antipathy forced dissolution of the medical establishment's legislative protections. Henceforth, not physicians, but the consumer would assert by their patronage their prerogative to define discomfort and indicate what treatment would be acceptable. The American medical societies, caught in a democratic upheaval within 50 years of their formation, were publicly humiliated by the revocation of their licensing authority.[11] The network of medical societies collapsed. The professional environment in America had been cleared of obscurantive medical dogma and of restrictive legislation regarding practice; now conditions encouraged innovation and experimentation, inventiveness and patents; worthy enterprise defined as the desires of society, would be rewarded with wealth.

During the 1830-1840 period, egalitarianism was achieved politically, but was lost in the economic sphere where society became increasingly stratified, with the emergence of a powerful "aristocracy of wealth." The financial panic of 1837, together with the ensuing depression and the mass immigration of European paupers, had by the mid-40's irrevocably widened the gap between impoverished laborers and financier capitalists. New York city alone had 21 individuals whose wealth exceeded a million dollars, and the term "millionaire" was coined. The image of the aristocrat had changed from the traditional agrarian patriarchal squire to the wealthy plutocrat, the city-centered merchant or industrialist who thrived under the laissez-faire economic conditions prevalent in Jacksonian America. Now EQUITY meant that all men "shall be free to become as unequal as they can."[13] An "aristocracy of wealth" was spawned — "creating a spirit of exclusion and persecution unknown in any other country."[13] Members of this " gilded society" were too self-centered, too conscious of their self-perceived distinctiveness to tolerate any remnants of the previous egalitarian medicine. The individualization of homeopathic practice suited their self-perceived unique status. Homeopathic practitioners had captured the top-scale market among the social, economic, and intellectual leaders of American society.

The absence of legitimate aristocratic tradition (one in which social rankings were unquestioned), made all Americans emphasize status. America's plutocratic self-centered and status-conscious society expected to be catered to. Position was asserted by means of "conspicuous consumption." No amplification of extravagance and luxury was too extreme: thus emerged a society pompous without dignity, gaudy without significance, lavish without taste, aristocratic without good manners. "Perhaps at no other time in American history were women so pampered as in mid-19th century America."[13] Not having domestic duties, nor being allowed to follow a profession or even a serious intellectual pursuit, aristocratic ladies gave an inordinate amount of attention to fashion. A commentator on women in America during the 1840-1850's noted; "The tendency to Orientalism is visible . . . woman as a being formed for no higher purpose than to be decorated, admired, and valued for her personal charm. Do we not see females in every fashionable circle who fill no loftier station in social life, and who live as idly and as uselessly as the gorgeously attired inmates of the harem. . . ."[13] The neck, and more, was bared. In any group the woman who was not décolleté was obviously the maid. Completely out of the question was the former medical practice of applying leeches, cupping, or lancing in the neck region! The ubiquitous fan was more utilitarian than merely a fashion statement. Concealment of the mouth was necessary in this era when decayed and lost teeth were a universal complaint; often the result of following the old-time medical prescription, "give mercury till toxic."[10] There was a need to invent the cult of Plastic Surgery!

For more than a century teeth had been transplanted from one person to another (a completely elective procedure that lasted into the 20th century). For ordinary prostheses, barrels of donor teeth were taken from the battlefields of the Napoleonic Wars and from the battlefields of the American Civil War. For wealthy VIPs to whom money was no obstacle in the search for cosmetic enhancement, there was a demand for young vigorous incisors from healthy people for direct transplant. Money was an inducement to be a donor; pain, however, was a potent inhibitor of this traffic in teeth. Morton with his factory capable of mass-producing artificial teeth had solved the donor problem, but was faced with the reluctance of those in need to submit to the pain of full mouth extractions. Pain was an impediment to the fortune to be made in dentures. There was a place for one ancillary aid to his dreams! Who else had an active tooth factory with employees and an extensive lucrative practice that had already made him wealthy, and which needed only one small additional device to expand and complete this capital enterprise? Four months before the actual success, Morton was able to confide to W.P. Leavitt, "I have got it now. I shall take my patients into the front room, and extract their teeth, and then take them into the back office and put in a new set, and send them off without their knowing anything about the operation."[8] Utilization of anesthesia was not the realization of an idealistic goal, but only a means to an entrepreneurial dream.

References

1. Greene NM: A consideration of factors in the discovery of anesthesia and their effects on its development. Anesthesiology; 35:515-522, 1971.
2. Vandam LD: The start of modern anesthesia. In: The History of Anaesthesia. Atkinson RS and Boulton TB, eds. Parthenon Press, 1988.
3. Caton D: The secularization of pain. Anesthesiology; 62:493-501, 1985.
4. Smith T: An Examination On The Question of Anaesthesia. New York: JA Gray, 1859.
5. Clarke EH: A Century of American Medicine 1776-1876. Philadelphia: Lea, 1886.
6. Patterson RW: The first human chloroformization. In: The History of Anaesthesia. Atkinson RS and TB Boulton, eds. Parthenon Press, 1988.
7. Guthrie O: Memoirs of Dr. Samuel Guthrie and the History of the Discovery of Chloroform. Chicago: Hazlett & Co., 1887.
8. Warren E: Some Account of the Letheon. 3rd Edition. Boston: Dutton and Wentworth, 1847.
9. Pernick MS: A Calculus of Suffering: Pain, Professionalism, and Anesthesia in Nineteenth Century America. New York: Columbia University Press, 1985.
10. Coulter HL: Divided Legacy. Vol III Science and Ethics in American Medicine. Washington, D.C.: McGrath Publishing Co., 1973.
11. Kett JF: The Formation of the American Medical Profession. New Haven and London: Yale University Press, 1968.
12. Eaton LK: Military surgery of the Battle of Tippecanoe. Bull Hist Med; 15:460-463, 1951.
13. Miller DT: Jacksonian Aristocracy. New York: Oxford University Press, 1967.

FRANZ KUHN
(October 12, 1866 — March 28, 1929)

Tribute to an outstanding surgeon on the occasion of the 125th anniversary of his birthday

MATTHIAS REINHARD[1] **and ELKE EBERHARDT**[2]
[1]*Department of Anesthesiology, Critical and Emergency Care, Städtisches Klinikum Fulde, Germany*
[2]*Department of Vascular Surgery at the Kurhessisches Diakonissenkrankenhaus Kassel, Germany*

The name of Franz Kuhn (1866-1929) is well known in the history of anesthesia. He tried unsuccessfully to establish endotracheal intubation and artificial positive pressure respiration as standard anesthetic techniques for a long time. His antagonist, Ferdinand Sauerbruch, at that time Germany's most famous surgeon, rejected the technique as being too dangerous. Instead, he promoted the use of his hypobaric chamber for the performance of intrathoracic surgery. As the dominating figure of the German surgical scene, Sauerbruch remained, as expected, the winner. Long-term, however, the idea of "pulmonary narcosis" was more convincing. Nevertheless, we first needed the comments of the British anesthetist, Noel A. Gillespie, in the year 1941 (German edition in 1953), to recall the name of Franz Kuhn and his outstanding contributions to modern anesthesia and surgery. But it was not until 1974 that he was given due recognition for his work by anesthetists in his native land, a plaque being unveiled outside the hospital in Kassel where he achieved so much.

Franz Kuhn, the pioneer of oral intubation, was born on October 12, 1866, in Aschaffenburg as the fifth child and only son of the farmer Michael Kuhn and his wife Marie. He began his medical studies in Würzburg and continued them in Berlin and Munich. He finally passed his boards back in Würzburg in 1890/91. He was also awarded his doctorate at the University of Würzburg in 1891 with a dissertation on "Morphological Contributions to Postmortem Putrefaction." In 1896 he published for the first time, in the Münchner Medizinische

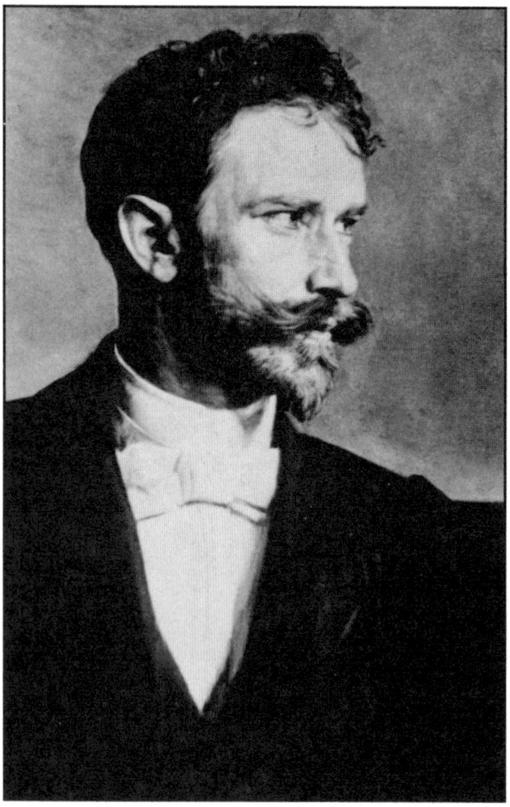

Fig. 1. Frans Kuhn (1866-1929).

Wochenschrift, his experiments with a metal spiral tube which he had developed and used as an aid for the performance of pyloric catheterization.

In 1897, a study trip took him to the United States where he received further stimulation for his work on intubation narcosis at clinics and institutes in New York, Philadelphia and Baltimore. Whether he also met Joseph P. O'Dwyer, a New York physician who was similarly occupied with the problems of oral intubation in connection with artificial positive pressure respiration for the therapy of asphyxia, opium and morphine poisoning, is rather doubtful. Nonetheless, Franz Kuhn was sure to have been inspired by his ideas.

In 1899, Franz Kuhn was appointed medical director of the newly built Elisabeth-Krankenhaus in Kassel. During this period (1899-1913) he developed the technique of orotracheal intubation to a matter of clinical routine. He published over 90 papers, 33 of which were concerned with intubation of the trachea and positive pressure ventilation. He used his flexible metal tube to treat asphyxia and to administer chloroform anesthesia, which he called "Pulmonale Narkose." The flexometallic tube consisted of a spiral of thin metal whose cross-section was s-shaped and wound so that the contiguous edges overlapped. At the distal end of the tube, which measured between 12 and 15 cm in length, was fixed a fenestrated cap reminiscent of the modern Murphy Eye. Above this was a cylindrical shoulder which prevented the tube being inserted too far into the trachea. At the proximal end, a protective shield was attached which prevented damage to the tube by the teeth. The tube was secured to the patient by means of a stout rubber band passed behind the head and fixed to a metal hook.

The great significance of his intubation narcosis in those days becomes clear when one considers that the great surgeon and Heidelberg Professor, Vinzenz Czerny, had Franz Kuhn travel from Kassel on January 13, 1905, in order that the first operation under intubation narcosis could be performed at the University Clinic. In 1911, his monograph about endotracheal intubation was published.

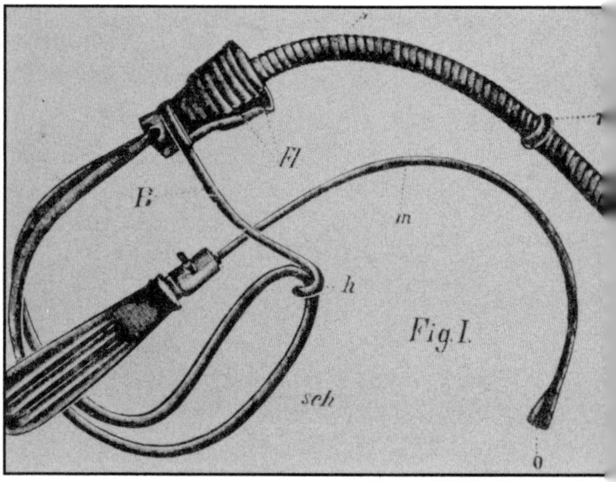

Fig. 2. Kuhn's tube which he called "Pulmonale Narkose."

Kuhn was also interested in thoracic surgery and in preventing the problems surrounding the production of a pneumothorax, which had confounded generations of surgeons before him. He became a central figure in the controversy which sprang up at the turn of the century as to how this problem should be best solved. In 1904, F. Sauerbruch, a 28-year-old surgeon working in Breslau invented a chamber into which the thorax of the patient was placed. The air was then partially sucked out the chamber while the patient continued to breathe spontaneously. In this way the problems caused by the pneumothorax which accompanied thoracotomy was avoided. This marked the beginning of the underpressure school of thoracic anesthesia. Kuhn, on the other hand, could appreciate that the key to successful thoracic anesthesia lay in simplicity. Instead of unwieldy pressure chambers, he recommended tracheal intubation, using his own tube, and the application of positive pressure directly to the end of the tube. For this purpose he developed, with the help of the Drager firm, several machines for thoracic surgery. Unfortunately, Sauerbruch had become such an influential figure, especially in Germany, that at the time Kuhn's novel ideas were met with hostility, and it is probably true to say that, through Sauerbruch, the further development of thoracic anesthesia was considerably delayed.

Because of the abundance of his medical duties and scientific work, it is quite astonishing how much time Kuhn devoted to the cultivation of social connections. As an illustrious member of society, he maintained active contact with distinguished personalities and groups disposed to the fine arts. Together with his friend Otto Fuhr, who had set up a practice as a general practitioner in Kassel, he was a member of the artists' group, "Pinselsruh," to which the tropical research Professor Menze and the painter Professor Knackfuss also belonged, among others. Incidentally, this portrait of Kuhn also was done by Knackfuss.

But Kuhn found rest and relaxation not only in social circles; his fondness for a rural lifestyle — he was a passionate rider and hiker — was always retained as a reputable surgeon. In Kassel, Kuhn also found his partner through life, who gave him two children, one of whom is a daughter who still lives in Berlin-Friedrichshagen.

Despite his love for Kassel, in 1913 Franz Kuhn assumed the directorship of the newly built St. Norbert Hospital in Berlin-Schönberg. As a competent surgeon and untiring scientist in possesssion of a marked talent for administration, he soon acquired a distinguished reputation in his new workplace. His passionate participation in all surgical congresses at home and abroad, as well as the consistent defense of his medical ideas, his reputation as a conscientious surgeon and self-sacrificing physician, and his calm and relaxed nature, allowed him to quickly gain a foothold in Berlin as well. In his private lifestyle, Franz Kuhn appears to us to have been a modern physician through and through, who instinctively practiced on himself the art of a natural autogenic training and thereby became what can be rightly said of him, without skeptical analysis of his character, a wonderful man and physician who not only wrestled with death, but could also valiantly face it. Specifically, although he suspected his own death, he put off his family and friends by saying it was rheumatic trouble. He did not allow himself to become bitter or resigned at his fate. Rather, he made a study trip in his weakened condition which took him to Egypt to the notorious Cairo slaughter houses.

Franz Kuhn was also responsible for the introduction of sterile catgut, in itself a monumental contribution to medical practice.

On March 24, 1929, he allowed his children to visit him on his deathbed in their Sunday clothes. On Maundy Thursday, March 28, 1929, Franz Kuhn died at age 63 of a lung carcinoma. So ended the life of a truly brilliant physician, characterized by high artistic and literary creativity, whose outstanding theoretical and practical achievements for medical science appeared for a long time to have sunken into darkness.

HENRY RUTH
MODERN ANESTHESIOLOGY'S UNHERALDED PIONEER

HENRY ROSENBERG and JEAN K. AXELROD
Professor and Chairman, Department of Anesthesiology,
Hahnemann University Hospital, Philadelphia, Pennsylvania, USA

The evolution of anesthesiology from a poor relation of surgery to equal acceptance in the galaxy of medical specialities is due to the unstinting efforts of such giants in the field, during the third and fourth decades of this century, as Lundy, Rovenstine, Waters, Tovell and Wood.

Henry Swartley Ruth, a 1923 graduate of Hahnemann University Hospital in Philadelphia, while not as well known, deserves recognition equal to those colleagues. Together they and a handful of other distinguished members of the field founded the American Board of Anesthetists in 1938 for the purpose of certifying anesthetists as specialists. Anesthesiology was reorganized as a separate major specialty board in 1941, and Ruth became President two years later.

Henry Ruth is probably best remembered as founder in 1941, and Editor for the next 15 years, of the journal "Anesthesiology," official publication of the American Society of Anesthesiologists and still the leading journal in the field.

During Ruth's student days and early career at Hahnemann, the homeopathic philosophy of gentle, natural healing was practiced. There was no conflict, however, with the use of powerful, potentially dangerous anesthetic agents when it came to life-saving surgical measures. Ruth quickly adopted this field, as much for its need for greater recognition and a solid organizational base as for its clinical challenges.

Following graduation Ruth worked as a staff medical anesthetist at both Philadelphia General Hospital (which with 2,200 beds and some 20,000 patients a year offered experience unavailable elsewhere) and at Hanemann. He became Chief of PGH's anesthesia division in 1933 and in the same year assumed the title of Clinical Professor of Anesthesia at Hahnemann Medical College.

Before Ruth's tenure at PGH, interns and technicians administered anesthetics due to fear that medical anesthetists would greatly increase overhead. Throughout his clinical and administrative careers he crusaded for hospitals, whatever their size, to establish anesthesia services; he was able to employ significant time- and cost-saving measures to convince many institutions to comply.

In 1936, Henry Ruth instituted the Anesthesia Study Commission of the Philadelphia County Medical Society to probe the cause of anesthetic fatalities and to improve anesthetic care.

Despite the strong editorial demands of a fledgling journal on Henry Ruth during the war years, his clinical and teaching responsibilities took on an added dimension. He was the driving force in Philadelphia behind requiring more military and naval officers to take a basic course in fundamental surgery to be followed by a curriculum in anesthesiology; he can be credited with bringing physicians into the specialty after World War II.

Ruth was first delegate from the Section of Anesthesiology of the House of Delegates of the American Medical Association. During his tenure (1941 to 1945) he often had to defend the position that anesthesia constituted a branch of medical practice. Because of his and his colleagues' persistence in countering the American Hospital Association, which considered anesthetists to be hospital employees and thus unable to bill for professional services, anesthesiologists can today submit professional fees and be reimbursed by the patient or a third party.

Among other honors and memberships: President of the American Society of Anesthetists, Inc. (1938) and recipient of the society's Distinguished Service Award in 1952; President of the Philadelphia Society of Anesthesiology (1947-48); President of the Pennsylvania Society of Anesthesiologists (1948-49). His bibliography, moreover, lists authorship of 54 articles, more than half of which dealt with clinical subjects. He also served as associate editor of the section on anesthesia in "Cyclopedia of Medicine" from 1939 to 1952.

Henry Ruth died following a fall at age 56, having retired the preceding year.

SIR HUMPHRY DAVY IN SLOVENIA
Neogenesis and the Girl from a Feverish Dream

JOSEPH RUPREHT* and D. SOBAN**
**Erasmus University Rotterdam, The Netherlands and the University of Ljubljana, Slovenia*
***University of Ljubljana, Slovenia*

Among anesthesiologists, Sir Humphry Davy (1778-1829) is generally known for his early work in the Pneumatic Institution and for his unique book on nitrous oxide. It is less appreciated, however, that Davy in his later years paid little attention to anesthesia and medicine in general. His distaste for surgery may have played a role, but it is probable that his poly-historic mind dealt with medicine as with just another of the many phenomena in the surrounding world. Davy is still famous as the pioneer of electrochemistry and for discovery of potassium, sodium, calcium, barium, magnesium, strontium and chlorine. He was a member of the Royal Society and its president from 1820 to 1828, the years when he visited Slovenia three times. It has been stated that Davy's greatest discovery was Michael Faraday. Another great Davy discovery, the miner's safety lamp, is well known.

Davy was also a poet, though he refrained from publishing his poetry. He was on friendly terms with the greatest English literary protagonists of his time: Coleridge, Wordsworth, Byron and Scott. His last work, *Consolations in Travel* or *The Last Days of a Philosopher,* written during his last travel in Europe (1828-1829), appeared soon after his death in 1829. It consists of six poetic and philosophic discourses among friends. In this book Davy describes the beauty of Slovenian Alpine valleys, the curious subterranean creature *Proteus anguinus,* and his grateful memories of the "Illyrian maid," the girl he met in Ljubljana, but was sure of having known her from a previous delirious fever.

Memorial Plate in Podkoren

After crossing the Pass of Podkoren, on his way from Carynthia to Carniola, Davy liked to lodge in a monumental Royal-Imperial Postal Station in Podkoren, now house number 63. The house has not changed since. During the time of Davy's visit to Slovenia, the owner was Alojz Razinger. In 1889, the Slovenian Section of the German-Austrian Alpine Association put a memorial plate on the house in Podkoren with an inscription in German: "In this house lodged the famous scientist Sir Humphrey Davy (born 1778, died 1829) who often visited this valley which he praised for its beauty to his contemporaries." The plate was removed between the two world wars and was re-installed on 5 May 1953, this time with the inscription in Slovenian. Supposedly, it is the same plate, the German inscription now behind, on the side attached to the wall.

The Human Fish, Proteus Anguinus and Neogenesis

The fourth dialogue in Davy's *Consolations in Travel* is titled, *The Proteus or Immortality,* and comprises over fifty pages. Part of this text contains all that was known about the human fish, *Proteus anguinus*, in Davy's time. Proteus had been described much earlier, in the seventeenth century, by Count J.W. Valvasor, resident of Carniola and also a member of the Royal Society. Proteus is a blind amphibious creature living in the cavern waters of Slovenia, deep under the earth. Its smooth and white skin gave rise to the nickname, "the human fish" or "poisson humain." Proteus is one of the greatest natural treasures of Slovenia and a biological rarity par excellence.

Davy started the fourth part of *The Consolations* by describing his trip from Tirol to Styria and Podkoren in Slovenia. There he stayed several days, "in this beautiful valley, in the heart of beauty." He then described the subterranean rivers of Illyria (Slovenia) and the particularly interesting Magdalen Cave, now known as the Black Cave. The dialogue about the Proteus takes place in the Magdalen Cave. Davy mentions that it was his third visit to Slovenia (Illyria). It was, indeed, also the last one of the three; 1818/19, 1827 and 1828 (Table 1). In the subterranean lake of the cave there were specimens of Proteus, which, Davy explained, could breathe under or above water. He introduced the concept of adaptation; in comparison to a polar bear, perfectly suited to arctic conditions, the Proteus was made for living in eternal darkness of subterranean waters. The interesting part of *Proteus or Immortality* is the discussion as to whether

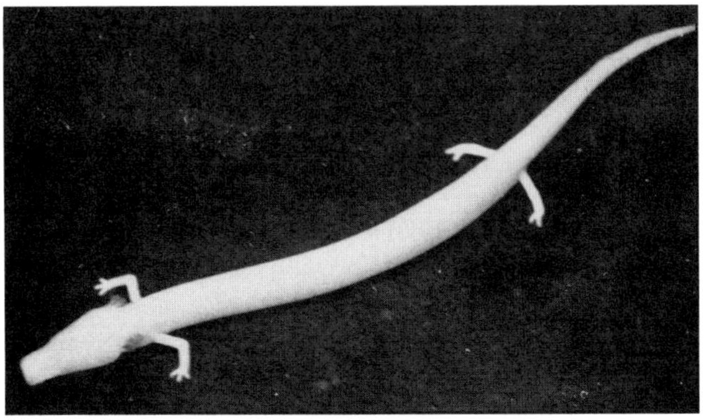

Fig. 1. *Proteus anguinus,* an amphibian subterranean creature of Slovenia which attracted S.H. Davy's scientific interest (photograph by A. Aljančič).

Proteus multiplies like all other creatures, or it simply is formed anew from the mud. Davy makes short steps with such a possibility, stating Harvey's rule "omne vivum ab ovo," that an egg precedes all life. Herewith, Davy also helped to bury the theory of neogenesis, or what was left of it in his time.

The Illyrian Maid

In the second part of *The Consolations,* Davy mentions the typhoid fever he had suffered from 25 years earlier, possibly contracted during his improvements of ventilation in a London jail. This disease followed very shortly his discovery of potassium and sodium in 1808. In his fever he repeatedly saw a beautiful woman, but not his future wife Jane Kerr. The girl was blue-eyed, had brown hair and rosy cheeks. For several days this appearance was quite clear to him, but would be forgotten when he recovered from the fever. Davy mentioned that all his feelings for this visionary girl were spiritual and elevated. Ten years later Davy travelled in Slovenia and was reminded of his old dream by a girl of about fourteen or fifteen years of age. Another ten years later, Davy goes on, he again met a person who looked like the woman of his vision. She nursed him during his illness and he considered her to be his guardian angel, the same as the vision of twenty years before.

Who was this "Illyrian maid," Davy's guardian angel? She certainly was not a product of fiction because he wrote to his brother John Davy, a military doctor in Malta, that he was ill and indebted greatly for his recovery to his lovely, small nurse (a letter of 21 December 1828). "The Illyrian maid" was also mentioned in Davy's letter from Ljubljana to his wife (5 October 1828). Davy's biographer, Anne Treneer, suggested the name Papina Dettela in the book, *The Mercurial Chemist.* Correct Slovenian spelling would be Pepina Detela, Pepina standing for "Josephine" and Detela for "Clover." In a book, "Inns of Old Ljubljana," an inn called "Pri Deteli" or "Pri Detelji" is recorded. It stood at the spot of the present hotel Union and was distinguished by a huge stone ball above the front entrance. The Slovenian writer and a judge in Ljubljana, I. Travcar, also mentioned the inn "Pri Deteli" and recorded that the owner's daughter was "an acquaintance" of the famous English scientist. In another booklet by A. Bauer, *Sir Humphry Davy in Oesterreich,* Josephine Dettela is also mentioned and, according to Bauer, Davy remembered Josephine in his last will with a considerable legacy.

No clarification has been forthcoming for Davy's first encounter in Ljubljana with a very young girl, and it is not clear whether he referred to his first or second visit to the Illyrian capital. There is no doubt that he met Josephine Detela on his last trip 1828/1829, when he first stayed in Podkoren from 20 August 1828 and arrived in Ljubljana on 30 August; he left Ljubljana on 31 October 1828. In Ljubljana he completed his Irish story, "The Last O'Donoghne."

Davy's wish to visit Ljubljana again, together with his brother John, in the spring of 1829, was not fulfilled. He wrote from Italy to his friend, Tom Pooley, to come and visit Revigo and Illyria, "the most famous part of Europe." But in March 1829, his health deteriorated badly. His brother came from Malta and his wife from London to accompany him back home. Davy arrived in Geneva on 28 May, 1829, and died one day later without being able to see again the valley from Podkoren to Ljubljana, "the most beautiful he saw in Europe."

Davy has never been forgotten in Slovenia where his admiration of the beauty of the country is highly appreciated. The contemporary Slovenian illustrated journal for natural sciences, *Proteus,* has published several accounts of Davy's scientific work and his sojourns in Slovenia, written by the great Slovenian naturalist, L. Cermelj (Proteus 23, 1960-61, pp 53-54; Proteus 26, 1963-64, pp 1-6 and 33-37). The Slovenian Medical Journal published reports of Davy's work on nitrous oxide and his visits to Slovenia (D. Soban, Humphrey Davy and his "laughing gas" in Slovenia, (in Slovene); Zdrav. Vestn. 47:601-6, 1978.

TABLE I
H. Davy's Travels to Slovenia

26 May 1818-1820	Flanders, Germany, Vienna, Hungary, Carniola, Italy, Pula, Napels, Rome; Carniola (1819), Italy (1820). Call on Byron.
January 1827	Ravenna (Italy); Ljubljana (19 April, 1827-23 May, 1827). Austria, Bavaria, Switzerland. Ljubljana (11 August-September)
29 March 1828 to 28 May 1829	France, Belgium, The Rhine, The Danube, Sturia, Illyria (Carniola): Podkoren (10 August); Ljubljana (20 August-6 October). Treiste, Ljubljana, Rome, Rovigo, Siena, Florence, Genoa, Turin, Susa, Mt. Cennis, Geneva (28 May 1829).

DUTCH NEWSPAPER REPORTS ON ANAESTHESIA IN EARLY 1847

J. RUPREHT, M. WALEBOER and M.J. van LIEBURG*

Department of Anaesthesiology and
**Department of History of Medicine*
Erasmus University Rotterdam, The Netherlands

Introduction

Dutch physicians embraced ether anesthesia only a few weeks after the well-documented applications of ether before surgery in London and Paris.[1] In medical circles there was the usual controversy about the merits of the new medical treatment, and there was no one to foresee the fundamental change in surgery brought about by anesthesia. University centers were not in the front line of application of anesthesia, although they provided useful reviews on the matter towards the end of 1847. From the study of medical journals, however, it was not possible to establish exactly how the news of anesthesia reached Dutch physicians. Physicians also failed to record the attitude of their patients and the reaction of the general public to the victory over surgical pain.

In addition to medical journals, the most convenient source of information about the early story of anesthesia is the public press, of which there has never been a shortage in the Netherlands. Information from the newspapers may be more rewarding although, admittedly, sometimes less reliable than professionally censored and inhibited reports in the professional medical press.

Dutch Public Press in 1846-1847

It can be estimated that there were about 40 Dutch dailies and weeklies printed in the Netherlands in 1846-1847. Of these, 36 were screened for availability of all issues between October, 1846 and May, 1847. Most of them have been preserved incomplete, or were discontinued between the two dates. Further selection as to the major cities and to the university towns left us with four complete newspapers for that period (Table I). There were four medical schools at that time in the Netherlands, at Amsterdam, Leiden, Utrecht and Groningen. All these cities were served by local newspapers.

TABLE I
Screened Issues of Dutch Newspapers between October 1846-May 1847

Newspaper	Days of Appearance
1. Amsterdamsche Courant	(Mon-Sun)
2. Utrechtsche Provinciale en Stads-Courant	(Mon, Wed, Fri)
3. Nieuwe Rotterdamsche Courant	(Mon-Sun)
4. Leydsche Courant	(Mon, Wed, Fri)

Usually, newspapers were divided into national and international sections and contained a few pages of advertisements. Reading these newspapers is rather difficult as the captions given refer only to a foreign country or city, followed by miscellaneous information — often no more than one sentence. Precise dates for events from abroad are usually absent as the correspondent sent in a collection of news items, dated on the day of writing, but the items were published several days later.

Reports of Anaesthesia. October 1846-May 1847

Thirty-nine reports on anesthesia were found, 28 being different items with 11 duplications. The earliest traced mention of anesthesia in the searched newspapers appeared in the Amsterdamsche Courant, on Wednesday 3 February 1847. The correspondent from Paris mentioned that several newspapers had reported successful applications of sulphuric-ether in France and Belgium. The news item also contained Malgaigne's communication to the Académie de Médicine that one must be very careful with ether in order to prevent an explosion, possibly also in the patient's chest. Reports peaked between 22 February and 12 March 1847; 95 percent of 39 reports appeared in this period. This peak falls only one week after the peak of reporting about anesthesia in German speaking countries.[2] Although the first reports dealt with anesthesia, most of the subsequent reporting concerned Dutch anesthetics (Table II).

TABLE II
Anesthetic Reports per Country of Origin

Country	Number
Netherlands	17
France	10
"Germany"	7
Britain	3
Italy	1
Belgium	1

Most reports, 16, appeared in the Nieuwe Rotterdamsche Courant; the other three newspapers dealt with anesthesia seven or eight times. Terminology for both anesthesia and for the type of anesthetic was variable and could be understood only in its context concerning surgery. "Ether" was spelled also "aether," likewise its vapor "etherdamp" or "aetherdamp." Very often "zwavel-ether" was the name for the agent described. Anesthesia produced by ether was called descriptively as "artificial sleep" or "under the influence," but also "sulphuric-aether-narcosis" or "aetherisation." Dutch journalists mentioned many French, German and Dutch physicians who practised anesthesia, but no English physicians: the only Anglo-Saxon who is mentioned in a somewhat erroneous context is Dr. Jackson for his "discovery."

Anesthesia in the News Items and Side Effects

Besides frequent description of the use of ether in dentistry, there is a surprising variety of medical procedures performed "under the influence," extending from oncologic surgery to trauma, urologic procedures, ophthalmologic operations, treatment of spasms or pain of delivery. Most interesting, perhaps, is the report on the use of ether in France to identify sham illness among military conscripts. Treatment of neuralgic pain was also successfully completed with ether. Anesthesia was also performed for animals.

Nine newspaper reports described side-effects and dangers of anesthesia with ether. Danger of explosion was mentioned, but there were also reports of lung disease, eventually lethal. Crying and unpleasant dreams caused by inhalation of ether were described. Inability to express pain during inhalation must, nowadays, be seen as an early record of inadequate anesthesia.

Origin of Untoward Anesthetic News

Dutch newspapers reported on the lethal outcome of anesthesia, but only from secondary sources. The only clear-cut case report of delayed death following surgery and anesthesia, but ascribed to damage of the lung by ether, was British. There were also French warnings against possible dangers, but no detailed lethal outcomes of anesthesia from Germany or the Netherlands. This may be due to the long British tradition of open discussion and reporting of medical complications. Otherwise, lack of reported deaths caused by ether may have been due to good luck and the significantly lower number of anesthetic procedures on the Continent. One is inclined to suppose that physicians on the Continent did see lethal outcomes of anesthesia because on 16 February, 1847, the local government in Franken officially limited administration of ether to physicians only. This early regulation was duly reported in the Netherlands in the Nieuwe Rotterdamsche Courant of 24 February, 1847.

Of interest is the refusal by patients to accept anesthesia. An item of anesthesia news from Paris reported that in March 1847, soldiers in Algiers refused to be anesthetized before operation because this would have indicated lack of courage to bear pain.

Dutch Journalists and Anesthesia in Early 1848

Regardless of Magendie's "masterly opposition" to the use of sulphuric ether, news was conveyed by the Amsterdamsche Courant of 27 February, journalists succeeding in a realistic presentation of anesthesia as it found its way on the Continent. There were equal numbers of enthusiastic news, sceptic warnings of untoward sequelae of anesthesia, and wider social information on anesthesia. Generally, journalists themselves, judging from the newspaper pages all anonymous, took great care to refrain from personal comments. However, a few times the correspondent clearly left trace in the news item. While reporting van Woerden's "trials" with ether in Utrecht (Utrechtsche Prov. en Stad-Courant, 3 March 1847), the journalist noted that, "in face of growing science to diminish human suffering it is an exceptional pleasure to report such facts." The news item of death following lithotomy under ether in Colchester, Essex, ended with the thought that one should not judge ether on basis of an exceptional event, but should consider also its "favourable record of fame." The positive attitude of Dutch journalists towards the new medical development became quite clear in a longer item on anesthesia, section "French Mail" of the Nieuwe Rotterdamsche Courant, 13 March 1847. Reporting on deliberations of the Academy of Sciences, the journalist wrote: "the result of ether is, regardless of side-effects, always the same, a complete destruction of the ability to feel pain. It has been said that ether may cause damage some time after the operation, because some patients died after the operation. However, to refute such false statements it is enough to examine the succumbed sufferers. Ether does prevent one to feel pain during a surgical procedure, but no one has ever claimed that it prevents a patient from dying."

References

1. Rupreht J: First years of anaesthesia in the Netherlands. In: the History of Anaesthesia. R.S. Atkinson and T.B. Boulton, Eds. Internat. Congress and Symposium Series 134, Royal Society of Medicine Services Ltd, London, 1989, pp 86-9.
2. Walser HH: Zur Einfuhrung der Äthernarkose im deutschen Sprachgebiet im Jahre 1847. Verlag H.R. Sauerländer & Co., Aarau, 1957, p. 9.

AN ERA OF DIETHYL ETHER ANALGESIA FOR MAJOR SURGERY IN ESTONIA

J. SAMARÜTEL
Tartu University, Tartu, Estonia

A decade after the first demonstration by J.F. Artusio in 1953 of feasibility to use extremely light levels of ether anesthesia, without loss of verbal contact with patient during major operations, this method enjoyed a brief period of popularity in Soviet Union and also in Estonia. It could be viewed as some kind of mental counteraction to previous broad use of "lytic cocktails" of French workers, with comparatively deep CNS and autonomic depression for protection of patient from surgical "shock." Unfortunately our followers of J.F. Artusio abandoned one important point of his technic — inhalation induction up to surgical plane of anesthesia permitting endotracheal intubation without relaxants. Here, after induction with barbiturate, the level of anesthesia was extremely light from the very beginning.

This was probably the main reason for unacceptable amount of patients' complaints of awareness, recollections of pain, etc. which after some years led to disappearance of the method. In Tartu University Hospital this technic was accidentally rediscovered (without knowledge of Artusio's original work) in 1963 and for some time we aimed in most endotracheal anesthesias for major surgery to achieve a state, when the patient reacted to questions and suggestions. For example, in 1964 among 780 endotracheal anesthesias in 53 it was documented, that for shorter or longer time the patient was verbally communicable.

It is interesting that commonly there were no serious hyperdynamic circulatory reactions. Some patients were able soon after operation to extubate themselves. At postoperative follow up 5/53 had recollections from operation, one of them felt severe pain. The main reason, what made us abandon this technic were frequent sleep disturbances in patients with complete amnesia about operation. During falling asleep, patients were wakened up by anesthesiologist's voice with words, told at operation most often "open your eyes." In no instance was there mentioned unusually intense complaints of postoperative pain, what could be deduced from modern pain theories. Our experience attests the feasibility of unconscious perception and retention of verbal suggestions at light levels of anesthesia.

THE HISTORY OF ANESTHESIA IN GUATEMALA

RICARDO A. SAMAYOA de LEÓN
Chief Anesthesia Service, Hospital Nuestra Senora del Pilar
Guatemala City,
Republic of Guatemala

Introduction

The history of Anesthesia in Guatemala starts with Mayan Empire 2,000 years B.C.; but emerges to actual concept on November 30, 1847 when Dr. José Luna first time employed ether for general anesthesia, only one year 34 days after Morton did in Boston.

During more than 30 years I studied historical documents, monographs, medical journals and theses, etc. and interviewed the physicians who started Anesthesia in Guatemala.

The development of Anesthesia in Guatemala can be divided in three periods, accordingly to my studies and experience:

1. **INITIAL: 1847-1947** All advances on new anesthetics, machines and technics were applied by General Surgeons and Physicians with interest to remove pain from surgical activities: *February 21, 1850:* Dr. José Luna employed chloroform for general anesthesia; *August 12, 1901*: Dr. Juan Ortega used rachianesthesia plus cocaine; *May 7, 1903*: Dr. Mario Wunderlich used Ombredanne apparatus plus ether; *June 23, 1930:* Dr. Mariano López used Gwathmey machine for nitrous oxide plus oxygen plus ether; and on *July 24, 1935*: he also used caudal anesthesia for delivery; *May 11, 1939*: Dr. Mario Wunderlich used Penthotal intravenously, and *July 12, 1945*: Dr. Eduardo Lizarralde used tracheal intubation for thyroidectomy with ether.

2. **DEVELOPMENT: 1948-1973** Was initiated by the first six Anesthesiologists specialized in: USA, France, Mexico and Chile and continued with the efforts and help of other 24 Colleagues, achieving in a short period of 25 years a substantial improvement in standards and level of efficiency of Anesthesia in Guatemala: *November 3, 1948:* Dr. Roberto Pérez starts Anesthesia Service in private Hospital Centro Médico; *July 2, 1949:* Dr. Gustavo Ordóñez is named Chief Anesthesia Service, General Hospital San Juan de Dios, followed (1956)

by Dr. Francisco Silva; *February 5, 1950:* Dr. Flaviano Velásquez is named Professor of Anesthesia in University of San Carlos and also Chief Anesthesia Service Traumatologic Hospital of Social Security Institute (SSI); *August 3, 1954:* Dr. Rafael Escamilla is named Chief Anesthesia Service, Obstetric Hospital of SSI; *February 2, 1958:* Dr. Ricardo Samayoa is named Chief Anesthesia Dept., Roosevelt Hospital, starting the Post-Graduate Course of Anes-thesia for Residents; and on *September 1, 1958:* the above mentioned six Anesthesiologists founded the Associación de Anestesiólogos de Guatemala (AGG), then the AAG is accepted like active member of CLASA on *May 4, 1968,* and of WFSA on *September 10, 1968,* with 33 years of adequate functioning.

3. **MODERN: 1974-1991**
Anesthesiology is recognized like a complete Medical Speciality, with eight good Anesthesia Depts., and three Post-Graduate Courses of Anesthesia, authorized by University; AGG grows to 50 active and 30 candidate members, organizes XV Latin American Congress of Anesthesiology; *August 26-31, 1979;* with Abstracts published by Excerpta Medica: ICS-490.

Summary:

During a period of 144 years development of anesthesia in Guatemala has been very satisfactory and always in accordance to the WFSA objective and theme: ANESTHESIA, SAFETY FOR ALL.

THE HISTORY OF LATIN AMERICAN CONFEDERATION OF SOCIETIES OF ANESTHESIOLOGY (CLASA) DURING 30 YEARS

RICARDO A. SAMAYOA de LEÓN
Guatemala City,
Republic of Guatemala

Introduction

When CLASA celebrated in Caracas, Venezuala its XXV anniversary on October 22, 1987, I was CLASA's General Secretary and I had the honor of giving a Conference about history of CLASA, and now I have completed this study.

Methods

Since 1960 I have attended Latin American Congresses of Anesthesiology and General Assemblies of CLASA, then I know all Abstracts and minutes of these Meetings; and also I have interviewed all Anesthesiologists related with the foundation, development and improvement of CLASA during its 30 years of functioning.

Results

The most important data and achievements are like follows:

1. **Congresses:** Argentenian Society organized first Latin American Congress Anesthesiology in Buenos Aires, *October 1949,* and Secretary Dr. José Delorme started the idea of CLASA, and continued with next Congresses: II in Sao Paulo *1954;* III in Bogotá, *1956;* IV in Viña del Mar, *1958,* and V in Mexico, *1960:* Dr. Zairo Vieira (Brazil) was elected Secretary; and during VI Congress in *Lima, Perú: October 22, 1962,* CLASA was founded by Delegates of: Argentina, Brazil, Bolivia, Colombia, Chile, Ecuador, Mexico, Perú, Uruguay and Venezuela; since then Latin American Congresses and General Assemblies of CLASA were realized every 2 years, with a change in 1967, until last XXI Congress and XVI Assembly: Río de Janeiro, *September 4-8, 1991;* achieving high standards of academic, scientific and gremial levels.

2. **General Secretaries of CLASA:** They were: Dr. Zairo Vieira, Brazil: *1962-64;* Dr. José Silva, Colombia: *1964-69;* Dr.

Juan Köster, Perú: *1969-71;* Dr. Carlos Castaños, Bolivia: *1971-79;* Dr. Jaime Herrera, Colombia: *1979-83;* Dr. Ricardo Samayoa, Guatemala: *1983-87;* Dr. Martin Marx, Uruguay: *1987-89;* and Dr. Virgilio Paez, Ecuador: *1989-91.*

3. **Teaching:** In 1984 General Secretary, Dr. Ricardo Samayoa (Guatemala) also member of Education Committee (CESA) of WFSA *(1980-88);* created the programmes GELAV-CLASA, similar to VET-WFSA, with financial aid of pharmaceuticals companies and WFSA, with excellent results: 1-2 programmes each year, 3-6 Professors, visiting 3-6 host Societies, during 3-6 weeks.

4. **Logo:** General Assembly of CLASA, in Río de Jaineiro: *October 12, 1971,* selected for CLASA the Logo designed by Dr. Juan Marín: a pioneer Anesthesiologist from Colombia; then Dr. Francis Foldes, President of WFSA suggested same Logo for the Presidential Medallion of WFSA, accepted during V-WCA in Kyoto, Japan: *September 1972,* and first worn by Dr. Otto Mayhoffer, when elected WFSA's President.

5. **WFSA:** Always CLASA maintained good relations with WFSA, and finally became a Regional Section of WFSA on *October 23, 1987* during XIV General Assembly in Caracas, Venezuala; due to the efforts of: Drs. Carlos Parsloe and Say Wan Lim, President and Chairman of WFSA, and Dr. Ricardo Samayoa, General Secretary (President) of CLASA.

Summary:

Today CLASA represents 20 Latin American Societies of Anesthesiology and 6,455 Anesthesiologists, working all together to maintain, improve and develope the level of efficiency of Anesthesia for all our Latin American Surgical patients.

THE DANISH INFLUENCE ON AMERICAN ANESTHESIA

OLE SECHER
Copenhagen, Denmark

When *Nikolai Ivanovich Pirogoff* (1810-81) wrote his book, "Recherches pratiques et physiologiques sur l'éthérisation," and published it in May-June 1847, he had given ether per rectum to 40 patients.[19] It is not known in how many patients he used his method, but in his description of the "Caucasian war" in the summer of 1847, "Rapport medical d'un voyage en Caucase," he mentions that he used rectal ether even for patients he operated on the battlefield. Shortly after his report from the war came out, chloroform was introduced and Pirogoff used this anaesthetic for the rest of his life.

The Danish military surgeon, later Professor *Oscar Wanscher* (1846-1906), wrote a small book in 1882, "On the use of ether for inhalation at surgical anaesthesia,"[27] in which he summarized evidence for the advantages of the use of ether, and the dangers of chloroform based on a literature study and his own experience. This was the start of the Danish part of the discussion of "ether contra chloroform," which took place all over Europe and in other places. Two years after the book came out, he published a short article about Pirogoff's methods of giving rectal ether.[28] In this article he mentions that he had found not more than one surgeon who had tried rectal ether vapor and that was the Swedish surgeon, General *Carl Johan Ekstrømer* (1793-1869) in Stockholm, who had used it in five cases in 1847.[24]

Wanscher, who had made a rather simple apparatus for the purpose (Fig. 2), had used the method 22 times in 20 patients and was quite satisfied with the results. He encountered only small problems. The same year, 1884, the Eighth International Congress for Medical Science was held in Copenhagen in August, and here Wanscher presented his results to the surgical section.[29]

In the same period Wanscher was trying out a mask to be used for inhalation anesthesia. Having tried other masks such as Ormsby's (*Lambert Hepenstel Orsmby*, 1850-1923),[17] he made a simple model, but he did not describe the mask before 1894. It was just a mask and a bag, into which was poured a bottle of ether which was then put onto the face of the patient.[30] It was essentially not worse or better than the Clover inhaler (*Joseph Thomas Clover* 1825-82) and other similar inhalers. Being a

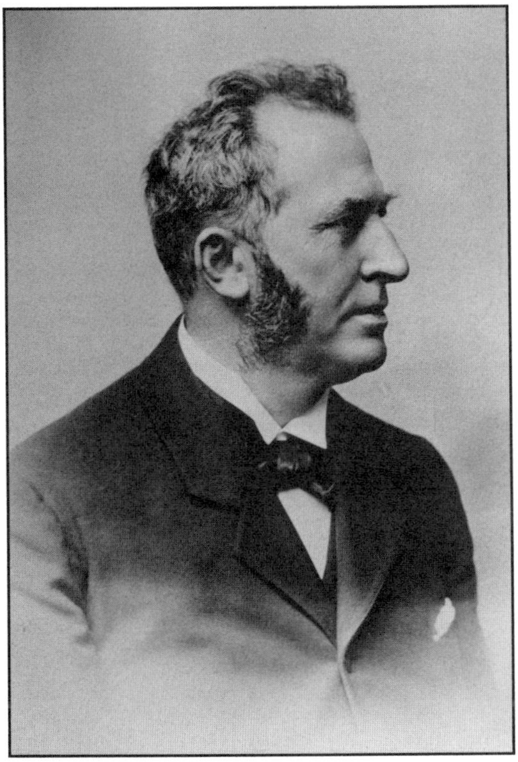

Fig. 1. Oskar Wanscher (1846-1906).

manic-depressive, Wanscher talked and wrote only a few times about ether anesthesia. He had difficulties convincing his colleagues that they should change from chloroform to ether. It was his colleague Professor, Thorkild Rovsing (1862-1927), who convinced most of the Danish surgeons about this change.[22]

In 1884, the Danish chief surgeon at the Municipal Hospital in Copenhagen, *Axel Iversen* (1844-92), visited the French Professor of surgery, *Daniel Mollière* (1848-90), at the l'Hôtel Dieu in Lyon. Lyon was the place where ether was used, Paris was the locale for chloroform. Iversen (often wrongly called Yverson) was an "ether-man" and convinced Mollière that he should use ether vapor per rectum as an alternative to ether inhalation. Mollière took up the method and published a paper about his experiences the same year.[16] This article was received with some interest in the U.S.A., where A. Post, Boston, tried the method and wrote a paper about his experiences with it, which was also published in 1884.[20] (Papers were published rapidly in those days.) Other Americans also tried the method.[26]

The issue of the Boston Medical and Surgical Journal, where Post's paper was published, also had an editorial about the administration of ether by rectum. Post mentions in his paper that the method came from Copenhagen, and the editorial mentions that Dr. Yverson (sic) had given the idea to Professor Mollière. How much the method was used in the U.S.A. is difficult to determine, but probably not much. In any case, the next American article of importance on the subject came in 1905, written by *John Henry Cunningham* (1877-1960) and *Frank Howard Lahey* (1880-1953) in Boston.[10] In this article, Wanscher, Iversen and Mollière are mentioned. The administration of rectal ether was likely used to some extent after this article because when *John Taylor Gwathmey* (1863-1944) published his book "Anesthesia" in 1914, it was *Walter S. Sutton* (?) from Kansas City who wrote the rather extensive chapter about rectal administration of ether.[26] He named the above-mentioned pioneers and had extensive literature references and descriptions of apparatus used.

In Denmark the rectal ether was used occasionally until about 1935.

As mentioned above, Oscar Wanscher also made a mask with a bag for ether administration, and it was Professor Thorkild Rovsing, who was the great advocate for the method he named, "morphine ether narkosis with Wanscher's mask."[22] This technique of administering ether was adopted in Norway, Iceland and some places in Sweden and Germany.

In the months May-July 1912, *Thorkild Rovsing* made a study tour to the U.S.A. to become acquainted with American surgery and anesthesia.[21] On this tour he went to Johns Hopkins Hospital in Baltimore, Philadelphia, New York, Boston and the Mayo Clinic in Rochester. Generally speaking, he was not impressed, neither with the surgery nor anesthesia. The best anesthetics he found were being given at the Mayo Clinic where they were

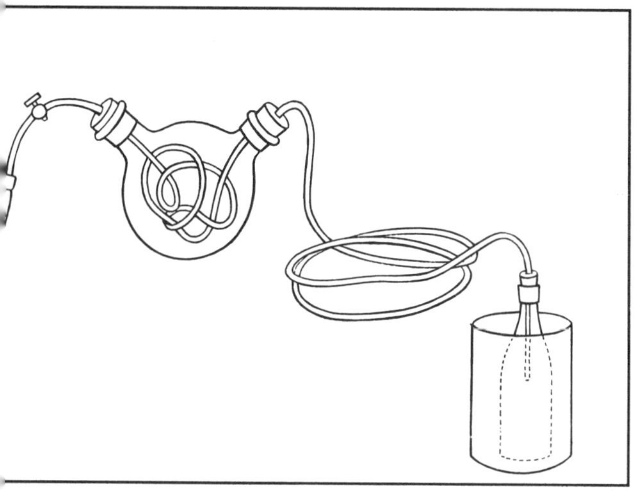

Fig. 2. Wanscher's apparatus for rectal ether vapour.

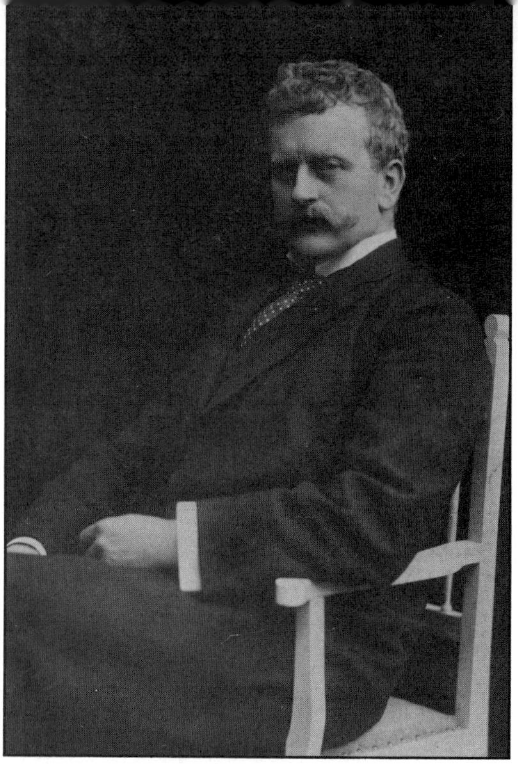

Fig. 3. Thorkild Rovsing (1862-1890).

administered by nurses.

While Rovsing was in Boston, he was asked to give a lecture at the Massachusetts General Hospital (MGH) in the "Ether Dome," and he talked about "Wanscher's etherisation method with demonstration for a very interested gathering of surgeons." As far as I know, he is the only Danish doctor who has talked in this historical place about ether anesthesia. Among the audience must have been the American physician, *Arthur Bryant* (1880-1935), who named himself "anaesthetist" due to the fact that he gave anesthetics at the MGH. In the period of 1912-14, Bryant spent time in Europe, and among other things he looked into surgical departments, and here he was particularly interested in anesthesia. He also came to Copenhagen and visited Rovsing's department at Rigshospitalet. When he came home he wrote a paper, together with the physiologist *Yandell Henderson* (1873-1944) at the Yale University. The paper was published in 1915, "Closed ether and a color sign."[7] The reason that he got together with Henderson must be that they both were interested in anesthesia and surgical shock. At that time Henderson had published his articles about CO_2 concentrations.[12] His theory was, in short, that high CO_2 concentrations in the patient prevented surgical shock, and that low concentrations stimulated its development. In the paper Bryant mentions that he had tried both high and low CO_2 concentrations during anesthesia and could confirm Henderson's theory in practice. In Europe he found the best anesthetics in France and Denmark. He said, "Nobody who once has seen a series of anaesthetics in his (Rovsing) clinic at the beautiful Rigshospital can forget or doubt the advantage, which can be obtained by the use of Wanscher's simple closed ether mask." The patients had a nice reddish color as a sign of good circulation due to CO_2 in inspiratory air. The pale color was due to bad circulation and low CO_2.

Bryant and Henderson's article was reviewed in the Danish medical literature by the internist, *Chresten Lundsgaard* (1883-1930). He wrote that we in Denmark should be very proud that Rovsing had developed and refined this excellent method. This of course developed a local discussion on the standard of anesthesia in Denmark, which by some was considered far behind.[14]

Lundsgaard later spent close to three years with *Donald Van Slyke* (1883-1971) at the Rockefeller Institute in New York and was involved in the fundamental work on cyanosis, which was summarized in the book of the same name.[15] Lundsgaard became Professor of

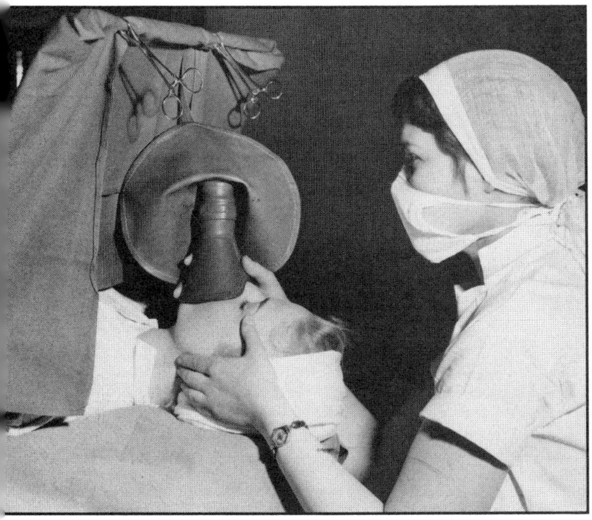

Fig. 4. Wanscher's mask in a late model of rubber only.

Internal Medicine in January 1924, at Rigshospitalet University Hospital, Copenhagen.

The Danish physiologist, *August Krogh* (1874-1945), Professor of Zoophysiology 1916-45, lecturer 1908, was a strong supporter of Henderson's theory. He presented Henderson's CO_2 investigations at a meeting in the Biological Society, Copenhagen, in 1910, "On CO_2 as a regulator in the organism and the causes of surgical shock,"[13] and the same year he became involved in a discussion with the Danish physiologist *Holger Møllgaard* (1885-1973), who became Professor at the Veterinary School in 1911 when he was 26 year of age.[25]

Møllgaard had constructed an anesthesia apparatus which gave a constant positive pressure independent of the respiratory phase. It was used for thoracic operations by the surgeon Rovsing. The apparatus had a motor blowing air into a system with a spirometer bell, an ether chamber, and a water-lock to regulate the pressure. Krogh claimed it was dangerous due to the washout of CO_2, and Møllgaard claimed the opposite. They never agreed.

When we tried the apparatus in 1961, it worked well even with low pCO_2 in the blood.[23]

Yandell Henderson's investigations on animals were rather convincing, but as we know they do not fit with our clinical experiences of today. This problem was brought to attention by Carlos Barsloe in 1987.[18] He pointed out that two Brazilian physiologists, brothers A. and M. Ozorio de Almeida, as a result of experiments in 1918, could prove that the hyperventilation of the animals which Henderson used produced cooling, which could explain the shock. Could the shock be explained by hypothermia and too high a mean pressure in the lungs?

August Krogh was awarded the Nobel Prize in 1920 for his investigations on and explanation of the capillary functions and influence on the circulation. Later, and also before this award, he was visited by a great number of scientists.

In 1926-27, a surgeon at the MGH, later

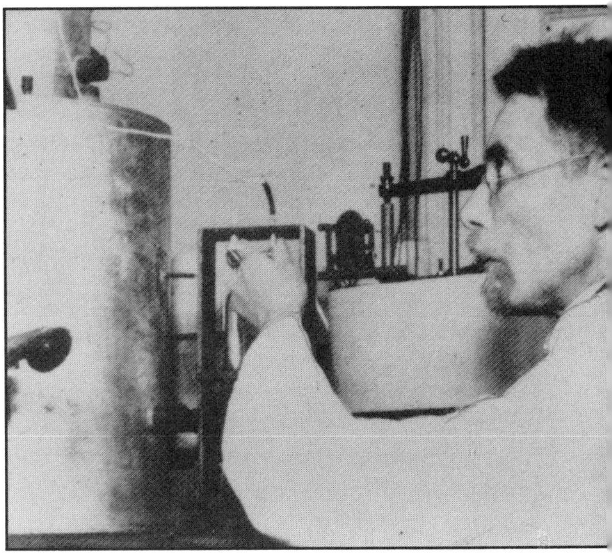

Fig. 5. August Krogh (1874-1945).

Professor *Edward Delos Churchill* (1895-1972), went on a long study tour to Europe. At that time the American physiologist, *Cecil Kurt Drinker* (1887-1956), Professor at Harvard University, spent a year with Krogh. Exchanging letters with Churchill, he suggested that he go to Copenhagen and work with Krogh. So he did, and from the beginning of February to the middle of May they worked together in Krogh's laboratory.[31] He used his time well, and when he had left he said, "I have put my name on two articles together with Drinker."[9,11]

When *Henry Knowles Beecher* (1904-76) had finished his three years of surgical residency in 1935, Churchill must have convinced him to go to August Krogh in Copenhagen for a year to study physiology.[8] He also used his time well because his name appeared on five articles published from Krogh's laboratory from 1935-36, and on two of them together with Krogh's. One article from 1937 was also based on investigations from Copenhagen.[1-6] Coming back to Boston in 1936, he became chief of anesthesia at the MGH, and in 1941 Professor. In 1938 his well-known and very fundamental book, "Physiology of Anesthesia" was published. It is dedicated to Professor August Krogh.

The Danish influence on American anesthesia has not been extensive and did not change circumstances. It is just an example of how ideas and information about anesthesia has been exchanged between countries.

References

1. Beecher HK: Note on distribution of platelets in peripheral blood. Acta med Scand; 87:311-12, 1935.
2. Beecher HK: Independent control of capillary circulation in mammal. Scand Arch Physiol; 73:1-6, 1936.
3. Beecher HK, Field ME and Krogh A: Method of measuring venous pressure in human leg during walking. Scand Arch Physiol; 73:7-16, 1936.
4. Beecher HK: Alive control of all parts of capillary wall by sympathetic nervous system. Scand Arch Physiol; 73:123-32, 1936.
5. Beecher HK, Field MR and Krogh A: Effect of walking on venous pressure at ankle. Scand Arch Physiol; 73:133-41, 1936.
6. Beecher HK: Adjustment of flow of tissue fluid in presence of localized sustained high venous pressure as found with varices of great saphenous system during walking. J Clin Invest; 16:733-39, 1937.
7. Bryant J and Henderson Y: Closed ether and a color sign. JAMA; 65:1-6, 1915.
8. Bunker J:P: Henry K. Beecher, in PP Volpitto, LD Vandam and J Adriani: The genesis of contemporary American anaesthesiology. Charles C. Thomas, Springfield Ill. U.S. 1982.
9. Churchill ED, Nakazawa F, Drinker C: The circulation of body fluids in the frog. J Physiol; 63:304, 1927.
10. Cunningham JH, Lahey FH: A method of producing ether narcosis by rectum with a report of forty-one cases. Boston Med Surg J; 152:450-9, 1905.
11. Drinker C, Churchill ED: Graphite suspension for intravital injections of capillaries. Proc Royal Soc Biology; 101:462, 1927.
12. Henderson Y: Acapnia on shock.
    I Am J Physiol; 21:126-56, 1908
    II Am J Physiol; 23:345-73, 1908-1909
    III Am J Physiol; 24:66-85, 1909.
13. Krogh A: On carbon dioxide as a regulator in the organisms and causes of surgical shock. A survey and some new investigations (Danish). Hosp Tid; 53:441-9, 1910.
14. Lundsgaard C: Closed or open ether narcosis? (Danish). Hosp Tid; 787:505-8, 1916.
15. Lundsgaard C, Van Slyke D: Cyanosis. Williams & Wilkins Co. 1923.
16. Milliere D: Note sur l'etherisation par la voie rectale. Lyon medicale; 14:419-22, 1884.
17. Ormsby LH: A new ether inhaler. Lancet; 1: 218, 1877.
18. Parsloe C: The contribution of two Brazilian physiologists to the introduction of carbon dioxide absorption into clinical anaesthesia. An Acknowledgement by Ralph M. Waters (1883-1979). In RS Atkinson & TB Boulton: The History of Anaesthesia. Royal Society of Medicine Services. Ltd. London 1989.
19. Pirogoff NI: Recherches pratiques et physiologiques sur l'etherisation. St. Petersbourg 1847.
20. Post A: Etherization by the rectum. Boston Med Surg J; 110:442-3, 1884.
21. Rovsing T: Impressions of a tour to America (Danish). Hosp Tid; 5.R.B.6:1188-96, 1227-36, 1913.
22. Secher O: Wanscher's bag or ether contra chloroform (Danish). Bibl Laeger; 153:435-60, 1961.
23. Secher O, Wandall H, Clemmensen T, Siverstsen U: The Mollgaard positive-pressure anaesthetic apparatus. Acta chir Scand; suppl 283:8-16, 1961.
24. Secher O: Introduction of ether into the Nordic countries.Acta anaesth Scand; 29:2-10, 1985.

25. Secher O: A Danish anaesthetic method in American spotlight (Danish). Danish Medical History Yearbook; 14:92-107, 1986.
26. Sutton WS: Anesthesia by colonic absorption of ether, in JT Gwathmey: Anesthesia, New York, 1914.
27. Wanscher O: On the use of ether as inhalation agent at surgical anesthesia (Danish). København 1882.
28. Wanscher O: Surgical anesthesia by ether vapour enema (Danish). Hosp Tid; 3.R.B.2: 553-6, 1884.
29. Wanscher O: Chirurgicale au moyen de lavement de vapeur d'éther. Compte-Rendu du Congrès périodique international Sciences Médicales 8me Session Tome 1. 5 section chirurgie 186-89. Copenhagen 1886.
30. Wanscher O: On ether narcosis (Danish). Ugeskr Læger; 5.R.B.4:770-1m 1894.
31. Wandall J: Personal communication 1991.

FROM EMPIRICAL CRAFT TO SCIENTIFIC DISCIPLINE
The Contributions of Claude-Bernard and John Snow to the Foundations of Anaesthesia

DAVID A.E. SHEPHARD
University of Saskatchewan,
Department of Anaesthesia
Regina, Saskatchewan
Canada

Because, in the earliest days of anesthesia a body of specific and unique knowledge was lacking, the administration of ether and chloroform was guided by personal experience and anecdotal information. The practice of anesthesia was an empirical craft, undertaken by individuals having no training in the new craft. This is not to disparage empiricism, which is a necessary starting point for any medical specialty, and one must admire the earliest etherizers and chloroformists for their courage as pioneers. But empiricism did not ensure reliability or safety, and too often, as Dudley Buxton suggested, the empiric trusted "to rule of thumb, scorns to learn the possible results of his actions, and possesses a courage born of ignorance."[1] Fortunately, soon after the practice of anesthesia was initiated, its nature and its problems came under the scrutiny of two men who shared the thinking of the scientist and who understood the limitations of empiricism. These two were Claude Bernard (1813-1878) in France, and John Snow (1813-1858) in England. Their work was of fundamental importance, and it was largely because of it that anesthesia evolved from empirical craft to scientific discipline and, eventually, to an independent medical specialty.

The contributions of Bernard and Snow to anesthesia are well known, and they need be no more than summarized here (Tables I and II). Less attention, however, has been given to the intellectual attributes that lay behind these contributions, and to the scientific vision that encouraged — even drove — them to commit so much of their careers to the research that came to lay the scientific foundations of anesthesia. In this paper, two aspects of the work of Bernard and two also of the work of Snow are discussed in this light.

TABLE I.

Claude Bernard's Contributions to the Scientific Foundation of Anaesthesia
Research
Physiology
Locus of Action of Anesthetic Agents (Theory of Anesthesia)
Pharmacology
Curare
Opium Alkaloids
Chloral
Physiological Thinking
Clinical Practice
Morphine as Premedicant
Education
Writing

TABLE II.

John Snow's Contributions to the Scientific Foundation of Anesthesia
Research
Respiratory Physiology
Oxygen Metabolism
Carbon Dioxide Metabolism
(Theory of Anesthesia)
Uptake and Elimination of Volatile Agents
Efficient Inhalers
Absorption
Rebreathing
Elimination
Pharmacology
Staging of Depth of Anesthesia (Antecedent of MAC)
Epidemiology
Cardiac Arrest with Chloroform
Clinical Practice
Guidelines for Administration
Education
Writing

Claude Bernard: Master Physiologist

Although Bernard never practiced anesthesia, he thought a great deal about its value in aiding him in his physiological research. Anesthesia was part of the experimental procedure; as he said, "to carry out truly physiological experimentation it is not enough simply to know how to administer anesthetics to animals, one must also be able to understand and explain the experiments one performs with their aid."[2] Though not strictly an anesthetic agent in the same category as ether or chloroform, curare suited his purposes well, for it immobilized his laboratory animals without immediately impairing or affecting physiological integrity. Bernard's research into the actions and properties of curare not only laid the scientific foundation of our knowledge of the pharmacology of muscle relaxants, but also illustrates the way he approached a scientific problem.

Bernard first acquired a sample of curare as early as 1844.[3] Many individuals, from Sir Walter Raleigh onwards, had been fascinated by the magic and mystery of the Central and South American poison, but no one had understood how it caused paralysis and death. Fascinated, too, by curare, Bernard determined to elucidate its action. But despite the earlier studies of individuals like Benjamin Brodie and Charles Waterton, he had to start from scratch, for, as he wrote:

> ... from the earlier observations, I could get no clear idea of the mechanism of death by curare; to get such an idea I had to make fresh observations as to the organic disturbance to which this organic poison might lead. I therefore made experiments to see things about which I had absolutely no preconceived idea.[4]

The use of the verb "to see" is interesting and illuminating, suggesting confidence in his ability to conceptualize a physiological mechanism.

Bernard studied the effects of curare in frogs, birds and animals immediately after their death.[5] He found that it had no effect on the heart or the circulation or the blood, and that it did not affect the sensory nerves and the muscles. But the *motor* nerves, and only the motor nerves, were affected, consistently failing to respond to mechanical or electrical stimulation.

Bernard's work on curare is of great interest

in the context of the need for a corpus of basic knowledge in anesthesia, even though curare was not first used clinically for another half century; but it is also of interest in illustrating his thinking as a physiologist. His reasoning is illustrated in the following excerpt from his great work, *An Introduction to the Study of Experimental Medicine:*

> In the case of curare, I reasoned in the following way: no phenomenon is without a cause, and consequently no poisoning without a physiological lesion peculiar or proper to the poison used; now, thought I, curare must cause death by an activity special to itself and by acting on certain definite organic parts. So, by poisoning an animal with curare and by examining the properties of its various tissues immediately after death, I can perhaps find and study the lesions peculiar to it.[6]

The site of action of ether and chloroform also attracted Bernard's attention. In considering where they exerted their effects, Bernard started from the common observation that anesthetic agents acted on the nervous system. Yet, he argued, however great the number of observations that might be made, this number was insufficient when the great need was to establish "more or less general properties" and to address "the root causes and inquire into the reasons for the things one observes."[7] The next step must be to experiment.

Bernard's experimental technique was simple yet elegant.[8] The essence of it was as follows: he filled two glass beakers with a 1:200 solution of chloroform in water, covering each with a rubber membrane. In one beaker he dunked a frog, head down and the upper half of the body immersed; in the other, a frog feet first and the lower half of the body immersed. The result: each frog became anesthetized all over because the chloroform had been absorbed through the skin and carried within the body by the circulation. But now, Bernard asked, what would happen if the circulation was obstructed? To answer this question, he ligated the aorta and the soft tissues, except for the lumbar nerves. Functionally, therefore, each frog so dissected was divided into two parts that were connected only by the nerves and spinal cord. Two frogs were now immersed in the chloroform solution as before. The result: anesthesia of the entire frog developed only in the frog whose upper half was placed in chloroform because it was in this half that the circulation was intact, even though the hind part had no contact with the chloroform, and, moreover, had no blood circulating through it. In other words, "it was not the blood which spread the anaesthesia since this route was barred by the ligature." The conclusion was clear: "It is the central nervous system which is the site of action of chloroform and ether" and "it is anaesthesia of the nerve centers which deprives them of their sensitivity."[9]

John Snow, Compleat Physician

If Bernard was the master physiologist, Snow was the master clinician. In much of the medical literature, Snow appears to have a dual nature; he is seen as an anesthetist by anesthetists and as an epidemiologist by epidemiologists. Rarely is he seen as he should be seen: as an unusually well-educated and versatile physician, with a profound understanding of chemistry and physics and of physiology and pathology. Only so rounded a physician and medical scientist would be able to solve some of the fundamental problems presented by anesthesia in its earliest phase, and so to lay much of the scientific foundation of anesthesia. Two of the problems in anesthesia that Snow solved, and that illustrate his approach as a medical scientist, concerned the effect of variations in ambient temperature on the volatilization of anesthetic agents, and the effect of blood solubility of volatile agents on the quantity required to induce anesthesia.

With respect to the importance of ambient temperature on the induction and maintenance of anesthesia, Snow appears to have understood the deficiencies in the earliest inhalers immediately on first witnessing ether being given at the end of 1846.[10] The inhalers, adapted from those used in respiratory medicine, such as Nooth's

Apparatus,[11] were not designed to permit control of dosage and of the temperature of a volatile anesthetic agent, which Snow realized was crucial to satisfactory and safe anesthesia. Ideally, he wrote, "the medical practitioner ought to be acquainted with the strength of the various compounds . . . and to be able to regulate their potency,"[12] but this was not possible with the earliest inhalers:

> Both glass and sponge being very indifferent conductors of caloric, the interior of the inhalers became very much reduced in temperature, the evaporation was very much checked, and the patient breathed air much colder than the freezing-point of ether. On this account, and through other defects in the inhalers, the patient was often very long in becoming insensible, and in not a few cases, he did not become affected beyond a degree of excitement and inebriety.[13]

The "other defects" were those that produced too great a resistance to breathing — the narrow caliber of those parts of the apparatus through which the patient had to breathe, the small inspiratory and expiatory valves, and the presence of objects like sponges.

Snow solved these problems by designing his own inhalers. As well as incorporating tubing that facilitated rather than impeded breathing, he ensured that the temperature of the volatile agent, and therefore its degree of volatilization and so its inspired concentration, would remain relatively constant — a principle that underlies the administration of volatile agents today.

Intensive and methodical research, which he described in a remarkable series of papers that he published from 1848 to 1851,[14] then led Snow to discover a second principle of timeless validity. In studying a series of volatile agents in order to determine their suitability as anesthetic agents, Snow came to formulate a relationship that similarly became part of the scientific foundation of anesthesia. This is the relationship between the amount of a volatile substance required to produce a certain depth of anesthesia and its solubility in the blood, which constituted an inverse ratio:

> . . . the quantity of each substance in the blood, in corresponding degrees of narcotism, bears a certain proportion to what the blood would dissolve — a proportion that is almost exactly the same for all of them. . . The actual quantity of the different substances in the blood, however, differs widely; being influenced by their solubility. When the amount of saturation in the blood is the same, then it follows that the quantity of vapour required to produce the effect must increase with the solubility, and the effect produced by a given quantity must be in the inverse ratio of their solubility. . .[15]

Discussion

Claude Bernard, one of the medicine's great philosophers, recognized that, while medicine in the middle years of the 19th century was "empirical in most cases" and having a complexity that would make it difficult to escape from empiricism, it was all the more important to apply the experimental method. Bernard stated that what was necessary was to rely on "direct and rigorous application of reasoning to the facts furnished us by observation and experiment"[16] — a dictum that John Snow, in his research on cholera,[17] as well as on anesthesia, would have wholeheartedly agreed. It is fortunate, therefore, that these two medical scientists should have concerned themselves with the problem of anesthesia in its earliest phase, when it was no more than an empirical craft, for as a result of their endeavors, and of their scientific thinking, anesthesia began to evolve from empirical craft to scientific discipline.

Bernard and Snow had much in common besides their vision of how medicine should evolve. Their work, on both anesthesia and other aspects of medicine, indicates that they shared a common view of the thinking and the work of the "true scientist":

The true scientist (wrote Bernard) is one whose work includes both experimental theory and experimental practice. 1) he notes a fact; 2) *a propos* of this fact, an idea is born in his mind; 3) in the light of this idea, he reasons, devises an experiment, imagines and brings to pass its material conditions; 4) from this experiment, new phenomena result which must be observed, and so on and so forth. The mind of a scientist is always placed, as it were, between two observations: one which serves as a starting point for reasoning, and the other which serves as conclusion.[18]

But, while Bernard and Snow shared the faculty of scientific reasoning — and many other faculties, such as open-mindedness, curiosity and especially a desire to find the "truth" — they also shared the most important quality of working through *doubt* to reach a scientific truth. This is well illustrated by the words of these two great medical scientists. Bernard put the importance of doubt to a scientist in forthright and certain terms. "The first condition," he wrote, "to be fulfilled by men of science, applying themselves to the investigation of natural phenomena, is to maintain absolute freedom of mind, based on philosophic doubt."[19] That was not to negate the value or the method of science; it was simply to ensure that the open mind would be free to accept or reject the outcome of rigorous scientific experimentation.

Likewise, for his part, Snow did precisely this in endeavoring to understand the manner in which cholera spread in human communities. At one key point in his investigation into cholera, in the summer of 1854, he realized that he could find the truth only by conducting field research on his own. As he explained, "I was desirous of making the investigation myself in order that I might have the most satisfactory proof of the truth or fallacy of the doctrine I had been advocating for the past five years."[20] His tenacity won the day; he was able to prove the "truth" of the hypothesis he had first formulated late in 1848, but he could only do so by accepting the existence of doubt.

The standards that Bernard and Snow set for themselves were very different from those of Buxton's empiric; neither trusted to rule of thumb, neither scorned the results of their actions, and the courage of each was based not on ignorance but on knowledge, which itself was attained by passing observations through the crucible of doubt. In this manner Bernard and Snow, sharing the approach of all true scientists, laid much of the scientific foundations of anesthesia.

Yet, Bernard and Snow had individual qualities that enabled each to work individual ways to facilitate the necessary evolution of anesthesia from an empirical craft to a scientific discipline. These also should be stressed, not only to emphasize the fact that contributions to the scientific foundations of anesthesia have always come from a partnership of basic science and clinical art, but also to illustrate the nature of scientific thinking. The work of Bernard and Snow illustrates this nicely, and it is appropriate to conclude by identifying the essence of the thinking of each man.

Consider Bernard, for example. As Fulton observed, Bernard's research on curare illustrated the impact of his thinking particularly well.[21] In elucidating its action, Bernard had to start from scratch conceptually and he could use only the simplest of laboratory equipment; as Fulton pointed out, "there were no galvanometers, no myographs — merely physiological thinking." Yet it was out of Bernard's *physiological thinking* that emerged knowledge that became part of the scientific foundation of anesthesia. It was by going from physiological observation to physiological observation, from idea to idea, and from experiment to experiment, that Bernard arrived at a body of factual knowledge that enabled him to formulate a valid concept of the action of curare, for example. Indeed, Bernard himself recognized the importance of his work on curare, stating that it showed "how the simplest single determinism. . . leads to secondary determinisms which grow more and more complicated till death ensues."[22] It was his knowledge of the action of so apparently simple a poison as curare that gave him not only insight into physiological mechanisms, but also a profound understanding of the method and the purpose of science in medicine.

For Snow, the clinician, the starting point in his research in anesthesia, and in cholera also, was clinical observation. As his laboratory work shows, he had an unusually clear understanding of the principles of the experimental method; but, in addition to being adept at research, he was a general practitioner with the training of an internist, and his daily task of diagnosis was enhanced by the Victorian naturalist's acuteness of observation. So the importance of observation as the step that precedes idea and then experiment was as evident to Snow as it was to Bernard — one of whose epigrams was that "observation shows, and experiment teaches."[23] Just one example of Snow's genius in this respect will suffice to illustrate Snow's faculty of *clinical thinking* and the intellectual chain that links observation, idea and experiment in the solution of clinical problems — the very essence, surely, of the art of medicine. This example is taken from the opening paragraph of his classic work on anesthesia:

> [The] process of inhaling smoke, as I first witnessed it in a gentleman connected with one of the eastern embassies. . . is very instructive, as showing that the lungs become emptied of their contents by three rather full expirations and inspirations. When this gentleman took the cigar from his mouth to speak, the smoke could be seen issuing thickly with each word till there was a momentary pause as he took a fresh inspiration, then the smoke could be seen issuing with each word as before, only not so thick, and after another inspiration, the smoke could be still perceived in the expired air, but in a very diluted state; but after a third inspiration, it could no longer be seen till he had resumed his cigar.[24]

Although Bernard knew that the complexity of medical phenomena would make it difficult for medicine to escape from empiricism, his work and that of Snow suggests that the secret of overcoming this complexity, and the way of science, lies through that simplicity of approach that only the greatest of scientists are able to fashion.

References and Notes

1. Buxton DW: Emprицism or science? — Anaesthetics, 1847-1897. *Lancet*; 2:1369-76, 1897.
2. Bernard C: *Leçons sur les anesthésiques et sur l'asphyxie*. Paris: J-B. Baillière et fils, 1875. This quotation is taken from the translation of this work by B. Raymond Fink, *Lectures on Anesthetics and Asphyxia*, Park Ridge, IL: Wood Library-Museum of Anesthesiology, 1989, p 33.
3. Bernard C: Etudes physiologiques sur quelques poisons americains. *Revue des deux mondes*; 53: 164-90, 1864. The quotation is taken from the translation of this work on page 1163 of *Foundations of Anesthesiology,* by A. Faulconer and T.E. Keys (Springfield, IL: Charles C. Thomas, 1965).
4. Bernard C: *An Introduction to the Study of Experimental Medicine.* Translated by J.C. Greene, New York: Dover Publications, Inc., 1957, p 157.
5. Bernard C: Etudes physiologiques sur quelques poisons américains. *Revue des deux mondes*; 53:164-90, 1864. The English translation appears on pages 1160-1182 of *Foundations of Anesthesiology* by A. Faulconer and T.E. Keys (Springfield, IL: Charles C. Thomas, 1965).
6. Bernard C: *An Introduction to the Study of Experimental Medicine*, 1957, p 157.
7. Bernard C: *Lectures on Anesthetics and Asphyxia*. 1989, - 72.
8. Bernard C: *Lectures on Anesthetics and Asphyxia*. 1989, pp 73-78.
9. Bernard C: *Lectures on Anesthetics and Asphyxia*. 1989, 76-77.
10. Ether was first used in England by James Robinson on Dec. 19, 1846, to facilitate extraction of a tooth. Two days later William Squire gave ether for Robert Liston, who performed an amputation. See, for example, R.H. Ellis, "Early ether anaesthesia: the news of anaesthesia spreads to the United Kingdom." In *The History of Anaesthesia* (R.S. Atkinson and

T.B. Boulton, eds.), London: The Parthenon Publishing Group Ltd., 1989, pp 69-76.
11. Duncum BM: *The Development of Inhalation Anaesthesia: With Special Reference to the Years 1846-1900*. London: The Wellcome Historical Medical Museum and Oxford University Press, 1947, p 133.
12. Snow J: *On the Inhalation of the Vapour of Ether*. Lond Med Gaz; 4:498-502, 1847.
13. Snow J: *On Chloroform and Other Anaesthetics; Their Action and Administration*. London: John Churchill, 1858, p 348.
14. Snow J: On Narcotism by the Inhalation of Vapours. This comprised a series of papers that were published in the *London Medical Gazette* from 1848 to 1851. They have been conveniently collected in a facsimile edition by R.J. Ellis (London: Royal Society of Medicine Services Ltd., 1991).
15. Snow J: On Narcotism by the Inhalation of Vapours, Part IV, *Lond Med Gaz*; 7:330-4, 1848.
16. Bernard C: *An Introduction to the Study of Experimental Medicine*, 1957, p 2.
17. Snow J: *On the Mode of Communication of Cholera*. (2nd edition) London: John Churchill, 1855.
18. Bernard C: *An Introduction to the Study of Experimental Medicine*, 1957, p 24.
19. Bernard C: *An Introduction to the Study of Experimental Medicine*, 1957, p 35.
20. Snow J: *On the Mode of Communication of Cholera* (2nd edition), 1855, p 76.
21. Fulton JF: Claude Bernard and the Future of Medicine. *Can Med Assoc J*; 27:427-32, 1932.
22. Bernard C: *An Introduction to the Study of Experimental Medicine*, 1957, p 88.
23. Bernard C: *An Introduction to the Study of Experimental Medicine*, 1957, p 5.
24. Snow J: *On Chloroform and Other Anaesthetics: Their Action and Administration*, 1858, p 25.

CREATING AN HISTORICAL NARRATIVE
Messages from the Life of Horace Wells

STEPHEN D. SMALL
Massachusetts General Hospital
Harvard Medical School
Boston, Massachusetts

A fascinating but disturbing gulf exists between the reality of Horace Wells and the paradigm, or new model, that he created, and the misinterpretation, truncation, and neglect of primary sources that has characterized the work of historians. Scholars of epistemology and the philosophy of science have not entered the field. Popular accounts of the discovery of anesthesia and the ensuring ether controversy have rarely attempted to provide more than a thin sentimentalized sketch of Wells. He remains stripped of deeper motivation and intellect, and his main contribution — "to push the inhalation much farther than for a mere exhibition for fun" — has been obscured. The genesis of this startling idea has never been closely examined.

This paper presents preliminary research into the life of Wells and his contemporaries and an analysis of his discovery. It also introduces a study in the historiography of anesthesia, or how history is constructed. New information on the death mask of Wells, and never before published annotations in his hand from his personal library, are included.

As the world draws near to the sesquicentennial celebration of the discovery of anesthesia, it is apropos to first consider how it is that we know what we think we know about it. In this age of proliferating information, new disciplines have arisen to represent and focus new perspectives on knowledge. Added to the sciences of metalanguage and metaanalysis, we have, not metahistory, but historiography — the study of the principles, theory and history of historical writing. "Who determines meaning, how, and what form does it take, and for what purposes?"[1] Marshall also writes, "whose history gets told? In whose name?"[2] A full analysis of the recording and telling of the history of anesthesia is the subject of a work in progress, but several points may be mentioned.

How is it possible that an expansive, Pulitzer Prize-winning book on *The Growth of*

American Thought, by a renowned historian, published in the year of the centennial of Well's discovery, and possessing a chapter called, "The Advance of Science and Technology," completely fails to mention Wells anywhere in the text or index?[3] Crawford Long, Morton, Charles Jackson, even the surgeon John Warren are there, but the man recognized by professional societies worldwide as the discoverer of anesthesia, with statues in Washington, D.C., Paris and Hartford, is neglected. Wells took great risks, catalyzed and galvanized scientists and physicians around him into expanding on his new paradigm, and was a Jacksonian American in every sense of the word. Yet this seminal book robs us of the essence of discovery, robs us of reality. We have been warned about anthologies and encyclopedias. "You will not be able to tell whether or not what you read is an *idée recue*, dead, dying or maintained by an effective pressure group. When you get to know some subject well, look it up and you'll see how incomplete and dangerous the account is. Right now you must start somewhere and run your risks. The older the edition the better."[4] An ongoing investigation into this history text will hopefully reveal its method of construction.

In 1848, the American Association for the Advancement of Science was founded. One of its objectives (stated on the letterhead of Science) is "to increase public understanding. . . of the methods of science in human progress." In 1848, the man who discovered anesthesia and served as the first experimental subject to undergo anesthesia, also became the first to commit suicide while under its influence. In 1847, the American Association for the Advancement of Science was incorporated. In that same year, a well-known sculptor, who was later to direct the study of modeling at the Massachusetts Institute of Technology for over two decades, was putting the finishing touches on a huge bronze statue. Cast in one piece in Paris, it represented the man who had been honored as the discoverer of anesthesia by the American Medical Association at its annual meeting in Washington, D.C. in 1870.

To read *Science* today, one would think that the sculptor, Truman Howe Bartlett, had labored over the visage of William Morton. In "Research News," the discussion of a new molecular theory of anesthesia was introduced by a nod to Morton and accompanied by a large reproduction of Morton stretching the frontiers of understanding.[5] Since information in *Science* is often abstracted for the lay press, it should be no surprise that the *Boston Globe* featured an article titled, "Customized Anesthetics," by a professor of physics a month later.[6] A different painting of Norton at work, a longer paeon to his accomplishments, and no mention of Wells accompanied the news.

Morton in fact was a student of the man who discovered anesthesia. There exists no evidence that he ever conceived of creating a surgical plane of insensibility before he met, studied and then consulted with Wells, and grasped what Wells had accomplished. The article in *Science* propagates popular misconceptions about how knowledge is created and why, and does disservice to an organ which proclaims to "increase public understanding of the methods of science in human progress." It serves as an excellent example of how the study of the process of learning and growth in thought can be manipulated through a combination of ignorance of fact, perpetuation of narratives preserved by controlling cultural interests, and access to media. Science editors declined to publish a letter clarifying the positions of Wells and Morton.

In an old classic, Miller jumbles manifest falsehoods with polemics and glib assumptions to create a readable but treacherous tale.[7] Wells is described as lacking the advantages of a skilled dentist, and he "therefore found it extremely difficult to make a livelihood in Hartford,[8] when the record shows he was well-respected, and operated on the Governor of Connecticut, his family, important religious figures and numerous professionals. Miller also has Wells "qualifying as a dentist in 1842."[9] Wells hung out his shingle in Hartford in 1836, after two years of study in Boston with an as yet unidentified master dentist. No schools existed to certify dentists until after 1840, and the first was in Baltimore. Miller fails to discuss any of the historical material detailing the conversations of Wells and Riggs in the night prior to their experiment, but spends an entire page relating the minutiae of Morton's wedding.[10]

When Nicholas Greene delivered the Benjamin H. Robbins Memorial Lecture at Vanderbilt University School of Medicine in 1970, he opened his talk on the discovery of anesthesia by moving from Long to Morton and then to an erudite discussion of great social movements that prepared man's consciousness for the inevitable progress of methods to relieve pain. Wells is mentioned briefly four pages later in an aside dealing with the special needs and observations of dentists. He states, "Morton had to solve the problem of the pain of the root extraction before the restorative procedure would achieve acceptance. He turned to ether, and while Wells had failed with nitrous oxide due to factors he had no control over, Morton's efforts were successful." Not only had Wells tried ether before Morton, but after his death over forty citizens of Hartford gave Congressional depositions attesting to Well's success with nitrous oxide. While Greene spends the entire first paragraph lauding Long, he admits futility of Long's work, and then does nothing to illustrate the seminal contribution of Wells.

In 1853, Senator Isaac Walker published a short pamphlet intended to debate the merits of the contestants in the ether controversy. It was in answer to Senator Truman Smith's publication supporting Wells, and it in turn supports Morton. Walker begins his salvo with a lengthy quote from a work on the history of anesthetic agents by James Y. Simpson, the discoverer of chloroform (1847).[12] He uses the quote to buttress his own belief that Wells did nothing original or creative. Yet there is a copy of one of Smith's works in which lies the inscription, "At the request of the Widow of Horace Wells, Discoverer (sic) of Anesthesia, to James Y. Simpson, 10 March, 1870." An accompanying leaflet and note indicates that Smith was addressing "The Ladies of Hartford, Connecticut," on the ether controversy. Young "had written an essay favoring Wells. . . Elizabeth Wells asked Smith to inscribe his book as a way of expressing their thanks for his support from abroad."[13]

Nathan Payson Rice's Trials of a Public Benefactor is the classic reference work on the life of Morton, and survives for the unwary as a mid-nineteenth century classic.[14] Rice never intended for his name to be on the frontispiece. Morton supplied much of the information himself, and published the book without Rice's consent initially. The twentieth century articles delineating the twisted circumstances of the book's production [15,16] have become as obscure as Rice's own published piece supporting Wells as the true discoverer of anesthesia.[17]

Numerous other examples of obfuscation of primary source material exist. One familiar with the information begins to detect an emerging pattern. Wells never studied medicine and was not an insider in any of the circles of power of his day. He came from Hartford, which did not yet have a hospital. A puzzling and complex man, easy to characterize as a depressive dilettante, he committed suicide in the Victorian age, when religious revivals were sweeping America and the taking of one's own life was unspeakable. He died young, poor and intestate.

At the turn of the century, Osler spoke out in favor of Morton, setting the tone for the next hundred years by declaring that whoever succeeded in gaining public acceptance for a new invention or idea deserved the credit. This myopic view of a complex phenomenon has limited understanding to the present. Ralph Waldo Emerson, whose sister had married Jackson, wrote in support of his role. This, along with Jackson's visibility in the international scientific community of his day and his long life and involvement in the national disputes of the ether controversy, served to fix his narrative in popular history. Horace faded from view, to surface occasionally in specialty journals in articles honoring him, publishing forgotten letters, or dissecting odds and ends of the war of attribution.

There exists a hoard of evidence that Wells was preoccupied with issues of suffering, compassion, pain, and spiritual redemption before he successfully demonstrated a new use for nitrous oxide.[18-22] Although Morton's contributions were substantial, they lie entirely within the framework of articulating the shocking new view of reality illuminated by Wells. The practice of normal science, as defined by Kuhn, depends on the assurance of the existence of a solution to the puzzle being solved.[23] Wells was working without certainty, without a model. His experiences provided his contemporaries with a new, defined shape for their problems

Some of Kuhn's remarks pertain directly to Humphry Davy's situation. "In the eighteenth century, for example, little attention was paid to the experiments that measured electrical attraction with devices like the pan balance. Because they yielded neither simple nor consistent results, they could not be used to articulate the paradigm from which they derived. Therefore, they remained mere facts, unrelated and unrelatable to the continuing progress of electrical research. Only in retrospect, possessed of a subsequent paradigm, can we see what characteristics of electrical phenomena they display."[24] There exists no evidence that Davy contributed to the rise of anesthesia past the popular dissemination of the exhilarating effects of nitrous oxide. The exact nature of Davy's influence in early nineteenth century America is the current subject of ongoing research, using rare medical student notes, catalogues of profesors' and physicians' libraries, journal articles and lectures.

This leads us to Wells's library.[25] In a measured, childish hand, Wells has written on the front end paper of a copy of Blair's *Grammar of Chemistry*, " Horace Wells, Jr. his book, 1831." There is also a simple doodle resembling a four-petaled flower on a stalk. He was sixteen. On page 107, paragraphs 369 and 370 are bracketed by hand. They read, respectively, "Nitrous oxide is procured by exposing nitrate of ammonia in a retort, to the heat of a lamp, until red hot. The oxide then rises in the form of a gas," and, "Nitrous oxide supports combustion better than atmospheric air. When breathed into the lungs, it communicates a pleasurable or intoxicating sensation." In the same ink and penmanship noted above, he has written in the margin to the second paragraph, "To sleep as in eternity." His father had died two years earlier, and Wells entered an academy in Amherst, Massachusetts, becoming converted and "uniting with the church. . . he even at one period though seriously of fitting for the ministry." The only reference to Davy in the chemistry text is in the preface to the first American edition, where B. Tucker has credited him with the observation that "heat is a property of matter." Multiple other bracketed passages dealing with the preparation and properties of nitrous oxide may be seen, but these are in pencil.

A copy of Joseph Black's Lectures on the *Elements of Chemistry* is another of the sixteen volumes in the Wells collection. It has no marginal annotations, but much material is bracketed between pages 32 and 37. On page 35, the word "acid" is crossed out and replaced with "ether" in Wells's hand, but it is impossible to date this.

In his *Paradise Lost*, by Milton, Wells had underlined, "Fallen cherub! to be weak is miserable!" He has also noted "Where all life dies, death lives, and nature breeds/Perverse, all monstrous, all prodigious things." There is finally a mark by the following, "Being as I am, why didst not thou, the head/command me absolutely to go/Going into such danger as thou saidst?"

Other revealing accents illuminate his copies of Hooker's, *The Doubting Christian* and *Hervey's Meditations*. Together they create a tantalizing mirage of a man who, perhaps like Faulkner's Quentin, "loved and lived in a deliberate and almost peprverted anticipation of death."[26] It perhaps becomes easier to visualize the man who, with a young wife and a five-year-old son, chose to inhale a relatively unknown gas to unconsciousness. It was the step that Humphry Davy was incapable of visualizing. It was the step that almost led Harvey Cushing to abandon the study and practice of medicine fifty years after Wells, when his first ether induction as a medical student failed and the patient abruptly died of massive aspiration.[27] A full account of Well's books and their notations is in progress, as is a study of the much larger library of his son, Charles, who probably acquired some of his father's books. A search to locate the last owner of the Wells library in 1974 will hopefully turn up more volumes or create new primary sources about his life.

The subject of death brings the focus around to John Riggs. He was a striking bachelor who knew how to run a farm and a forge, had finished seminary school, and then became a dentist, probably studying with Wells and then opening an office in the same building.[28] While at college, he adopted the middle initial "M." When asked what it stood for by his father, he would only say "Mankey," and failed to offer any explanation. The only meaning ascribed to mankey in English usage and, curiously, dating to the early nineteenth century, is "an ancient kind of worsted stuff, much glazed, worn by females." [29] Rigg's role as the dental surgeon who extracted Wells's molar during the first anesthetic experiment is well-known. It is less often appreciated that Riggs has supplied the most interesting account of the evening before the experiment, however, when he and Wells "canvassed till near midnight the whole subject as to its safety and the degree of inhalation. As we had resovled to push the inhalation much farther. . . the chances of the death of said patient confronting us, Dr. Wells volunteered to be the patient and to make the trial on himself, charging me to stand by and care for him."[30] In another letter, Riggs states they had no way of knowing "to what point the inhalation was to be carried — the result was painfully problematical to us, but the great law of Nature, hitherto unknown, was kind to us. . ."[31]

When Wells killed himself four years later, Riggs was there again. The death mask of Wells, photographed and published by Archer in 1944, has been an enigma until this year. A study of the three editions of Truman Smith's book on Wells revealed a previously unappreciated annotation in a copy of the third edition.[32] A man named Bartlett stated in 1887, along with his gift of the book, that the death mask of Horace Wells had been made by John M. Riggs, dentist, three weeks after death. In addition, he went on, a bronze statue of Wells was erected in Bushnell Park in Hartford in 1875. Assistant Librarian Edwin Brigham's report to the Boston Medical Library Association in 1888 identified the benefactor as F.H. Bartlett.[33] No one by that name could be identified until a random search of the Dictionary of American Biography disclosed a T.H. Bartlett under the entry for Paul Wayland Bartlett, a famous American sculptor. Truman Howe, his father, it noted, was also a sculptor, known for his large monument to Horace Wells in Hartford.

The origin of the metal mask still eludes full characterization. It appears to have been sand cast. A compositional analysis has not been helpful in deciding if Riggs had a hand in it here in America, or if Bartlett had it made in Paris at the Gruet foundry as a model aid for the creation of the Wells monument.[34] Study of voluminous Bartlett papers has yet to yield pertinent information,[35] but Truman Bartlett had a wonderful sense of history, gifting pieces of Americana and natural history objects to libraries, museums and historical societies, and it is hoped he will have kept some notes on Wells.

Some additional information on Wells's contemporaries has surfaced during a close reading of Koch's *History of Dental Surgery*. While it has been assumed since Archer in 1944 that Wells could only have been trained by N.C. Keep, T.W. Parsons, W.F. Flagg, or D. Harwood (based on city directories listing surgeon-dentists in 1834), the biography of Joshua Tucker quotes his "Reminiscences on Dentistry" and mentions nine practicing dentists in Boston besides himself in 1834, the year Tucker returned from his adventures in Cuba.[36] John Randall, one of these nine, had a son two years older than Wells and with similar interests in natural history. Randall died the year before Wells's discovery in 1844.[37] This would account for the puzzling fact that no Boston dentist ever took credit for training Wells after the importance of inhalation anesthesia became known. It is a curiosity that Randall married a woman by the name of Elizabeth Wells — the identical name of Wells's wife, whose maiden name was Wales.

Of interest also is the fact that Tucker reports training with an excellent dentist in Charleston, South Carolina, by the name of C. Starr Brewster.[38] Little information about the mysterious Parisian expatriate dentist who helped Wells advance his claims in France has been available. Perhaps this will prove a fruitful lead.

In the end, history is about human beings. Their complex motivations and interlocking activities resist closure, as do the struggles of writers and scholars.As we more fully assimilate the great stories of our traditions, the characterizations of our patterns of learning and methods of acquiring knowledge will help us to dig deeper into ourselves.

Acknowledgements

The author is indebted to Richard J. Wolfe, Curator of Rare Books and Manuscripts in the Francis A. Countway Library of Medicine, and Joseph Garland, Librarian of the Boston Medical Library, for his support and useful conversations. Leonard Menczer, Curator of the Hartford Medical and Dental Museum, played an essential role also. Some of the ideas for this paper were formed during a 1991 Paul Wood Fellowship granted by the Wood-Library Museum, Park Ridge, Illinois. Patrick Sim, librarian, was extremely helpful.

References

1. Marshall BK: Teaching the Postmodern: Fiction and Theory. New York and London: Rutledge, 1992, p 4.
2. ibid., p 47.
3. Curti M: The Growth of American Thought. New Brunswick and London: Transaction Book, 1987.
4. Miller V in Pound E and Spann M ed: Confucius to Cummings. New York: New Directions, 1964, p. 330.
5. Matthews R: Science 255: 156, 1992.
6. The Boston Globe, Monday February 10, 1992, p 30.
7. Fulop-Miller R: Triumph Over Pain. New York: The Literary Guild of America, Inc., 1938.
8. ibid., p 108.
9. ibid., p 107.
10. ibid, p 113-114.
11. Greene NM: A consideration of factors in the discovery of anesthesia and their effects on its development. Anesthesiology, 35: 515, 1970.
12. Walker Hon IP: Answer to "An Examination of the Question of Anesthesia." Washington: Lemuel Towers, 1853, p 4.
13. The Wells Collection, Hartford Public Library, Hartford, Connecticut.
14. Rice NP: Trials of a Public Benefactor. New York: Pudney Russell, 1859.
15. Viets HR: Nathan R. Rice, M.D. and his Trials of a Public Benefactor, New York, 1859. BullHist Med 20: 232, 1946.
16. Beecher HK, Ford C: Nathan P. Rice's Trials of a Public Benefactor - A Commentary. J Hist Med, April 1960, p 170.
17. Rice NP: A grain of wheat from a bushel of chaff. The Knickerbocker or New York Monthly Magazine; 53; 133, 1859.
18. Archer WH: Life and Letters of Horace Wells, Discoverer of Anesthesia. J Am Coll Dent; 11: 81, 1944.
19. Wells H: An Essay on Teeth. Hartford: Case, Tiffany and Co., 1838.
20. An Examination of the Question of Anaesthesia Arising on the Memorial of Charles Thomas Wells, Presented to the US Senate, 2nd Session, 32nd Congress, and referred to a Select Committee, of which the Hon. Isaac Walker is Chairman. Prepared for the Information of Said Committee. Francis A. Countway Library, Boston, Massachusetts.
21. Smith Hon T: An Examination of the Question of Anaesthesia. New York: John A. Gray, 1958.
22. Smith Hon T.: An Inquiry into the Origin of Modern Anesthesia. Hartford: Brown and Gross, 1867.
23. Kuhn TS: The Structure of Scientific Revolutions Chicago: University of Chicago Press, 1970, p 37.
24. ibid., p 35.
25. op.cit., 13.
26. Faulkner W: The Sound and the Fury. New York: Random House, 1954, p 411.

27. Beecher HK: The first anesthesia records. Surg Gyn Ob 1940, p 689.
28. Lee B in Koch ed: The History of Dental Surgery, vol. II. Chicago: The National Art Publ. Co., 19099, p 345-352.
29. The Oxford English Dictionary, unabridged, 1984.
30. Trumbull JH ed: The Memorial History of Hartford County, Connecticut, vol I. Boston: Edward L Osgood, 1886, p 147.
31. Riggs JM: Letter addressed to Drs. Hasbrouch and Howland in New York, 1872, reproduced in part in Nakahara S. The Father of Anesthesia - Dr. Horace Wells. Japan, 1991.
32. Rare Books, Francis A. Countway Library, Boston, Massachusetts.
33. Twelfth and Thirteenth Annual Reports made to the Boston Medical Library Association, by Edwin H. Brigham, M.D. (ibid).
34. Lie H: Conservator of Objects and Sculpture, Harvard Art Museums, commissioned report.

ARTHUR GUEST AND THE "GUEST CANNULA"

BRIAN H. SMITH
Featherstone Department of Anaesthetics
Queen Elizabeth Hospital
Edgbaston
Birmingham,
United Kingdom

It is now just over 50 years since Arthur Guest, writing from the Queen's Hospital in Birmingham, described his cannula. The article was published in the British Medical Journal of December 20, 1941, in the section headed "Preparations and Appliances," and filled just one column. It was to revolutionize transfusion techniques, to the benefit of both patients and anesthesiologists. Appearing just one month after the Japanese attack on Pearl Harbour, which escalated the war and its casualties, the article was, moreover, timely.

Britain had a National Blood Transfusion Service from the start of the war in 1939, supplied then as now by volunteer donors. The usual transfusion technique consisted of exposing a vein through a short incision, most often the saphenous at the ankle, passing two ligatures beneath it, and tying off the lower end. A blunt cannula connected to the transfusion set was then introduced through a small lateral incision in the vein wall and was tied in place with the higher ligature before the wound was closed. This procedure, carried out usually by inexperienced junior doctors, sometimes under field conditions, was time consuming and sacrificed a large vein. Complications in the pre-antibiotic era were frequent and included thromophlebitis, sepsis, thrombosis and embolism. These gave both morbidity and mortality.

From the summer of 1940 onwards, Birmingham suffered a number of heavy air raids, and many wounded were treated at the Queen's Hospital, where Arthur Guest, qualified just three years, was a resident medical officer. His experience there led him to develop the cannula. In his article, Guest illustrated his device, attached to a 2 ml. Record syringe, by a line drawing. The point was illustrated, and the cannula also shown disassembled.

The details he gave were: The cannula (gauge 17 SWG) is fitted with a hollow needle instead of a solid stylet. This inner needle is of standard pattern, the length being such that, when fully inserted into the cannula, the bevel point protrudes just beyond the blunt end of the cannula. He wrote: "I have adopted the following procedure;[1] a small intracutaneous bleb of 2 percent procaine is introduced through a fine hypodermic needle at the chosen site.[2] After a light tourniquet has been applied, the cannula, with syringe attached, is introduced and the vein is sought and just entered.[3] After confirming entry by drawing back blood, the inner needle is withdrawn about an eighth of an inch whilst the cannula is held steady.[4] The cannula now has no projecting point, and may be pushed firmly up the vein to the hilt, without danger of it piercing the wall of the vein.[5] The syringe, still attached to the inner needle, is completely withdrawn.[6] The standard adapter on the tubing from the blood reservoir is then firmly attached to the cannula.[7] Two strips of surgical tape are applied parallel to and over the wings of the cannula to prevent slipping."

On originality he also wrote: "It is not claimed that the instrument is entirely original in conception. A similar, but narrower type of cannula, and with a solid stylet instead of a hollow needle, has long been in use at the Children's Hospital in Birmingham. I have not seen a blunt transfusion cannula with a sharp hollow introducer to which a standard syringe can be attached."

I myself remember the small cannula well. It had a solid stylet with a rounded end, and was inserted through a small incision in a vein wall into an infant's vein, which had been exposed by cutting down.

For his cannula, Arthur Guest went to Philip Harris & Co, in Edmund Street, Birmingham, and the cannula could subsequently be obtained from them. I am grateful to their present Managing Director, Mr. David Linney, for the information that the cannulae were manufactured for them by Shrimpton and Fletcher, at Redditch, fifteen miles south of Birmingham, and the center of the British needle industry.

The ethos of the day, in Britain at least, was that medical advances were not patented. Such a simple invention was rapidly copied worldwide and came into a widespread use. However, by the early sixties it had been replaced by a whole range of similar devices, mostly with cannulae made of modern plastic materials, and production of the actual Guest Cannula ceased.

Though in no small measure forgotten in Britain, the name "Guest Cannula" has lived on widely as a collective term for a whole range of generic successors using its principle The last time I was in an operating room in the United States, in 1988, I heard an anesthesiologist in his twenties ask for a "Guest Cannula."

The widespread copying of the cannula ensured that Philip Harris made little money from it. However, the firm has gone from strength to strength as suppliers of medical and scientific equipment, much for educational purposes in third world countries.

The Queen's Hospital, the home of the cannula, was founded in 1839, the first hospital in Britain built specifically for the education of medical students. With the opening of the new Queen Elizabeth Hospital in Edgbaston in 1938, it became beyond the resources of the Board of Governors of the United Birmingham Hospitals to maintain it, and industry took over its finance until the National Health Service was founded. It was renamed the Birmingham Accident Hospital in 1942. It will astonish those unfamiliar with the parsimony applied by successive British Governments of both political parties to the National Health Service to see the original 1840 building still there after 150 years. Plans to replace it have existed all my working life.

It is more important to speak of the man himself. Isidore Arthur Guest was born in Edgbaston, Birmingham, in 1911. In later life he seldom used his first name, and in the Medical Directory it was, unusually, enclosed in brackets at his request.

He won a scholarship to King Edwards School, Birmingham, founded in 1552 by Edward VIth, son of Henry VIIIth by Jane Seymour. Then, as now, King Edwards took the brightest boys from a population of over one million. Former pupils who shortly preceded him include J.R. Tolkien, the author of the trilogy, "The Lord of the Rings," and also Henry

Featherstone, the first president of the Association of Anaesthetists of Great Britain and Ireland.

From King Edwards Guest went to Cambridge, taking the B.A. in the basic medical sciences in 1934. At Cambridge it is still common practice for medical students to complete their clinical training elsewhere, and he returned to Birmingham for this purpose, graduating M.B., B.Chir (Cantab) in 1937. He intended to train to become a consultant physician, and to this end remained in hospital residence, completing the Membership Examination of the Royal College of Physicians only three years after qualifying, and well below par for the course.

He described his cannula in 1941.

The war was subsequently spent in the Royal Army Medical Corps, where he reached the rank of major,and was employed on research on motion sickness, an important subject in view of the forthcoming seaborne invasions. In the postwar period, he trained as a neurologist at the National Hospital, and Cambridge M.D. in 1950, and became a Fellow of the Royal College of Physicians in 1970.

Elected in 1945, the new Labour Government planned to create the National Health Service in 1948. In 1947, Birmingham City Council shrewdly realized that it would not for long have to pay the salaries of new medical appointments made to the staffs of its municipal Hospitals, and it doubled those staffs. Guest was appointed a consultant physician, with a special interest in neurology, to the staff of Selly Oak Hospital. He subsequently also joined the staff of the Midland Center for Neurosurgery at Smethwick.

As a Birmingham medical graduate, I knew him by reputation, and when I had completed my anesthetic training in Professor William Mushin's Department in Cardiff, my first appointment had sessions at Smethwick, and I had opportunities to discuss his cannula with Arthur. He was a pleasant, modest man who never received a penny for the cannula that bears his name. Sadly, he died in August, 1976, shortly after retirement. He is survived by his wife, who still lives in Edgbaston, and I am grateful to her for her help and his photograph.

GARDNER QUINCY COLTON
The Laughing Gas Man

GARY B. SMITH
Consultant in Intensive Therapy & Anesthesia,
Queen Alexandra Hospital, Portsmouth, United Kingdom

The contribution of the Hartford dentist, Horace Wells, to the story of the introduction of nitrous oxide as an anesthetic agent is well known. However, it has been said that, had there been no Gardner Quincy Colton, there would have been no Horace Wells, and it is possible that nitrous oxide may not have found its current popular position in the armamenterium of every anesthesiologist.

Gardner Quincy Colton was born in Georgia, Vermont, a small village on the shores of Lake Champlain, on February 7, 1814. His family was descended from Quartermaster George Colton, who had sailed from England in the early 1600's and had settled in Springfield, Massachussetts. Gardner was the youngest of 12 children and suffered a hard early life. Having spent time working in his youth on a farm as an apprentice chairmaker and as a bell-ringer, Gardner married Eleanor Pomeroy Colton on November 28, 1839. Their only child, Ellen Kathleen, was born on September 21, 1840. Sadly, his wife Eleanor died only five months later. Colton's older brothers then offered to help him through medical school.

Colton entered the Crosby Street College of Physicians and Surgeons in New York in 1842. He studied under Robert Watts Jr., Professor of Anatomy and Physiology, and Willard Parker, Professor of Surgery. After only two years at medical school, Colton decided to "...throw physic to the dogs..." and went off to lecture on chemistry and natural philosophy. Before doing so, Colton became interested in the properties of nitrous oxide and, as well as making the gas for medical student colleagues, he put on shows in New York. One of them, at the Broadway Tabernacle in the spring of 1844, resulted in a profit of $400.00. The success of this spurred Colton on to further similar exhibitions throughout New England.

On Tuesday December 10, 1844, Colton gave a show at the Union Hall in Hartford, Connecticut. The legendary events of that evening are well known the world over. Colton administered nitrous oxide to Samuel A.

Cooley, a druggist's assistant who, under its influence, began to dance and jump about. He ran against some wooden benches on the stage and bruised his shins badly. As the effect of the gas wore off, he took his seat next to a local dentist, Horace Wells, who was astonished to find that Cooley had not felt pain until the effects of the gas had passed off. The next day Colton and Wells met at Well's office where a neighboring dentist, John Riggs, extracted a tooth from Wells. On recovering, and finding his tooth out, Dr. Wells apparently exclaimed "It is the greatest discovery ever made. I didn't feel it so much as the prick of a pin!"

After the success of the tooth pulling, Colton taught Wells how to manufacture nitrous oxide and, with the assistance of Riggs, Wells used it for both dentistry and surgery. Unfortunately, Wells' abortive attempt to demonstrate the anesthetic qualities of nitrous oxide in Boston in January, 1845, and the introduction of ether, soon ousted memories of nitrous oxide. Meanwhile Colton continued his lectures.

Over the next few years Colton became involved in two major scientific inventions. He became friends with Samuel Morse, inventor of the telegraph, and was involved in the first telegraph message to be received in New York. Morse instructed Colton in the use of the telegraph and gave permission for Colton to lecture on the subject. While lecturing on the telegraph, Colton, using the principles of the electromagnet, conceived the idea of an electric engine that could be driven on a track. It was one of the first motors in electric railroad history and is now displayed in the Smithsonian Institute in Washington, D.C.

In 1849, after his brother Walter's appointment as Civil Governor of California, Gardner sailed to join him. He arrived in San Francisco on May 10, 1849, and immediately became involved in the gold rush of that year. During the rainy season it was impossible to work the mines, and he returned to San Francisco where he set up a hospital. Only months later he was able to send $10,000 to his second wife, Emily, in New York.

In the late fall of 1849, despite having no legal background, Colton was appointed as the first Justice of the Peace for San Francisco by Governor Riley and Perfect Horace Hawes. As a result, he found himself in charge of the coroner's business, minor legal trials and the controversial matter of the sale of town lots in the city. After the formation of the State of California in November, 1848, a great deal of confusion existed regarding the ownership of land in San Francisco. However, acting under the powers that he believed had been granted to him, Colton commenced selling lots, often at bargain prices. The Town Council thought differently and directed a city attorney, Archibald Peachy, to institute legal proceedings against Colton, A public notice was issued on December 21, 1849, and declared all grants of town lots made and signed by G.Q. Colton void and of no effect. Colton contended that the cases brought against him were abandoned before trial, but confusion continued to reign in San Francisco for some time afterward over ownership of land titles known thereafter as the "Colton Grants." Colton left California a rich man, and history is blurred as to whether he ever made any accounts of the proceeds of lands sold by him.

After arriving home, Colton spent time in Boston, writing for the Boston Transcript. About this time, he invested much of his money in the ill-fated Salt Works of Syracuse. Having rapidly lost his investment, he resumed his lectures and laughing gas exhibitions.

After Well's death, the use of nitrous oxide for all anesthetic purposes ceased; Colton was solely responsible for its reintroduction. In one of his writings, Colton comments that he was persuaded to administer nitrous oxide for dental surgery to a lady in New Britain, Connecticut, in the summer of 1862. It is reputed that, when Colton returned to New Britain in 1863, he found that the local dentist, later identified as Dr. R.C. Dunham, had subsequently administered the gas to more than 600 patients. Colton states that he and Dunham then joined forces with another dentist, one Joseph H. Smith of New Haven, Connecticut, for 3 weeks in the summer of 1863. In Colton's other writings, his story is somewhat different. These other versions allege that in June, 1863, Colton visited New Haven for another of his exhibitions. He invited a number of gentlemen to attend a private preliminary entertainment at which he gave a history of the discovery of anesthesia, stating also that he had never been able to encourage a dentist to try the gas. A local dentist, Joseph H. Smith of Olive Street, New Haven, who was present, agreed to try the gas provided that Colton administered it. The next day they extracted seven teeth from a well-known wealthy lady using nitrous oxide as the anesthetic.

Colton then abandoned the "Exhibition" business and agreed on a partnership with Smith. Colton would provide and administer nitrous oxide for one week and Smith would extract the teeth. They were so successful that they continued for 23 days, during which time they extracted "a little over 3,000 teeth." Colton then decided to return to New York where, in July, 1863, with the help of two eminent New York City dentists, Dr. John Allen and his son William, he set up the Colton Dental Association, an institution devoted exclusively to the extraction of teeth under nitrous oxide gas. Initially, Colton and his colleagues were the target of ridicule, sarcasm and misrepresentation, and it is alleged that in the first year Colton spent $8,000 in advertising, advocating, and defending "his invention." Gradually, business and support increased, and over the next few years nearly all the leading dentists of New York sent patients requiring an anesthetic to Colton. According to The New York Times, his office was known to "seven out of every ten New Yorkers who had ever lost sleep from troublesome grinders." From the commencement of records on February 4, 1864, until 1897, more than 193,800 patients, ranging in age from 3 to 90 years, were recorded as having had nitrous oxide at the Colton Dental Association. There were apparently no fatalities. The Colton Dental Association was based at No. 19 Cooper Union in New York. A poster produced by the Association advertised tooth extractions at a rate of $2 for the first and $1 for each subsequent extraction. In a manner similar to today's newspaper advertisements, it contained complimentary remarks by satisfied customers, such as:

> A pleasure instead of pain
> This beats my chloroform!
> No more old fashioned dentistry for me!
> and
> Ought to erect a statue to the inventor.

Colton also used nitrous oxide during three surgical operations — a mastectomy and two limb amputations — performed by J.M. Carnochan. Despite Colton's background in medicine and chemistry, and his unrivaled expertise in the administration of nitrous oxide, he remained unaware of the true chemical and physiological effects of the gas. I quote from his writings:

> . . .It is composed of precisely the same elements — oxygen and nitrogen — as the common air, only the proportions are different. . . In this gas there is half oxygen and half nitrogen, or by volume, one of oxygen to two of nitrogen. Oxygen is the life giving principle of the air and in the gas we have more of it; a person lives a little faster while under its influence. . . The laughing gas acts as an exhilarant, as by supplying an extra supply of oxygen to the lungs, the pulse is increased 15 to 20 beats to the minute.

Indeed, so convinced was Colton of the beneficial effects of nitrous oxide that he repeatedly inhaled the gas himself and also advocated its use as resuscitative therapy in asphyxia.

At this time Colton almost certainly used a version of the White nitrous oxide bag. Although initially using the standard two-liter version, Colton later employed one of up to thirty liters. Later still, Colton administered the gas direct to the patient from an apparatus designed by Mr. A.W. Sprague of Boston.

In the spring of 1867, Colton visited Europe and brought his experience to England. He traveled to London and on Friday, June 5, addressed a meeting of dental and medical practitioners at the house of Mr. C.J. Fox, a dental practitioner. He then administered the gas to four patients with complete success and repeated his address five days later. Fox later championed the cause of nitrous oxide in England.

Colton returned home in 1868 and opened dental offices in St. Louis, Chicago, Brooklyn, Cincinnati, Boston, Baltimore and Philadelphia, all of which operated simultaneously. He continued to practice dental anesthesia until on August 10, 1898, he died in Geneva, Switzerland. His body was returned to New York where it was cremated and his ashes buried in the Aurora Hill plot of Woodlawn Cemetery in the Bronx, New York.

Gardner Quincy Colton's life was varied in its extreme. To the activities already described one can add an interest in geology, death and circuses (he was a good friend of P.T. Barnum). He was a devout Christian and a prolific author of many pamphlets, books and letters on varied topics. However, without doubt, his greatest legacy to humanity has been the gift of nitrous oxide anesthesia. Without Colton, it is unclear if this agent would ever have found the position in modern anesthesia that it now holds.

This abstract is reprinted in this form with permission from the International Anesthesia Research Society (Anesthesia & Analgesia 1991; 72:382-91.)

Reference

1. Smith GB, Hirsch NP: Gardner Quincy Colton: Pioneer of nitrous oxide anaesthesia. Anesth Analg; 72:382-91, 1991.

ALFRED KIRSTEIN
Pioneer of Direct Laryngoscopy

GARY B. SMITH
Consultant in Intensive Therapy & Anaesthesia,
Queen Alexandra Hospital, Portsmouth, United Kingdom

In April 23, 1895, in Berlin, Alfred Kirstein performed the first direct examination of the interior of the larynx. Until then laryngologists had been content with the technique of indirect laryngoscopy using mirrors — a method popularized by Garcia, Turck and Czermak. Indeed, before Kirstein's discovery, it was felt that a direct view of the larynx was impossible due to the geometric relationship between the mouth and the vocal cords. However, Kirstein learned from a colleague, Rosenheim, that a scope intended to be passed into the esophagus had accidentally slipped into the trachea and, much to the surgeon's surprise, a perfect view of the bronchial bifurcation was obtained. Armed with this knowledge, Kirstein worked furiously to devise a method of direct laryngoscopy, but also laid down those principles which are still in clinical practice throughout the world today.

Alfred Kirstein was born on June 25, 1863, in Berlin. He studied medicine in Freiburg, Strasbourg and Berlin. In 1886, he was awarded a doctorate for his thesis titled, "Concerning the part played by tuberculosis in the aetiology of chronic septic infections of the urinary tract." Following short periods working in Jena and Cologne, he returned to Berlin to the Institute for Legal Medicine, from where he published an important work concerning, "The Diffusion of Poisons from the Corpse."

In 1895, Kirstein became interested in obtaining a direct view of the larynx. Following Mikulicz's invention of esophagoscopy, and Rosenheim's subsequent modification of Mikulicz's esophagoscope into a lightweight handy instrument, Kirstein undertook many esophagoscopies, often without topical anesthesia. Following Rosenheim's revelation, Kirstein set about devising a reproducible method of viewing the larynx directly. His early attempts were unsuccessful and resulted only in views of part of the epiglottis, something he acknowledged had been easily achieved by many others. His initial technique involved placing an esophagoscope into the esophagus, and following topical cocaine, passing a similar but shorter 25cm instrument into the larynx. Using the upper incisors as a fulcrum, he obtained a view of the larynx by firmly displacing the root of the tongue and elevating the epiglottis in an anterior direction.

The question of illumination was a problem. Traditional methods of indirect laryngoscopy had used a head mirror and an incandescent light source. Kirstein found this to be inadequate for direct examination, as he felt that the cone of reflected light must come from a source attached to the observer. He resolved the problem by employing electrical methods of illumination. Initially, he modified the head mirror and invented the "forehead lamp for reflected light." Electric rays from a lamp on the head were collected by a convex mirror and deflected at a right angle by a small perforated mirror, through which the observer was able to view the subject. Although he found this method of illumination satisfactory, he used the electric light source in a second way, one that is of great importance to the anesthetist. He employed an electric hand lamp, termed the "electroscope," which had been devised by Caspar for examination of the urethra. The light rays from this lamp were collected by a lens and deflected through 90 degrees by a prism. This hand lamp was used as a handle to which the 25cm esophagoscope was attached. He named the combination of the electroscope and esophagoscope, "The Autoscope," and direct examination of the larynx he termed "Autoscopy." Twenty-three days after his first view of the larynx, Kirstein gave a comprehensive demonstration of autoscopy to the Berlin Medical Association. At this point he had already abandoned the need for the initial esophagoscopy, but still undertook the procedure with the patient lying horizontally, the head extended over the edge of a table.

Despite the infancy of autoscopy and the autoscope, Kirstein already recognized the potential of his new discovery, suggesting that it would allow the removal of foreign bodies from the trachea and permit catheterization of the bronchi. Of particular interest is the fact that Kirstein's autoscope was held in the left hand, thereby freeing the right for surgery.

Despite success with autoscopy, Kirstein was aware of a number of problems associated with the method. He was concerned about the pressure exerted by the autoscope on the upper incisors, and also the need for the marked extension of the neck. Furthermore, he considered cocaine to be poisonous. He therefore directed his attention to overcoming these disadvantages, and one month after his demonstration in Berlin he presented a report of a modified autoscope. The handle of the instrument remained the same, but in place of the esophagoscope was attached one of two different designs of blade. The standard blade was 14 cm long and was designed with a slight downward curve to elevate the epiglottis by anterior pressure on the base of the tongue and in the valleculae. The tip of the blade was thickened and well-rounded in order to avoid injury to the mucus membranes. It was also notched to receive the median glosso-epiglottic fold. The intra-laryngeal blade was introduced beneath the laryngeal surface of the epiglottis. Forward and upward movement of the blade elevated the epiglottis, revealing the larynx. The blade formed a perfectly straight groove which ended in a thin convex border. Lateral ribs on each blade were designed to house hoods which served to keep the upper lip and even moustaches from the operator's field of vision. Each blade was made of nickel-plated silver and bore a striking resemblance to those laryngoscopes currently in use today.

On June 15, 1895, Kirstein reported in the German Medical Journal that the patient could be sat on a chair with their head comfortably extended. Although he initially continued to use the autoscope previously described, by June 26 Kirstein had modified the technique so that he now stood in front of the patient who sat in a chair in a usual upright position. Initially, the autoscope was used as a standard tongue depressor, then it was slid backwards and the handle lifted to allow visualization of the anterior aspect of the epiglottis Finally, the autoscope handle was further elevated until, with slight movement of the patient's head forward, the larynx, trachea and posterior epiglottis were viewed.

With the introduction of his modified autoscope, Kirstein found that he had overcome those problems which concerned him. Pressure on the upper incisors could easily be avoided and, in many cases, prior use of topical cocaine was unnecessary, especially when the standard blade was used. Furthermore, he now found that extreme extension of the neck was not required for the procedure. In describing the best position for obtaining a direct view of the larynx, he reported that:

> . . .the body must be placed in such a position as that imaginary continuation of the laryngo-tracheal tube would fall within the opening of the mouth. . ."
>
> "When the military position is assumed, the continuation of the windpipe would strike somewhere in the neighborhood of the root of the nose. . ."
>
> ". . .when the head is bent comfortably backward, as in looking aloft, it would about strike the chin. . ."
>
> ". . .the position adopted for autoscopy must therefore be somewhere between the two positions just mentioned, and can be easily obtained by gently tilting the head upwards until the axis of vision forms with the axis of the trunk an angle of about 135 degrees. . ."
>
> "This tilting movement of the head is a rotation on the atlanto-occipital articulation. . .

Therefore, Kirstein fully appreciated the importance of the rotation at the atlanto-occipital articulation and was almost certainly the first to describe what Magill termed some 20 years later as the "sniffing the morning air" position for intubation.

Surprisingly, within one year of its invention, the use of the autoscope was abandoned by Kirstein. His undoubted skill at performing direct laryngoscopy from in front of the patient, without topical anesthesia, made it easy for him to adapt his technique to one which incorporated the use of a tongue depressor of his own design and his own electric head lamp. Ironically, this ability may have led to his technique of direct laryngoscopy passing into history, only to be rediscovered some years later by others.

(Reprinted with the consent of the editor of the journal *Anaesthesia*. Anaesthesia 1986; 41;42-45).

Reference

1. Hirsch NP, Smith GB, Hirsch PO: Alfred Kirstein: Pioneer of direct laryngoscopy. Anaesthesia; 41:42-45, 1986

HENRY S. RUTH
A Mentor and Pioneer

C.R. STEPHEN
Chesterfield, Missouri, USA

Henry Swartley Ruth was born in 1899 in Philadelphia and never moved from his home base. The fact that he was an only child and was brought up in a reasonably affluent atmosphere may have colored some of his later behavior, namely, that of a somewhat austere character who was known as a stern taskmaster and who was not willing to take "no" as an answer to a problem. He attended Swarthmore College in 1917-18 and then Hahnemann School of Science, being awarded a BS degree in 1919. He then entered the Hahnemann Medical College and received the MD degree in 1923.

The name Hahnemann is inextricably linked to Samuel Hahnemann (1755-1843), a German physician who founded the school of homeopathy. The basic principles of homeopathy are two fold: first, that the cure of disease is effected by drugs that are capable of producing in a healthy person symptoms similar to those of the disease to be treated, e.g., the use of quinine to treat malaria: and second, that the action of minute doses of a drug, smaller than those used conventionally, have curative powers. Hahnemann's theories were not widely accepted in Germany and he eventually moved to Paris to continue his practice. His philosophy spread throughout the world. However, in the United States, although the name which is synonymous with homeopathy has persisted, the American Institute of Homeopathy has adopted the following resolution:

> "A homeopathic physician is one who adds to his knowledge of medicine a special knowledge of homeopathic therapeutics. All that pertains to the great field of medical learning is his by tradition, by inheritance, by right."

After graduation from medical school in 1923, Dr. Ruth began the practice of anesthesia at Hahnemann Hospital, where he remained until his untimely death in 1956 at the age of 57. There were no formal residency programs in those days and one learned the arts of anesthesia administration by observation, probing the knowledge of others, and by the trial and error method. Eventually, Dr. Ruth became Professor of Anesthesia at the Hahnemann Medical College, a post that he retained during his lifetime. An indication of his influence on the development of anesthesia practice in the Philadelphia area is the fact that at various times he was also Chief of Anesthesia at the Philadelphia General Hospital and Consultant to the St. Christopher Hospital, St. Luke's Hospital, and Children's Hospital.

In 1929, at the behest of Dr. John Lundy, and with the blessing of Dr. Ralph Waters, Dr. Ruth was invited to become a founding member of the Travel Club, which was composed of some 15 anesthesiologists from United States and Canada, and which met annually in various places on the continent to present discussions and exchange ideas about the burgeoning specialty. Being a member of this group led to a close friendship with Dr. Lundy and provided associations which let to a sharpening of anesthetic abilities and involvement in organizational affairs. For example, it was probably at these meetings that Dr. Ruth was first made aware of the value of cyclopropane as an anesthetic, as first used clinically by Dr. Waters in 1932 or 1933, and of the introduction of thiopental by Dr. Lundy in 1935. Except for the World War II years, the Travel Club met annually until 1952 when it was expanded into the present Academy of Anesthesiology. In this new organization Dr. Ruth was named the official historian.

Also in 1929, primarily due to the stimulus of Dr. Ruth, one of the earliest residency training programs in anesthesia was instituted at Hahnemann.

A few years later, in 1935, Dr. Ruth is credited with beginning the first Anesthesia Study Commission in the country under the aegis of the Philadelphia County Medical Society, acting as Chairman. Reports of patients who had died within 24 hours of receiving an anesthetic were discussed freely at regular meetings, after which votes were taken as to whether the fatality was preventable or non-preventable, the probable cause of death was decided, and recommendations made regarding possible better management. All cases were brought to the commission for discussion on a voluntary basis by anesthesiologists from the metropolitan area hospitals. In 1947, in a report published in the JAMA, Dr. Ruth and colleagues presented an analysis of the results of 306 fatalities which had been discussed up to that time. Of these 306 patients, 47 percent had been classified as preventable. These efforts to enhance the safety of anesthetic administrations soon spread to other localities and today the Anesthesia Patient Safety Foundation exemplifies nationally the ongoing efforts to reduce anesthesia hazards.

It was during the 1930's and 1940's that anesthesia really came into its own as a specialty. Much of the impetus for a national society came from Dr. Paul Wood who, in a dramatic plea in 1936 at a meeting of the New York Society of Anesthetists, urged that the name of the Society be changed to the American Society of Anesthetists. His exhortations were successful and the new society became an entity with 487 members and annual dues of $5.00. A short time later it officially became the American Society of Anesthesiologists (ASA). In 1938, Dr. Ruth was elected as the third President of the ASA, a task which undoubtedly was associated with many burdens.

At the same time a campaign was underway to create a specialty board of anesthesia, of which several had already been established in other disciplines. Dr. Lundy was appointed as a negotiator in this process and succeeded in 1938 in establishing the American Board of Anesthesiology (ABA) as an affiliate of the American Board of Surgery. Dr. Ruth was one of the members of this original Board and was its President in 1943-44. By December of 1939, there were 87 Diplomates certified by the ABA. In 1941 it was approved as a separate and independent Board.

Still another struggle, led primarily by Dr. Lundy, had been ongoing for a number of years. It was the fond hope among many anesthesiologists that a separate Section of Anesthesia could be established in the American Medical Association (AMA), which at that time was the major force in organized medicine in the country. Eventually, in 1940, the House of Delegates of the AMA voted unanimously to establish a Section of Anesthesiology. The first Secretary of the Section was Dr. Lundy, in which capacity he remained for 17 years, and the first delegate to the Section, representing the ASA, was Dr. Ruth, a position which he occupied ably until 1955.

During his tenure as delegate to the AMA, Dr. Ruth fought long an hard to establish the principle that the administration of anesthetics was indeed the practice of medicine. Today, of course, such practice is a *sine qua non,* but it might not have been had Dr. Ruth not labored so hard and so assiduously. The American Hospital Association was trying to claim that all who administered anesthesia, including physicians, be classified as hospital employees and thus, not being practitioners of medicine, not able to bill for the professional services rendered. After arduous and at times exhausting discussions, the House of Delegates of the AMA decreed, in passing the so-called Hess Report, that the practice of anesthesia was indeed the practice of medicine. We are all indebted to Dr. Ruth for his perseverance in overcoming one of the obstacles to the proper practice of our specialty.

There is still another feather in the cap of Dr. Ruth for which we must all be thankful. With the organization of the ASA as a national body, there were increasing suggestions and requests that there should be a journal in which scientific advances in the specialty could be published. Through the joint efforts of Dr. Ruth as Editor and Dr. Paul Wood as Business Editor, the first issue of Anesthesiology was published in 1940 and sent to 568 members of the ASA and to 300 additional subscribers. Dr. Ruth remained as Editor through 1955, guiding this fledgling publication through its formative years. Today our journal is recognized as the leading publication of anesthesiology in the world. Not content with this enormous task, Dr. Ruth was also an Associate Editor of the American Journal of Surgery for a number of years.

So one can see that, in the formative, organizational stages of our specialty, Dr. Henry Ruth was wearing a number of hats simultaneously: as President of the ASA in 1938, as a member of the ABE beginning in 1938, assuming its presidency in 1943; as the first delegate of the ASA to the AMA beginning in 1941; and as the first Editor of the journal, Anesthesiology, beginning in 1940. For these multiple responsibilities which he carried out so thoroughly and faithfully, he was honored by the ASA in 1952 by receiving the Distinguished Service Award, which he richly deserved.

Meanwhile, one must have been wondering what was going on at home in Philadelphia. Evidence suggests that Dr. Ruth was not idle. In 1942, for example, he organized a three month course of instruction on anesthesiology for medical officers, six at a time. The first two weeks, as required by the Surgeon General's office, was a basic course outlining the fundamentals of surgery. This was followed immediately by the curriculum in anesthesiology, which consisted of clinical work, conferences, seminars, lectures, and attendance at local medical meetings. Headquarters for the course was at Hahnemann Hospital, and cooperating in the instruction were Drs. Robert D. Dripps of the University of Pennsylvania, Philip D. Woodbridge of Temple University Hospital, and Frederick P. Haugen of Presbyterian Hospital.

Clinical work was provided in all types of anesthesia: inhalation with all the agents and methods in common use, including endotracheal; regional blocks, including spinal; rectal; intravenous; supportive measures; therapeutic, diagnostic and prognostic nerve blocks; and resuscitation. This list is indeed comprehensive, but one wonders how the officers felt when they completed the course and found that they were not permitted to use cyclopropane at military posts in the field.

One formal conference was held each week, consisting of discussions of interesting cases and of any fatalities that occurred. Lectures, held every day, were delivered primarily by anesthesiologists in the metropolitan area and covered a wide range of topics. Each officer presented a seminar on an assigned topic during the course of instruction. In addition, each student was required to abstract and report on one article a week from the current literature.

There is one other facet of accomplishment which Dr. Ruth has left for posterity, and it is his contributions to the literature. His publications began to appear as early as 1929 and they continued until a new years before his death. From 1936 through 1950 he authored on an annual basis the Section on Anesthetics in the revision service volume of the Cyclopedia of Medicine, Surgery and Specialties, indeed a no mean accomplishment. He even delved into scientific exhibits, presenting one on Anesthesiology as a specialty at the 1952 meeting of the American Medical Association.

What kind of a man was this who played so many roles — physician, teacher, editor, author, medical politician — so effectively? A few episodes from his personal life may be revealing. Dr. Ruth married in 1924, a year after receiving his medical degree. He had met his wife at a musical contest at which each was competing as a pianist. In due time two children were added to the family. In view of his many activities, which often took him out of town, one wonders how much time he was able to spend with his family.

In 1938, one of his interesting extracurricular activities was participation with fellow Rotarians in a minstrel show. To those of you who are unfamiliar with this form of entertainment, it consists of a group of men who sing, tell jokes and occasionally dance. The interlocutor is in the center and he announces numbers and initiates lead-in questions to the "end-men," of whom there are two at each end. They are black-faced and supply the wit, humor and antics to the show. Minstrel shows were always a lot of fun for both participants and the audience. We do not know what role Dr. Ruth played in the Rotarian show. An accomplished pianist, which Ruth certainly was, is a vital necessity for such a show, and this may have been his role. On the other hand, it would appear that Ruth would make an excellent interlocutor, who by character is somewhat aloof, but suave, worldly, and master of the situation. Dr. Ruth liked to drive big cars and he did not like to drive behind other cars. Therefore, there was a frequent tendency to exceed the speed limit, which occasionally aroused sirens along the way. It was said that he was reasonably well known for these foibles by the Philadelphia traffic force.

There were some personal characteristics that tended to make Dr. Ruth stand out in a crowd. He was always immaculately dressed in public, and perhaps this was a form of one-upmanship which could be used to advantage at times. All of his clothes were made by a tailor who would come by his home in the evening, show samples of cloth, make measurements, and then return subsequently for fitting. This flair for the best, and also for personal privacy, extended to barbering, for he never went to a barber shop — the barber came to his home where tonsorial perfection could be achieved in peace and quiet.

One more anecdote tends to reveal something of the character of Dr. Ruth. He was somewhat particular about how he was addressed by people: by those who were personal friends he liked to be called "Hen;" by those he had known for a long time but of whom he was not particularly fond, he preferred to be called "Henry;" to anyone not fitting the above categories he was Dr. Ruth. One of his residents, Dr. Kenneth Keown, felt he had passed a milestone when one day Dr. Ruth said: "Kenny, you may now call me Hen."

Well, here is a portrait, dim as it may be, of a man who by his multifaceted, unselfish efforts helped immeasurably to make our specialty what it is today. May each of us be encouraged to follow in at least some of his footsteps.

CHRISTOPHER LANGTON HEWER AND ETHANESAL

JOHN B. STETSON
Professor, Emeritus
Department of Anesthesiology
Rush Medical College, Chicago, Illinois, USA

The Beginning: Some of the People Involved

Christopher Langton Hewer's (C.L.H.) grandfather, father, and great uncle (John Langton) qualified in medicine. All qualified from St. Bartholomew's Hospital Medical College, London.[1] John Langton became the hospital's "Administrator of Chloroform." C.L.H. followed in the family tradition and qualified from "Barts," "the best medical school in London,"[2] in 1918. He received the MB BS London degree (distinction in Physiology). His later distinctions were many. He became the Anaesthetist in charge of Department, St. Bartholomew's Hospital, Honorary FFARCS, Secretary of the Anaesthetic Section of the Royal Society of Medicine 1930 and 1931, President 1936-37, Vice President of the Association of Anaesthetists of Great Britain and Ireland, Founder Editor of *Anaesthesia* (1946-1966), Advisory Editor (1966-1976), then Editor Emeritus. He was awarded both the Henry Hill Hickman and John Snow medals in 1966. In 1932 he founded the series, *Recent Advances in Anaesthesia and Analgesia.*

Hewer had administered anesthetics as a clerk before entering the army. In the army, he had the good fortune of being placed in training with Dr. Torrance Thomson. Thomson was a leading specialist in Edinburgh. When Thompson entered military service, he brought his own Gwathmey apparatus with him. In 1919, Hewer returned to St. Bartholomew's, was a resident Anaesthetist for six months, and was then appointed to the hospital staff. Henry Edmund Gaskin Boyle, OBE, DA, FRCS (Honorary), was Anaesthetist at Bart's, 1905-1940. He and Hewer worked together and were co-editors of the text, *Practical Anaesthetics* (1923). Boyle became an Ethanesal enthusiast and presented talks on its clinical use during a 1921 North American junket. An earlier Boyle achievement is worth noting. Boyle persuaded the Coxeter company, an English firm, to construct a replica of Gwathmey's American continuous-flow gas oxygen apparatus. Hewer wrote, "I well remember the excitement of unpacking the machine at Bart's and getting it

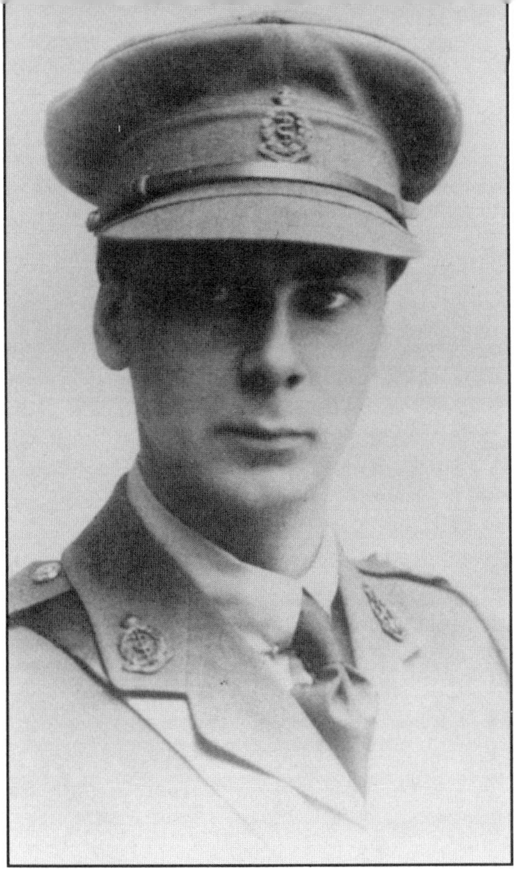

Fig. 1. Christopher Langton Hewer, about 1918, in his Royal Army Medical uniform.

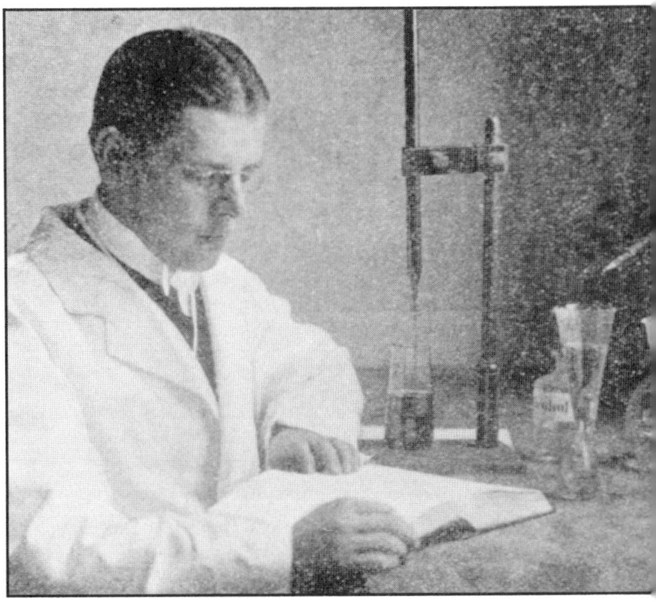

Fig. 2. Robert Lauder Mackenzie Wallis. Date of picture not known. Wallis died in 1929, age 43.

ready for an afternoon operating session."[2] The machine was a success and the British Army Medical Corps ordered a large number of the machines; many were sent to France and used in Casualty Clearing Stations. The action of the British Army is in contrast to the U.S. Army Medical Corps. Dennis E. Jackson designed an anesthesia machine for U.S. Army use, but army officials rejected it as it was too complicated.[3] This comparison of responses to use of a device (anesthesia machine) that would improve patient safety (ability to administer oxygen) was a portent of the development of anesthetic practice between the "Great Wars," professional with physicians in the U.K., professional and technician in the U.S.

Robert Lauder Mackenzie Wallis (Fig. 2) received his BA from Downing College, Cambridge (first class in the Natural Sciences Tripos). He became Lecturer in Chemical Physiology at University College, Cardiff; in 1911 he went to Bart's and in 1912 was appointed Demonstrator in Chemical Pathology. He studied medicine while working at Bart's and obtained the diploma of LMSSA in 1913. After the war he obtained the Cambridge MD in 1919. His obituary noted he received the Horton Simthe Prize for his thesis, but the title is not noted (it would indeed the interesting if the thesis concerned his experiments with ether). He died at the age of 43 in 1929. The obituary did not mention his military service nor interest in ether.[4]

The biographical data concerning Dr. Hadfield was included because he worked at Bart's and was active in the section of the Royal Society of Medicine, where Hewer and Wallis presented their first talk on Ethanesal, April 1, 1921.[5] Twenty years later, Hadfield referred the trichloroethylene project to CLH.

Publications About Ethanesal-Favorable

The Wallis-Hewer talk noted above was not published for some months. In the interval, Hewer published a short note in his hospital's journal.[6] In the note, C.L.H. reported that as of May of 1921, he had used Ethanesal 300 times. Ethanesal was described as a purified ether (mercaptans removed), a small quantity of ketones "fairly high up in the series" was added to the ether, as was ethylene and carbon dioxide (the carbon dioxide rendered the preparation stable). The advantages were listed; less toxic, less irritating, less vomiting, less after-taste, and pulse-pressure remained higher than with either or chloroform.

Ethanesal must have made a stir in London as the Wallis-Hewer address of April 1 was printed in *The Lancet* for June 4, 1921.[7] This issue also contained an editorial[9] that noted the article by Wallis and Hewer in the issue, as well as Cotton's work in Canada (see James Henry Cotton and Cotton Process Ether, this volume). Cotton also claimed pure ether was not an anesthetic; rather it was the carrier for the necessary analgesics — ethylene and carbon dioxide. Wallis took the Cotton theory a step further by adding ketones.

Wallis gave the first part of the presentation at the Royal Society. He reported his work in India, where he had prepared pure ether and found that it had no anesthetic effect on animals. Permanganate was used to remove mercaptans; anhydrous copper sulphate removed the remaining impurities. On returning to Bart's, he made pure ether for Hewer who found it had no anesthetic effect. They knew of the work of Cotton and found their pure ether absorbed "large amounts of carbon dioxide and ethylene." Ethylene was prepared by two methods, ethyl alcohol mixed with either sulphuric acid or with phosphoric acid. The sulphuric acid method yielded a pleasant and more potent ethylene. While Hewer had written that the ketones added were "high up in the series,"[6] Wallis reported, "The ketones used comprise those in the middle of the series,. . . loose chemical combination between these substances and the carbon dioxide and ethylene. . . .[7]

At the Royal Society, C.L.H. reported 200 uses of Ethanesal (April 1). He felt its action was between that of ether and that of chloroform. Pulse pressure remained wide; graphs to demonstrate this feature were presented. Hewer was able to obtain ether analgesia, and only 52 percent of the patients vomited.

C.L.H. used a multitude of combinations of inhalation drugs. In some cases, induction was with ether or Ethanesal in a Clover's inhaler, then open drop Ethanesal. In other patients, open ethyl chloride was followed by open drop Ethanesal (Hewer used 20 layers of gauze on his mask). In children, tincture of orange was employed prior to the anesthetics. The Boyle's apparatus was employed (gas-oxygen-ethanesal) as well as intratracheal insufflation, especially, ". . .when both pleural cavities's may be opened simultaneously."

All the patients received atropine. Morphine was not used unless the patient was "very excitable or nervous." Hewer did administer morphine "just before the patient regains consciousness." The relationship of morphine to nausea and emesis was not noted. Induction time averaged 4.1 minutes. At the time *The Lancet* went to press, C.L.H. had used Ethanesal on 500 patients. Hewer ended *The Lancet* article with ". . .thanks to those surgeons who have afforded me opportunities for taking blood-pressure reading, and to Mr. B. B. Sharp, late resident anaesthetist to St. Bartholomew's Hospital, for his help in taking the readings."

The Royal Society of Medicine Proceedings[5] report included discussions. Dr. H.E.G. Boyle reported that Dr. Hewer had administered ethanesal to him when he had had an operation on his hand and he had done well. Boyle had employed ethanesal about a dozen times (April 1, 1921). One of the discussants noted that when Dr. Wallis had spoken before the Medico-legal Society he attributed the anesthetic properties of ether to the ethylene contained in it (ketones not mentioned).

H. Edmund G. Boyle, OBE, MRCS, LRCP, was the representative of the Anaesthetic Section of the Royal Society of Medicine at the Joint Meeting of the Canadian, Interstate and New York Anesthetists. He gave the Honorary Chairman's Address before this group. ". . .as well as before the Nose and Throat Section of the Ontario Medical Association," Hotel Clifton, Niagara Falls, Canada, June 1-3, 1921 (two months after his comment at the Royal Society of Medicine). The title of his address was, "Gas-Oxygen-Ethanesal-Chloroform (Figs. 3a, 4a) combined anesthesia for Nose and Throat and Abdominal Surgery."[8] He also read

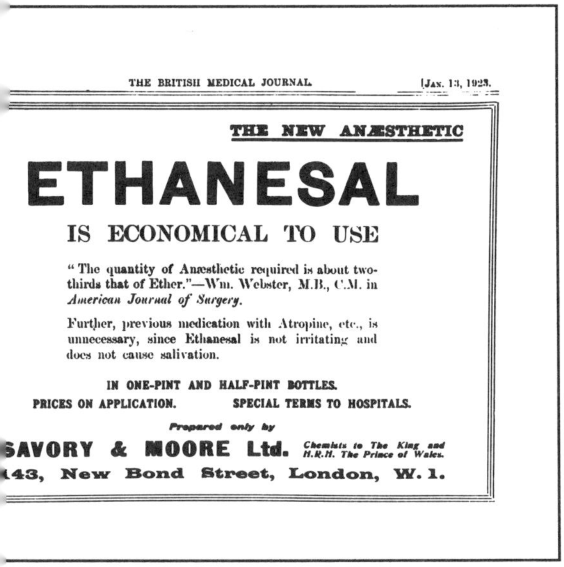

Fig. 3a. Advertisement, February 19, 1922, British Medical Journal.

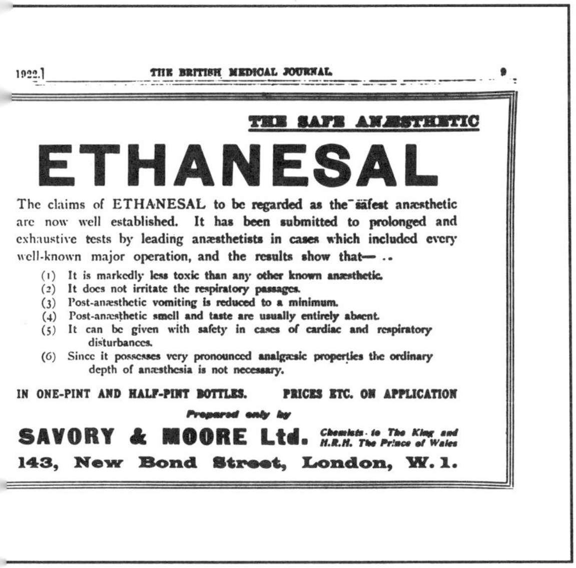

Fig. 3b. Advertisement, January 12, 1923, British Medical Journal.

this paper before the Anesthesia Session of the A.M.A. Section on Miscellaneous Topics, Boston, June 8, 1921. An abstract of the talk was published in the *British Medical Journal*;[9] a similar talk was given at the Section of Anaesthetics, British Medical Association, Portsmouth, July, 1923. For induction, Boyle used 10:1 nitrous oxide: oxygen, the vapors (ethanesal and/or chloroform) were added for surgical depth. After the incision the vapors were shut off (unless needed for relaxation). The patients were to be kept "pink," 4:1 gas:oxygen was used when "anesthesia had been established." If the pupils became widely dilated, the bag was to be rapidly emptied, refilled with oxygen, and the mask applied to the face. Either Dr. Boyle liked to talk and write about his drug combinations, or audiences like to hear him (or read his articles or abstracts), or there was a dearth of speakers, as anesthetics was a new specialty.

Questions began to appear. K.B. Pinson reported that he had used ethanesal on 32 patients (in 30 he used the warm ether "bomb"). He had a favorable impression, but found 16 percent more ethanesal than ether was necessary. He also wished to know, ". . .what quantity of ketones, and how much CO_2 and ethylene, are added to the ether. . ."[10] Wallis and Hewer had always been vague on these matters.

The abstract of Boyle's Canadian talk, published in the British Medical Journal,[9] prompted a comment[11] by Dr. Stock of Clifton. He agreed with all of Boyle's points except the use of chloroform for relaxation. The use of diathermy was an exception; if diathermy was in use, chloroform was indicated. Boyle's article was published October 15, Stock's letter was dated the 26th and published November 5!

Perhaps the most interesting article concerning ethanesal in the year 1921 came from South Africa. The May issue of *The Medical Journal of South Africa* contained "A Short Note on an Ether Representing Ethanesal."[12] The first sentence of the "note" was almost a paragraph:

> "Many of you may have noticed a paragraph in the lay Press some two months or so ago, to the effect that a new perfectly safe anesthetic was being used in London, to which the name "Ethanesal" has been given and which the paragraph described as being a chemically pure ether."

As the Wallis-Hewer presentation at the Royal Society of Medicine was on April 1, it would indicate lay press coverage (the *Sunday Times* was named) prior to April 1. The author notes that "pure ether" is a poor anesthetic (he was another Cotton-Wallis) and that he had had an ether saturated with carbon dioxide and ethylene made for him prior to seeing a resume of the Wallis-Hewer paper on "Ethanesal" in the British Medical Journal (I missed this reference in my paging through the 1921 BMJ). Considering travel (mail) time to South Africa in 1921, the report is remarkable. Cotton and Cotton Process Ether is not mentioned by the South African; Wallis was aware of Cotton when he put together ethanesal. The South African doctor use his ether for a hernia, an appendectomy, a tonsils and adenoids, and a dental case. The cost of production precluded further trials, and he had ". . .cabled for a small supply of ethanesal. . . ." It is hoped a follow-up article can be located.

Articles concerning Ethanesal published in 1922 were not located. Hewer had a letter[13] in the British Medical Journal in response to an article that had reported spinal anesthesia safer than gas-oxygen-ethanesal. In the letter, C.L.H. bristled, but he did it politely.

Although not an "ethanesal" article, Hewer had a short note on "The Effects of Vagal Trauma on the Anaesthetized patient" in the 1922-23 volume of the Proceedings of the Royal Society of Medicine. Two case reports were presented. The second patient was a 20 year old girl with chronic left-sided empyema. "She was induced with ethanesal in a Clover's inhaler, and anaesthesia was maintained by gas and oxygen given through an endotracheal catheter."

By 1923, five years after qualifying in medicine, Hewer was in full swing. His article on endotracheal anesthesia for major surgery[14] was far ahead of contemporary practice in the United States. Phillip Woodbridge performed the first endotracheal intubation done at the Mayo Clinic in 1928.[18] C.L.H. had done a thousand intubations; the first 150 were "serious" operations, the next 850 routine. There were no anesthetic deaths. Hewer used a Boyle's machine; the small standard bottle was used for chloroform, a large tin container with pressure gauge for Ethanesal. Hewer felt Ethanesal was superior to ether. He also felt ". . .that the endotracheal administration of ethylene-oxygen is superior. . ." to gas-oxygen ethanesal. Thirty-six years later he wrote, "Ethylene proved to be a disappointing anaesthetic and it was surprising that it attained such popularity in the United States."[2]

In 1926 there was a joint meeting of the Associated Anesthetists of the United States and Canada and the International Anesthesia Research Society in Joint Meeting with the Sections on Surgery and Anaesthetics of the British Medical Association, in Nottingham, England. Hewer spoke on "Endotracheal Nitrous Oxide [sic] Oxygen-Ether Anaesthesia in Gastric Surgery;"[15] there was *no* mention of Ethanesal. He wrote, ". . .best results of all in gastric surgery; this consists of administering a mixture of nitrous oxide-oxygen and ether through a tracheal catheter. I have now employed this method as a routine for five years in about 3,500 cases, of which about 1,100 were for upper abdominal operations." Five years before would have been 1921, when Hewer was touting Ethanesal! One wonders, in 1926, did Hewer consider his Ethanesal anesthetics as ether anesthetics and lump them together?

Hewer had published, "Anaesthesia in Children," in 1923.[16] This may be the first book on the subject. He noted, "The chapter on Ethanesal is largely an account of the painstaking researches of my friend and colleague, Dr. R.L. Mackenzie Wallis." In the Ethanesal chapter toxic impurities were identified. Mercaptans, especially methyl mercaptan, were the worst. These were removed by distilling with potassium permanganate. The pure ether produced was a poor anesthetic. The researches of Dr. J.H. Cotton, ". . .in America. . ." (in the early 1920's many in England still looked upon Canada and the United States as one large colony) were noted. The results of adding ethylene and carbon dioxide were noted. Wallis then found that a "mixture of the middle. . ." ketones added to the ethylene-carbon dioxide treated ether produced the best anesthetic, it also possessed marked analgesic properties. Pure ether was being used as a vehicle, and Wallis claimed other vehicles had been used with success! The rest of the chapter was similar to earlier reports.[5,7] Hewer added a drop feed for "open" mask anesthesia (flannel was used as a cover rather than gauze).

Hewer co-edited Boyle's text, *Practice Anaesthetics,* Third Edition, 1923. Chapter IX dealt with "Modification of Ether." Cotton's researches were noted, as were those of Wallis. It was written of Wallis, "He had evolved a preparation of mixed ketones dissolved in purified ether to the strength of 5 percent, and this preparation is sold under the name of "Ethanesal." The virtues of ethanesal were listed, less irritation, quieter respirations, pulse rate does not rise as high as with ether, more analgesia, and less after-taste.

Ross had a short favorable report on ethanesal in the second edition of his handbook (1923),[18] but there was no mention of the drug in the third edition (1929).

Charles Hirsch, anaesthetist for the Epilepsy and Paralysis Hospital, Maida Vale, and the West End Nerve Hospital, had a letter in *The Lancet*[19] (". . .Ethanesal gives better results than ordinary anaesthetic ether."). His article on anesthesia for cerebellar operations was delightful, and the instructions as good (or better) than those I received thirty years later when a trainee (with the exception that we used intravenous fluids, he used a rectal drip of saline).[20] He pumped air or bubbled oxygen either over or through ethanesal in a Wolf bottle (fancier than the Richardson bottle used in Boston) and passed the vapor through a worm in a thermos flask of boiling water (no information on how the water was kept boiling). The apparatus was marketed by Messrs. Coxeter and Sons.

A surgeon, Sir Crisp English of London, ". . .had tried Ethanesal for two years with admirable results." His anesthetist (if present) was not asked his opinion.[21]

The most recent (last) clinical mention of Ethanesal I could locate was by Boyle and Hewer. They used gas-oxygen-ethanesal-chloroform by endotracheal catheter for major pelvic surgery with patients in the Trendelenburg position.[22]

This publication is tedious reading, but is done on the chance that it may save some future medical historian the onerous task of locating the scattered references.

Publications About Ethanesal, Neutral

J. Blomfield, OBE, MD, wrote a short review on recent work on anesthetics in 1922.[27] A few years later, Blomfield was the editor of *The British Journal of Anaesthesia.* In the 1922 review, Blomfield quaintly noted that Hewer did not administer Ethanesal alone; it was always preceded by or given in conjunction with gas and/or other anesthetics.

"This makes judgment of the actual properties of the new anaesthetic more difficult. . . ."

Charles F. Hadfield, mentioned above, authored a beginner's text published in 1923.[28] He noted the expense of ethanesal and that he could not obtain the results Hewer claimed for the drug. He modestly concluded, "As this is so opposed to Hewer's experience, it is probably due to faulty technique."

Publications About Ethanesal, Negative

After Hewitt died, the fifth edition of his book was edited by Henry Robinson.[29] He was unable to discover any advantage of Ethanesal over ether and noted it was more expensive. He saw more vomiting after Ethanesal than after ether.

A year after his article in *The Practitioner,* [27] Blomfield had moved from neutral to negative, as he felt that Ethanesal was quite potent in causing mucous and salivary secretion.[30]

In Canada, Colonel Webster pointed out that doubt had been thrown on the findings of Cotton, and Wallis and Hewer. He listed reliable researchers who had proved pure ether was an anesthetic.[31]

R.P. Beebe of Kalamazoo, Michigan, tried ethanesal.[32] The first sixteen patients were done with bottles from one lot of drug and were satisfactory. The next eight patients were done with the drug from another lot and respiratory irritation and other "sequels" were very aggravated.

His report was given in June, 1924, published January, 1925. Ethanesal was at the end of its tenure.

A 1932 Australian publication noted, ". . .Ethanesal has passed out of vogue."[33]

Savory and Moore

It is not known why Wallis picked Savory & Moore to manufacture his improved ether. Savory & Moore is now part of McCarthy's. Inquiry to their headquarters in Leighton Buzzard, Bedfordshire, earned the reply, ". . .company has changed hands a number of times over the years and no information is available regarding the history of many of the products."

The 1923, Volume I, of *The British Medical Journal* carries advertisements for ethanesal (Figs. 3a and 3b) and of Savory & Moore's food. The food "is *not* a substitute for new milk it is a supplement and aids its digestibility." Savory & Moore were located at 143, New Bond Street, London, W.I. It is an attractive structure, now occupied by Polo-Ralph Lauren, a gentlemen's clothing emporium. The name Savory & Moore is very visible on the marquee (Fig. 4). Advertising of Ethanesal prompted competitors (J.F. MacFarlan & Co, Duncan Flockhart & Co, Wellcome, and Boots) to advertise their anesthetics. The trade war was soon terminated.

The Lancet carried an analytical report on Ethanesal.[34] It was found to be anhydrous, free from sulfur, and with a neutral reaction. Part of Ethanesal had a higher boiling point than regular ether. It was assumed this change in boiling point was due to the ketones said to be added to the ether.

Martindale, *The Extra-Pharmacopeia,* is published by the Royal Pharmaceutical Society of Great Britain. A paragraph on Ethanesal was present in the 18th edition (1924), 19th edition (1928) and 20th edition (1932). The non-complimentary article by Dale, King and Hadfield is noted in the three editions (this article will be reviewed in the section on pure ethers).

The British and Colonial Pharmacist's Diary for 1925 contains an entry on Ethanesal. The column with space for composition is blank. The paragraph on "Therapeutic Uses" is glowing (obviously written by the manufacturer).

It is not known when Savory & Moore ceased manufacture of pharmaceuticals. Their

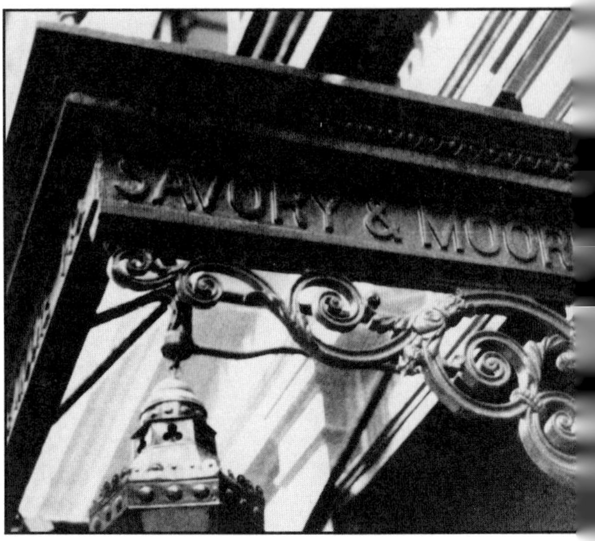

Fig. 4. Savory & Moore, 143, New Bond Street, London (Polo-Ralph Lauren, men's furnishings, now occupy the building).

retail stores in the London area have closed (or were sold). There are operating stores in the Oxford area and, from the company letterhead, one would assume in other parts of England and in Scotland. The Savory & Moore name is said to be common on toiletries sold in their stores.

Pure Ethers

Three centers in different countries produced pure ether, each by a different method. The three centers reported that pure ether was an anesthetic. Two centers also performed analysis of Ethanesal to determine its composition. There were also exchanges of letters and other indications of interest in pure anesthetic drugs, as shown by editorial comments in medical journals.

Cotton demonstrated his Cotton Process Ether (pure ether with 2 percent ethylene, .05 percent carbon dioxide, 1 percent ethyl alcohol) at the Royal Victoria Hospital, Montreal (1917). The first rebuttal came from the same center. Wesley Bourne, the anesthesiologist (he received the Henry Hill Hickman medal of the Royal Society of Medicine in 1935) and the pharmacologist R.L. Stehle, produced a pure ether by combining sodium ethylate with ethyl iodide. They tested their pure ether on animals and it worked well. Five surgical and one obstetric patient received the pure ether. No premedication was employed; nor were induction drugs or gas used. All patients were anesthetized with ease and there was nothing to suggest pure ether was not an excellent anesthetic drug. The pure ether was tested for ethylene content; it was less than 0.04 percent. The nails were being driven into the coffin to hold Ethanesal (and Cotton Process Ether).

The January 13, 1923, issue of *The British Medical Journal* carried a half-column report on J.F. MacFarlan & Co's chloroform and ether.[36] The editorial-type article reported, "The problem of ether has been complicated by the conclusions of Cotton and of Wallis. . .," and ". . .Stehle an Bourne prepared highly pure ether. . .it had the same anaesthetic power as ordinary ether. . .," another nail driven. MacFarlan did not use ethyl alcohol as their starting material (it was heavily taxed), therefore, they could make pure drugs at about a third of the former cost.

The March 3, 1923, issue of *The Lancet* carried a powerful article by H.H. Dale, C.F. Hadfield (assistant anaesthetist, St. Bartholomew's Hospital, Fig. 5) and H. King.[37] Dalen and King worked at the National Institute for Medical Research. King prepared ether by the ethyl alcohol-sulfuric acid method, then

Fig. 5. Drs. Dale and Hadfield at St. Bartholomew's Hospital, 1902.

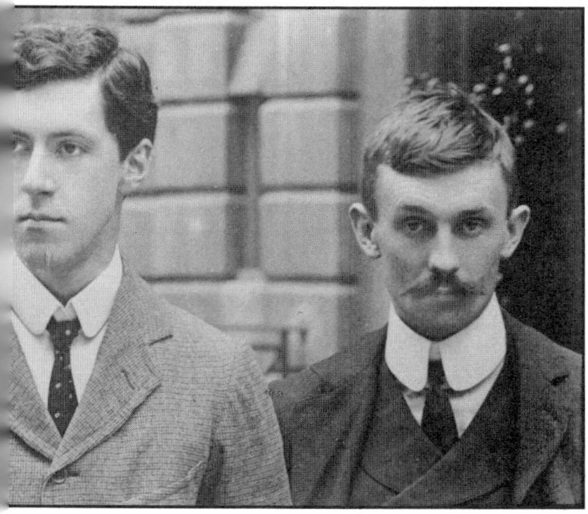

subjected it to multiple re-distillations and washings. King took the pure ether and used it on animals and the results were as with ordinary ether. Hadfield then used the pure ether on eight surgical patients and all had a normal anesthetic response. Dr. King then obtained commercial samples of Ethanesal and examined them. He found Ethanesal to be 95.55 ether, 4 percent n-butyl alcohol, 0.5 percent ". . .a mixture of ethyl alcohol and aldehyde. . .," but *no* ketones. Comments by Drs. Wallis and Hewer were appended to the report (it is assumed they were invited by the editor). Dr. Wallis took a half page, Dr. Hewer a full page for their responses. Dr. Wallis, ". . .was quite at a loss to explain" Dr. King's finding. He reported the first Ethanesal contained 2 percent ketones, but the ketone content was raised to 5 percent. He did "admit that certain forms of pure ether have an 'anaesthetic action'. . .," but ether-ketone mixture is better and has a different action. Dr. Hewer spoke extensively, but said little. He reviewed "a recent American paper" concerning Cotton Process Ether and the bubbling off of ethylene. Dale gave Hewer some of the pure ether and C.L.H. anesthetized a lady of 24 years of age. The pure ether worked, but it was not as good as Ethanesal. C.L.H. had, ". . .no doubt of the accuracy of the work of Dale and his colleagues. . .," but could not explain the discrepancies from his theory. He finished with the comment he had used Ethanesal over 4000 times and "it gives on the average, better results than any anaesthetic ether that I have tried." Others may have had doubts, but Hewer was still firm in his belief.

In the United States, *Current Researchers in Anesthesia & Analgesia,* in its second year of publication, carried an editorial concerning the need for pure anesthetics.[38] The investigator was Professor Allan Winter Rowe of the Evans Memorial Department of the Massachusetts Homeopathic Hospital (now the Evans Memorial Hospital of Boston University School of Medicine). There was no mention of Cotton, Wallis nor Bourne.

The lid was probably placed on Ethanesal's coffin March 7, 1924. Professor W. Storm van Leeuwen of Leiden, Holland, accepted an invitation to speak at the Royal Society of Medicine, "On the Narcotic Action of Purest Ether."[39] The talk was on the seventh; eight days later both *The Lancet*[40] and *The British Medical Journal*[41] carried extensive editorials. The Professor used benzidine which crystallized with ether. The cooled crystals were then heated and a very pure ether driven off. In animals and man, the pure ether was an excellent anesthetic. Comments from the discussions were included in the editorials. Dr. Wallis spoke of his early research findings; Dr. Hadfield wished to know the exact composition of Ethanesal as he had read three different formulae; it was recommended the high tax on ethyl alcohol (in the U.K.) should be removed when used for the manufacture of ether; Dr. Boyle produced a chart of 10,000 anesthetics done with Ethanesal; C.L.H. responded, but his words had little significance; Dr. Shipway drew attention to Stehle and Bourne's[35] research; Dr. Dale invited Dr. Wallis to prepare some pure ether by his method, bring it to Dale's Laboratory and they could examine and test it together; finally, Dr. Blomfield declared the discussion had degenerated into a sort of clinical fog, with vague impressions being counted as fact with little definite evidence. One bit of evidence that Professor van Leeuwen had presented concerned ketones. The Professor had prepared pure ether and added measured amounts of specific ketones to the ether. The mixtures were administered to cats; some of the ketones Wallis had reported as beneficial proved to be either without effect, or deleterious, or were toxic!

The feud was not over. The May 10, 1924 issue of *The Lancet* carried a letter from Professor van Leeuwen.[42] He restated what he had said at the Royal Society of Medicine; he agreed with Dale that there were no ketones in Ethanesal, but rather n-butylalcohol. As a final insult, he noted that 5 percent methylethylketone added to pure ether made an anesthetic that proved fatal to cats (hemorrhage into the lungs, liver and kidneys). His letter concluded, concerning an ether containing 5 percent methylethylketone, ". . .its use in therapeutics would be criminal."

The next week saw Hewer's response in print.[43] He noted that toxicity of a drug to an animal did not indicate it would be toxic to man. He then repeated an earlier comment by Wallis that anesthesia could be had with ketones alone without ether. His report is so unusual, it is worth quoting: "Pure ketones were next tried with no added ether, and an extremely good anaesthetic resulted. None of these patients vomited at all or exhibited any other after-effects whatever, and the method was only discontinued because some difficulty was experienced in obtaining a suitable vaporizer. The apparatus used consisted of a perforated aluminum plate heated by a resistance coil. . ." ". . .the ketones used. . .were purchased direct from British and foreign chemical manufacturers. . ." Hewer ended with the comment that van Leeuwen's statement that the use of 5 percent methyethylketone "would be criminal," was, ". . .to say the least, somewhat exaggerated." All one can do now, nearly seventy years later, is try to imagine what Hewer did, the ketones employed, and wonder why further investigations were not performed years later. What did Hewer vaporize on the hot metal plate? Was the aluminum a catalyst?

The memory of the pure ether controversy lingered and was recalled in 1927.[44] A letter to the editor of *The Lancet* reviewed the old feud and added the question of peroxides. A remark by a coroner prompted the letter. Late in the year an editorial reviewed the problem of peroxides in ether.[45]

In Canada, Bourne continued his studies. In 1926 he published his studies on acetaldehyde, ether peroxide, ethyl mercaptan, ethyl sulphide, di-ethyl ketone, acetone, and ethyl methyl ketone.[46] Bourne used dogs placed in a glass box as experimental subjects (van Leeuwen had used tracheotomized cats). He found the ketones, ". . .apparently indifferent in concentrations up to 5 percent." Hewer was vindicated in relation to van Leeuwen's claims, but in a sense he was humiliated. Hewer should have investigated the action of ketones in the manner Bourne did. The ether centennial issue of *Anesthesiology,* (November, 1946) had as its lead article, "Pure Ether and Impurities: A Review," authored by Wesley Bourne.[47] Bourne brought the circle around, not to the beginning, but to a sensible level. He wrote that an ether that met USP requirements could have some impurities, the drug could be delivered in large containers, and ether could be used from containers that had been open a few days. Minor amounts of impurities did not add to, nor subtract from the anesthetic properties of ether.

A decade had elapsed from the start of Cotton's and Wallis' investigations, their claims that pure ether was not an anesthetic, the need for specific additives, the problems that could be caused by some impurities, and finally, a reasonable resolution. Ether was an anesthetic, it should be reasonably pure, but absolute purity was not essential. Cotton Process Ether was gone, ethanesal was gone, Hewer employed selective memory and went on to other accomplishments. Wallis died at an early age in 1929; one must wonder how the Ethanesal fiasco affected him and if he became depressed and went into a decline.

Selective Forgetting

C.L.H. continued with his usual vigor, trying new things, writing, editing, organizing, being a leader in his field. Some examples of his selective memory have been cited. Only two more examples will be given.

Two years after being an Ethanesal enthusiast, C.L.H. was an ethylene enthusiast.[48] When Wallis and C.L.H. made ethylene to add to ether they used the sulfuric acid method as previously noted, the gas was sweeter and made a more potent mix with ether. When it came time to try ethylene-oxygen anesthesia, the gas was prepared for him using phosphoric acid. In his article on the subject, C.L.H. wrote, "The recent observation that ethylene dissolved in pure ether alters its anesthetic properties revived interest in the gas. . . ." The absence of his name, the name of Wallis, or mention of ethanesal is striking. The ethylene was given by "to and fro," with complete rebreathing. There is an illustration of a Waters system,[49] but the name Waters does not appear; C.L.H. was using "to and fro" within a year of its introduction. In 1925 he felt ethylene had. . . "certain advantages over the other anesthetics at present in use, . . .;" his negative feelings towards ethylene in 1959 were noted above.

The series, *Recent Advances in Anaesthesia and Analgesia,*[50] was introduced in 1932. The chapter on ether opened with the comment that there would be no discussion on whether or not absolutely pure freshly prepared ether was an anesthetic. He did not mention his role in the question, nor Wallis, nor Ethanesal. The van Leeuwen exchanges were eight years in the past.

Hadfield and Hewer forgot their earlier differences, and with the outbreak of World War II they were both on the Joint Committee of the Medical Research Council and the Section of Anaesthetics of the Royal Society of Medicine. Hadfield was secretary of the committee and a letter about trichlorethylene (from a Mr. Chalmers of Muswell Hill, whose further identity seems to be lost to history) was passed to Hadfield from the editor of *The Lancet.* Hadfield passed it on to C.L.H. who investigated the drug.[51] Hewer delineated the drug's virtues, how to use it, the danger of poor soda-lime in a closed circuit, and so on. Anesthesiologists who use trichlorethylene found it of value. The author feels the drug was especially suited for obstetric anesthesia practice and neurosurgical procedures (especially hind brain procedures because the patient could continue spontaneous ventilation); he also feels it disappeared from the market because it was so inexpensive there was no incentive to the pharmaceutical companies to market it.

Hewer did a marvelous job of introducing the drug after Dennis Jackson failed,[3] and outside forces removed it. Ethanesal and trichlorethylene are a contrast, a generation apart, in Hewer's career.

Conclusions

Hewer was young, he believed in Ethanesal; with maturity, he wiped it from his memory. *Libenter homines id quod volunt credunt* (Men freely believe that which they desire). (Caesar. De bello gallico, Book III, 18:6)

References

1. Boulton TB: Editorial, Anaesthesia 41:5469-71, 1986.
2. Hewer CL: Forty years on, Anaesthesia 14(4): 311-30, 1959.
3. Stetson JB: Dennis Emerson Jackson (1878-1980), Atkinson RS and Boulton TB eds. The History of Anaesthesia, Royal Society of Medicine, International Congress and Symposium Series Number 134 London, pp. 564-71, 1989.
4. Obituary: RL Mackenzie Wallis, MA, MD. St. Bartholomew's Hospital Journal p. 118, May, 1929.
5. Wallis RLM, Hewer CL: A new general anaesthetic: its theory and practice. Proceedings of the Royal Society of Medicine. Section of Anaesthetics. 14:37-47, 1921.
6. Hewer CL: A few points about ethanesal. S Bartholomew's Hospital Journal, p. 124, May, 1921.
7. Wallis RLM, Hewer CL: A new general anaesthetic: its theory and practice. Lancet i: 1173-8, 1921.
8. Boyle HEG: Gas-oxygen – Ethanesal-chloroform combined anesthesia for nose and throat and abdominal surgery. American Journal of Surgery, Anesthesia Supplement, 36:17-21, 1922.
9. Boyle HEG: Anaesthesia for nose, throat, and abdominal surgery by the nitrous oxide-oxygen-C.E. combination. British Medical Journal ii: 591, 1921.
10. Pinson KB: The properties and composition of ethanesal. Lancet i: 1382, 1921.
11. Stock SV: Methods of Anaesthesia. British Medical Journal, ii:769, 1921.
12. Hall TG: A short note on an ether representing ethanesal. The Medical Journal of South Africa, 17:191-2, 1921.
13. Hewer CL: Spinal analgesia and general anaesthesia. British Medical Journal, i:190-1, 1922.
14. Hewer CL: The endo-tracheal administration of nitrous oxide-oxygen-ethanesal as the routine anaesthetic of choice for major surgery. British Journal of Anaesthesia i:113-22, 1923.
15. Hewer CL: Endotracheal nitrous oxid oxygen-ether anesthesia in gastric surgery, Anesthesia & Analgesia, 5:303-5, 1926 (also published in the British Medical Journal).
16. Hewer CL: Anaesthesia in Children. HK Lewis & Co, London, 1923. In the United States, Paul B Hoeber, Inc, New York, 1923.
17. Boyle HEG, Hewer CL: Practical Anaesthetics, Third edition, Henry Frowde and Hodder & Stoughton, London, 1923.
18. Ross JS: Handbook of Anaesthetics, Second edition, E & S Livingstone, Edinburgh, 1923.
19. Hirsch CTW: Experiences with ethanesal. Lancet ii: 42, 1923.
20. Hirsch CTW: Anaesthesia for cerebellar operations-some points in technique. Medical Press & Circular (London), p. 377, May 9, 1923.
21. English C: Discussions (Anaesthetic from the Surgeon's Point of View) Lancet, ii:302, 1923.
22. Boyle HEG, Hewer CL: Recent Work in Anaesthesia for Gynaecology and Obstetrics. Journal of Obstetrics and Gynecology of the British Empire, 31:264-6, 1924.
27. Blomfield J: Recent Work on Anaesthetics. Practitioner, p. 163, January-June, 1922.
28. Hadfield CF: Practical Anaesthetics. Bailliere, Tindall and Cox, London, 1923.
29. Robinson H: Anaesthetics and Their Administration (Hewitt), Fifth edition. Henry Frowde and Hodder & Stoughton London, 1922.
30. Blomfield J: Anaesthetics in Practice and Theory. Chicago Medical Book Co., Chicago, 1923 (the English publisher was probably Wm. Heinemann Medical Books, London).
31. Webster W: The Science and Art of Anesthesia. C.M. Mosby Company, St. Louis, 1924.
32. Beebe RP: Clinical experiences with ethanesal anesthesia. American Journal of Surgery. Anesthesia Supplement, 39(1):12-14, 1925.
33. Brydon AG, Hallows, BR, Hughes M, Kaye G, et al: Practical Anaesthetics. Australian Medical Publishing Company, Glebe, p. 67, 1932.
34. Ethanesal. Lancet. i:1309, 1921.
35. Stehle RL, Bourne W: The Anesthetic properties of pure ether. JAMA, 79 (5):375-6, 1922.
36. Reports on Drugs. Chloroform and ether. British Medical Journal i:83, 1923.
37. Dale HH, Hadfield CF, King H: The anaesthetic action of pure ether. Lancet, i:424-9, 1923.
38. Editorial. Purity of Anesthetics. Anesthesia & Analgesia 2 (3):81-2, 1923.
39. van Leeuwen WS: On the Narcotic action of purest ether. Proceedings of the Royal Society of Medicine. Anaesthesia Section. 17(9):17-34 1924.
40. Editorial. Pure ether. Lancet i:561-2, 1924.
41. Editorial. Anaesthetic properties of ether. British Medical Journal i:471-2, 1924.
42. van Leeuwen S: The Narcotic action of pure ether. Lancet i:975, 1924.

43. Hewer CL: The Narcotic action of pure ether. Lancet i:1026, 1924.
44. Laws HE: Anaesthetic ether. Lancet i:788-9, 1927.
45. Editorial. Impurities in ether. Lancet ii:1305-6, 1927.
46. Bourne W: On the effects of acetaldehyde, ether peroxide, ethyl mercapton, ethyl sulphide, and several ketones-di-methyl ethyl methyl and di-ethyl – when added to anaesthetic ether. Journal of Pharmacology and Experimental Therapeutics. 28(3):409-32, 1926.
47. Bourne W: Pure ether and impurities: a review. Anesthesiology 7:509-605, 1946.
48. Hewer CL: Ethylene anesthesia with observations on 120 administrations. American Journal of Surgery. Anesthesia supplement. 39:119-22, 1925.
49. Walters RM: Clinical scope and utility of carbon dioxide filtration in inhalation anesthesia. Anesthesia & Analgesia. 3:20-2, 1924.
50. Hewer CL: Recent advances in anesthesia and analgesia. Churchill, London, 1932.
51. Hewer CL, Hadfield CF: Trichlorethylene as an inhalation anaesthetic. British Medical Journal, i:924-7, 1941.

WILLIAM E. CLARKE AND HIS 1842 USE OF ETHER

JOHN B. STETSON
Professor Emeritus
Department of Anesthesiology
Rush Medical College, Chicago, Illinois, USA

Introduction

Henry Munson Lyman, A.M., M.D. was "Professor of Physiology and of the Diseases of the Nervous System," Rush Medical College, and "Professor of Theory and Practice of Medicine" The Woman's Medical College, both of Chicago, Illinois. In 1881, Lyman's book, "Artificial Anaesthesia and Anaesthetics" was published by William Wood and Company.[1] Books about other medical subjects, in identical bindings, published by Wood, have been seen suggested that Lyman's volume was part of a subscription or popular medical series. The book contains a very complete historical introductory section. The contents of the book appear to have been well researched and information is documented. The book is an excellent historical reference source.

A Provocative Paragraph in Lyman's Book

> In like manner, during the year 1839, a young student of chemistry, in the city of Rochester, N.Y., William E. Clarke by name, now a veteran physician in Chicago, was in the habit of entertaining his companions with inhalations of ether. Among the participants in these frolics was another young man, named William T.G. Morton, who afterward became a dentist. At the Berkshire Medical College, during the winter of 1841-42, Clarke diligently propagated this convivial method among his fellow-students. Emboldened by these experiences, in January, 1842, having returned to Rochester, he administered ether, from a towel, to a young woman named Hobbie, and one of her teeth was then extracted without pain by a dentist named Elijah Pope.

Who were the people named by Lyman? Could Lyman's account be verified? Did Clarke publish an account of his use of ether? How did Lyman (Figs. 1,2) know about Clarke and his use of ether?

Some Answers

Named in the paragraph are Clarke, William T.G. Morton, Miss Hobbie, and Elijah Pope. Discussion of Clarke will be skipped until

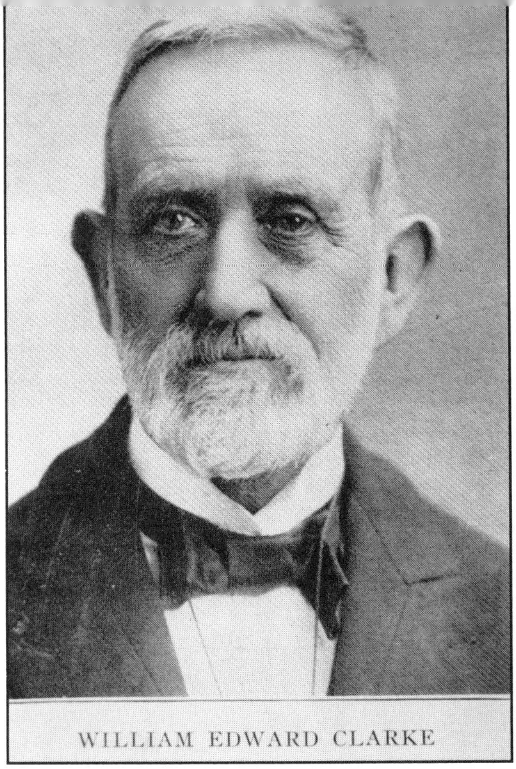

Fig. 1. William Edward Clark.

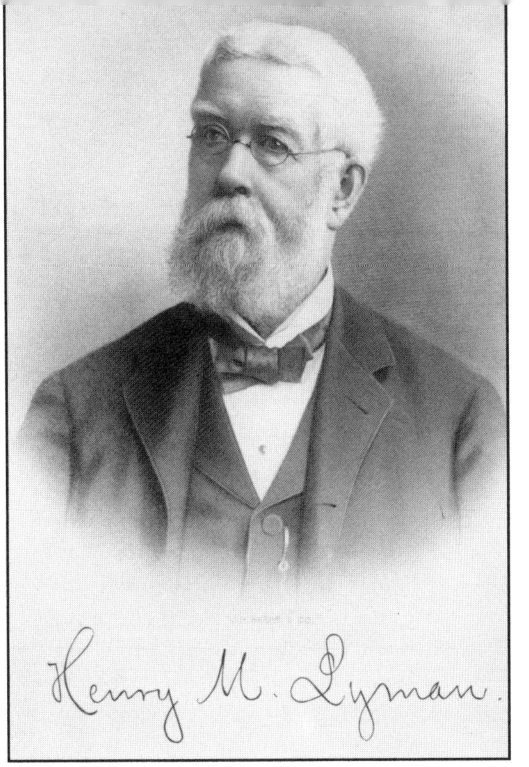

Fig. 2. Henry M. Lyman.

later and we will start with Morton.

Morton's successful demonstration of ether anesthesia at The Massachusetts General Hospital, October 16, 1846 (Professor John Collins Warren, surgeon) is so well known, further comment is not necessary. Confirming Morton's presence at the Berkshire Medical College or in Rochester, N.Y., has not been possible. There was railroad service from Rochester to Auburn, New York, and connections there to parts of New England. Morton may have traveled seeking employment, a preceptorship, or educational opportunity. During 1841-2 he visited Wells in Hartford several times, and a few years later with an office on Tremont Row in Boston, he used the train to commute from his home in Wellesley.

Lyman read a paper entitled "The Discovery of Anaesthesia" before the Mississippi Valley Medical Society, Quincy, Illinois, July 14, 1886.[2] Information similar to the quoted book paragraph was included. Morton's purported visit or visits to Clarke were mentioned three times in this article. It should be noted Morton died following "an apoplectic attack" in Central Park, New York City, eighteen years prior to the Quincy talk.

Morton was also mentioned in an article entitled, "Was William E. Clarke of Rochester the First American to Use Ether for Surgical Anesthesia?"[3] The clue to this article was a 1965 newspaper article![4] The newspaper article was entitled, "Another Medical First for Rochester." The author of the article quoted from ". . .'The History of Surgical Anesthesia,' just published by Dover Publications of New York." The book quoted was the "paper-back" edition of Thomas Keys' well known book. Keys included a shortened version of Lyman's account in his book (properly referenced). The article's author (the newspaper's Science Writer) interviewed the Rochester, N.Y., city historian who ". . .cited a paper written on the subject in 1950 for the Rochester Historical Society by Phyllis Allen Richmond, then a graduate student." In his article,[3] William E. Clarke remains without a middle name, only the initial, "E." Concerning Morton, she wrote, ". . .among the young men participating in these adventures was William T.G. Morton, who was then in Rochester and may have picked up the idea of using ether as an anesthetic from these experiences." Ms. Richmond gave no references in her article. Was she quoting Lyman or did she have other sources? In her article, she mentions reviewing the Edward Mott Moore letters in the University of Rochester Library, and the problems of reading Dr. Pope's letters (he attempted to change the spelling of the English language), but the location of the Pope letters is not noted, nor if they contained mention of Morton. The University of Rochester Alumni Office has no record of Ms. Richmond, another mystery!

Next, we will comment on Miss Hobbie (Lyman), or Miss Hobby (Richmond). She has not been identified, but the 1844 Rochester City Directory lists Joseph C. Hobbie as a "medical student." The 1845-46 directory lists him as a "dentist." A list of the students and graduates of the Vermont Medical College contains the name of Joseph C. Hobbey (the third way of spelling) of Rochester, N.Y., as enrolled in 1845.[5] One can probably assume that Joseph C. Hobbie and Joseph C. Hobbey are the same person. Allen Hobby of New York (city or town not identified) attended (or graduated from) the Castleton (Vermont) Medical College the summer session of 1845.[6] Was Clarke's Miss Hobbie (Hobby) related to one (or both) of these medical (dental) students? William Edwin (Edwin, not "E.") Clarke of Rochester, N.Y., is listed as graduating from the Vermont Medical College in 1845.[7] Joseph C. Hobbie and Clarke were in Rochester, N.Y., at the same time, and at Vermont Medical College at the same time. If Miss Hobbie was related, there is a connection with Clarke. There is no evidence of a romantic connection between Dr. Clarke and Miss Hobbie. Chauncey D. Leake, inventor of divinyl ether, wrote *Letheon, The Cadenced Story of Anesthesia*.[8] Leake employed poetic license when he termed the person etherized as Clarke's fiancée (Figs. 3a, 3b).

It is not known if J.C. Hobbie attended the Berkshire Medical College (in Massachusetts). Clarke is reported to have attended for one lecture session (lecture courses were generally fourteen to sixteen weeks in length). The student rolls are probably available, but as yet I have not located a source.

The third person identified is Elijah Pope. The 1841 Rochester City Directory describes him as a "student;" in 1844 he has progressed to "surgeon-dentist." The 1845-46 Directory lists him as a "manufacturer of surgical instruments." Pope was enrolled in the Vermont Medical

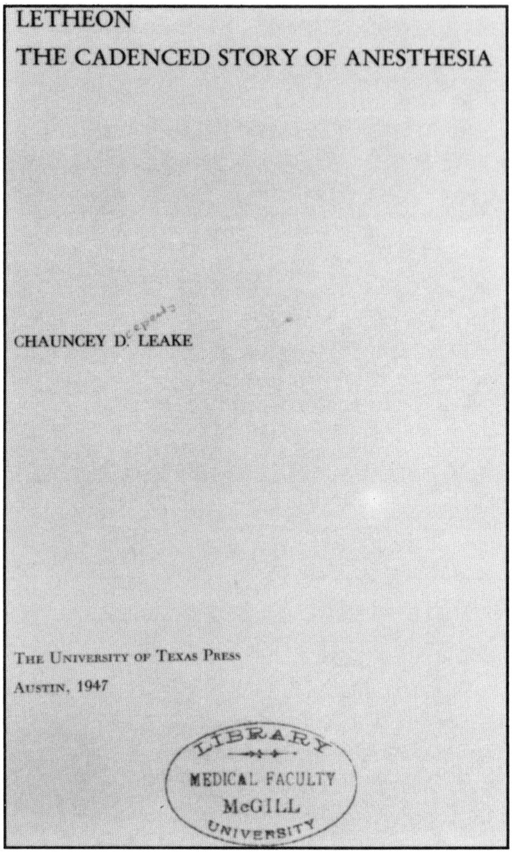
LETHEON
THE CADENCED STORY OF ANESTHESIA

CHAUNCEY D. LEAKE

THE UNIVERSITY OF TEXAS PRESS
AUSTIN, 1947

Figs. 3a and 3b.

In Boston, Collins Warren thought
of ether inhalations for relief
in pulmonary inflammation,
and many younger medicos had learned
to sniff at laughing gas and ether
for a frolic.
William Clarke of Rochester
was one of these.
His sympathy for pain
in tooch-ache in his fiancé
suggested ether sniffing while
the tooth was pulled.
No pain was felt.

But Clarke thought little further on it, and
said nothing more about it.
Yet, he'd used the ether first for
pain relief in surgery!

College in 1843.[9] Although Pope could not be found in the Rochester directories for 1847-48 or 1849-50, Richmond wrote: "Dr. Pope remained in Rochester for many years, practicing dentistry and selling medical instruments. . . .[3] Richmond thought it odd that Pope had been as reticent as Clarke about the ether episode. Pope may have been similar to Dr. John M. Riggs, the dentist who pulled Horace Wells' molar tooth after Gardner Quincy Colton administered nitrous oxide to Wells. Riggs never sought any acclaim or credit. A second thought is that Pope felt humbled by his failure to have ether employed on any of his patients other than Miss Hobbie. Professor Moore's warning to Clarke may have silenced him.

Two biographical sketches of Clarke (W.E.C.) have been located. The first was published four years before his death.[10a] His name is listed William E. (letter only), and there is no mention of ether. The book also contains a biography of Crawford W. Long.[10b] The Long biography is about nine column inches in length and half of the article is dedicated to information about Clarke! It is evident the editor gathered his information "first hand." On the subject of the first person to use ether, ". . .the editor of this work desires to call attention to the apparent justness of the claims of one who is still living, and whose biographical sketch is printed on another page of this volume. He now refers to the venerable Dr. William E. Clarke of Chicago." It is noted the young woman resisted the efforts of a dentist to extract a diseased tooth. Clarke gave ether, she became "seemingly unconscious" and the tooth was extracted without pain. Clarke's preceptor was Professor E.M. Moore, who, ". . .recently stated that at that time he was of the opinion, that the woman in a hysterical freak feigned unconsciousness, and for that reason advised his pupil to make no more experiments in that direction, and that his advice was unfortunately followed." We now have a better description of the operation on Miss Hobbie than of the operation on Mr. Venable. We also have the reason why Clarke did not continue his ether trials.

The second biography[11] was published twenty-four years following his death. It is titled William Edward (not Edwin) Clarke. The second biography begins: "That he was the first to discover the value of ether as an anaesthetic is the claim made for Dr. William Edward Clarke [W.E.C.], who was president of the Chicago Medical Society, 1875-76. It is said that Dr. Clarke administered ether for the extraction of a tooth in January, 1842."

W.E.C. was the son of Dr. Thaddeus and Deborah Baker Clarke. He was born February 22, 1819, in Lebanon, Conn. Both his grandfathers were medical officers in the Revolutionary War. In one biography, Thaddeus is listed as the "first resident [sic]" of the Connecticut Medical Society. Connecticut State Medical Society records do not confirm this honor. Thaddeus did represent Windham County at the October, 1797 convention of the state medical society and was on the "Examining Committee" for Windham County.

W.E.C.'s early education was under the supervision of his mother, ". . .a highly cultivated woman of decided Christian character." She was a descendant of Jonathan Edwards (1703-58) the noted preacher and president of Princeton College.[11] There is a question of Clarke's middle name, Edward or Edwin, or was it originally Edwards after Jonathan? It is not known if the Clarke family moved from Connecticut to Rochester or if W.E.C. came to Rochester alone. In the late 1830's he entered Rochester Collegiate Institute (R.C.I.). The Reverend Doctor Chester Dewey (1784-1867) was Principal of the R.C.I., 1835-50. Dewey, a Williams College graduate, was a well known Congregational minister and educator. In 1822 he joined the faculty at Berkshire Medical College (Pittsfield, Massachusetts) as Professor of Chemistry and Medicinal Botany. In 1823 he organized the first anti-slavery society in Massachusetts. From 1842-1849 he held academic positions at Woodstock Medical College in Vermont. W.E.C. attended Berkshire Medical College for one course of lectures (probably 1843) and was an assistant to Dewey at both R.C.I. and Berkshire (number of years not known). In adult years, in Chicago, W.E.C. was a deacon of the First Congregational Church for twenty-seven years. It is not known if Clarke's family were congregationalists or if his interest can be traced to Dewey. Jonathan Edwards was a Calvinist, and later, evangelical.

In Rochester, before attending Berkshire Medical College, W.E.C. began the study of medicine about 1840, in private classes, with Edward Mott Moore (1814-1902) and Frank Hastings Hamilton (1813-1886). His studies with Moore in Rochester and at the Vermont Medical College, continued five years. Moore's negative influence on Clarke in relation to the use of ether has been noted. Moore had a general medical practice in Rochester and taught the Principles and Practice of surgery at Vermont Medical College (Woodstock, 1842-1853). Moore trained at the university of Pennsylvania (M.D., 1838, one year ahead of Crawford Long). He moved to Rochester in 1840 and W.E.C. became his student. W.E.C.'s choice of V.M.C. (M.D. in 1845) was probably influenced by Moore. In 1853, (After W.E.C. had left Rochester and moved West) Moore left V.M.C. and became Professor of Surgery at Berkshire Medical College. Moore was an outstanding teacher (as was Dewey) and prominent in medicine (President New York State Medical Society, American Surgical Society, the American Medical Association) and civic activities (First President, New York Board of Health; President, Rochester Park Commission; Board of Trustees, University of Rochester).

Frank Hastings Hamilton was educated at Union College. He took Chair of Surgery at Geneva Medical College, August 10,1840. He left for a visit to Britain and Europe, 1843-4. It is assumed that while he was at Geneva he came to Rochester for the classes W.E.C. attended (or W.E.C. went to Geneva). Hamilton was Professor of Surgery at the University of Buffalo, 1846-1858. He was a consultant in the care of President Garfield after he was shot. After Garfield died, Hamilton penned a report on the ". . .true causes of the embarrassments in treatment, as revealed by the necropsy,. . . ." Hamilton moved to Brooklyn, entered the Union Army in 1861 and rose to the rank of Medical Inspector. He was one of the founders of Bellevue Hospital Medical College and his obituary termed him ". . .the greatest surgeon that city had ever known. . . ."

As noted above, W.E.C. took one course of lectures at Berkshire Medical College, two at Vermont Medical College (M.D., 1845) and had outstanding teachers. He returned to Rochester in 1845 and entered into practice with Dr. Moore. The 1847-48 Rochester city directory lists W.E.C.'s office address as "over 4 and 6 Buffalo street" and his boarding address as 73 Fitzhugh Street. He had probably left Rochester prior to publication of these addresses. Richmond wrote; "after graduation Clarke seems to have applied unsuccessfully for a military appointment."[3] The source of this information is not listed.

From Rochester, Clarke moved to Cold Water, Michigan, where he settled in the fall of 1847. He married Miss Harriet H. Hale of Kalamazoo[10a] or of Marshall, Michigan.[11] In 1852, they moved to Chicago where he was surgeon for both the Michigan Central and Michigan Southern railroads. "The climate of Chicago proving too severe for the health of Mrs. Clarke, the doctor was obliged to relinquish his position in Chicago, and after spending some time in travel he returned to Michigan, and remained, doing a major part of the surgical practice for a large section of the country, till the spring of 1861, when he was reappointed surgeon of the Fourth Regiment Michigan Volunteers."[10a] Clarke saw much action in the field. When the Nineteenth Michigan Infantry was raised under his cousin, Colonel N.C. Gilbert, he transferred to that regiment. He again saw much field duty, was captured by the confederates, but exchanged after two weeks. Due to severe illness, he resigned his commission in July, 1863. After recuperation, he received an appointment that put him in charge of the Carver General Hospital in Washington, D.C. (Fig. 4). Perhaps his old teacher, Frank Hastings Hamilton, then the Medical Inspector for the Union Army, had a hand in the appointment. Mrs. Clarke accompanied her husband and did ". . .faithful and efficient duty among the sick and wounded, but at last the health of Mrs. Clarke compelled him to leave with her for their home. . . ."[10a] Mrs. Clarke died on the way home and W.E.C. returned to duty and remained until the close of the war.

Clarke then returned to Chicago and medical practice and marriage in 1865 to Miss Mary L. Reed of Lake Forest[11] or Chicago.[10a] He was a consultant to the Hospital for Women and Children, and Mary Thompson Hospitals, and consulting gynecologist to the Presbyterian Hospital. In 1975-76, he was President of the Chicago Medical Society. He was a delegate to the Illinois State Medical Society in 1852, 1874, and 1890. Henry Lyman was also a delegate in 1874 and both W.E.C. and Lyman took part in the discussions concerning vaccination.

Clarke died at River Forest, Illinois March 22, 1898. There were two children by the second marriage, William E. Clarke, Jr., an attorney, and Grace who married Glenn E. Plumb. The children (grandchildren), have not been traced as yet. It is hoped they can be traced and that family papers are available that will shed further light on the tale.

Summary and Conclusions

Clarke used ether in January, 1842. His teacher, Professor Moore (Fig. 5), misjudged the patient's condition and there were no further trials. Clarke did not seek "lay" recognition of his use of ether. Henry Lyman, a recognized authority, wrote of Clarke's successful trial. Professor Moore gave a statement to R. French Stone, the editor of a popular information source concerning American physicians and surgeons

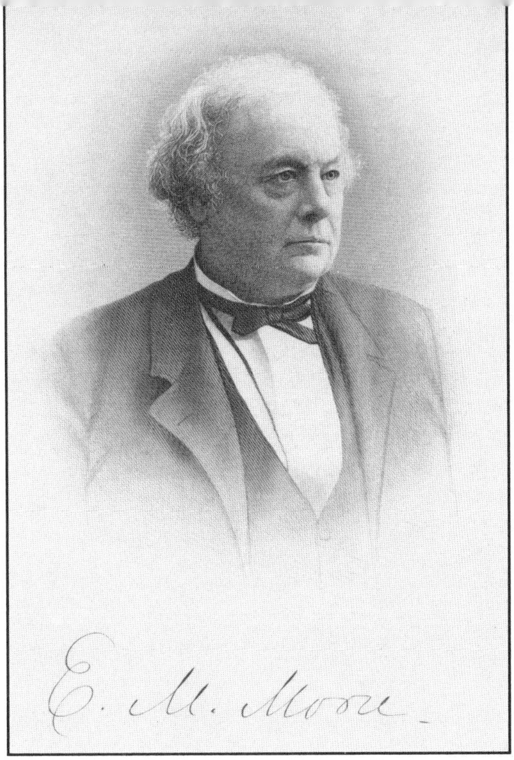

Fig. 5. E.M. Moore.

confirming Clarke's trial of ether and why trials were not continued.

One can compare Clarke and Crawford Long. Long's grandfather was an educated immigrant from Ulster and he fought in the Revolutionary War (with Lafayette's troops). Both of Clarke's grandfathers were medical officers in the Revolutionary War. Long's father was a very prosperous plantation-slave-business owner, W.E.C.'s father was a physician. Both were well educated; Long at Franklin College (University of Georgia), Transylvania University, University of Pennsylvania (M.D., 1839), and walking the hospitals in New York City; Clarke at Rochester Collegiate Institute, private classes, Berkshire Medical College, and Vermont Medical College (M.D., 1845). Long

Fig. 4. A Civil War field hospital.

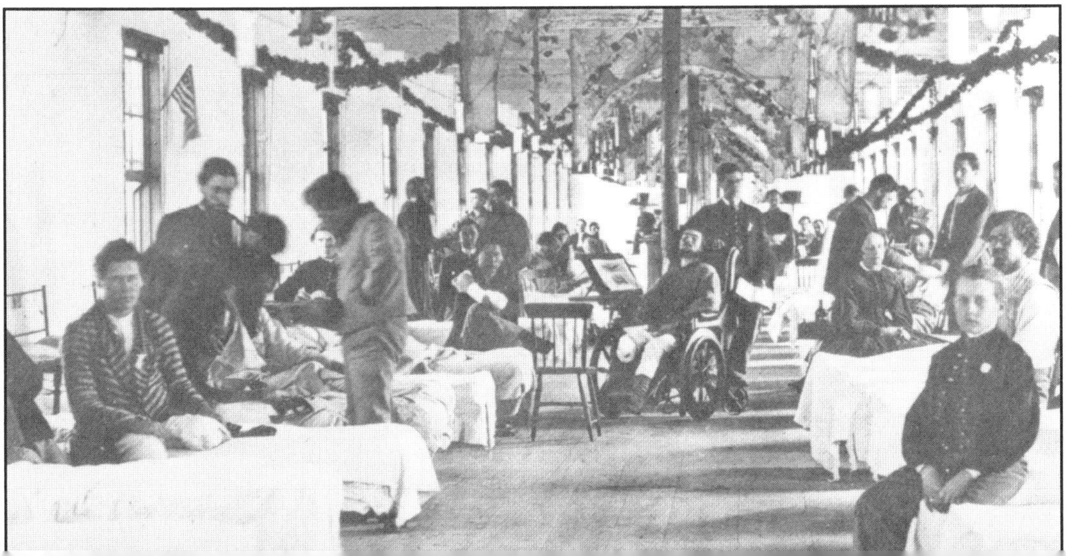

inherited plantations, slaves, and had an active general medical practice. Clarke practiced with Dr. Moore in Rochester, moved to Michigan, then Chicago, then back to Michigan, practicing surgery. During the Civil War Long was in charge of the hospital in his home town of Athens, Georgia (his services were retained by the Union Army when they took charge), and decorated by the United Daughters of the Confederacy.

Clarke was an active battle field surgeon at many engagements, was in charge (by biography) of the Carver Hospital in Washington, D.C. After the Civil War, Long continued his medical practice, still had a plantation, but was reduced in wealth. His 1849 publication concerning his 1842, 3, 4 use of ether was forgotten.

Clarke returned to Chicago after the Civil War and had a surgical and gynecologic practice. In 1877, J. Marion Sims, published his article bringing Long's claim to fame back to life.[12] Long died in 1878 and has been honored since death as a southern hero. Clarke, as noted, did not publish a note concerning his use of ether, but his colleague Henry Munson Lyman did.[1,2] Clarke had active field duty with the Union Army (the winning side), was President of the Chicago Medical Society, and a consultant to prominent Chicago hospitals. There was no emotional need for family members or other area physicians to elevate Clarke's memory to fill a void.

Although Clarke and Long employed ether, it was Morton's public demonstration, newspaper accounts, telegraphic news transmission, articles in medical journals (especially the Boston Medical and Surgical Journal), and letters written by Professor Warren that propelled the use of ether around the world. Clarke and Long are reminders that one must have an alert mind and the will to champion one's own observations.

Acknowledgments

Mr. Christopher Hoolihan of the Edward G. Miner Library of the University of Rochester has been extremely generous in affording valuable assistance. Mr. Robert J. Brunell of the Connecticut State Medical Society, Mr. Mark T. Dolan of Ruth Medical College, and Ms. Pamela Sheffel of Rochester Public Library also rendered valuable assistance.

Addendum

Dr. Genevieve Miller kindly supplied Dr. Richmond's address. A copy of Dr. Richmond's article[3] was sent to her, but she was unable to remember the source of her information concerning the presence of W.T.G. Morton in Rochester, N.Y. She believed the information concerning Dr. Pope was located at the Rochester Museum of Arts and Sciences.

Three further sources of information about Dr. Clarke were located. His obituary in the *JAMA* (30:807, 1898) used the middle initial "E," but the family name was spelled without an "e," that is, Clark! Clarke was ill for two weeks before his death on March 22, 1898. Relatives listed were, ". . .Grace Greenwood, the Washington authoress, and Major Charles E. Clark, a prominent retired army officer of Washington." As a Civil War veteran, Clarke was mustered into the Grand Army of the Republic, March 28, 1884. His service is listed in the "Personal War Sketches of the Members of the Phil Sheridan Post No. 615 (Oak Park, Illinois)," p. 163. His portrait is on page 34. Although a note at the Chicago Historical Society indicated that Dr. Clarke had been decorated, the name of the medal could not be located. The "Memorials of Deceased Companions of the Commandery of the State of Illinois, Military Order of the Loyal Legion of the United States" (published by the Commandery, 320 Ashland Block, Chicago, 1901) contains a photograph and complete biography (pp. 361-364). His middle name was Edwin. His parents did move to Rochester, N.Y., when he was a youth. Information about his education is confirmed and Lyman's report[1] is quoted. His rank in the Civil War was Major and Surgeon, Nineteenth Michigan Infantry. He served in the Peninsular Campaign under General McClellan and was later "in charge of Carver United States General Hospital in Washington." His son's obituary is contained in the same volume (pp. 202-203). William Edwin Clarke, Jr., was born in Chicago, May 7, 1867, and died there October 6, 1894. He graduated from Amherst College and Northwestern University Law School (1891). One great-grandfather, Joseph Baker, a surgeon on General Putnam's staff in the Revolution is noted. No marriage is recorded.

References

1. Lyman HM: Artificial Anaesthesia and Anaesthetics. New York, William Wood & Co., p. 6, 1881.
2. Lyman HM: The Discovery of Anaesthesia Virginia Medical Monthly, 13 (6) 369-392, 1886.
3. Richmond PA: Was William E. Clarke of Rochester the First American to Use Ether for Surgical Anesthesia? "Scrapbook," The Rochester Historical Society, 1:11-13, 1950.
4. Van Buren J: Another Medical "First" for Rochester? Democrat & Chronicle, Rochester, N.Y., January 20, 1965.
5. Waite FC: The Story of a Country Medical College, Vermont Historical Society, Montpelier, Vt., p. 189, 1945.
6. Waite FC: The First Medical College in Vermont, Castleton, 1818-1862, Vermont Historical Society, Montpelier, Vt., p. 214, 1949.
7. Waite FC: The Story of a Country Medical College, Vermont Historical Society, Montpelier, Vt., p. 161, 1945.
8. Leake CK: Letheon: The Cadenced Story of Anesthesia. The University of Texas Press, Austin, 1947.
9. Waite FC: The Story of a Country Medical College, Vermont Historical Society, Montpelier, Vt., p. 196, 1945.

10a. Stone RF: Biography of Eminent American Physicians and Surgeons, Carlon & Hollenbeck, Indianapolis, p. 89, 1894.

10b. ibid, p. 286.

11. Council of the Chicago Medical Society, History of Medicine and Surgery and Physicians and Surgeons of Chicago, Biographical Publishing Corp., Chicago, p. 54, 1992.
12. Sims JM: The Discovery of Anaesthesia, Virginia Medical Monthly, 4(2):81-100, (May) 1877.

JAMES HENRY COTTON AND COTTON PROCESS ETHER

JOHN B. STETSON
Professor, Emeritus
Department of Anesthesiology
Rush Medical College
Chicago, Illinois, USA

Introduction

Ether has been used for 150 years to induce analgesia-anesthesia to alleviate the pain of surgical procedures. Seventy-five years ago, James Henry Cotton, Jr. (1891-1952), put forth the thesis: "absolute gas-free ethyl-ether is not an anaesthetic."[1] How did Cotton's counter-theory begin, exist, end?

Cotton (Fig. 1) was the son of J.H. Cotton, Sr., "One of the best known surgeons in Canada."[2] The Cottons were "old" Canadians (J.H.C., Jr. was a *4th* or *5th* generation Canadian). Father and son were both graduates of the University of Toronto, J.H.C., Jr., was not accepted for military service in WWI (the reason has not been identified). To atone for this failure he put his energies into developing a better analgesic-anesthetic to help the "boys" who had been wounded. He felt carbon dioxide and ethylene must be suspended (under pressure) in pure ether to produce anesthetic mix (truly, the champagne of anesthetics!). His theory influenced Hewer and Wallis in England (see "Christopher Langton Hewer and Ethanesal," page 388, this volume). In 1920, E.I. DuPont De Nemours & Co., the chemical giant, placed Cotton Process Ether (C.P.E.) on sale (in a limited market) with much press coverage. Studies confirming the anesthetic properties of pure ether began to appear in 1922.[3] The American Medical Association labeled the claims made for C.P.E. and Ethanesal quackery, and DuPont quietly slipped C.P.E. off the market.

In 1923, Arno Luckhardt of the University of Chicago introduced ethylene anesthesia;[4] he started his prolonged investigations following identification of ethylene as a greenhouse villain (prevented the opening of buds). Also in 1923, William Easson Brown of the University of Toronto and the Toronto General Hospital reported on the anesthetic properties of ethylene.[5] Brown noted he began his investigations

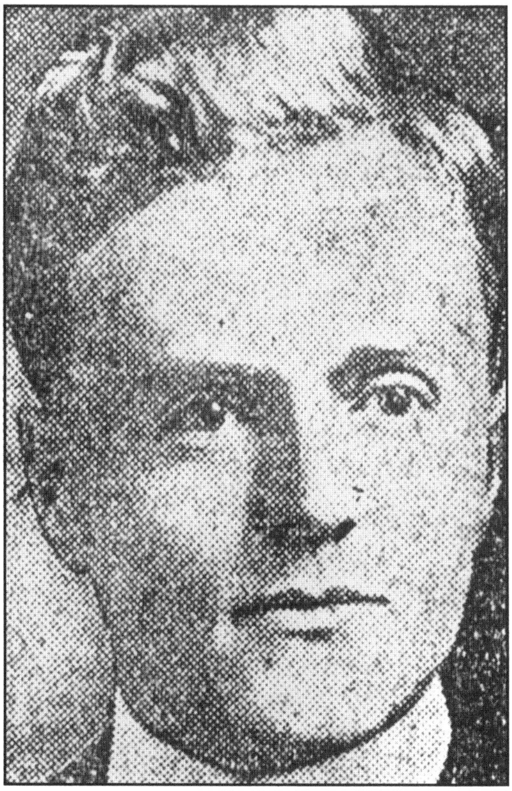

Fig. 1. This photograph of Cotton was used by Toronto newspapers in the many articles dealing with him.

because ethylene was a component of a "new" ether being touted at that time (he did not identify the drug as C.P.E. or Ethanesal, or both). Brown seemed to be a "golden boy;" he was Canadian Inter-Collegiate all-around champion, 1912; track captain, 1914; a Captain in the Royal Canadian Army Medical Corps with overseas service; his classmate, Dr. Fred G. Banting, the "discoverer" of insulin, ". . .was, at his own request, the first human subject to have ethylene administered."[6] By contrast, Cotton, although well connected, an excellent student and chemist, handsome (newspaper photograph, Fig. 1), and active, seemed to be an outsider. Cotton claimed the credit for the introduction of ethylene anesthesia should be his, and received support for this claim from Francis H. McMechan (see section on the "James H. Cotton Fund of the International Anesthesia Research Foundation").

J.H.C. Jr. married Ruby Long (stage name, Mlle. Audrie Rubanni, a coloratura soprano), January 25, 1919. Both were colorful and the subjects of numerous newspaper articles. In 1937, the pair took a month-long 600 mile horseback tour from Toronto to Limberlost and back. It seemed to be their swan song at an early age. J.H.C. Jr. died November 21, 1952, "after an illness of three months." His obituary contained the eulogy that he had "received acclaim for his discovery of ethylene. . ."[7] His widow survived him; no children were mentioned.

Cotton Process Ether-Clinical Introduction

The Place: Academy of Medicine, Toronto. Date: Tuesday, April 10, 1917: "8:30 o'clock." The section of medicine held their meeting, a "Clinical Evening." Part II of the meeting was, "Demonstration of Anesthesia with a Purified Ether — J.H. Cotton (by invitation)." A copy of the minutes were kindly supplied by the Academy. Legibility is poor; the essence of the notes are that J.H. Cotton, by a process of his own, can free commercial ether from aldehydes and obtain a perfectly pure ether. "To this is added CO_2 and he obtains an anaesthetic which produces analgesia without general narcosis." "Two cats were anaesthetized, one with ordinary ether and the other with Dr. Cotton's anaesthetic and it was evident that the second cat went under more rapidly and easily and recovered much more quickly. A patient was then given a sufficient amount of ether (+) and Dr. ____ extracted a number of teeth."

On June 14, 1917, Cotton gave a demonstration before the Canadian Medical Association at the Royal Victoria Hospital, Montreal.[1a] He restated his thesis that absolute di-ethyl ether was not an anesthetic, that carbon dioxide absolute ether (as demonstration in Toronto) produced an anesthesia similar to nitrous oxide, and that ethylene when added to absolute ether produced an analgesic mixture. Again, there was a cat demonstration. This was followed by a clinical demonstration. A middle aged Chinaman received "Absolute ether, carbon dioxide." "He had an infected upper arm;" "eight incisions were made over biceps," "Patient free from sensation but not at all unconscious." The second patient was a middle aged Englishman. The anesthetic was "Absolute ether-ethylene." The operation was: "Resection splintered bone from elbow. Patient capable of carrying on active conversation and yet was entirely free from sensation." It would seem that Dr. Cotton was gifted at administering ether analgesia. His conclusions were that ethyl-ether "is not an anaesthetic," rather it is a vehicle for analgesic gases (carbon dioxide, ethylene, other gases).

J.H.C.'s clinical demonstration impressed the audience, so much so that an editorial concerning his demonstration appeared in the same issue of *The Canadian Medical Association Journal* as his paper.[1b] The editorial ended with the comment that marketing of an ether of the type recommended was eagerly awaited. Cotton reported only two surgical patients (plus the cats). One does not know if further demonstrations of C.P.E. were made in Montreal. It is startling the editor did not request further information on the methods of producing C.P.E. and further clinical demonstrations before enthusiastic endorsement.

A year later, September 25-27, 1918, Cotton spoke at the Joint Session of the Interstate Association of Anesthetists and Indiana State Medical Association, Claypool Hotel, Indianapolis, Indiana. Cotton was preceded on the program by Lieutenant Arthur E. Guedel, M.C., U.S. Army. Guedel's paper, the "Auscultatory Control of Anesthesia for operation under the Fluoroscope" was read by proxy, so Guedel may not have been present. Cotton's address concerned C.P.E. and ether analgesia.[9] The report indicates Cotton was an acute clinician. He noted, ". . .alcoholics required from 25 to 75 percent more ether than did the non-alcoholics." A chart correlating the depression of special senses, the C.N.S., sympathetic nervous systems, antonomic nervous system, and spinal cord with the stages of anesthesia was presented (Fig. 2). Cotton reviewed his research work (but did not delineate his method of preparing pure ether) and how he discovered that carbon dioxide and ethylene (both under pressure) must be added to pure ether to obtain an analgesic mixture. The product (C.P.E.) was supplied in one ounce

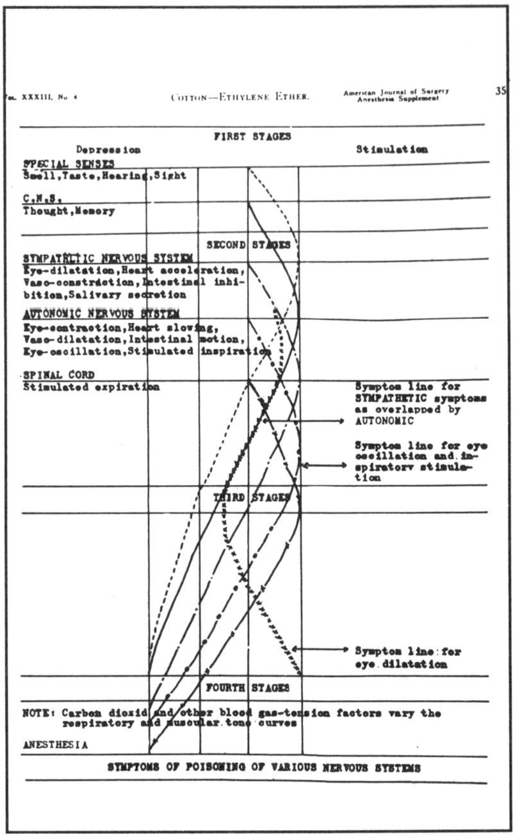

Fig. 2. Cotton's chart of the response of the various parts of the nervous system to increasing "depths" of ether. The chart was shown at a meeting, September 25-27, 1918. Arthur Guedel preceded Cotton on the program, but his paper was "read by proxy." If Guedel knew of Cotton's chart, it may have been an influence in his decision to publish and eye sign chart (reported a year later).

ampules and used with a device similar to an ethyl chloride dripper (Fig. 3). Cotton used C.P.E. "semi-closed" with Rice's "perfected method" and a Gwathmey apparatus. He claimed C.P.E. did not cause nausea.

A very interesting paragraph in the report described a closed system made by filling the ether container ". . . with caustic potash sticks in order to absorb any accumulation of carbon dioxide." An excess of oxygen was given, 10 to 20 liters per hour. . ." If oxygen consumption was 250ml/minute, 15 liters per hour, there were

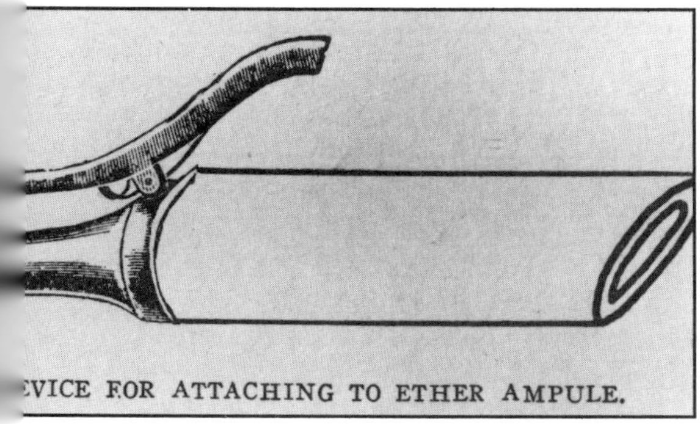

Fig. 3. Ampule of Cotton Process Ether (one or two ounces) with dripper attachment. DuPont marketed Cotton Process Ether in standard quarter pound cans. At a later date Cotton commented that the ethylene content of C.P.E. had to be reduced from 5 percent to 2 percent as the DuPont cans would not withstand the pressure generated by 5 percent ethylene.

no leaks and efficient carbon dioxide absorption, would keep the bag full (closed system anesthesia). As the caustic potash would absorb the carbon dioxide suspended in the C.P.E., one can argue that Cotton was defeating his own theory. The ethylene bubbling out of the C.P.E. would fill the closed system and speed induction (and perhaps afford ethylene-oxygen-ether analgesia).

Cotton described "Analgesia with ethylene ether." The patients received "Open Mask Administration direct from Ampule." An 18 year-old-male had a tubercular mass resected from his abdomen. "He was given a small meal while the surgeons were operating on him. Abdomen was completely relaxed, except at one time when he insisted upon kissing the nurse." One is reminded of Crawford Long's letter to a friend requesting ether for a "frolic" so he could collect sweet kisses from the young ladies. As noted above, Cotton must have been a master at administering ether analgesia. He notes ". . .anesthesia is a specialty requiring the highest possible education in both chemistry and physiology." He also noted, ". . .for major surgery a great deal more knowledge of the intricacies of anesthesia is required for its (C.P.E.) use than has heretofore been necessary." Cotton ended his talk with the comment that his research was undertaken ". . .to make things more bearable for the boys at the Front. . ." when they needed painful dressings.

In his September, 1919, talk, Cotton spoke of one ounce ampules of C.P.E.. The December, 1919, issue of the DuPont Magazine contained an article about "The New Ether" and a picture of a quarter pound can of DuPont Anesthesia Ether (Cotton Process).[10] The DuPont article reviewed Cotton's work, printed sample case reports (analgesia and anesthesia), placed emphasis on rapid induction and recovery with C.P.E. plus the lack of nausea. The DuPont article did not mention either carbon dioxide nor ethylene and the formulation was not listed on the can. DuPont put news of their wonderful anesthetic before the newspapers. "News" articles soon appeared in the lay press. The American Medical Association headquarters received newspaper clippings from members and a four year skirmish between DuPont and the AMA (see section, "The A.M.A. and C.P.E.") began.

The 1920 Edition, Sales Department, E.I. DuPont De Nemours & Company, Inc., lists "Ether-Cotton Process" on page 99. The one paragraph description notes, ". . .it provides quicker induction. . ., more rapid recovery and practical freedom from troublesome after effects, such as nausea, etc." The paragraph is followed by: "(Note): At present solicitation is confined to a limited territory. Notification will be given when general solicitation is desired."

Although there seemed to be problems in communication between the AMA and DuPont seventy years ago, the author wishes to thank the Hagley Museum and Library of Wilmington, Delaware, for their kind cooperation (the Hagley Museum is the repository for DuPont records.)

The first non-Cotton authored report about C.P.E. appears to be that of Lumbard.[11] Lumbard reported he had used C.P.E. 400 times and had difficulty obtaining ether analgesia as some patients ". . .passed into surgical anesthesia before any analgesic stage could be demonstrated." He felt C.P.E. was stronger than other ethers during induction, the same as other ethers during maintenance,and that recovery seemed less disturbed. Lumbard appended the "opinion and conclusions of others" to his report. C.C.McLean of Dayton, Ohio, had used C.P.E. 400 times and had been able to obtain ether analgesia. The evaluations were fairly favorable when C.P.E. had been used in a closed or semi-closed system. Lumbard reported that C.P.E. contained 2 percent ethylene by volume, "1/2 volume of carbon dioxide and 1 percent by weight of ethyl alcohol."

Dr. Cotton gave a talk and clinical demonstrations before the Dental Society of the State of New York, Albany, May 13, 14 and 15, 1920. The lecture and discussions were published in 1921.[12] The content of the talk was similar to his Indianapolis presentation of 1919, J.H.C. wrote: "With ethylene plus ether, nausea after the patient awakens has not as yet occurred. . ." He also noted, ". . .it is also well to bear in mind the following two facts: 1) Post-operative nausea rarely occurs in old people, especially when they are suffering from any degree of blood pressure. 2) A certain class of operations having to do with the intestines, especially the gallbladder, will of themselves give rise to nausea." The "two facts" listed were proof of J.H.C.'s clinical acumen (especially true in the 1920's, with ether anesthesia; the "facts" may seem quaint to recent medical graduates). During the discussion period Cotton stated, ". . .we have done an operation for appendicitis, and had the patient eating his breakfast at the same time." This could be termed the acme of ether analgesia. Artusio described ether analgesia and its employment for cardiac surgery.[13] Artusio brought the patients to stage III, plane 1, and then lightened the patients to stage I, plane 3. Cotton seemed to be able to go directly to the analgesic state (the meager description of Long's use of ether on James Venable, and of some of Morton's first anesthetics, also suggest ether analgesia). After its introduction (or re-introduction) by Artusio, ether analgesia was in common use for cardiac surgery in the 1950's. Artusio's technique was not used for abdominal surgery. Perhaps stupidity and bias prevented those of us who used Artusio's technique from repeating Cotton's successes.

Dr. William J. Lederer of New York added a strong note of caution and safety to the Albany discussion. He questioned the idea that the average dentist had the ability to obtain the results demonstrated by J.H.C. It was also obvious from his comments that one of the patients who had received C.P.E. had "carried on" in the dental chair.

Paul Cassidy, a dentist in Cincinnati, Ohio, did a very thoughtful study of C.P.E.. He recorded the rate of loss of ethylene from C.P.E. after the tin was opened. There was 2.24 percent ethylene in C.P.E. when the tin was opened. Fifteen minutes after opening the tin, ethylene content had dropped to 1.12 percent and at a half-hour after opening, 0.30 percent. Cassidy devised a system that allowed opening of the C.P.E. tin can within a closed anesthesia machine. Again, the ethylene bubbled off and reached the patient before the ether vapor when the "exit valve" was opened. Cassidy devised a sealed light bulb chamber within the vaporizer and used the heat of the light bulb to keep the ethylene-ether mixture consistent. Cassidy found C.P.E. treated patients did very well when his system was used (this system also included added carbon dioxide or rebreathing). His report ". . .endeavored to reawaken our interest in a product which has been very badly marketed." The paper was read by proxy at the joint Canadian-American meeting held at the Hotel Clifton, Niagara Falls, Canada, June 1-3,1921. H. Edmund G. Boyle, of St. Bartholomew's Hospital, London, was on a North American junket in 1921 and was Honorary Chairman of the meeting. Boyle's address was titled, "Gas-Oxygen-Ethanesal-Chloroform Combined Anesthesia for Nose and Throat and Abdominal Surgery."[14] Cassidy's talk was published in both of the journals edited by F.H. McMechan.[15,16] Those in attendance at the meeting heard about both C.P.E. and Ethanesal — two "improved ethers" on the verge of extinction.

The first volume of *Anesthesia and Analgesia* was published in 1922; F.H. McMechan, Editor. McMechan also edited the Anesthesia Supplements of the American Journal of Surgery (the supplements began in 1914). Articles from the supplements were gathered by McMechan and published as "Year Books." McMechan, the father of Anesthesia Journals, can also be considered the father of The International Anesthesia Research Society. The December, 1922, issue of *Anesthesia and Analgesia* carried a full page advertisement for C.P.E. (Fig. 4).

Although Cotton was a Canadian, there is a dearth of articles about C.P.E. and Ethanesal at the Manitoba Medical Association meeting, November 10, 1921, and it was published in Canada.[17] An almost identical paper was presented before the Manitoba Hospital Association in 1922, and published by McMechan.[18] Webster saw no advantage in the use of C.P.E.; he was slightly more impressed by Ethanesal.

Webster's textbook was published in 1924. The three page section on "New Anesthetic Ethers" reviewed C.P.E. and Ethanesal.[19] Cassidy's chart on the disappearance of ethylene was included. The then new research work of Bourne and Stehle in Canada,[3] and Dale, Hadfield and King[20] in England was noted. Both groups proved pure ether was an anesthetic. The days of C.P.E. and Ethanesal were numbered.

One of the last, if not the last, clinical article about C.P.E. was that of C.C. McLean.[21] The footnote with the article notes it as read "during the National Anesthesia Research Society Congress Hotel Deshler, Columbus, Ohio, October 30-November 1,1923.: It was published in the June, 1923, issue of *Anesthesia and Analgesia*. It is not known if there is a printing error (date), or if the June issue was printed five months late. McLean administered C.P.E. with the "Ben Morgan Ether Apparatus." He was able to carry the patients in a very light plane (or stage) of anesthesia.

Cotton spoke at the First Annual Meeting of the Eastern Society of Anesthetist, Hotel McAlpin, New York City, October 20-24, 1924.[22] He still felt that "...our ethylene was an analgesic gas which could be administered in ...ether... with analgesic results." He reviewed his development of techniques for the purification of ether and the purification of ethylene.

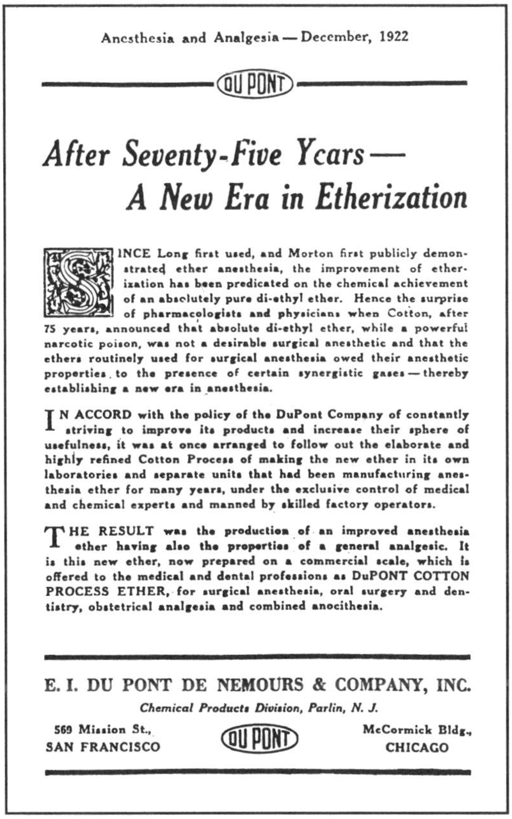
Anesthesia and Analgesia — December, 1922

DU PONT

After Seventy-Five Years —
A New Era in Etherization

SINCE Long first used, and Morton first publicly demonstrated ether anesthesia, the improvement of etherization has been predicated on the chemical achievement of an absolutely pure di-ethyl ether. Hence the surprise of pharmacologists and physicians when Cotton, after 75 years, announced that absolute di-ethyl ether, while a powerful narcotic poison, was not a desirable surgical anesthetic and that the ethers routinely used for surgical anesthesia owed their anesthetic properties to the presence of certain synergistic gases — thereby establishing a new era in anesthesia.

IN ACCORD with the policy of the DuPont Company of constantly striving to improve its products and increase their sphere of usefulness, it was at once arranged to follow out the elaborate and highly refined Cotton Process of making the new ether in its own laboratories and separate units that had been manufacturing anesthesia ether for many years, under the exclusive control of medical and chemical experts and manned by skilled factory operators.

THE RESULT was the production of an improved anesthesia ether having also the properties of a general analgesic. It is this new ether, now prepared on a commercial scale, which is offered to the medical and dental professions as DuPONT COTTON PROCESS ETHER, for surgical anesthesia, oral surgery and dentistry, obstetrical analgesia and combined anocithesia.

E. I. DU PONT DE NEMOURS & COMPANY, INC.
Chemical Products Division, Parlin, N. J.
569 Mission St., SAN FRANCISCO — DU PONT — McCormick Bldg., CHICAGO

Fig. 4. A 1922 DuPont advertisement of Cotton Process Ether.

His excuse for not offering technical details in 1917-1919 with his clinical reports, was "war work." Cotton Process Ethylene was manufactured by the Cheney Chemical Company of Cleveland.[23] A 1926 advertisement in *Anesthesia & Analgesic* was headed "Cheney Perfected Ethylene," Cotton's name was not mentioned (Fig. 5).

Dr. Cotton was elected a member of the Associated Anesthetists of the United States and Canada in 1925. Other Canadian members that year were: Executive Committee: Edith McKay Ross, Winnipeg; Advisory council: Charles La Rocque, Montreal and H.H. Shields, Toronto; Council on Teaching and Hospital Service: William Webster, Winnipeg,and W. Easson Brown, Toronto. The associated anesthetists were the "parent" of the International Anesthesia Research Society (I.A.R.S.).

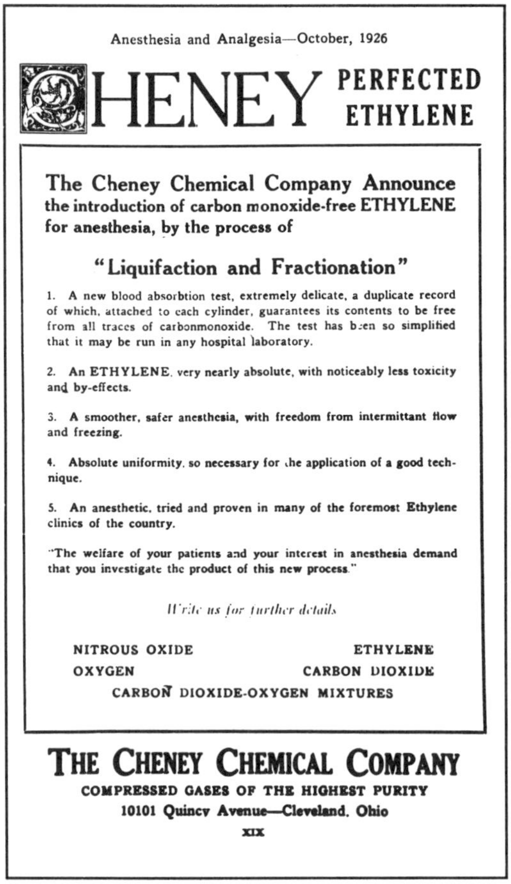

Fig. 5. The Cheney Chemical Company was incorporated in 1924 (or 1925) and had a capitalization of $15,000 ($75,000 reported in 1927). Merle B. Cheney was the President and Treasurer, Morris S. Cheney Vice-President, and Ray T. Miller, Secretary. In 1929, the company's address changed to 2929 E. 67th Street (Cleveland). Morris moved to New York City in 1931, Merle in 1936, but the company address remained in Cleveland. If Cheney used Cotton's method in the manufacture of his ethylene, it is not noted in the advertisement. It is not known how much money the Cheney Co. gave the IARS for the Cheney Fund, nor the fate of the money.

The James H. Cotton Fund

At the 1925 (First Annual) Meeting of the Eastern Society of Anesthetists in New York City, Dr. F.H. McMechan, the Secretary General of the Associated Anesthetists of the United States and Canada, announced the establishment of the International Anesthesia Research Foundation. Dr. Cotton "...placed all patents and processes covering his years of research work in trust to the I.A.R.S..." "...royalties could be used in establishing the James H. Cotton Fund..."[24,25] Mr. Cheney, the Cleveland chemist, also gave his patents and processes in trust. The Cotton Fund is mentioned in Toronto newspaper articles about J.H.C. and in his obituary. Attempts to obtain information about the Fund have been futile. There is a void in the I.A.R.S. archives prior to 1930. It is thought "...most of Dr. McMechan's original documentation was moved with Mrs. McMechan to California many years ago"[26] It is hoped information concerning the location of these records will surface.

In the editorial, Dr. McMechan,[24,25] wrote: "It will be recalled that Dr. James H. Cotton of Toronto, Canada, re-introduced ethylene into the field of anesthesia in 1917, before meetings of the Canadian Medical Association and the Interstate Anesthetists." The term "re-introduced" was in deference to the reports of Nunneley and others (Ref. 22, -p 79). The 1917 Canadian meeting article is Reference 1; the Interstate Anesthetists meeting was 1918, not 1917, (Ref. 9). The initials "McM" follow one of the editorials,[25] the other[24] is unsigned but almost identical. With Dr. McMechan's credit to him in print, Dr. Cotton probably felt justified in listing himself as the modern discoverer of ethylene. This action probably did not endear J.H.C. to colleagues in Toronto where W. Easson Brown was granted this honor.

Pure Ether Does Produce Anesthesia

Stehle and Bourne of Montreal (site of Cotton's 1917 demonstration) proved pure ether is an anesthetic.[3] In London, Dale, Hadfield and King did the same.[20] Hadfield was one of Hewer's seniors at St. Bartholomew's Hospital. Professor W. Storm van Leeuwen of Leyden, Holland, also proved "purest ether" had narcotic action.[27] A more complete review of this subject is included in the essay on Christopher Langton Hewer and Ethanesal (page 388, this volume). The research groups each used different chemical methods for the production of their pure ether. These exacting reports in 1922, 1923, and 1924, sealed the coffins of C.P.E. and Ethanesal.

The A.M.A. and C.P.E.

The JAMA carried the note: "About January 20, 1920, the 'News Service' of the "E.I. DuPont De Nemours and Co., Inc. circularized the press of the country with what it was pleased to term a 'good filler.'"[28] The JAMA note contained J.H.C.'s name, reported lack of specific data on the composition of C.P.E., and lack of corroboration of results of its use. The last paragraph of the note warned, ". . .use of a therapeutic agent of unknown composition is unscientific. . ." ". . .it is many times more serious for a physician to employ a secret or semi-secret substance as an anesthetic. A physician using such a semi-secret substance would have little defense if the patient should die."

Three months later an even shorter note appeared in the JAMA.[29] The DuPont Company had decided to present Cotton Process Ether to the Council on Pharmacy and Chemistry of the American Medical Association (AMA) for "consideration." C.P.E. was defined as" "An improved anesthesia ether consisting of highly refined diethyl oxid ($(C_2H_5)_2O$), plus approximately two volumes of ethylene (C_2H_4), 1/2 volume of carbon dioxide (CO_2), and 1 percent by weight of ethyl alcohol." Ethyl alcohol was added to anesthetic ethers to reduce frosting when used on "open drop" masks.

The two short reports noted above were reprinted in a 1922 AMA publication.[29] In 1923, the JAMA carried a full page article on the "So-Called Improved Ethers." Cotton and C.P.E., Hewer and Ethanesal, were both politely ridiculed. H.E.G. Boyle's addresses in America, such as the one at Niagara Falls,[14] were noted without comment, other than reference to the work of Stehle and Bourne,[3] and Dale, Hadfield and King.[20] The subtitle of the article was: "Claim that Pure Ether Has No Anesthetic Properties, Without Foundation." The last clause of the article was: ". . .the theory of ether anesthesia is still unchanged."[30] Cotton Process Ether was dead.

James Henry Cotton — Biographical Information

J.H. Cotton, Sr. was born at Garafaxa, Ontario, July 20, 1849. He graduated from the University of Toronto in 1874, went to Edinburgh and gained a medical degree in 1876, then later took graduate training in New York City. J.H.C., Sr was reported, in Toronto Newspaper obituaries, to have been a founder of both Western Hospital and Grace Hospital. He was active on the staffs of both hospital and obituaries noted him as "One of the best known surgeons in Canada." He retired about 1915 because of failing health, and died suddenly of "heart failure" on January 9, 1917. His widow, Anne Maude Christopher Cotton, died September 23, 1922. J.H.C., Jr. was born in 1891. When J.H.C., Jr. died, the newspapers did not feature extensive obituaries (or I failed to find them), therefore exact date of birth was not identified. J.H.C., Jr. had two sisters, Mrs. Arthur W. Treble, of Hamilton, and Marguerite S., who married Clifford Marshall, December 29, 1926. The baptismal name of Mrs. Treble is not known, nor the age of either sister. J.H.C., Sr. would have been 41 or 42 when J.H.C., Jr. was born, Marguerite may have been in her thirties when she married. The Treble and Marshall families are still being traced.

J.H.C., Jr. attended Harbord Collegiate (so did W. Easson Brown), was A.B. University of Toronto, 1912, M.A. 1914, M.B. 1915 (Brown was 1916) and M.D. 1916. The title of his Master's thesis was, "Multiple Astatic Rectangular-Field Galvanometers;" of his M.D. thesis, "The Chemistry of Ether and its Numerous Impurities Relative to Anaesthesia." It is hoped a copy of the 1916 thesis can be obtained for review.

J.H.C., Jr. married Ruby Long, of Toronto, January 25, 1919. She was born in Bond Head, Simcoe County, Ontario. Miss Long was a coloratura soprano (stage name, Mlle. Audrie Rubanni). They were married by Rev. Dr. James A. Long (it is not known if he was a relative). The couple took a wedding tour to Washington, D.C., Baltimore, New York, Philadelphia and Atlantic City. The couple were said to have met at a military hospital; Mlle. was entertaining after a cross continent tour, J.H.C., Jr. was doing medical work.

After medical qualification in 1915, J.H.C., Jr. worked as an anesthetist at Toronto General Hospital. He used his improved ether, with success, on a young girl with extensive burns. His demonstrations at the Academy of Medicine and the Royal Victoria Hospital in 1917 are reported above. Three Toronto newspapers (Star, Globe and Telegram) carried articles about J.H.C. and C.P.E. on January 27, 1920. DuPont is mentioned and the date would fit the American Medical Association report. (See section: The AMA and C.P.E.)

The Toronto Star for May 5, 1921, reported J.H.C. had addressed the Ontario Dental Association. On May 10, the Star reported C.P.E. had a "truth telling" effect; people could not tell lies during C.P.E. analgesia. The demonstration of 1920 in Albany[12] was detailed and C.P.E. was termed "ethylene-ether."

In 1923, the character of the stories changed. Luckhardt had reported on the use of ethylene in Chicago,[4] and Easson Brown had reported from Toronto.[5] Articles now appeared in Toronto newspapers supporting Cotton's claim for credit for the introduction of ethylene anesthesia. Cotton had champions, and an attempt was made to obtain a Provincial reward. Banting was voted $10,000 for his work on insulin; the same amount was requested for Cotton. The grant was to be from the Provincial government, not the Canadian Confederation. To add spice to the stew, Cotton pointed out that Toronto General Hospital (TGH, University of Toronto) used Franco-American ether, and that Mr. Macdonald, the hospital chemist, was the Franco-American representative and distributor. Mr Samuel Johnston, chief anesthetist at TGH, claimed Franco-American was chosen after blinded samples of different ethers were tested. A long article in The Star, Mary 5, 1923, noted the work of Wesley Bounce on pure ether,[3] and that Easson Brown had employed pure ethylene,[5] while Cotton used ethylene suspended in ether. A May 12 article quoted Dr. W.D. Howell, chief anesthetist of the Royal Victoria Hospital (Bourne's hospital) that was complimentary to Cotton.

In 1925, with the advent of the Cotton Fund of the IARS, J.H.C. was again in the news. The August 26, 1925, Telegram carried pictures of him "then" (four years of age) and "now." J.H.C. was interviewed about the germ that causes cancer; J.H.C. said credit should be given to Dr. Glover of Toronto, now working in New York City, for this discovery.

Cotton's name was found in medical articles in the Toronto Glove, Mail, and Telegram for 1925,1926 and 1927. His endeavors were linked to other medical stores. It was reported he had refused $135/day or $150/day to go to the Untied States and work for a private company — the rights for C.P.E. were not for sale, but for mankind.

With 1927 came new articles. J.H.C. was the Grand 1*st* Vice President of the Native Sons of Canada and his talks received newspaper coverage. He was again consulted by a newspaper re: use of serum made from blood of a recovered infantile paralysis patient. J.H.C. pointed out that by the stage of disease when infantile paralysis is recognized (and the serum given), "the damage has been done." He recommended ". . .keeping the surrounding muscles fit until the nerve can grow again."

In 1928, Cotton became President of the Native Sons and he spoke out "Against Unrestricted Entry of Settlers." The immigrants were to come from Great Britain, *no* thought of immigrants from other countries, and be settled "on the land." J.H.C. feared the immigrants would drift to the cities and drive Canadian born to the United States for employment.

In the 1920's, J.H.C. had reported sleeping on one's back could cause diabetes, in the 1930's that cancer could be treated with sodium phosphate. He also attacked the appointment system at the University of Toronto Medical School (UT). Local hospitals had become UT-affiliated and Cotton claimed older clinicians, often those who had worked with the founders of the hospital, had been forced out and been replaced by UT appointees. He also alleged the appointments were made based upon family or social connections. One wonders if J.H.C. was forced out of Western or Grace (or another) hospital. In 1925 he moved from Toronto to Willowdale, a Toronto suburb.

Cotton also called for keeping statistics on all operations performed by Toronto surgeons to reduce unnecessary surgery and weed out the incompetent (in 1992 this idea was put forth by Dr. C.E. Koop, former Surgeon General of the United States).

J.H.C. felt farmers often had poor diets, that bad teeth caused systemic disease, carbon monoxide from smoking was injurous (true), that relief payments to physicians (Canadian version of Medicaid) were not sufficient to cover expenses, that a specific murder conviction was in error, careless tuberculosis testing of cattle by some veterinarians caused needless killing of cattle, and other topics I have omitted or missed. The newspapers found J.H.C. a ready talker.

In 1936, J.H.C. resigned from The Native Sons because he felt they were distributing anti-British Empire literature.

During these years Mrs. Cotton was not idle. She was a candidate for the "Board of control," Toronto, 1931. She had made here debut in Steinway Hall, New York (but the report was not clear as to date). She felt "domestics" should eat the same food as the lady of the house, and ". . .have stipulated hours of work just as should a business girl." For a successful marriage, there must be "mutual interests." "If a man goes out duck-hunting, his wife should go too." She criticized Canadian men for looking upon women as inferior. J.H.C. was a good partner for his wife. He stated, "You cannot base marriage on sentiment. That is evanescent. If two people are trained to respect one another, they could get along, even without sentiment, more happily than 90 percent of the people now married." (Star, September 29, 1934).

In 1934, Mrs. Cotton caused "fireworks" at the Ward Four Women's Liberal-Conservative Association. The Toronto Mail for July 14, 1934, devoted thirteen column inches of type to the vituperating of Mrs. Cotton and officers of the association. Mrs. Cotton's tongue was obviously good for more than soprano singing.

On August 25, 1937, the Toronto Globe carried the story of the Cotton horseback trip. Mrs. Cotton had great empathy for the cabin dwellers they met in the woods. She reported, ". . .the plight of old folks who, unable to afford an automobile and afraid to travel the highways by buggy because of the fast traffic. . . were obliged to stay home from even the nearest village." Others met were poor people, perhaps a wounded ex-serviceman and wife, making do with what they raised and the little they earned.

It is not known when J.H.C. stopped practice, or the type of practice he had. He and his wife were obviously intelligent, gifted people. Unfortunately, he was not capable of accepting his error about pure ether and the fact that he had "missed the boat" on ethylene. Caesar recognized this personality defect:

libenter homines id quod volunt credunt.
Men freely believe that which they desire
—*Caesar De bello gallico; Book II*: 18:6

References

1a. Cotton JH: Anaesthesia from commercial ether — administration and what it is due to. Can Med Assoc; 7:769-77, 1917.

1b. Editorial. Doctor Cotton's paper on the causation of ether anaesthesia. ibid pages 825-6.

2. Obituary, Toronto World, January 10, 1917.
3. Stehle RL, Bourne W: The anesthetic properties of pure ether. JAMA; 79:375-6, 1922.
4. Stetson JB: Arno Benedict Luckhardt and the introduction of ethylene. The History of Anaesthesia. Ed: Atkinson RS, Boulton TB, Royal Society of Medicine, International Congress and Symposium Series, Number 134, pp 595-601.
5. Brown WE: Preliminary report: Experiments with ethylene as a general anaesthetic. Can Med Assoc J; 13:210, 1923.
6. Anon. Toronto Globe, April 25, 1923.
7. Obituary, Can Med Assoc J; 68: 184, 1953.
8. Symposium on Anesthesia in War Surgery, JAMA; 71:1606-7, 1918.
9. Cotton JH: Cotton Process Ether and Ether Analgesia. Am J Surg, Anesthesia Supplement; 33:34-43, 1919.

10. Anon. The New Ether. DuPont Magazine, December, 1919, pp 13-15.
11. Lumbard JE: Remarks on Cotton Process Ether from personal experience and the reports of other observers. Am J Surg, Anesthesia Supplement; 34:118-21, 1920.
12. Cotton J: Cotton process ether for dental operations. Dental Cosmos, January, 1921.
13. Artusio JF: Di-ethyl ether analgesia: a detailed description of the first state of ether anesthesia in man. J Pharmacol Exper Ther; 3:343-8, 1954.
14. Boyle HEG: Gas-oxygen-ethanesal chloroform combined anesthesia for nose and throat and abdominal surgery. Am J Surg, Anesthesia Supplement; 36:17-21, 1922.
15. Cassidy P: Experimental and Clinical Observation on Cotton Process Ether. Anesth Analg 1:10-2, 1922.
16. Cassidy P: Experimental and Clinical Observations on Cotton Process Ether. Am J Surg, Anesthesia Supplement; 36:73-5, 1922.
17. Webster W: Some new anaesthetic ethers. Can Med Assoc J; 12(n.s.):15-6, 1933.
18. Webster W: Some new anesthetic ethers. Am J Surg, Anesthesia Supplement, 36:71-3, 1922.
19. Webster W: The Science and Art of Anesthesia. St. Louis C.V. Mosby, 1924, pp 81-84.
20. Dale HH, Hadfield CF, King H: The anaesthetic action of pure ether. Lancet, i:424-9, 1923.
21. McLean CC: Scope and utility of Cotton Process Ether. Anesth Analg; 2:88-90, 1923.
22. Cotton JH: Some technicalities of research dealing with the purification of ether and the introduction of pure ethylene into the anesthetic field in 1917. Anesth Analg; 4:51-60, 1925.
23. Cheney MB, Michalske AI: Further purification of nitrous oxide by finely divided metals. II The manufacture of Cotton Process Ethylene. Anesth Analg; 4:252-6, 1925.
24. International Anesthesia Research Foundation. Anesth Analg; 4:p 2, p 60.
25. McM. International Anesthesia Research Foundation. Am J Surg, Anesthesia Supplement; 39:29, 1925.
26. Maggiore AF: Letter dated November 20, 1991.
27. van Leeuwen WS: On the narcotic action for the purest ether. Proceedings of the Royal Society of Medicine, Section of Anaesthetics; 17:17-33, 1924.
28. Queries and Minor Notes. "The New DuPont Ether." JAMA; 74:544, 1920.
29. Anon. The Propaganda For Reform in Proprietary Medicines. Vol. 2, p 421-422, Chicago, Press of American Medical Association, 1922.
30. Anon. So Called "Improved" Ethers. JAMA; 81:1040, 1923.

THE FIRST SUCCESSFUL OPEN-HEART PROCEDURE DONE WITH THE HEART-LUNG EXTRACORPOREAL PUMP

ARTHUR B. TARROW

This procedure became of interest when I reported to Thomas Jefferson University as Professor Anesthesiology in 1970, after serving in the U.S. Air Force for 27 years. I found cardiac surgery in full bloom. I knew that Thomas Jefferson University had been one of the pioneers in heart surgery and that the first successful heart procedure employing the extracorporeal pump had been done there. I also realized that, if I were to be accepted as an erudite professor, I would have to master this procedure.

Besides working in the cardiac operating rooms on actual patients, I began a study of the background of cardiac surgery in order to accumulate lecture material. To my surprise, there were no records of the original or other early procedures in the Medical Records Library. When I discussed this with the cardiac surgeons, they were evasive. After probing many sources unsuccessfully, it was suggested that I talk with Mrs. John T. Gibbon, whose husband had been the surgeon who had completed the first successful procedure. She lived on a farm near Philadelphia. Unfortunately, Dr. John T. Gibbon had died so that I could not speak with him. I met with Mrs. Gibbon, who told me about her life with Dr. Gibbon and about his work.

Dr. John T. Gibbon Jr.'s father had been the Professor of Surgery at Thomas Jefferson University. John Jr., after receiving his medical degree and interning, had chosen surgery as his specialty. He obtained a position as a "Fellow" with Dr. Edward Churchill at Harvard in 1929. After the death of a patient from a massive pulmonary embolism, he began to experiment with several types of machines which could be used to bypass the heart and lungs. He tried all kinds of oxygenators which had evolved from the experiments of many scientists, which will be mentioned in the next portion of this paper. Dr. Gibbon was not successful, and all of his mentors suggested that he work in more lucrative surgical fields to accumulate a better curriculum vitae so that he could go unto academic medicine. Dr. Gibbon persisted.

While in Boston, Dr. Gibbon met Mary Hutchinson, the socialite daughter of a famous portrait painter. Mary knew little about research, but she knew that she wanted to marry Dr. Gibbon. She volunteered to work in his laboratory. They were married soon after.

After a four-year period back in Philadelphia, where Dr. Gibbon practiced surgery and also did some experimental work at the University of Pennsylvania, he was granted another "Research Fellowship" at Harvard. He began in earnest to develop a successful extracorporeal pump. He devised a barrel which rotated as the blood was introduced. The blood filmed over the inner surface of the barrel and the oxygen was added to it. Beginning with cats, he progressed to larger animals and was able to maintain them for a reasonable time.

World War II interrupted Dr. Gibbon's experimental work. He served in the CBI for five years and returned to Jefferson. He became the first Professor of Experimental Surgery and Head of the Surgical Research Laboratory. This laboratory became world-famous, and Dr. Gibbon shared willingly all of his findings on extracorporeal circulation. The University of Minnesota and the Mayo Clinic were constantly in touch.

On May 6, 1953, Dr. Gibbon completed the first successful open heart procedure, employing a new pump-oxygenator with screens instead of bubbles, over which the blood filmed. An 18-year-old girl with a large interauricular septal defect had become almost moribund. Her parents allowed Dr. Gibbon to operate on her as a last resort. This procedure will be explained in detail.

Why, then, were there no records in the Medical Records Library? Mrs. Gibbon explained that Dr. Gibbon had become disenchanted with the politics of choosing his successor and had removed all his experimental and clinical records. They were in the attic of his farmhouse. I then began to realize why everyone had been so evasive. The old-timers were loyal to the memory of Dr. Gibbon. Several of the group had been left out in the political conflicts.

After considerable search, Mrs. Gibbon and I found the original record of this world-renowned event. Mrs. Gibbon agreed to bring this record to Thomas Jefferson University. At the request of the President, I arranged a luncheon at the Faculty Club. After lunch and the presentation, Mrs. Gibbon allowed the president's secretary to make two copies of this record — one for the archives and one for me. She retained the original for a book she planned to write.

THE HISTORY OF ANESTHESIA AT THE NEW YORK HOSPITAL
Cornell Medical Center

ALAN VAN POZNAK and ADELE A. LERNER
The New York Hospital/Cornell Medical Center
New York, New York
USA

Chartered in 1771 during the reign of King George III of England, The New York Hospital is the second oldest hospital in the United States (Figs. 1,2). Medical case records extend continuously from 1808 to present; thus it is possible to read descriptions of surgery performed on unanesthetized patients prior to the first public demonstration of ether anesthesia in Boston on October 16, 1846. Although the Charter for the New York Hospital was granted in 1771, construction on the first building did not begin until the late 1780's. The first hospital building burned on the eve of completion and had to be rebuilt. It opened for patients on January 3, 1791, and was situated on Broadway opposite Pearl Street in lower Manhattan. One of the earliest extant pictures of the hospital, known as the Murray print, shows an engraving of an imposing stone building with a large front yard containing a few cows. A pump is visible on the edge of the sidewalk at the curb line. We have only engravings of the hospital since photography was not developed by Daguerre until 1839. Imagine what it must have been to conduct surgery in a hospital of this sort. There was no running water, lighting was poor, operations were carried out usually on the uppermost floor so that light could come through a skylight and also so that the patients' screams of agony would be less likely to be heard by passers-by in the street below.

Patients' charts as such did not exist at this time. Instead, case books were kept by the house officers. These case books were compiled at the end of the year from notes which had been kept by the house officer during his time of service to the institution. These books are quite legible and are divided into medical and surgical cases selected from the wards of The New York Hospital.

Surgeons of the day had to work with great speed since anesthesia had not been developed. The only remedies to control pain were alcohol, either in the form of brandy, rum or whiskey,

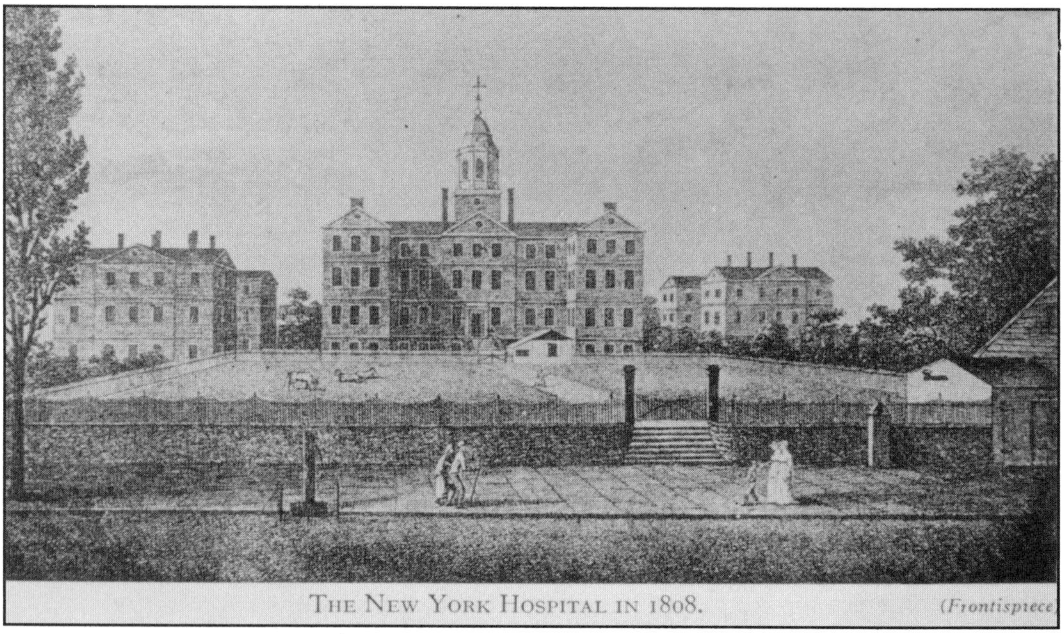

Fig. 1. The first building of the New York Hospital.

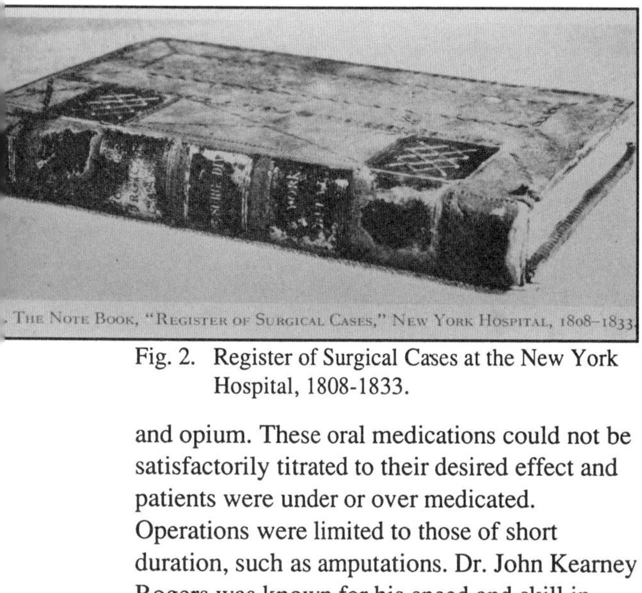

Fig. 2. Register of Surgical Cases at the New York Hospital, 1808-1833.

and opium. These oral medications could not be satisfactorily titrated to their desired effect and patients were under or over medicated. Operations were limited to those of short duration, such as amputations. Dr. John Kearney Rogers was known for his speed and skill in amputating a leg. He could complete an amputation in less than 90 seconds as measured by an observer's watch. Early records from the hospital also attest to social conditions of the times; for example, a bill in our records indicates services rendered to a slave. Food and medical care for three days' costs were $1.31. Funeral expenses were $5. This bill was rendered in 1801.

October 16, 1846, the first public demonstration of ether anesthesia was given by Dr. William Thomas Green Morton in Boston, Massachusetts. Reports of this extraordinary event rapidly passed around the entire world. It would be interesting to know how the news about ether reached New York City. The first record of ether administration for anesthetic purposes at The New York Hospital is dated Dec. 4, 1846, approximately one and one-half months after the announcement of the administration of ether in Boston. This administration of ether at The New York Hospital was for the control of pain occasioned by the burning of a camphur moxa on the abdomen of a patient; it was successful for its intended purpose. Reports of the use of ether for surgical operations began to appear with increasing frequency after this time. In early 1847 there is a report of a leg amputation in which ether was administered and no pain experienced. Nevertheless, ether was not used routinely until many years later.

A very recent discovery from records in the medical archives of The New York Hospital/ Cornell Medical Center is that nitrous oxide was

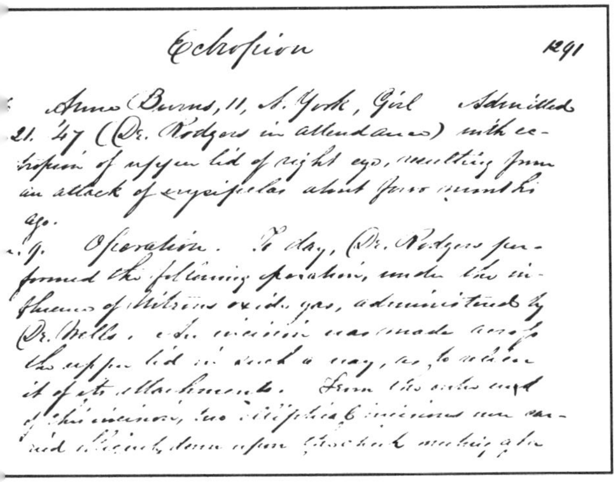
Ectropion 1291

Anna Burns, 11, N. York, Girl Admitted 21. '47 (Dr. Rodgers in attendance) with ectropion of upper lid of right eye, resulting from an attack of erysipelas about four months ago.

9. Operation. To day, Dr. Rodgers performed the following operation, under the influence of Nitrous oxide gas, administered by Dr. Wells. An incision was made across the upper lid in such a way, as to ... it of its attachments. From the extremities of this incision, two ... incisions were carried downward, down upon ...

Fig. 3. Record of administration of nitrous oxide by Horace Wells at the New York Hospital, January 9, 1848.

administered here by Horace Wells on Jan. 9, 1848 (Fig. 3), not many days before his suicide in the Tombs Prison on Jan. 23, 1848. The records speak of a patient named Anna Burns, a girl of 11 years of age from New York, who was "admitted on Dec. 21, 1847, with Dr. Rogers in attendance. She had an ectropion of her upper lid of her right eye which had resulted from an attack of erysipelas about 4 months previously. On Jan. 9 an operation was performed. Today Dr. Rogers performed the following operation under the influence of nitrous oxide gas administered by Dr. Wells."

I have searched the hospital records trying to find out how and under what conditions Dr. Wells was permitted on our staff. Thus far we have not been able to determine who it was who recommended him to administer anesthesia at The New York Hospital. His sad story is so well known that it needs little repetition. Following his failure to demonstrate adequate analgesia for extraction of a tooth in Boston in 1844, Horace Wells came to New York and set up dental practice at 120 Chambers Street in Manhattan. He had become increasingly addicted to the use of the substances which he used professionally. He had inhaled nitrous oxide many times without knowing the necessity for adding oxygen to it. He had also become addicted to the inhalation of chloroform vapor. About the middle of Jan. 1848, he formed a most unfortunate association with a young man who wanted sulfuric acid to throw on a young woman who had spurned his advances. Wells provided the sulfuric acid and a bottle from which to dispense it, and was in the company of the young man as he sprinkled the sulfuric acid on the young lady's clothing. Following this adventure, Wells returned to his room and inhaled chloroform until he felt greatly exhilarated by it. In this deranged state he went out to the street by himself and sprinkled sulfuric acid on women he saw walking on Broadway at night. He was arrested for this action and placed in the Tombs Prison. When it was learned who he was, he was permitted to return to his room in the company of a guard in order to secure certain personal effects. He brought back to his prison cell not only his razor and the knife but a bottle of chloroform. He subsequently wrote several suicide notes, inhaled the chloroform until he was intoxicated, and then with his straight razor laid open the flesh on his left thigh down to the bone, severing the femoral artery completely. He bled to death in his cell and was discovered by the guard some time later. He was 33 years old at the time and left a wife and a son aged 9 years. This tragic loss of a talented young man should be remembered forever by the practitioners of our profession as an example of the terrible dangers that follow upon the misuse of the very potent pharmacologic agents we are privileged to administer.

There are two letters in The New York Hospital Medical Archives concerning Dr. Morton's involvement in the Ether Controversy. One is written by New York Hospital surgeon Gurdon Buck, known for his contributions to urology, plastic surgery and treatment of fractures. In this letter dated July 3, 1858, Dr. Buck proposes the establishment of a fund for the welfare of Dr. Morton. The other letter is from attorneys representing Dr. Morton, pleading to the hospital as a beneficiary of the blessing of anesthesia for funds to help Dr. Morton in his impoverished state.

With the rapid advances in medicine during the 1800's, the old building quickly became outmoded and was superseded by a new building located uptown near 6th Ave. between west 15th and 16th streets. Completed in 1877, this building was six stories high and had not only gas and electric lighting, but elevators and a ventilation system which was intended to draw away the vile disease-laden air and replace it with fresh clean air. Running water and improved sanitation helped make this building a great advance over its predecessor. By the early part of the 20th century we also boasted an ambulance service, first horse-drawn and then driven by the internal combustion engine. Scenes in the operating room show the administration of open drop ether under bare electric bulb illumination (Fig. 4). Surgeons wore rubber gloves, caps and masks. The anesthetist did not wear a mask, nor did other observers in the operating room. Anesthesia administration was principally open drop ether by mask, although nitrous oxide as an inducing agent was also well known in the early part of the 20th century. Surgical speed was comparable to that which we see today.

It would be interesting to know under what conditions anesthesia was first given in the hospital and by whom. Early records state only that the vapor of sulfuric ether was administered. To what extent the anesthetist was part of the surgical staff, the nursing staff or other personnel is not known. We are in the process of tracing the beginning of anesthesia records at The New York Hospital and their evolution into their present form. Payment for the anesthetist is a subject of some interest. We have a letter dated Oct. 8, 1904, to the Executive Committee of The New York Hospital signed by six of our leading surgeons, as follows:

"Gentlemen: Since the opening of the private patient's building the feature of the administration of anesthetics in connection with the surgical operations has been assuming constantly increasing importance and we believe the time has come when the position of the anesthetist and his skill should receive proper recognition.

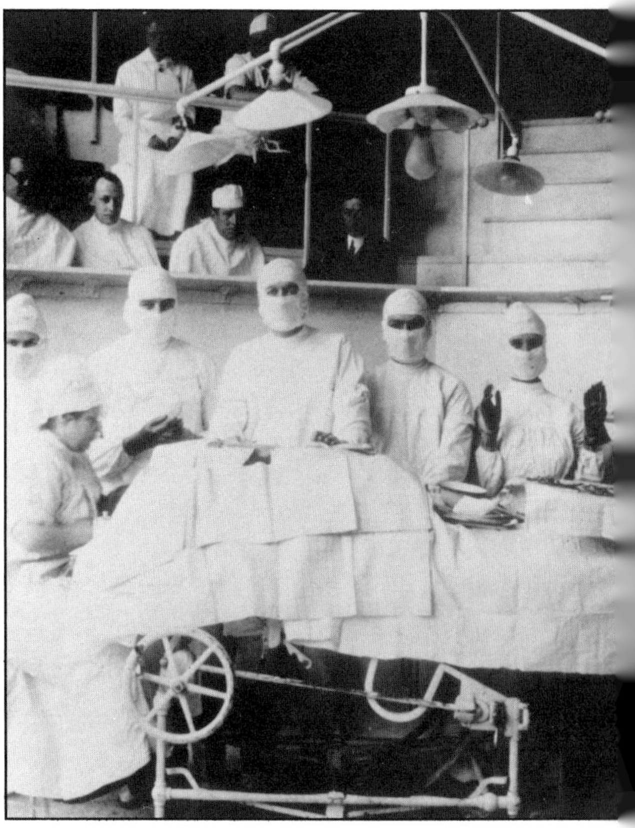

Fig. 4. Operating room of the New York Hospital, Dr. Mann, Anesthetist.

"Under existing circumstances his fee of $3 is paid by the hospital. We believe this is wholly inadequate in amount and not a proper charge upon the hospital and that in accordance with the custom generally prevailing in private operations a proper amount should be fixed upon and the fee paid by the patient as an essential part of the operating expenses. The service should be placed upon a similar level to the operation itself.

"Accordingly, we would suggest that the existing custom be discontinued that the minimum fee of the anesthetist be $10.

"And furthermore that the anesthetist render his account to the patient in the same manner as is now done in the case of the surgeon's fee.

"If this meets with your approval we would suggest that the date of Oct. 1, 1904 be fixed for it to be put in force. Signed Charles Mc Burney,

C.R. Bolton, Frank Hartley, Francis H. Markoe, Louis A. Stimson and Alexander V. Johnson."

In the time the second hospital building became inadequate and it was necessary to move further uptown to the present location at York Ave. and 68th Street. This building was begun in 1929 and opened for patients in 1932. It was originally intended to be a self-sufficient city of healing with its own power supply independent of the danger of electrical power failure in New York City.

Anesthesia in this new building was largely administered by a staff of nurse anesthetists. There were two staffs of anesthetists, one under the control of the chief of the department of surgery (Fig. 5) and the other under the control of the chief of the department of obstetrics and gynecology. These staffs were merged when Dr. Joseph Artusio became the first full-time chief of anesthesiology at The New York Hospital/ Cornell Medical Center. Much encouragement and protection of this new division was given by Dr. Frank Glenn, our former chief of surgery, to whom a great deal of credit is due for his wisdom and foresight in believing that anesthesiology should become a separate department, not only within the hospital but also within the medical college. Though this took years to accomplish, eventually both of these goals were realized.

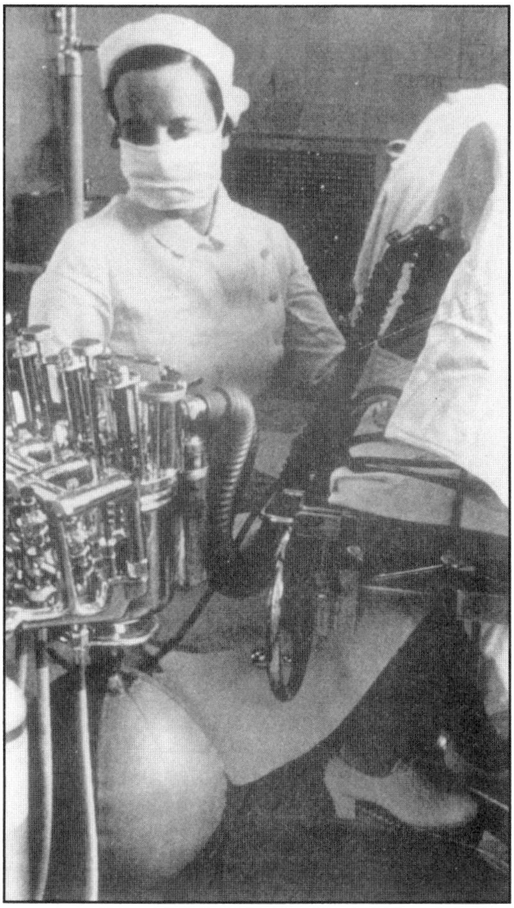

Fig. 5. Chief nurse anesthetist Ella Hediger, the New York Hospital, 1930's.

Other contributions to the advancement of anesthesiology made from this institution include the development of the neuromuscular block reversing agent, edrophonium, which was developed by Drs. Walter F. Riker, Joseph F. Artusio and Clarke Wescoe. Dr. Riker has also demonstrated pre-junctional effects of many facilitatory and blocking drugs of the neuromuscular junction. Dr. Artusio has demonstrated and redefined the first stage of ether analgesia and has clearly demonstrated that surgical operations can be performed in a partially conscious patient under diethyl ether analgesia. We have also been interested in the design and testing of non-flammable inhalation anesthetics, and from this were were able to perform clinical trials on the first non-flammable ether anesthetic, methoxyflurane. We have also attempted to produce anesthesia by electrical means and have helped in developing the concept of the metabolism of inhalation anesthetics.

Under the leadership of our new chairman, Dr. John Savarese, we hope to continue the progress in anesthesia which started in 1846. Dr. Savarese's interest in the development of new neuromuscular blocking drugs is an appropriate and happy extension of the many years of work which Dr. Walter Riker has done in our pharmacology and anesthesiology laboratories. We are proud that both Dr. Artusio and Dr. Riker, though emeritus, continue actively in our

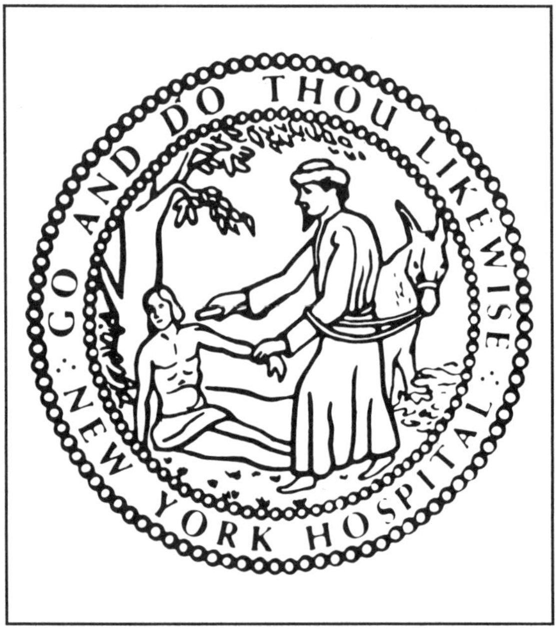

Fig. 6. The seal of The New York Hospital.

laboratories. We hope to continue our progress in the spirit of and under the sign of The New York Hospital, the seal of the Good Samaritan (Fig. 6) which ever urges us to "Go and do thou likewise."

Acknowledgement

We would like to express special thanks to Robert M. Sorlin, D.M.D., for generously providing a copy of *The Life and Letters of Horace Wells*.

BENJAMIN PERLEY POORE AND HIS HISTORICAL MATERIALS FOR A BIOGRAPHY OF W.T.G. MORTON, M.D.

LEROY D. VANDAM
Brigham and Women's Hospital
Harvard Medical School
Boston, Massachusetts, USA

Of all the claimants to the discovery of anesthesia, only one has been distinguished by an official biography, William Thomas Green Morton, who gave the first public demonstration on October 16, 1846, at Boston. As compiled by Nathan Payson Rice, the biography was instigated by a committee of New York City physicians who sought to aid Morton in his protracted efforts to procure monetary reward from the U.S. government.[1] At the suggestion of the committee, N.P. Rice M.D., Harvard Medical graduate, none too successful, New York City surgeon and a scrivener of sorts, was accepted by Morton, previously unknown to him, to produce the biography. The details of the arrangement as given by Rice were that on June 6, 1858, an agreement was drawn up between him and Morton, and that two days later he went to work at Morton's cottage in West Needham, Massachusetts. By dint of prodigious effort, while constantly under the critical eye of Morton, Rice completed the first portion of the work, delivered to Morton's hands on August 8, and by September the remainder was ready for Morton's approval, ultimately a volume of 460 pages, completed in three months.[2]

On closer analysis, however, Rice's accomplishment might not have been Herculean as it seemed, for he had as reference two bound volumes which form the gist of the biography: Statements Supported by Evidence of William T.G. Morton,M.D., on his claim to the Discovery of the Anaesthetic Properties of Ether: U.S. 30th Congress, 2nd Session, 1853;[3] and Benjamin Perley Poore's Historical Materials for a Biography of W.T.G. Morton M.D.[4] (Fig. 1)

"Materials" derived from a great mass of information previously gathered by Poore had

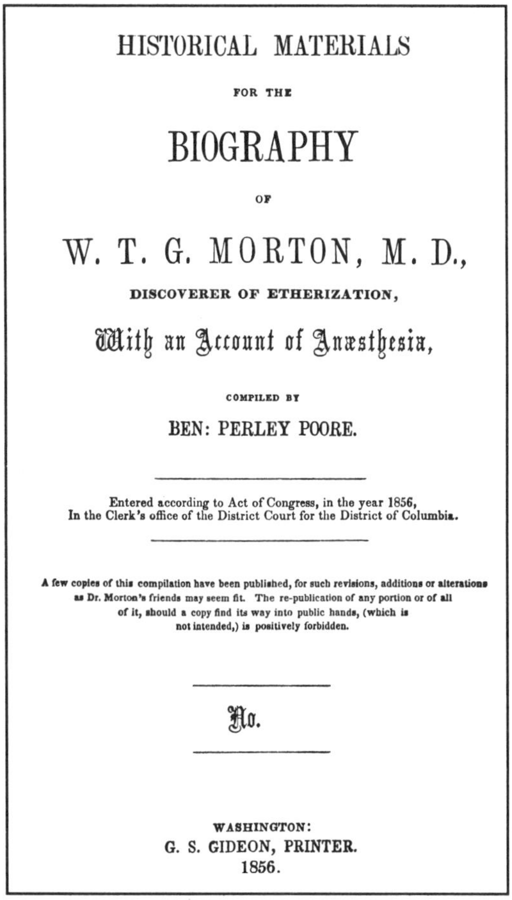
HISTORICAL MATERIALS

FOR THE

BIOGRAPHY

OF

W. T. G. MORTON, M. D.,

DISCOVERER OF ETHERIZATION,

With an Account of Anæsthesia,

COMPILED BY

BEN: PERLEY POORE.

Entered according to Act of Congress, in the year 1856,
In the Clerk's office of the District Court for the District of Columbia.

A few copies of this compilation have been published, for such revisions, additions or alterations as Dr. Morton's friends may seem fit. The re-publication of any portion or of all of it, should a copy find its way into public hands, (which is not intended,) is positively forbidden.

No.

WASHINGTON:
G. S. GIDEON, PRINTER.
1856.

Fig. 1. Benjamin Perley Poore's Historical Materials for a Biography of W.T.G. Morton, M.D.

already been printed in preliminary form in 1856, a work of 114 pages, issued interleaved, "A few copies of this compilation have been published for such revisions, additions or alterations as Dr. Morton's friends may seem fit." There was also a warning that, "The republication of any portion or of all of it, should a copy find its way into public hands (which is not intended), is positively forbidden." The few copies must indeed have been in Morton's possession, as no restrictions were placed on Rice in repeating large segments of Poore's commentary. There is a place for numbering the copies on the title page, but numbers are not found on the three copies extant: one in the Osler Library at McGill University, and two in the Boston Medical Library, Francis A. Countway Library of Medicine. G.S. Gideon was the printer in Washington, D.C. where Poore resided at the time, and copyright was issued in 1856, presumably to Poore, but no individual is designated. As an indication of affairs probably amiss between Morton and Poore, the latter does not mention the work in his two volume autobiography, "Perley's Reminiscences of Sixty Years in the National Metropolis," and "Materials" is not cited in the account on Poore in the Dictionary of American Biography. Why the interleaving on the alternate pages, a simple printing process? Probably Morton's idea, but a risky one in that he might have received many an unfavorable comment in the ongoing controversy at that time. There are no comments in the two copies reviewed by me.

Who was Poore and how did Morton make his acquaintance? A well-traveled New Englander, Poore in 1854 was the Washington correspondent for the Boston Journal, and a popular columnist writing under the sobriquet of Perley. On January 20, 1853, he had testified before the U.S. Congress about his knowledge, gathered while he was in Paris, of the ether demonstration and expressed sympathy for Morton, then under scurrilous attack by Charles T. Jackson. Thus, it was only natural that Morton should ask this seasoned writer to compile the official biography.

In spite of Perley's vast editorial experience, his effort seems careless in many spots. For example, he erred in giving Morton's birthplace as Charlton, Massachusetts and probably the wrong day of birth, the 9th rather than 19 August, 1819. Not only does he misspell Morton's mother's given name as Rebecca (it was Rebeckah), but he cites her maiden name as Needham, whereas it was Stevens. John Stevens was her father and I have the deed for the property on which the Morton house stood in Charlton. He also repeats the lie that Morton was a student in 1840 at the Baltimore College of Dentistry. He also misspells the name of George Hayward. No doubt some of the misinformation was the result of Morton's counsel.

However, there are two fascinating paragraphs in "Materials" which are not repeated in Rice, again suggestive of Morton's paranoia. A paragraph on page 7 states, "Another professional friend of Dr. Morton's, at this stage of his career (1830s) was Dr. Horace Wells, who had met him on a professional visit at Mr. James Morton's beautiful residence, years previous, when that gentleman was giving his son that intellectual training of which we have spoken. When young Morton returned to the North, the acquaintance was renewed, and it resulted in an association of their names for the practice of dental surgery in Boston (the capital of Dr. Morton's native state) where Dr. Wells had previously been professionally located, though he had since gone to Hartford." This is a fascinating comment because it sheds some light on Wells' early career. It has been assumed that he might have been tutored by one of the eminent Boston dentists in the 1830;s. Now it seems that he was then an itinerant dental practitioner.

Then on page 57 of "Materials" there's a note from J.Y. Simpson.

> Mr dear Sir: I have much pleasure in offering, for your kind acceptance, the accompanying pamphlet. Since it was published we have had various other operations performed here, equally successful. I have a note from Mr. Liston telling me also of its perfect success in London. Its rapidity and depth are amazing.
>
> In the monthly Journal of Medical Science for September, I have a long article on etherization, vindicating your claims over those of Jackson.
>
> Of course, the great thought is that of producing insensibility and for that the world, is, I think, indebted to you.
>
> I read a paper lately to our society, showing that it was recommended by Pliny, etc in old times.
>
> With very great esteem for you, allow me to subscribe myself,
>
> Yours very faithfully,
>
> Edinburgh, 19th Nov. 1847
>
> "J.Y. Simpson"

Why was there no further circulation of Perley's work? Possibly from Morton's biased viewpoint, Perley was too honest, not flattering enough, and too brief in the account. They might have had a falling out just as Morton and Rice would later part ways. Nevertheless, on June 18, 1864, eight years later, Ben Perley Poore wrote a friendly letter to Morton from Washington, D.C. concerning a proposition he'd had from Dr. Jackson, to share in any remuneration Morton might receive from Congress.

References

1. Viets HR: Nathan P. Rice and his Trials of a Public Benefactor, New York, 1859 Bull Hist Med; 20:232-43, 1946.
2. Rice NP: Trials of a Public Benefactor, as Illustrated in the Discovery of Etherization. New York: Pudney and Russell, 1859, pp 460.
3. U.S. — U.S. Congress, 2nd session. Statements supported by Evidence of WTG Morton, M.D., on the Claim to the Discovery of the Anaesthetic Properties of Ether. Washington, D.C., 1853, pp 582.
4. Historical Materials for the Biography of WTG Morton, M.D. Discoverer of Etherization, With an Account of Anaesthesia, compiled by Ben Perley Poore. Washington, D.C.: G.S. Gideon, Printer, pp 114, Interleaved.

THE ST. ELISABETH'S HOSPITAL IN STAD DELDEN, THE NETHERLANDS (1903-1963)
Anaesthetic Considerations

M. van WIJHE and L. QUAK

Introduction

Delden is a town in an area called Twente in the eastern Netherlands close to the German border. It had a population of 1940 people in 1900, growing to 3839 in 1951, and over 7000 today. The town serves as a center to the surrounding rural areas, with about as many inhabitants.

The St. Elisabeth Hospital was founded in 1903, at a time when the advantages of institutional medical care had become clear, and all the larger towns in the Netherlands had hospitals. Eight beds were enough initially, but by the time of closure in 1963 there were 92, including the separate tuberculosis ward.

In Delden, as in many smaller towns, the church took the initiative to found the local hospital in which "the sick and suffering" could be properly treated close to home. This was beneficial, especially for the poor who suffered from cramped living conditions and poverty in addition to their sickness.

Staff

Sisters of the Congregation of St. Joseph at Mersfoort managed the hospital. During its entire existence the sisters were the backbone of the organization. They worked very long hours; one long-retired sister tells of having fallen over during prayers once, overcome with sleep. Local staff cared for the building and terrain maintenance and the kitchen, and there were numerous local nurses aides.

The Roman Catholic denomination of the hospital did not play a role in patient selection or referral. Although the practices of the general practitioners were divided more or less along Protestant-Catholic lines, the hospital accepted everyone.

The local general practitioners had the day-to-day medical responsibility for the patients, obtaining a small fee (10 cents) per patient per day for the daily ward rounds. They also performed elective minor operations and attended emergency cases brought to the hospital. If necessary, a patient could be referred to a larger institution in nearby Hengelo (6 km).

There was no medical staff. A surgeon from Hengelo had an operating session in Delden on Monday and Tuesday mornings, returning later in the week to check on his patients and to see outpatients. Similarly, a gynecologist from Almelo (15 km away) treated and operated on patients in Delden. Both specialists had their main practice elsewhere. A radiologist came regularly, but other specialists rarely saw patients in Delden.

Patients

A number of admissions books and operating theater books are still available, giving an impression of the kind of pathology presenting and the surgery performed (1930-1963). For example, the admission diagnoses of patients in the year 1951 (total 383 patients) are listed in Table 1.

Operations were mainly minor procedures such as biopsies, abscess drainage, inserting nails for skeletal traction of fractures, removal of superficial tumors, corrective procedures on the extremities, appendectomy, all kinds of hernia and elective minor gynecologic procedures. Only rarely was major surgery performed; resection of bowel,[2] parotoid tumor,[1] meningomyelocele,[1] cesarean section.[3] These cases were either emergencies or unexpectedly complicated.

Separate from the hospital, a tuberculosis ward was opened in 1952 which served a much larger area; it was supervised by a chest physician from Almelo.

Anesthesia

In 1951, there were 185 operations, of which 129 were done using an ether inhalation anesthetic; of these, 90 received an inhalation ethyl chloride and 33 and intravenous Kemithal induction. A total of 38 patients had local infiltration anesthesia, 14 were done with Kemithal only, and 3 received no anesthetic at all.

The anesthetic was administered by a nurse. Her duties consisted of dispensing ether from a dropping bottle on to the gauze face mask (Julliard type) after induction with ethyl chloride, or "Doctor had injected something into the vein of the patient." Another nurse could take the pulse rate and measure the blood pressure if the surgeon so requested. The theater nurses were general nurses with no anesthetic training, but did have extensive practical experience.

From the available theater books the following highlights could be distilled: in the 1930's, ether, sometimes preceded by ethyl chloride, was the sole anesthetic used for adults; children sometimes received chloroform. Hexobarbital was first used for intravenous induction of anesthesia in April, 1948, Kemithal in September, 1950. By 1956 Kemithal was the most popular induction agent, always being used by the surgeon Boelens. The gynecologist Van der Loo preferred hexobarbital, even using it for such lengthy procedures such as portio amputation and uterine prolapse: 1000 to 2000 mg were given to such patients in the course of an operation; this practice was discontinued in 1959.

In March, 1959, a 30 year old woman died undergoing a D&C for abortion, three minutes after receiving hexobarbital, 1000 mg. Allegedly, she was rather anemic. The gynecologist operated on three other patients the next day, however, again using only hexobarbital (1000, 500 and 2000 mg doses).[1]

Similar problems recurred: cardiac arrest in a healthy patient undergoing a minor procedure on her foot; luckily she was successfully resuscitated (not recorded in the theater book, but clearly remembered by her retired G.P.).[2]

Reportedly, vomiting during the operation was not a problem.[3] Contraindications to anesthesia were "general poor condition" and the probability of a blood transfusion being necessary.

Each year between 120 and 180 patients were operated on, the procedures being basically the same as in 1951.

Discussion

St. Elisabeth's Hospital served the local community according to its statutory purpose, offering local hospital care to all in need of it.[4] The hospital's policy was to limit admission to those patients who could be handled; that this was successful is reflected by the municipal population registers. Elderly persons and neonates died in the municipality, whereas children died in Hengelo (presumably after timely referral), and young adults occasionally died of accidents elsewhere in the Netherlands.[5] The quality of care was never the subject of public concern.

The simple anesthetic techniques in use were common in small Dutch hospitals.[6] Amongst surgeons intravenous anesthesia with only hexobarbital had enthusiastic proponents.[7] In most hospitals just after the Second World War, there were no, or only a single, anesthetist, and the anesthetic was still the surgeon's territory. The availability of newer, better and safer techniques was becoming generally known, however, as well as the acceptance of anesthesiology as a new discipline.[8] More and more warnings appeared in the journals stressing the dangers of new intravenous anesthetic techniques in the hands of the unqualified.[9] As more anesthetists became available in the 1950's and 1960's, the surgeons gave up their responsibility for the anesthetic. It appears that there were some accidents in Delden too which can be attributed to the anesthetic.

The local population greatly appreciated hospital care close to home and had considerable difficulty accepting the impending closure of the institution in 1963. Many similar small country hospitals were closed at that time, due to opposition from the government medical inspectorate, on grounds of inadequate quality of care and the growing rivalry of larger institutions in nearby large towns which were better equipped and staffed. This situation also applied to Delden, where the absence of a specialist medical staff and the limited operative possibilities without a proper anesthetist were no longer acceptable to the licensing authority. In 1963 the hospital was closed and replaced by a nursing home.

In summary, we have described the nature of operating theater activities in a typical Dutch country hospital in the first half of this century. Inadequate quality of medical care in the changing times, especially concerning anesthetic care, led to its closure.

References

1. Theater and admission books, St. Elisabeth's Hospital, Delden.
2. van Beusekom W: Personal communication.
3. Sr. Serafina: Personal communication.
4. Anonymous. Zilveren Jubileum van het R. K. Ziekenhuis "St. Elisabeth" te Delden. Nieuwe Hengelose Courant, 21 Nov. 1928.
5. Gemeente archief Stad Delden.
6. de Zwaan J: Moderne Narcose. Keesings Medisch Archief; 1783-5, 1791-3, 1947.
7. Stuyt CLM: Narcose met Hexobarbiton. Ned Tijdschr Geneeskd; 93 IV: 3440-2, 1949.
8. Nierstrasz JL: Moderne Narcose. Ned Tijdschr Geneeskd; 96 IV: 2955-9 & 97 II: 1548-52, 1953.
9. Wolff JDP: Gevaar van intraveneuze narcotica. Ned Tijdschr Geneeskd; 98 I: 729, 1954.

VIDEOTAPED INTERVIEW OF HERR OBERINGENIEUR JOSEF HAUPT AND PROF. LESLIE RENDELL-BAKER On October 7 and 8, 1990

CARL F. WALLROTH
Drägerwerk AG, Lübeck, Germany

On October 7 and 8, 1990 Professor Leslie Rendell-Baker met with Oberingenieur Josef Haupt at the "historical corner" of the exhibition hall of the Drägerwerk AG in Lübeck, Germany. Herr Haupt had been the chief design engineer from 1936 through 1979 for Dräger anaesthesia equipment and knew Professor Rendell-Baker for more than a decade from international standard development meetings.

The author used the opportunity to interview these two pioneers who left their fingerprints in the design and standardization of safety features for anaesthesia equipment. The interview was performed in front of historical and modern equipment, which both gentlemen used to demonstrate the evolutionary design development process of anaesthesia equipment from the turn of the century through 1990, to reflect on their international standard development efforts and on their lives.

The idea of the interview was presented to the author by Professor Rod Calverley of San Diego during an earlier visit to Lübeck and to the "historical corner" and is based on the Wood Library "living history of anaesthesiology" series.

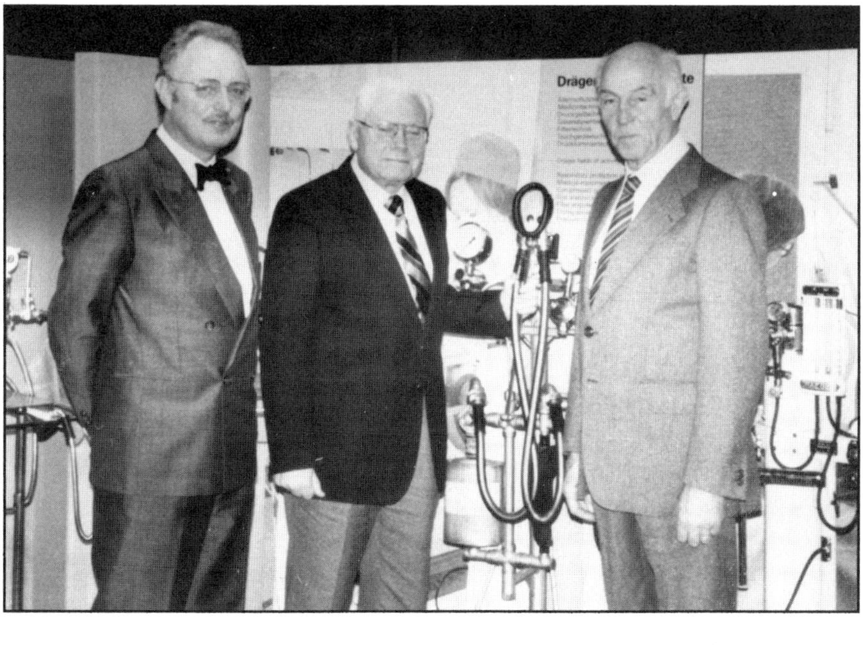

Fig. 1.
Far left, Dr. Ing. Carl F. Wallroth, born 1941, July 12.
Middle, Prof. Leslie Rendell-Baker, M.D., born 1917, March 27.
Left, Herr Oberingenieur Josef Haupt, born 1914, July 8.

THE DECADE OF THE 1840'S IN GEORGIA

JUDSON WARD
929 Vistavia Circle, Decatur, Georgia, USA

Crawford W. Long practiced medicine in Jefferson, Georgia, from 1841 until 1850 when he moved to Athens. This was a decade of significant development as Georgia came to be known as the Empire State of the South.

The Indian question having been settled by the removal of the Cherokees in 1838, land hungry settlers quickly moved into the northwestern corner of the state. Cotton was the principal product of the rich Piedmont plateau cultivated largely by slave labor; but textile mills began to make their first appearance in a few Georgia towns. At the same time, a railroad system, centered in the village of Atlanta, provided outlets for cotton on the Eastern seaboard, and profitable connections with Kentucky and Tennessee via Chattanooga.

The politics the early political factions allied themselves with the national Democratic and Whig parties, giving Georgia two distinct parties. Although the Democrats dominated, the Whigs won the governorship and the majority in both houses of the state legislature in 1843; and they established a State Supreme Court in 1845.

Savannah continued to be the only large city, but Augusta, Athens, Milledgeville (the capital), Macon and Columbus located along the fall line began to grow. Lively newspapers were published, and a merchant class began to emerge.

Efforts to establish a system of public schools failed, but higher education was available at the University of Georgia, where Long graduated, and at the newly founded denominational colleges of Oglethorpe, Emory Wesleyan, and Mercer. The Baptist and Methodist preachers won many converts and thus their denominations dominated religious life.

Material prosperity characterized the economy as population increased, but illiteracy was widespread, and Georgia's contributions to literature, drama, art and music were minimal as was characteristic of the predominantly rural life of most of the nation.

Crawford Long lived and practiced his profession in the rapidly developing Piedmont section of middle Georgia which dominated Georgia politically, financially and culturally during the decades prior to the Civil War. Acquaintance with the major developments of this period should give added insight into the life and labors of Dr. Long.

THE INTRODUCTION OF A MOBILE RESUSCITATION SERVICE — 1918

ROD WESTHORPE
Honorary Curator, Geoffrey Kaye Museum of Anaesthetic History, Melbourne, Australia

The treatment of severely wounded soldiers has posed a problem for military doctors since they were first recruited to the battlefield as barber-surgeons in the 14th century. Napoleon's chief surgeon, Baron Dominique Larrey, was the first to introduce a retrieval system, moving wounded soldiers away from the battlefront by horse-drawn cart, so beginning the first established ambulance service. The concept had been introduced on an occasional basis as early as 1487 during the siege of Malaga by Ferdinand, King of Aragon.[1,2]

By the time of the First World War, a so-called "classic" system of evacuation of wounded had been developed. Wounded were provided with basic first-aid at an Advanced Dressing Station, having been carried there by fellows or stretcher bearers. They were then transported by stretcher or ambulance to the Main Dressing Station and on to the Casualty Clearing Station, where there were facilities for surgery, anesthesia and transfusion. After definitive treatment, soldiers were then sent by road or train to the Base Hospital.

As weaponry and ballistics became more advanced and destructive, so the distances travelled by the severely wounded began to play a greater role in determining mortality. This problem was compounded by the reduced mobility of the Casualty Clearing Stations as the war progressed. The distance from the battlefront to the Casualty Clearing Station, by the end of World War I, was often 25 to 35 kilometers. It was frequently 4 to 6 hours before the wounded arrived at the Main Dressing Station, and 2 to 3 hours more before casualties arrived at the Casualty Clearing Station.[3,4]

The Director of Medical Services of the Australian Imperial Forces, Major Neville Howse, estimated in 1918 that, of all the wounded arriving at Casualty Clearing Stations, 85 percent had suffered no appreciable hardship from their journey, 10 percent arrived in recoverable shock, and the remaining 5 percent were so shocked that their condition was "hopeless."[3]

A survey of 79 "non-transportable" cases in 1917, reported by the U.S. Army Medical Department,[3] revealed the following relationship:

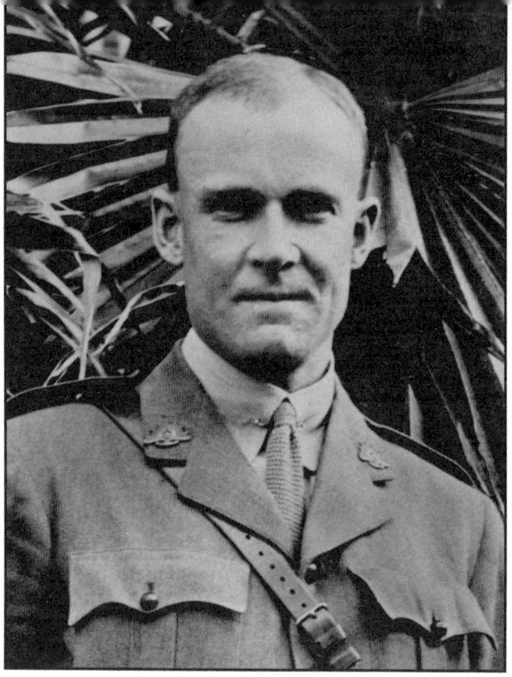

Fig. 1. Dr. A.W. Holmes á Court

Time between injury and treatment	**Mortality**
less than 3 hours	11 percent
3 to 6 hours	37 percent
8 to 10 hours	75 percent

In May 1917, in Paris, an Interallied Congress of Surgeons was held and M. Duval, one of the leading French Military surgeons of the time, proclaimed, "It is impossible that the wounded man should go in search of a surgeon; it follows then that the surgeon must betake himself to the wounded man."[3]

It was a young Australian doctor who took up this idea and instituted what was probably the first established mobile resuscitation service. Having graduated in Sydney in 1911, Dr. Alan W. Holmes á Court joined the Australian Army Medical Corps in 1916 at the age of 29 (Fig. 1). By January 1918, he had been promoted to Major and was attached to the 4th Australian Field Ambulance on the Western Front in France.[5,6,7]

Major Holmes á Court had undoubtedly seen and experienced the developments in treatment of shocked and wounded soldiers which had occurred by this stage of the war. Throughout the First World War, warmth and rest were considered of primary importance in the treatment of shock, and morphia was often available as an adjunct. Intravenous infusions were used, saline and bicarbonate solutions in the early years, largely supplanted by solutions of Gum Acacia solution, consisting of 6 percent Gum Arabic (a dried gum exudate from Acacia Senegal) in 0.9 percent saline, together with 0.05 percent KC1 and 0.05 percent $CaCl_2$, had a similar viscosity and osmotic pressure to blood and did not exude so rapidly into the tissues as saline or bicarbonate. This first plasma substitute was later found to be hepatotoxic and to coat erthrocytes, reducing their oxygen carrying capacity and causing agglutination.[10] Despite causing some deaths, in the absence of anything better, its use undoubtedly saved many lives. (It is interesting to note that the use of Gum Acacia solution was still advocated in manuals of military medicine published at the time of outbreak of the Second World War.) The entry of America into the War in 1917 greatly enhanced the use of blood transfusion, which eventually, when available, replaced Gum infusions.

In early 1918, at the No. 3 British Casualty Clearing Station at Gezaincourt, a "shock center" was established.[3] This was within easy access to the Australian sector and many of the Medical Corps officers visited or worked at the center. It was probably from this experience that Holmes á Court conceived the idea of the field ambulance resuscitation teams.

In May 1918, Lieut. Col. Thompson set up a temporary operating theater at a Main Dressing Station for urgent haemorrhagic and abdominal cases, performing 30 operations in 2 weeks. He in turn recommended that such a facility be instituted at each Main Dressing Station, but his plea received little support.[3]

In late June, Holmes á Court and his colleagues in the 4th Field Ambulance began applying resuscitation measures in their work and soon received unofficial permission by their Commanding Officer to establish a "transfusion team." One important factor in facilitating this establishment was the experience of Col. Morley, an Assistant Director of Medical Services. He was wounded in the leg on June 24, severing the posterior tibial artery in the upper third. Under existing conditions at the 4th Field Ambulance, no effort could be made to ligate the artery, and evacuation a further 18 kilometers with a tourniquet in place resulted in eventual amputation.[3]

The "transfusion" or "resuscitation team"

was then ready for the battle of Hamel on July 4, having collected equipment from various sources, including serum for blood typing, and gum and glucose solutions from a British Casualty Clearing Station.

In the first 15 hours, 30 cases demanded the immediate attention of Homes á Court and his team, prompting Col. McGregor to write, "The results achieved were such as to impel him to recommend a 'special transfusion team' with each division." The achievements of the team during the battle and subsequently were such that, 7 weeks later, and after a visit by Major General Howse, and later by the Consulting Surgeon of the British Expeditionary Forces Sir Anthony Bowlby, the team was given official approval. Teams were instituted as permanent establishments in each of the 5 Australian divisions and renamed the Corps Resuscitation Teams.[3,4,8]

Personnel in each team were 2 medical officers, one designated in charge and expert in performing rapid urgent surgery, blood transfusion and general resuscitation; the second medical officer was experienced in nitrous oxide/oxygen anesthesia, resuscitation, and classification of blood donors. The medical officers were assisted by 4 others, one non-commissioned officer and 3 orderlies trained in theater and resuscitation work.[4,5,8]

Their equipment included the following: Surgical instruments as per the No. 1 Field Service Pannier; Gas-oxygen apparatus; Blood transfusion set, including blood grouping apparatus, 6 Kimpton-Brown flasks, one Robertson's bottle, and sodium citrate; Gum infusion set including 18 doses of gum; other surgical requirements including bowls, dressings etc.; rechauffement box, for rewarming the wounded soldier, together with other sundry equipment, all packed in a Field Service Basket Panneir.

Each team had the use of a motor ambulance and was attached for duty to a Main or Advanced Dressing Station as required.

The primary role of the resuscitation teams was to treat soldiers suffering from:

Severe shock — treated with warmth, and blood or gum infusions;

Hemorrhage — where large vessels required ligation so eliminating the need for long term tourniquets;

Shattered limbs — requiring amputation, minimizing the risk of infection and gangrene.

The use of nitrous oxide/oxygen anesthesia enabled emergency surgery to be performed, with minimal depression of the circulation and rapid recovery for subsequent evacuation.

Blood transfusion was frequently performed by the "direct-indirect" method with blood from lightly wounded casualties after blood typing. The apparatus used was the Kimpton-Brown flask, enabling both collection and administration of blood. Coagulation was prevented by careful coating of the whole vessel with a thin layer of paraffin wax. This was usually done by heating the flask with a ball of wax inside, rotating the flask until all the glass was coated. Major Holmes á Court devised a much simpler method, whereby he dissolved flakes of wax in ether. The liquid was then poured into the flask, allowing the wax to leave a thin coat on all surfaces as the ether evaporated.[11]

The citrate method was introduced by Oswald Robertson from the U.S. during 1917.[9] This allowed easier collection and delivery of blood, as well as storage for up to 2 hours. Preserved blood was prepared by allowing citrated blood to settle, the supernatant then being replaced with a 2.5 percent gelatine in saline solution. It was advocated for use in the Advanced Dressing Stations, but was found to be fraught with practical difficulties related to transport, storage and asepsis.

The teams furnished a report on 14 October[3,4,8] detailing the results of their activities during August and September. In addition to other general resuscitation, closure of penetrating chest wounds, major dressings, etc., they performed 948 operations, 52 blood transfusions and 62 gum and other intravenous infusions.

The report also included the following comment: "Many limbs were saved by the early removal of tourniquets and it is found that severely shocked patients arrive at the Casualty Clearing Station in much better condition after resuscitation, transfusion, etc. than would otherwise be the case."[4]

The Consulting Surgeon of the 4th Army, Major G. Gordon-Taylor, wrote, "Several months' experience in the Casualty Clearing zone behind the Australian Corps has enabled me to form an estimate of the excellent work of the resuscitation teams of that Corps. There can be no room for doubt that very many lives have been saved by the work of Major Holmes a`Court and the members of the other resuscitation teams."[4,8]

Following receipt of this report and accompanying letters of support, The General Headquarters of the British Expeditionary Forces issued the following memorandum to the Directors of Medical Services in all Armies:

"The attached report on the organization and work accomplished by Divisional Resuscitation Teams Australian Corps, is forwarded for your information and consideration with your Consulting Surgeon. . . . Where circumstances are such that the maximum good is likely to result by the employment of teams as indicated in the report, you will no doubt be able to bring the principle into operation."[3]

Peace came with the Armistice just 11 days later, and the place of resuscitation teams seems to have been forgotten in the planning of medical services for subsequent armed conflict. In the Spanish Civil War, mobile operating theaters with a staff of 14, and fully equipped with folding beds,[12] worked close to the battlefront and this principle was continued into the Second World War.

Later in World War II, and more especially in the Korean War, the principle of emergency resuscitation in the field, with subsequent evacuation to hospital, was again established, reaching its height of development in the Vietnam conflict.

Although he was awarded the Médaille des èpidémies (en argent) and promoted to Lieut. Colonel, Dr. Holmes á Court's foresight in establishing the first mobile resuscitation service has been largely unrecognized by modern historians.

After the War he proceeded to London where he forsook a continuing career in surgery and became a Member of the Royal College of Physicians in 1919. He then returned to Australia and was awarded an M.D. for his thesis titled, "Intravenous Injections in the Treatment of Haemorrhage and Shock," based largely on his experiences in the resuscitation team during the war.[11]

He was appointed as a transfusionist to Sydney Hospital and, together with Dr. George Bell, established the principle of intravenous infusions and performed the first blood transfusion there. He had a distinguished career as clinician, teacher and examiner. He was a foundation fellow of the Royal Australasian College of Physicians, serving as President from 1952 to 1954, and was chairman of the editorial committee of the *Australian Annals of Medicine* until his death in 1957.[5,6,7]

References

1. Richardson, AG: Larrey: Surgeon to Napoleon's Imperial Guard. London: John Murray, 1974.
2. Trueta J: The Principles and Practice of War Surgery. London: Heinemann, 1943.
3. Butler AG: Official History of the Australian Army Medical Services 1914-1918, Vol II, The Western Front. Canberra: Australian War Memorial, 1940.
4. Australian War Memorial Document File, AWM; 25:921/6.
5. Obituary: Alan Worsley Holmes á Court. Medical Journal of Australia; 2:145-147, 1957.
6. Robertson TI: Alan Worsley Holmes á Court. in: Roll of The Royal Australasian College of Physicians.
7. Mitchell AM: Alan Worsley Holmes á Court. in: Australian Dictionary of Biography, Vol. 9, 351-352.
8. Australian War Memorial Document File, AWM; 25:921/11.
9. Keynes G: Blood Transfusion. London: Oxford Medical Publications, 1922.
10. Gordon-Taylor G: The Abdominal Injuries of Warfare. Bristol: John Wright, 1939.
11. Holmes a`Court AW: Intravenous injections in the treatment of haemorrhage and shock. Medical Journal of Australia, 2:25-30; 49-56, 1920.
12. Jolly DW: Field Surgery in Total War. London: Hamish Hamilton, 1940.

ARTHUR LÄWEN
The Use of Muscle Relaxants in Anaesthesia in 1912

D. J. WILKINSON
Department of Anaesthesia
St. Bartholomew's Hospital
London, England, United Kingdom

Introduction

The role played by Griffith and Johnson in the introduction of muscle relaxants into clinical anesthesia in 1942 in Montreal is unchallenged.[1] This was undoubtedly the spur for subsequent enthusiasm for the drug and its general acceptance worldwide. It is now apparent, however, that other workers experimented with the drug many years before this, and despite their publication of the work no notice was taken by the anesthetic community. This poses some intriguing questions.

Early Reports on Curare

The early reports of the action, and the subsequent use, of curare in a variety of medical conditions has been exhaustively reviewed by McIntyre[2] and by Thomas.[3] The early experimenters determined that animals could be kept alive after the administration of the drug, in paralyzing dosages, by artificial ventilation. Others then tried the drug in lesser doses in man to try to treat a wide variety of conditions in which muscular spasms were a major clinical feature; these included its use in hydrophobia, strychnine poisoning and in tetanus. Over a period of some 200 years, a variety of isolated attempts were made to use the drug, mainly in France and England. They were all eventually abandoned because of the inability to produce a standard concentration of curare which would permit reproducible results.

Curare in Anesthesia

In England

The use of curare by de Caux in England, in 1928, was an isolated incident, was not published at the time, and did nothing to influence our specialty as a whole. It does, however, represent the first use of the drug in England for anesthetic purposes.

de Caux used an aqueous extract of the drug, which was prepared by the hospital pharmacy from an unknown source, on eight patients at the North Middlesex Hospital in London. He was attempting to facilitate muscle relaxation during nitrous oxide and oxygen anesthesia (often just 'gas and air'), a technique which, despite his undoubted mastery, proved to be a poor one for many major abdominal cases. Like many before and after him, he abandoned his work with curare due to lack of drug and an inability to standardize the concentration used.[4]

In Germany

However, in Leipzig in 1912, Arthur Läwen used an extract of curare during surgical operations with great success, and published his findings in a major scientific journal.[5] (de Caux was fluent in German and travelled extensively on the continent during the first three decades of this century, and its interesting to speculate whether he heard of Läwen's attempts and thus instituted his experiments.)

Läwen's early life and medical training has been reviewed in detail by Goerig et al.[6] Born in Waldheim in February 1876, he was to train as a surgeon with some of the great men of German medicine of that era, like Trendelenburg and Payr. Having worked extensively with Braun investigating local anesthetics, he moved to the Surgical Department of the University of Leipzig where he met Boehm, chairman of the Pharmacology Department, who at that time was purifying and experimenting with curare.

Boehm published his work on the isolation of curarine in 1897.[7] He wrote; *I would like to retain the old name "Curarin" for the effective main component of the Calabash Curare. The isolation of it has proved to be best in the method first described in 1886.. . . . The finely pulverized Curare is mixed with 25 times the amount of water in a retort and left standing for 8 days in normal temperatures, shaking it frequently. Having filtered the extract, one treats the undissolved sediment twice more, the third time with the addition of some dilute sulphuric acid with the same amount of water.*

He continues to describe over several pages of text the extraction process in great detail, a process which involved multiple filtrations, dissolving of sediments in alcohol, washing in hyrochloric acid, ammonia, ether, and then in chloroform. Eventually he was left with a concentrated extract of the original calabash curare which had to be of a certain standard. *These procedures have to be repeated to the point where the "Curarin" proves its effect in the test: 0.34 mg. per Kg. should kill a rabbit. He added, To produce Curarin it has not been advisable to work with quantities larger than the contents of one Calabash at a time.* This was the purified substance that Läwen used successfully in the treatment of tetanus in 1906.[8] He followed this with experiments during anesthesia in 1912.[5]

Läwen wrote, *A great problem with light anaesthesia is the fact that the patients tighten up their abdominal muscles during the suturing of the abdomen. This makes a normal layering of sutures very difficult. The tension in these abdominal muscles can often be avoided if a local anaesthetic is used — however there is a failure rate.* He was aware of the actions of curare on musculature from work he had performed in the laboratory, *as we know from experiments in the laboratory it is possible to paralyse the respiratory muscles and keep the animals alive with artificial respiration. One is able to perfectly control as well as eliminate the Curarin intoxication. .. . . one can sit and wait for the Curarin to be excreted and the function of the respiratory muscles to be resumed.* With this in mind, he decided to use Boehm's Curarin in anesthetic practice, *I have done some experiments to avoid tension of the abdominal muscles by other means. I have used Curarin, a substance produced by Boehm from curare-preparation. Curarin has the great advantage over curare drugs that the dosage can be so precise that it will always produce the same result. I would not have had the courage to use the ordinary curare drugs in humans, as there is no control over the way it works due to the variable contents of the curare.*

He was interested in the analogy between the effects of local anesthetics producing muscle relaxation and that of the curarine having a similar effect, but was well aware that different mechanisms of action were involved. *My intention was to bring the effect of local anaesthesia and that of Curarin closer together*, he wrote, *The former results in a reduction of sensory stimulation and motor impulses. The latter acts as a block between motor nerve endings and striped muscles thereby producing a barrier for the weaker innervation stimulus which can only produce a very weak muscle contraction if any. There is no danger of intoxication as the necessary dosage of Curarine to reach this point is not very big.*

Here is perhaps where the story becomes even more intriguing as Läwen describes the dose he gives to produce effective muscle relaxation. *I have given the Curarine drugs, to adults either subcutaneously or intramuscularly in a concentration of 2 percent in the biggest dosage of 0.8 mg. The effect of this dosage was most evident and pleasing during the suturing of the abdominal walls. However I believe that this dose could and should be increased.* Once again, however, we come to the problem that bedeviled all the early workers with these drugs, and that was the lack of supplies.

One gets results with a smaller dosage given intravenously. Unfortunately it is not possible to obtain sufficient quantities of curare drugs. I was therefore not able to establish the Curarin dosage for the above mentioned purpose due to lack of substance. He fully realized the value of this drug in this situation and summed it up, *By restricting inhalational anaesthesia we lessen an important factor in the aetiology of complications. The good physical condition of the patients after operation is the best evidence of the efficacy of the method.*

So further use of muscle relaxants was delayed for many more decades until a large supply of curare was brought back by Gill in the 1930's,[9] which would in turn give rise to the work by Griffith and Johnson. Läwen's contribution has been largely overlooked because it was never translated into English, although some have made passing reference to his study.[10,11]

What drug did Lawen use?

What remains interesting speculation is what the actual drug injected by Läwen was? From the dosage given, and the clinical effects observed, together with the source of the drug, one may conjecture that it was not curare that was administered, but another relaxant. In 1963, Foldes et al described the use of alcuronium in anesthetic practice.[12] The drug is synthesized from calabash curare by a complex process. I believe that Boehm's complicated extraction of Curarine produced a similar product some 80 years previously. Alcuronium is currently marketed by Roche, who have not been able to confirm or deny this theory.

Conclusions

Whatever the drug used by Läwen, he undoubtedly used a curare extract to facilitate abdominal closure during laparotomies. The work did not receive widespread publicity, but may have been the spur for de Caux's work a decade later. The plaudits for the introduction of muscle relaxants are quite correctly given to Griffith and Johnson for their work in the 1940's, which changed the face of clinical anesthesia for all time.

Acknowledgements

I am most grateful for the help provided in the research for this paper by the late J. Alfred Lee from Southend, and Michael Goerig of Hamburg. The research would have been impossible without the generous assistance of Mrs. Inge Newton who translated the German texts for me.

References

1. Griffith HR, Johnson GE: The use of curare in general anesthesia. *Anesthesiology*; 3: 418-20, 1942.
2. McIntyre AR: *Curare: Its History, Nature, and Clinical Use*. University of Chicago Press. Chicago. 1947.
3. Thomas KB: *Curare: Its History and Usage*. Pitman Medical Publishing Co. Ltd. London. 1964.
4. Wilkinson DJ: Dr. F.P. de Caux — the first user of curare for anaesthesia in England. *Anaesthesia*; 46: 49-51, 1991.

5. Läwen A: Ueber die Verbindug der Lokalanasthesie mit der narkose, über hohe Extraduralanasethesie und epidurale Injectionen anästhesierender Lösungen bei tabischen Magenkrisen. *Beitrage klin Chir*; 80: 168-89, 1912.
6. Goerig M, Schulte am Esch J: Reminiscences on Arthur Läwen — an extraordinary pioneer in anesthesia. *Proceedings of the Third International Symposium on the History of Anaesthesia.* 1992.
7. Boehm R: Ueber Curare und Curarealkaloide. *Arch der Pharmacie;* 235: 660-84, 1896-7.
8. Frey R: Obituary, Arthur Läwen. *Der Anaesthetist*; 7: S 128, 1958.
9. Gill RC: *White Water and Black Magic.* Victor Gollancz Ltd. London. 1941.
10. Scurr CF: A comparative review of the relaxants. *Bri J Anaesth;* 23: 103-16, 1951.
11. Lee JA, Atkinson, RS: *A Synopsis of Anaesthesia.* John Wright and Sons Ltd. Bristol. 7th Edition. 1973.
12. Foldes FF, Brown IM, Lunn JN, Moore J, Duncalf D: The neuromuscular effects of diallylnortoxiferine in anesthetized subjects. *Anesth Analg*; 42: 177-87, 1963.

KEEPING THE AIRWAY OPEN:
Esmarch's Manoeuvre or Heiberg's Heave?

D. J. WILKINSON
Department of Anaesthesia
St. Bartholomew's Hospital
London, England, United Kingdom

Introduction

In the first months after the introduction of ether anaesthesia, surgical operations were often performed under what would be regarded today as extremely light planes of anaesthesia. Movement during operations, and even vocalization, were the normal rather than the unusual in practice.[1] These light planes of anaesthesia were obviously a great improvement for patient and surgeon alike. However, as experience with ether and then chloroform developed, the full potential of the drugs was realised, and what we would regard as full surgical anaesthesia became the usual practice. This increasing depth of unconsciousness produced increasing problems with maintaining the airway.

John Snow

It is interesting to review how this great scientist failed to appreciate the potential problems that this progressive loss of the airway might provoke. He certainly recorded the effects of this obstruction and referred to stertorous and rattling respiration as an indicator of depth of anaesthesia, but seemed to make no attempt to alleviate the problem, but merely lightened the anaesthetic. He wrote, *If there is the least snoring I always leave off the vapour entirely, . . . The snoring now and then increases for a quarter or half a minute after the inhalation is left off, the breathing becoming deep, accompanied with heaving of the chest, and sometimes blowing of the lips; but this stertorous breathing always subsides again in a minute or two, and need therefore excite no alarm; it should, however, always be looked on as an indication for discontinuing the ether for a time.*[1]

In his text on chloroform, published posthumously, he adds, *Falling back of the tongue. It has been alleged that the falling back of the tongue into the throat, under the deep influence of chloroform, might be the cause of death by suffocation; but this appears to be an error; for the muscles of the larynx and neighbouring parts preserve their action as long as the diaphragm, and contract contemporaneously with it. When the breathing has ceased, the tongue is indeed liable to fall backwards, if the person in a state of suspended animation is lying on the back, and this circumstance requires to be attended to in performing artificial respiration.*[2]

It was unusual for Snow to miss an aspect of care so entirely.

Friedrich von Esmarch

Without doubt one of the greatest surgeons of his era, Esmarch, produced a wide variety of anaesthetic and surgical apparatus. In response to a competition initiated by the Empress of Germany under the auspices of the Red Cross, he wrote a textbook of military surgery that won first prize, and which was intended to be a pocket reference handbook for the surgeon on the battlefield.[3]

There is a section on operative surgery which advocates the use of chloroform for this type of surgery. He writes, *In every major operation, and for every prolonged examination, the patient should be rendered anaesthetic by inhalation of chloroform. Under some circumstances, however, this wonderful drug may be dangerous to life, therefore certain prudential rules are to be observed in its administration.* He believed that patients should be fasted for at least four hours, that they should be anaesthetised on their back, and not in a sitting position which might make them faint, and that premedication with morphine was of benefit. He continued, *During the administration of the chloroform, pulse and respiration must be kept under observation.* He designed and provided illustrations of his dropper bottle and wire frame mask and then, having detailed the signs and stages of an inhalation induction, proceeded to outline some of the problems that could arise during anaesthesia. *In asphyxia, open the mouth at once, and press the lower jaw forwards with both hands by placing the forefingers behind the ascending ramus, so that the lower teeth project in front of the upper (partial dislocation). By this movement the hyoid bone and root of the tongue, and the epiglottis are drawn forwards, and the entrance to the larynx is thus freed from obstruction.*

Esmarch realised that this was sometimes difficult to manage and provided further advice, *If this cannot be accomplished because of convulsive contraction of the muscles, separate the teeth with a dilator, seize the end of the tongue with the fingers, or with a tongue forceps, and draw it out of the mouth as far as possible.* Line drawings in his text illustrate these two manoeuvers well. He continued, *If in spite of this, the respiration is difficult and rattling, the cause may be the presence of mucus or blood in the region of the glottis. Remove this with a sponge, carried down to the area on a dressing forceps.* This was a time, after all, before the introduction of suction apparatus. Finally, if things continued to deteriorate, *If respiration ceases entirely, artificial respiration should be instigated at once— and preferably by Sylvester's Method.*

It is not therefore surprising that, on the European continent, and certainly in Germany, this simple jaw-thrust manipulation to preserve the airway became known as Esmarch's manoeuvre.

Jacob Heiberg

Jacob Heiberg was the son of Johan Frikner Heiberg, a general surgeon from Christiana (Oslo) in Norway. Jacob was born on 12 June, 1843, in Christiana. He trained as a doctor in Berlin under Professor Reichert, and consolidated that training in Rostock under Professor Keonig. After further studies with Schoenborn in Konigsberg, he returned to Norway in 1873. While working at the University he published a paper in a London Journal which predates Esmarch by some 3 years.[4] His ideas were almost identical with those later propounded by the German surgeon, . . . *there are several circumstances which may occur during the administration of chloroform, and cause anxiety to the operator and his assistants. These cases are chiefly associated with incomplete, rattling respiration, pale livid colour of the face, feeble pulse, etc. It is especially the imperfect respiration which causes anxiety, and gives the impression that the entrance to the trachea is, as it were, closed by a valve. As a remedy for this evil, which is, so to say, of daily occurrence in every surgical infirmary, a special treatment has been methodised. A peculiar gag is applied, with a screw which forces the teeth apart, and the tongue is then drawn out with forceps or with pointed muscle hooks.*

Heiberg was not impressed with this technique, *I do not know whether it has occurred to others, as it has to me, that there is something unsympathetic in this process, although I have myself many times been obliged to employ it. I have had three special objections, namely — First: It gives to the whole operation an appearance of uneasiness and anxiety, which is not at all desirable. Second: The patient's teeth are not infrequently broken; the tongue is often so much injured by the manipulation, that the patient, . . . is inconvenienced for many days, speaks badly, or swallows with difficulty. Thirdly: The narcosis is prolonged by this expedient, . . .*

He then places his ideas even further back from Esmarch, *Two years and a half ago I hit on an expedient, which in my opinion is available for the avoidance of all the inconveniences referred to. This consists in drawing forward the under jaw in toto.* His description of the jaw-thrust is very vivid, *When the rattling, incomplete respiration begins — that is to say, in all those cases in which the teeth are otherwise forced apart, and the tongue drawn out — I draw the under jaw forward by the following means. Standing preferably behind the reclining patient, the operator places both his thumbs on the symphysis of the lower jaw, presses the second joint of the bent forefingers behind the posterior margin of the rami ascendentes of the under-jaw, and thus holding the whole bone fast between the two hands, draws it forcibly upwards (anatomically speaking).*

He continues, *. . . the head of the jaw slips forward over the tuberculum with an appreciable jerk, the whole under-jaw slides forward, . . . and the patient's countenance takes the appearance which the Danes called "under-jawed" and the French called "ganache." When the experiment is successful, a deep complete respiration will immediately take place, and will be continued as long as the jaw is kept "luxated" forward.*

He had tried this on over 1,000 consecutive chloroform anaesthetics and had not needed any other instrumental intervention. He believed that others should now try the technique to further validate his method. His interests in anaesthesia then obviously waned as he became Professor of Anatomy at the University of Christiana (Oslo). He continued to publish a series of papers and books on anatomic matters, and was Editor of one of the most prestigious Norwegian Journals. His health failed at a relatively young age and he died on 30 April, 1888, aged 45.[5]

Joseph T. Clover

Almost exactly a month after Heiberg's paper appeared in the English journal, Clover wrote on anaesthesia in the British Medical Journal, *When ether or chloroform is inhaled, the throat is stimulated; coughing and movements of deglutition commonly occur. . . The act of swallowing is usually performed well enough; but, . . . then the deglutition may be delayed at the moment when the epiglottis covers the larynx, . . . raising the chin, and pulling it as far as possible away from the sternum, is usually sufficient to obviate this source of obstruction.*[6]

These ideas were gradually incorporated into the major anaesthetic texts of that era, often with illustrations,[7,8] and the procedure became normal practice. The introduction of the oral airway[9] did not alter the need for this process, nor did the development of tracheal intubation. It may be that it is only the advent of the Brain laryngeal mask that will see the end of this simple manoeuvre for which generations of anaesthetists have been grateful.

Conclusions

The preservation of the airway during anaesthesia by lifting the lower jaw forward is often ascribed to Esmarch. However, the true accolades should be given to the Norwegian doctor and anatomist, Jacob Heiberg, who described the manoeuvre many years before Esmarch.

Acknowledgments

I am most grateful to Professor Ole Secher for setting me on the right path for this research project.

References

1. Snow J: *On the inhalation of the vapour of ether in surgical operations.* John Churchill. London. 1847.
2. Snow J: *On chloroform and other anaesthetics: their action and administration.* John Churchill. London. 1858.
3. Esmarch F: *Handbuch der kriegschirurgischen Technik.* Carl Rumpler. Hanover. 1877.
4. Heiberg J: A new expedient in administering chloroform. *Medical and Surgical Gazette*; 1: 36, 1874.
5. Guldberg GA: Obituary of Professor Dr. Jacob Munch Heiberg. *International Monatschrift fur Anatomie und Physiologie, Leipzig* 5: 431-2, 1888.
6. Clover JT: Remarks on the production of sleep during surgical operations. *British Medical Journal*; 1: 200-203, 1874.
7. Hewitt FW: *Anaesthetics and their administration.* Macmillan and Co. Ltd. London. 2nd Edition. 1901.
8. Gwathmey JT, Baskerville C: *Anesthesia.* D. Appelton and Company. New York. 1914.
9. Hewitt FW: An artificial "airway" for use during anaesthetisation. *Lancet;* 1: 490-1, 1908.

BENJAMIN PAUL BLOOD
Anesthesia's Philosopher and Mystic

A. J. WRIGHT
Clinical Librarian, Department of Anesthesiology Library
University of Alabama at Birmingham
Birmingham, Alabama, USA

Introduction

> *. . .with the most intense belief and prophetic manner I exclaimed to Dr. Kinglake, "Nothing exists but thoughts! The universe is composed of impressions, ideas, pleasures and pains."*
>
> Humphry Davy

> *With anesthetic agents we seem to have a tool for producing and holding at will, and at little risk, different levels of consciousness — a tool that promises to be of great help in studies of mental phenomenon.*
>
> Henry K. Beecher

Almost a century before Beecher's comment was published,[1] New Yorker Benjamin Paul Blood began fourteen years of experimentation into the nature of "mental phenomenon" using ether and nitrous oxide. Blood eventually developed these experiences into a complex mysticism which he attempted to articulate in books, pamphlets, journal articles and newspaper correspondence. Thus, he may be the only patient in history whose experience with anesthesia led to the formulation of an entire philosophy.

Blood's Biography

The most significant outward events of Blood's life are noted by his entry in the venerable *Dictionary of American Biography*.[2] He was born in Amsterdam, New York, on November 21, 1832. Blood attended Amsterdam Academy and made one of his few trips away from that town to briefly study at Union College. He married twice and had two daughters and a son. Blood died in the city of his birth on January 15, 1919.

Despite his lack of travel far from home, Blood was quite active. An only child, he inherited the 700 acre farm developed by his father along the Mohawk River, but seems to have been an indifferent farmer. At one time or another, Blood was a boxer, weight-lifter, gambler, business speculator, mill worker and inventor. Among his inventions were a swathing reaper and a safety side-saddle for female horseback riders.[3]

In a letter to William James in June 1887, Blood confessed that he only farmed "'in a way,' that in his youth he had been a successful gambler, but had thrown the money away, that he had been a 'fancy gymnast' and had had some 'heavy fights.' Blood accompanied the letter with a picture of himself after he had lifted 1160 pounds." A decade later, in a June 1896 letter to James, "Blood stated that he had been working ten hours a day in a mill."[4]

By the time he was eighteen, Blood was also a published author, and over his long life produced a "million or more words of writing" in the form of books, pamphlets, journal articles and a vast number of letters and poems to local newspapers. His topics included religion, local and national politics, philosophy and linguistics.[5] "He is an author only when the fit strikes him," William James wrote of his friend,"and short spurts at a time; shy, moreover, to the point of publishing his compositions only as private tracts, or in letters to such far-from-reverberant organs of publicity as the *Gazette* or the *Recorder* of his native Amsterdam. . . Odd places for such subtle efforts to appear in. . ."[6]

In 1860, Blood was given ether for a dental procedure, and there in the dentist's office had an experience he would spend the rest of his life attempting to articulate — the Anaesthetic Revelation, "unutterable by any, yet accessible to all, and of singular interest if not of novel instance."[7] For the next thirteen years, Blood experimented with this revelation via ether and nitrous oxide inhalations, and finally described the philosophical results in a thirty-seven page pamphlet he published privately in 1874, *The Anaesthetic Revelation and the Gist of Philosophy.*

The number of copies Blood had printed is unknown, but he seems to have scattered them to numerous individuals in the United States and Europe. Among the recipients were such luminaries as Alfred Lord Tennyson and William James. The copy I have seen was marked "A. Winchell/8 April 1874/From the Author." How Blood picked these particular people is also unknown, although in the case of James a personal connection may have been the factor. "The first man of genius I ever saw alive was Henry James." Blood wrote to James about his father in August 1882. "He preached at the Presbyterian church here."[8]

At the time he received his copy of Blood's work, James was early in his illustrious career, having received an M.D. from Harvard Medical School in 1869 and become an instructor in physiology and anatomy at that institution in 1872. About this same time he began publishing a number of book reviews.[9] In the spring of 1874, James must have received Blood's pamphlet just after his return from Italy, where he had gone to recover from a recurrence of the poor health he had suffered from 1869 to 1872.[10] James published an anonymous review of *The Anaesthetic Revelation for Atlantic Monthly*, in which he said "we shall not howl with the wolves or join the multitude in jeering at it." Although James' initial reaction was not entirely enthusiastic, he recommended it to readers as ". . .thoroughly original and very suggestive."[11]

In 1882, Blood and James began a correspondence which continued intermittently until the latter's death in 1910. The two met only once, in June, 1895, a meeting of the minds described by a local Amsterdam paper as "concerning the possibility, feasibility, and the advisability of attempting a further and better expression of the anaesthetic revelation. . ."[12] The letters between these two philosophers were personal and friendly. James, who suffered bouts of depression throughout his life, confided to Blood in June, 1896, "I take it that no man is educated who has ever dallied with the thought of suicide."[13] Blood's biographer has noted about this correspondence, "There are various remarks that Blood had not pushed the experience to its limit, nor fully articulated the implications."[12] That observation James made in a letter to Blood just after their 1895 meeting; James thanked Blood for sending him some clippings of his articles and said, ". . .they are good but the cosmic stuff is better. So do, like a good boy, sit down and have a crack at the anaesthetic revelation again. Squeeze it tight. . ."[14]

Blood claimed, "The hundreds of letters that came to me after the distribution of my pamphlet in 1874 gave a feeling. . .as if 'all the books in the world were written by one man.'"[15] Tennyson's letter, written from the Isle of Wright and dated May 7, 1874, informed Blood, "I have to thank you for your essay. . . It is a very notable sketch of metaphysic, ending yet once more, apparently, in the strange history of human thought, with the placid Buddha, as verified by nineteenth century anaesthetics. . . I have never had any revelations through anaesthetics.. . ." As Blood himself noted, Tennyson was being disingenuous; a rough draft of this letter, later published in his memoirs, contains an account of just such an experience. As he was emerging from his only surgical anesthetic, a friend who was present informed Tennyson that the poet had ". . .blurted out a long metaphysical term which he could not reword for me." Blood stated confidently that "Had Tennyson repeated the experience he would have recalled this expression."[16]

However, others who responded to Blood's pamphlet seem to have had similar problems articulating their revelation. Edmund Gurney (1847-1888), a British psychical researcher, wrote Blood in January, 1883. "I had this extraordinary experience myself last year, under nitrous oxide, harmonizing with your description; but the result was almost ludicrously disappointing. For half a minute or more after I had come to, I was quite sure that the problem was solved and that when I could I would tell the dentist about it, and that it had something to do with time. When I got my breath I found that I could not get it out. . ."[17]

With the exception of a political pamphlet, two major journal articles, a few poems, and numerous letters to newspapers and James and other correspondents, Blood published little else before he died in 1919. Although his biographer does not mention them, Blood apparently issued other pamphlets on his revelation. William James, in one of the lectures he gave in Edinburgh in 1901-1902, and which were published as *The Varieties of Religious Experience*, alludes to Blood's "pamphlets of rare literary distinction" and "in his latest pamphlet, *'Tennyson's Trances and the Anaesthetic Revelation,'* Mr. Blood. . ."[18] During his last decade Blood wrote the manuscript for *Pluriverse*, a final summation of his thinking that appeared the year after his death. The Amsterdam philosopher, who had flirted with renown in certain intellectual circles during his lifetime, slipped back into the obscurity from which he had appeared in 1874, and where he has more or less remained ever since.

Blood's Philosophy

Despite his physical isolation in a tiny New York town, Blood became a student of intellectual trends early in his life. His pre-revelation work includes two important essays. *The Philosophy of Justice* (1851) "was a youthful essay on religion, which marked a transition from an adolescent atheism to a peculiarly personal interpretation of Christianity." Nine years later, another pamphlet, *Optimism: The Lesson of the Ages* (1860) "illustrated the subtlety of Blood's mind, his skill at logic, the sweep of his rhetoric" in its consideration of God, purpose and evil.[19]

As Blood's thought was maturing in mid-century, he entered the stream of American intellectual development at "a period in which philosophy's perennial problems are treated in a framework no longer theological in structure. . . the emphasis here was shifted from problems of conscience to those concerning the relations of appearance to reality and the One to the Many." His philosophy of later years combined his anesthetic experiences and his readings from the influential American *Journal of Speculative Philosophy*" of translations of Kant, Fichte, Schelling, and Hegel. . ." and ". . . attempted to relate the philosophic problems inherent in German idealism to the primacy of experience. . ."[20] In essence, Blood's thinking progressed from one stage to its opposite. The first, monism, was the idea that the universe and God are knowable through reason, and one which Blood still supported in *The Anaesthetic Revelation.* Blood's philosophy after that pamphlet developed into a pluralism, acknowledging creation as too large for a single explanation via man's logic — philosophy he finally developed in his posthumous work, *Pluriverse.*

The linchpin of Blood's development was the experience he had during emergence from anesthesia — at first the accidental result of ether in a dentist's office, but thereafter repeated during more than a decade's self-experimentation with nitrous oxide. Although he admitted other routes to this state of mind were possible, Blood stated that anesthetic gas was for him the trigger. "Of this condition, although it may have been attained otherwise, I know only by the use of anaesthetic agents. After experiments ranging over nearly fourteen years I affirm — what any man may prove at will — that there is an invariable and reliable condition (or uncondition) ensuing about the instant of recall from anaesthetic stupor to sensible observation, or 'coming to,' in which the genius of being is revealed; but because it cannot be remembered in the normal condition it is lost altogether through the infrequency of anaesthetic treatment. . ."[21]

The emotional impact of his revelation must have been fierce in this weight-lifting inventor-farmer who had struggled for years attempting to reason his way through mysteries of existence. "My first experiences of this revelation had many varieties of emotion. . ." which Blood listed as sadness, solemnity, serenity, "ancient" peace, majesty and supremacy "unspeakable". . ."so am I now not only firm and familiar in this once weird condition, but triumphant — divine."[22]

Blood was not hesitant in making claims based on his experimentation ". . .in those brief seconds of instant recall from stupor to recognition, each patient discovers something grotesque and unutterable about his own nature, the genius of being is revealed, and the mystery of life is understood at last as but a common thing. . . By this revelation we enter to the sadness and majesty of Jesus — to the solemn mystery which inspired the prophets of every generation. By some accident of being they entered to this condition."[22]

Blood also made efforts to discuss this experience with other people. "Yet I have warned others to expect this wonder on entering the anaesthetic slumber, and none so cautioned has failed to report of it in terms which assured me of its realization. I have spoken with various persons also who induce anesthesia professionally (dentists, surgeons, etc.) who had observed that many patients at the moment of recall seem as having made a startling, yet somehow matter-of-course (and even grotesque) discovery in their own nature, and try to speak of it, but invariably fail in a lost mood of introspection."[22]

Blood's biographer, Marks, has neatly summarized the transition between his two major philosophical works. "It is in *The Anaesthetic Revelation* that Blood first comes to grips with solid philosophical ideas. Here Blood develops a mature metaphysical argument which posits design as an outcome of process, and which in itself gives no evidence of purpose. His metaphysics is completed in Pluriverse, where he disavows monism, holding that the universe is too great either for a personal God or any unitary Absolute. Cosmic 'cause,' he argues here, may be nothing more than a system effect, a concatenation of force patterns. All necessary and possible explanation of cause and design is perhaps to be found in the perceptual flux as it is experienced here and now."[23]

Blood wrote a dense, mesmerizing prose that draws in even the reader who may not understand it all. "The revelation, for us, is of sanity at its utmost tension and interest, realizing at once the effort and the fatuous incongruity and impossibility of self-vision, and having a clear and unquestionable consciousness that this condition and this effort realize the genius of being, and effect the process of time; but above all is a sense of admonition — perhaps an afterglow from our religious associations — that this is the secret of the world, inevitably such; no other account of it can be mentionable in the same connection."[24]

Blood's decades-long attempt to articulate his revelation reflects the kind of difficulties faced by any mystic who tries to describe the infinite using the limited resources of language.

Other "Anaesthetic" Mystics

Man's search for meaning through the millennia has included a group of experiences labeled as "mystical" and appearing in numerous cultures and time periods. O'Brien has noted three generic elements of the mystical experience: "[1]. The object confronted in mystic experience is thought by the mystic to be somehow ultimate. . .[2] The manner of confrontation is immediate, direct. . .[3]. The confrontation is always different from the familiar exercise of either sense perception or of reasoning."[25]

Fischer discusses the relationship of mystical awareness to the continuum of human conscious experience in his "cartography" of ecstatic and meditative states.[26] Methods of reaching this state have ranged from serendipity to fasting, self-flagellation, ritual dancing and drug use. A surprising number of mystical awareness reports stem from anesthetic use.

Reports of mystical experiences relating to anesthetic agents group naturally into two categories, "incidental" and "deliberate." The first group consists of individuals whose experience occurs during the normal course of anesthetic administration for surgery, etc. The second group of experiences may or may not originate in the first, but the individual continues anesthetic use in a non-clinical context in order to either repeat the experience or to induce it initially.

Incidental reports: Within months after Morton's public demonstration of surgical anesthesia in October, 1846, British physician Francis Plomley described the reaction of a fourteen year-old boy emerging from ether anesthesia given for strabismus surgery: ". . . he exclaimed in a high tone of voice, and with great energy, 'I have been going to heaven; I have been seeing the angels, and I don't know what all! I have been going to heaven, that's all I know about it! Angels and trumpets are blowing!' He continued to talk in this strain for ten minutes. . ."[27]

On December 8, 1846, A.L. Cox of New York City tested on himself some of Morton's "letheon" to determine its nature; he suspected it might be ether, a substance he had apparently inhaled at frolics since 1822. His suspicion confirmed, Cox also noted in his published account, "I felt, on recovering, as if I had been in a beautiful vision."[28]

Other nineteenth century accounts include one by English writer and poet John Addington Symonds (1840-1893) describing his experience in the dentist's office in February 1873. "On Tuesday I was put under the influence of chloroform and laughing gas together. I felt no pain, but my consciousness seemed complete. . . After the choking and stifling of the chloroform had passed away, I seemed in a state of utter blackness: then came flashes of intense light, alternating with blackness, and with a keen vision of what was going on in the room around me. . . I thought that I was near death; when, suddenly, my soul became aware of God, who was manifestly dealing with me, handling me, so to speak, in an intense personal present reality I felt Him streaming in like light upon me. . . I cannot describe the ecstasy I felt. . ."[29]

After his ether anesthesia for nasal surgery in the mid-1880's, George E. Shoemaker reported, "Swiftly running auras or waves (that) seemed to follow one another rapidly from within outward over the limbs, and the 'Ego' was gone. . . The strange impressions took a deep hold upon me and, matter-of-fact and unimaginative as I am by nature, it took days to shake off the feeling that I had a glimpse of another phase of existence.. . ."[30]

An Englishman wrote to William James about his only anesthetic given late May or early June, 1895, for a tooth removal. One researcher has identified this Englishman as none other than Oscar Wilde.[31] "The next experience I became aware of, who shall relate! My God! *I knew everything*. A vast inrush of obvious and absolutely satisfying solutions to all possible problems. . . an all-embracing unification of hitherto contending and apparently diverse aspects of truth took possession of my soul by force. . . Then, in a flash, this state of intellectual ecstasy was succeeded by one that I shall never forget. . . a state of moral ecstasy. I was seized with an immense yearning to take back this truth to the feeble, sorrowing, struggling world in which I had lived."[32]

Another report documented around 1900 by William James was that of "a gifted woman. . . (who). . . was taking ether for a surgical operation." The Englishwoman described in detail her encounter with "A great Being or Power. . ." who showed her that "Knowledge and Love are One" and "The eternal necessity of suffering these things may seem to you delusions. . . but for me they are dark truths, and the power to put them into even such words as these has been given me by another dream."[33]

Incidental reports have continued into this century. Irish playwright J.M. Synge, under surgical ether, observed, "I seemed to traverse whole epochs of desolation and bliss. All secrets were open before me, and simple as the universe to its God."[34] A Columbia, South Carolina, physician recorded "The Throngs of broken, brilliant image (that) struggle for expression. . . It seemed that the corporal part of me was being borne. . . far beyond the infinity of blue."[35] Englishman D.I. Evans described a vision of circles: "These retracting and advancing circles suggested themselves to me as the final explanation of life. The eternal problems of both God and man were all resolved into this fantastically simple equation."[36] Bergstrom et al reported a patient who described "The sensation turned to belief that she had solved the question of life, and she felt humble."[37]

Deliberate reports: Comments by William James, no doubt based on his personal experiences with nitrous oxide, perhaps explain why individuals have used anesthetics in seeking mystical experience. "With me, as with every other person of whom I have heard, the keynote of the experience is the tremendously exciting sense of an intense metaphysical illumination. Truth lies open to the view in depth beneath depth of almost blinding evidence." James himself became aware that "unbroken continuity is of the essence of being, and that we are literally in the midst of *an infinite*, to perceive the existence of which is the utmost we can attain." James apparently experimented with nitrous oxide on more than one occasion; he mentions the "sheet after sheet of phrases dictated or written during the intoxication." Acknowledging that the writings which might be "drivel" to others, "at the moment of transcribing (they) were fused in the fire of infinite rationality." James was convinced of the usefulness of this experience; "I strongly urge others to repeat the experiment. . ."[38]

The feeling that the revelation has slipped into nonsense after emergence from anesthesia is common. Physician-author Logan Clendening preserved an interesting anecdote of this type. ". . .Mr. Carl Van Vechten has told me of a fellow-novelist who became so obsessed with the elusive nature of this experience that he had a tank of nitrous oxide installed in his basement and employed a nurse to give it to him. He took it day after day. Each time he firmly decided to remember the real secret of the universe. Each time he went under, the mystic and awful explanation was vouchsafed him. But invariably when he regained consciousness, he could no longer remember what it was."[39]

Oliver Wendell Holmes also had this experience. "I once inhaled a pretty full dose of ether, with the determination to put on record, at the earliest moment of regaining consciousness, the thought I should find uppermost in my mind. . . The one great truth which underlies all human experience, and is the key to all the mysteries that philosophy has sought in vain to solve, flashed upon me in a sudden revelation... As my natural condition returned. . . I wrote. . . A strong sense of turpentine prevails throughout."[40] Holmes made a second attempt to discover the secret, and wrote, "Put Jesus Christ into a Brahma press and that's what you will get."[41]

During the 1880s, two anesthetic experiments were almost as persistent in their search for the revelation as Blood himself. The mysterious Xenos Clark was apparently known to both Blood and James, who described him as "a philosopher, who died young at Amherst in the '80s, much lamented by those who knew him, (and) was also impressed by the revelation." James has quoted extensively from a letter to him from Clark. "The real secret would be the formula by which the 'now' keeps exfoliating out of itself, yet never escapes... You walk, as it were, round yourself in the revelation... So the present is already a foregone conclusion, and I am never too late to understand it. But at the moment of recovery from anaesthesis (sic), just then, *before starting on life*, I catch, so to speak, a glimpse of my heels, a glimpse of the eternal process just in the act of starting..."[42] Clark is known to have published one book, *Animal Music, Its Nature and Origin* (Philadelphia, 1879); nothing else has been discovered about him.

In *Pluriverse*, Blood quotes extensively from William Ramsay, who began experimenting with various anesthetics around 1880 and published his observations in 1893 in the *Journal* of Britain's Society for Psychical Research. "An overwhelming impression forced itself upon me that the state in which I then was, was reality; that now I had reached the true solution of the secret of the universe..."[43] In May, 1911, Ramsay wrote Blood, "It is interesting to find that your experiences under anaesthetics have been similar to mine. I fancy that a good many people are thus affected. I have been at least fifty times..."[44]

After discussing Ramsay, Blood then describes what must be the only conference ever held of anesthesia mystics.

> About ten years after the publication of these experiences of Sir William Ramsay there was held a symposium of persons who had been led by his example to test the anaesthetic vision for themselves, at No. 20 Hanover Square, London, June 24, 1904. The gathering comprised representatives of quite distinguished literary and social eminence, and the current discussion of the topic had the advantage of not only frank and ingenuous expression but of scientific and historical criticism. A considerable number of the associates related their individual experiences, which, however various in seemingly temperamental details, fell generally under the summing-up of Mr. Ernest Dunbar, the lecturer of the evening:
>
> "After the first effects of ether have passed off, there comes a time of profound intellectual stimulation, during which the mind reasons with astonishing rapidity, choosing, in some individuals, transcendent lines, appearing to solve, *once and for all*, the mystery of the universe."[45]

Dunbar himself had published an account of his experiments with numerous drugs, including such anesthetics as chloroform, ethyl bromide and iodide and ether. "Then by degrees I began to realize that I was the One," Dunbar wrote, "and the universe of which I was the principle was balancing itself into completeness."[46] This impression sounds like one of Blood's insights: "Philosophy proposes a weird partnership or equation between men and the world, is subject and object, and these two prove strangely convertible and interwoven."[47]

Anecdotal literature and one research study document the relationship between mystical experience and nitrous oxide.[48-52] One group of researchers even reported an organized use: "contact was made with a 'mystical-religious' group that used the gas to accelerate arriving at their transcendental meditative state of choice."53 Marcia Moore and Howard Altounian have extensively documented their 19970's ketamine research, which was an effort to study its "higher consciousness" potential.[54]

Blood and James

The friendship that developed between these two men is easy to understand, given their similarities. Blood was a farmer, inventor, physical culturist, author and philosopher who spent most of his life trying to understand a revelation delivered to him by anesthetics. Painter, physician, physiologist James became a psychologist and proponent of pragmatism with an interest in altered states of perception — everything from mysticism to hysterical blindness, telekinesis and automatic writing. Marks wrote about Blood, "... he was persistently absorbed with the relation of appearance to reality. It was perhaps this common concern which drew Blood and James so closely together."[55]

Both men had a healthy skepticism about philosophy. James felt that "Philosophy is a queer thing — at once the most sublime and yet the most contemptible of human occupations;"[56] on of his intellectual biographers has noted "...his refusal to join the sect of 'the knights of the razor.'"[57] Blood had similar ideas. "A definition of philosophy would be apt to make an end of it. The difficulty is in the question rather than the in the answer," he wrote in 1886.[58] Ten years earlier he had conjured up the amusing vision, "What could be more ridiculous than two philosophers with their heads together, cooing and congratulating over an interior revelation which neither could tell the other or anybody else?""[59]

Biographers of these men have noted another similarity. "It is therefore my contention," Seigfried observes, "that a literal recounting of James' position is impossible. His writings cannot be read for long — five minutes will do — without encountering contradiction." Marks says, "In the sixty-five years or more of Blood's philosophical activities he evidence considerable shifts in point of view. . ."[61]

The most obvious evidence of the relationship between Blood and James in the latter's lengthy essay, "A Pluralistic Mystic." This homage to Blood was written by James near the end of his life and was published just one month before his death in August, 1910. James seems to be paying an intellectual debt to Blood, as well as drawing attention to his thought and what James may have considered his ephemeral publications. "Now for years my own taste, literary as well as philosophic, has been exquisitely titillated by a writer the name of whom I think must be unknown to the readers of this article, so I no longer continue silent about the merits of BENJAMIN PAUL BLOOD."[62]

Talking about Blood's 1874 pamphlet, James reported, "I forget how it fell into my hands, but it fascinated me so 'weirdly' that I am conscious of its having been one of the stepping-stones of my thinking ever since. . . it ends in a trumpet-blast of oracular mysticism, straight from the insight wrought by anaesthetics — of all things in the world! — and unlike anything one ever heard before."[63] James quotes liberally from the *Anaesthetic Revelation*: "I am using my scissors somewhat at random on my author's paragraphs, since one place is as good as another for entering a ring by. . ."[64] James even acknowledged he might misinterpret Blood: "... and I am not quite unprepared to hear him say, in casc hc cvcr reads these pages, that I have entirely missed his point. No matter, I will proceed."[65]

In June, 1910, James wrote Blood from Switzerland to warn him of the essay's appearance and to state overtly his purpose in writing it. "About the time you receive this, you will also be surprised by receiving the *Hibbert Journal* for July, with an article signed by me, but written mainly by yourself. Tired of waiting for your final synthetic *procunciamento*, and fearing I might be cut off ere it came, I took time by the forelock, and at the risk of making ducks and drakes of your thought, I resolved to save at any rate some of your rhetoric, and the result is what you see. Forgive! Forgive! Forgive!" James in his letter assured Blood the essay would make him famous.[66]

"In the last letters to James," Marks wrote, "Blood chanted a ceaseless refrain: philosophy is dead, there is only the Revelation."[67] Perhaps as he neared the end of his life, James agreed that the mystery was beyond man's intellect, if not his acceptance. He chose to end his essay on Blood with a quote any mystic might accept: "Let *my* last word. . . be *his* word — 'There is no conclusion. What has concluded, that we might conclude in regard to it? There are no fortunes to be told, and there is no advice to be given — Farewell!'"

Conclusion

Ignoring his advice for the moment, what can we conclude about Benjamin Paul Blood and his Anaesthetic Revelation? Is he just an eccentric footnote to anesthesia history, or does his life's work have meaning beyond the trivial?

Blood's relationship with James would seem to be reason enough to rescue the former from obscurity. Their intellectual friendship of some 35 years duration cast Blood in the role of mentor, and James in that of student. James' final essay was a tribute to and public acknowledgment of this status. Yet Blood rates only brief mentions in the various biographies of his friend; researchers have essentially ignored the man their subject identified as a major influence. A physical lifetime spent in a tiny New York town, and a writing life spent primarily in obscure newspapers and pamphlets has left Blood with a low profile indeed.

Another prominent American writer who felt a kinship with Blood was Theodore Dreiser. Although best known for such novels as *Sister Carrie* and *An American Tragedy*, Dreiser was a playwright early in his career. His one-act play, "Laughing Gas," describes the mystical experience of a physician while he undergoes nitrous oxide/oxygen anesthesia for surgery. The play was unproduced in Dreiser's lifetime, although it was published in *The Smart Set* magazine in February, 1915. According to Dreiser, two months later he became familiar with Blood's 1874 pamphlet and James' essay, "On Some Hegleisms." Dreiser was impressed enough with Blood's work to append it and James' comments to the 1916 second printing and 1926 republication of a drama collection which included "Laughing Gas."[68-69]

Robert Walter Marks' 1953 dissertation on Blood, written at New York City's New School for Social Research, was the first and so far only attempt to consider Blood's life and work in any depth. Marks differentiates Blood and James by describing the former as oracular and the latter is more of a "system-builder."[70] Marks notes Blood's geographic and intellectual isolation in Amsterdam and concludes, "What is remarkable in Blood. . . is that with so little to start. . . he should have persisted so long in his philosophical speculations, and that in isolation and loneliness he should have accomplished so much. Despite his philosophical shortcomings, his critical acumen towers over that of most of his American contemporaries including. . . Brockmeyer, Bronson, Alcott and Emerson. . ."[71]

Mystical revelation has been a consistent component of anesthesia history for almost two centuries, an ironic counterpart to anesthesia's practical value in giving relief from surgical pain.[31] Benjamin Paul Blood was the most articulate promoter of this use of anesthetics and one of its most tireless.

References

1. Beecher HK: Anesthesia's second power: probing the mind. *Science* 105: 164-6, 1947.
2. Bates ES: Blood, Benjamin Paul. In: Allen Johnson, ed. *Dictionary of American Biography*, vol. 2. New York: Scribner's, 1957, pp 383-84.
3. Marks RW: The Philosophic Faith of Benjamin Paul Blood: A Study of the Thought and Times of an American Mystic. Ph.D. dissertation, New School for Social Research, 1953, pp 19-24.
4. James W: A pluralistic mystic. In: *Essays in Philosophy*. Cambridge: Harvard University Press, 1978, p 228.
5. Marks, *op cit*, pp 28-41.
6. James, *op cit*, p 172.
7. Blood BP: *The Anaesthetic Revelation and the Gist of Philosophy*. Amsterdam, New York: privately printed, 1874, p 3
8. Perry RB: *The Thought and Character of William James*. Briefer version. Cambridge, Mass.: Harvard Univ Press, 1948, p 211
9. Myers GE: *William James: His Life and Thought*. New Have: Yale Univ Press, 1986, p 5.
10. *Ibid*, p xvii.
11. James W: Anonymours Review of Benjamin Paul Blood's *Anaesthetic Revelation. Atlantic Monthly*; 34: 627-9, 1874.
12. Marks, *op cit*, p 48.
13. Myers, *op cit*, p 46.
14. Marks, *op cit*, p 49.
15. Blood BP: *Pluriverse: An Essay in the philosophy of Pluralism*. 1920. Rep. New Yor:k: Arno, 1976, p 225.
16. *Ibid*, pp 216-7.
17. *Ibid*, - 229.
18. James W: *The Varieties of Religious Experience*. New York: Modern Library, 1936, pp 380-1.
19. Marks, *op cit*, p 29.
20. Marks, *op cit*, pp 16-7.
21. Blood, *Anaesthetic Revelation*, pp 33-4.
22. *Ibid*, p 34-6.
23. Marks, *op cit*, pp 143-4.
24. Blood, *Pluriverse*, pp 238-9.

25. O'Brien E: *Varieties of Mystic Experience: An Anthology and Interpreation.* New York: New American Library; 1965, pp 14-5.
26. Fischer R: A cartography of the ecstatic and meditative states. *Science*; 174:897-904, 1971.
27. Plomley F: Operations upon the eye. *Lancet*; 1:134-5, 1847.
28. Cox AL: Experiments with the letheon in New York. *Boston Med Surg J;* 35:456-9, 1846.
29. Brown HF: *John Addington Symonds: A Biograrphy.* London: Smith, Elder, 1903, pp 292-4.
30. Shoemaker GE: Recollections after ether-inhalation — psychical and physiological. *Therap Gazette*, 3rd ser., 2:521-6, 1886.
31. Smith PB: *Chemical Glimpses of Paradise.* Springfield, Illinois: C.C. Thomas, 1972, p 38.
32. James W: Consciousness under nitrous oxide. *Psycholog Rev*; 5:194-6, 1898.
33. James W: *Varieties...* pp 383-4.
34. Synge JM: Under ether: personal experiences during an operation. *Interstate Med J*; 23:45-9, 1916.
35. G RW: Broken dreams: an ether experience. *J South Carolina Med Assoc*; 24:136-7, 1928.
36. Evans DI: A layman's account of "going under." *Brit J Anaesth*; 18:119-25, 1942-43.
37. Bergstrom H, Bersteing K: Psychic reactions after analgesia with nitrous oxide for caesarean section. *Lancet*; 2:541-2, 1968.
38. James W: On some Hegelisms. In: *The Will to Believe and Other Essays in Popular Philosophy.* New York: Dover, 1956, pp 294-5.
39. Clendening L: *Behind the Doctor.* New York: Alfred A. Knopf, 1933, p 313.
40. Holmes, Oliver Wendell: "Mechanism in Thought and Morals." In: *Pages from an Old Volume of Life: A Collection of Essays*, 1857-1881. Boston: Houghton, Mifflin, 1950, p 283.
41. Blood, *Pluriverse*, pp 230-1.
42. James, *Varieties*, pp 380.
43. Blood, *Pluriverse*, p 217.
44. *Ibid*, p 224.
45. *Ibid*, p 225.
46. Dunbar E: The light thrown on psychological processes by the action of drugs. *Proceedings Soc Psychic Res*, London; 19:62-77, 1904-1905.
47. Blood, *op cit*, p 2.
48. Brillliant L: Nitrous oxide as a psychedelic drug. *N Engl J Med*; 283:1522, 1970.
49. Green R: Nitrous Oxide. *Rolling Stone*, 1990:48-51, 74, 1975.
50. Shedlin M, Wallenchinsky D, Salyer S: *Laughing Gas: Nitrous Oxide.* Berkeley, And/Or Press, 1973.
51. Lazar J: The 50 cent, one minute high. *Esquire*; 90:65, September 12, 1978.
52. Atkinson RM, Green JD, Chenoweth DE, Atkinson H: Subjective effects of nitrous oxide: Cognitive, emotional, perceptual and trascendental experiences. *J Psychedelic Drugs;* 11:317-30, 1979.
53. Lynn EJ, Walter RG, Harris LA, Dendy R, James M: Nitrous oxide: It's a gas. *J Psychedelic Drugs*; 5:1-7, 1972.
54. Moore M, Altounian H: *Journeys into the Bright World.* Rockport, Massachusetts: Para Research, 1978.
55. Myers, *op cit*, p 76.
56. Myers, *op cit*, p 45.
57. Seigfried CH: *William James's Radical Reconstruction of Philosophy.* Albany: State University of New York Press, 1990, p 392.
58. Blood BP: Philosophical reveries. *J Speculative Philosophy*; 20:1-53, 1886.
59. Blood BP: What is truth? *J Speculative Philosophy*; 10:89-94, 1876.
60. Seigfried, *op cit*, pp 7-8.
61. Marks, *op cit*, p i.
62. James W: "A Pluralistic Mystic," p 172.
63. *Ibid*, p 173.
64. *Ibid*, pp 176-7.
65. *Ibid*, p 174.
66. Marks, *op cit*, pp 53-4.
67. *Ibid*, p 158.
68. Wright AJ: Theodore Dreiser's "Laughing Gas." *Anesth Analg*; 69:391-2, 1989.
69. Boren LS: William James, Theodore Dreiser and the "anaesthetic revelation." *Am Studies;* 24:5-17, 1983.
70. Marks, *op cit*, p 159.
71. *Ibid*, p 156.

SELF-EXPERIMENTATION IN ANESTHESIA

A. J. WRIGHT
Clinical Librarian, Department of Anesthesiology Library,
University of Alabama at Birmingham
Birmingham, Alabama, USA

The researcher's use of his own body as an experimental subject has been widespread and often well known in the history of medicine. (Altman, *Who Goes First?* 1987) Less prominent have been the numerous examples of self-experimentation in anesthesia.

Many of these efforts fall into seven periods that can be termed "chronological cluster." ***1. Before 1846***: Between April and July 1799, Humphrey Davy, Research Director at Thomas Beddoes' Pneumatic Institute in Bristol, England, created a self-experimentation salon at which such luminaries of the age as Samuel Taylor Coleridge, Robert Southey, Peter Mark Roget, James Watt as well as Beddoes and Davy inhaled frequent doses of nitrous oxide and described their reactions. Other self-experimenters of this period include Allen (N_2O, 1800), Barton (N_2O, 1807), Serturner (morphine, 1817) and such ether experimenters as Cox (1822), Collyer (1835), Long (1841), Jackson (1841) and Wells (1844). ***2. Ether and chloroform*** (1846-1848): Ether self-experimenters in this cluster include Morton, Cox and Bigelow (U.S., 1846); Squire, Young and Plomley (Great Britain, 1846-1847); Barboza (Portugal) and Benavente and group (Spain). Simpson and group (Edinburgh) and Gerdy and group (Paris) experimented with chloroform. ***3. Ether - chloroform substitutes (1847-1870)***: This large cluster includes Simpson and group (iodoform, benzene, aldehyde, etc., 1847-1848), Nunneley (chloride of acetylic, 1849), Snow (amylene, 1856), Sprague and Clover (N_2O, 1860s), Bigelow (kerosolene, 1861) and Amory and Colton (N_2O, 1870). ***4. Cocaine (1884)***: In 1884 alone at least twelve individuals self-experimented with cocaine, including Koller in Vienna; Halsted, Hall, Busworth, Knapp and Jackson in New York City; Tiffany in Kansas City; Williams in Boston; Shakespeare and Turnbull in Philadelphia; and Benson in Dublin. ***5. Cocaine substitutes (1880s-1920s)***: This cluster includes Dawbarn (sterile air, 1885), Ogston and Middleton (drumine, stimulation, 1912) and Allen (apothesine, 1916). ***6. Pain sensation (1930s-1950s)***: This self-experimentation cluster includes Lewis and Kellgren (1930s), Hardy and group (1936, 1939, 1948-1949), Jackson (1950) and Hanger and Livingston (1952). ***7. Muscle relaxants (1944-1952):*** included in this cluster are Prescott and Smith (d-tubocurarine, 1944 and 1946), Sadove and group (curariform agents, ca. 1949), Paton and group (decane and pentane diiodide, 1948) and Mayrhofer (succinylcholine, 1952).

Numerous examples of anesthesia self-experimentation do not fit within these chronological clusters. Some of these instances fall within two subject areas. ***8. Memory-hearing:*** This group includes Jones (chloroform, 1907), Crila (N_2O/oxygen, 1908), Erickson (ether, 1932) and Loftus (N_2O-oxygen-isoflurane, 1985). ***9. Non-clinical:*** This area includes the work of Blood and James (N_2O, 1860s and 1870s), Symonds (chloroform), Altounian and Moore (ketamine) and Gregory (ketamine).

Self-experimentation has been used since the earliest days of anesthesia research and continues in use today.

SIR WINSTON CHURCHILL AND ANESTHESIA

GERALD L. ZEITLIN
Department of Anesthesia,
Brigham and Women's Hospital
Boston, Massachusetts, USA

Sir Winston Churchill was born on November 30, 1874, and died 90 years later on January 24, 1965. He played many roles and led a life of an almost unimaginable variety of achievements, and also failures. He had many accidents, illnesses and operations. For most of the operations he was anesthetized, but for some he was not. When I submitted the abstract for this paper I had no idea of the scope and variety of these episodes, so I will describe a few of them briefly and recount only two in greater detail.

In 1898 he travelled to the Sudan and, at the battle of Omdurman, led a troop of Lancers in the last cavalry charge by the British army. He survived unscathed and attributed this to the fact that, because of his recurring dislocation of the shoulder, he could not wield a sword. He found his pistol much more effective.

I wondered whether he used his pistol in the same way he played polo — with his arm strapped to his side. In his book, "My Early Life," Churchill issued a stern warning to young people to be careful of their shoulders, and he leaves the impression that when necessary he replaced it by himself without benefit of analgesia or anesthesia he continued to play polo thus handicapped until the age of 52.

After the battle of Omdurman he came across a doctor treating a fellow officer who had suffered a severe sword cut. The doctor said a skin graft would be necessary and asked for a donor. Churchill rolled up his sleeve. The doctor warned him he would feel as though he were being flayed alive, and Churchill later recalled, "My sensations as he sawed the razor slowly to and fro fully justified his description of the ordeal."

In 1908 the then Home Secretary, Mr.. Gladstone, set up a Commission of Enquiry into Deaths under Anaesthetics. This was the latest, but is the least known, of several similar commissions, including of course the well-known Hyderabad Commission on Chloroform. The Report was completed and published in March, 1910, by which time Churchill was Home Secretary. The Commission was the result of a major controversy between a number of groups with conflicting interests. These were: the desire of coroners for more power and influence; the anger of members of Parliament whose constituents were dying under anesthesia with monotonous regularity; the rights of dentists to give anesthesia for general surgery; the reactionary influence of the General Medical Council; and the almost desperate pleas of leading professional anesthetists such as Frederick Hewitt and Bellamy Gardner for better training of medical students in anesthesia and their attempt to have an Anaesthetics Bill passed by Parliament.

Because of the position he held, Churchill became involved — in a way that I believe was not to his credit. The only reference I have been able to find about this Commission in any of the standard anesthesia history texts is a brief mention in Keys' History of Surgical Anesthesia. Research into this complex episode will, I hope, be presented in a future forum similar to this one.

We now move forward to October, 1922, when the Coalition Government that Lloyd George had put together during the Great War was collapsing. Churchill, who was Secretary for the Colonies, was intimately involved. On Sunday evening October 15, he invited the leaders of both the Liberal and Conservative parties to his house in Sussex Square for dinner and discussion. The next morning he complained of abdominal pain and on Tuesday, the 17th, he was moved to a nursing home in Dorset Square. Nursing Homes were private hospitals, used by the middle and upper classes of society and often owned by entrepreneurial nurses. On the night of the 17th Churchill underwent an appendectomy. The King's surgeon, Lord Dawson, probably performed the operation, and the consulting physician was Sir Crisp English. A Dr. Hartigan was also involved — this according to Martin Gilbert, who is Churchill's leading biographer. I have found no information about Dr. Hartigan. Was he the anesthetist? And what anesthetic was used? So I consulted two of my former chiefs in England.

Dr. J. Alfred Lee, who, sadly, died two years ago, wrote as follows; "Now as to Churchill's appendectomy. Almost certainly this took place in a nursing home and I will eat my hat if records are available. Such places would provide a slightly modified bedroom with a portable tin table and the anesthetic would almost certainly have been open chloroform followed by open drop ether. I was a medical student in 1922 and lived through this period."

Dr. Peter Dinnick, now retired as Chief of Anaesthesia at the Middlesex Hospital in London wrote: "It is almost certain that nursing homes had no anaesthetic machines — all anaesthetists carried their own equipment. My guess would be that this was certainly a Hewitt's wide bore modification of the Clover as the basic induction weapon — aided by small, foot-operated $N_20/0_2$ cylinders. If it was only a quick operation there might have been enough gas to maintain anaesthesia using a Shipway or a Boyle — but if a long session was anticipated a switch to open ether was a common practice and one on which I was introduced to the specialty as a student."

I also have a letter from Dr. "Bobby" Roberts who was Dr. Dinnick's chief during the second World War. He wrote; "From 1936 to 1939 I was in practice in London and there was indeed a "nursing home" in Dorset Square. I gave a few anaesthetics there between 1936 and 1939 and all I can remember was that it had a reputation of encouraging surgeons to work there, by giving them a complimentary whisky before leaving. As for the type of anaesthetic he received — I can only assume that as anaesthetics did not progress much between 1880 and 1933 he must have had ether or chloroform with an induction of, a) nitrous oxide/ether with a Clover inhaler, or b) ethyl chloride/ether on a Bellamy Gardner mask."

The only direct evidence available, which suggests that ether was used, comes from the diary of Maurice Hankey, the Secretary of the Cabinet. He noted; "Masterson Smith told us a characteristic story of Winston Churchill. On coming to from his anaesthetic he immediately cried, 'Who has got in for Newport? Give me a newspaper.' The doctor told him he could not have it and must keep quiet. Shortly after the doctor returned and found Winston unconscious again with four or five newspapers lying on the bed."

His recovery was very slow. Perhaps he had an appendix abscess. Three weeks later he travelled to his own constituency in Dundee in Scotland to campaign for reelection. He was so weak he had to be carried into the hall and had to sit while speaking — to largely hostile audiences. When the votes were counted, he had lost his seat in the House of Commons for the first time since 1901. As he said himself, "I am without an office, without a seat, without a party and without an appendix."

We will move forward again to December 11, 1931, when Sir Winston arrived in New York to begin a long lecture tour. In part this was to shore up his financial position — he had lost a great deal of money during the Wall Street crash. Two days later, having settled in an apartment in the Waldorf Tower, he received a phone call that evening from Bernard Baruch, the financier, inviting him to come over to his apartment on Fifth Avenue. Churchill forgot to ask for directions and, after trying for some time to recognize the correct block through the cab window, told the driver to deposit him on the Park side of Fifth Avenue, saying he would do better on foot. He paid the driver and stepped onto the roadway. When he reached the middle, he looked the wrong way — the English way — to the left. Almost immediately he was struck by another taxi travelling uptown at 30 miles an hour. He lay there dazed and bleeding freely; the temperature was 40 degrees Fahrenheit. He later described how he had no feeling and no movement from the shoulders on down, but soon after his hands started tingling and sensation and the power to move rapidly returned. Was he temporarily quadriplegic from a contusion to the spinal cord? It's hard to tell, but it's equally hard to believe that Churchill could have imagined this.

The cab driver, an unemployed mechanic named Mario Constasino, was distraught. The traffic stopped, a crowd gathered, the police arrived, and he was lifted into the taxi that had knocked him down and taken round the corner to the Lenox Hill Hospital. Churchill told the police that Constasino was not to blame, and indeed Constasino came to visit him in hospital several days later.

Churchill himself tells the story in an article he wrote about the accident for the London Daily Mail — for 600 pounds Sterling — a very large sum. "Then came the blow. I felt it on my forehead and across the thighs. But besides the blow there was an impact, a shock, a concussion indescribably violent. I do not understand why I was not broken like an eggshell or crushed like a gooseberry. I certainly must be very tough or very lucky or both."

Several days later, while recovering, he cabled to London to his scientist friend Frederick Lindemann, asking him to calculate the shock to a stationary body weighing 200 lbs., of a car weighing 2400 lbs. and travelling at 30 miles an hour. Lindemann cabled back, "Collision equivalent falling 30 feet on pavement. Or equivalent stopping 10 lb. brick dropped 600 feet. Rate inversely proportional thickness cushion surrounding skeleton and give of frame. Congratulations on preparing suitable cushion, and skill in bump."

Churchill continues, "At last we arrive at the hospital. A wheeled chair is brought. I am carried into it. By now I feel battered but perfectly competent. They said afterwards I was confused, but I did not feel so."

"Are you prepared to pay for a private room and doctor?" asked a clerk. "Yes, bring all the best you have. Take me to a private room. Where is your telephone? Give me the Waldorf Astoria."

He continues, "Not for a moment had I felt up to the present any sensation of faintness, but now I said, "Give me sal volatile or something like that." Soon I am on a bed. Presently come keen, comprehending eyes and deft firm fingers. "We shall have to dress that scalp wound at once. It is cut to the bone." "Will it hurt?" "Yes." "I do not wish to be hurt any more. Give me chloroform or something." "The anaesthetist is already on the way."

His description continues; "More lifting and wheeling. The operation room. White glaring lights. The mask of a nitrous oxide inhaler. Whenever I have taken gas or chloroform I always follow this rule. I imagine myself sitting on a chair with my back to a lovely swimming bath into which I am to be tilted, and throw myself backwards; or again, as if one were throwing own's self back after a tiring day into a vast armchair. This helps the process of anaesthesia wonderfully. A few deep breaths and one has no longer the power to speak to the world. With me the nitrous oxide trance takes this form; the sanctum is occupied by alien powers. I see the absolute truth and explanation of things, but something is left out which upsets the whole. So by a larger sweep of the mind I have to see a greater truth and a more complete explanation which comprises the erring element. Nevertheless there is still something left out. So we have to take a still wider sweep. This almost breaks mortal comprehension. It is beyond anything the human mind was ever meant to master. The process continues inexorably. Depth beyond depth of unendurable truth opens. I have always therefore regarded the nitrous oxide trance as a mere substitution of mental for physical pain. Pain it certainly is; but suddenly these poignant experiences end, and without a perceptible interval consciousness returns. Reassuring words are spoken. I see a beloved face. My wife is smiling."

After leaving hospital, Churchill went to the Bahamas to recuperate. While there he had an attack of the depression that recurred many times in his life. He called it his Black Dog. His wife Clementine wrote to their son, "He is terribly depressed at the slowness of his recovery and last night was very sad."

I will end by showing my favorite slide of Sir Winston and add a speculation. Is it possible that he thought of anesthesia as a way to escape the stresses of his life or even to alleviate his depressions? For example, at a time of great controversy about Irish independence when hatreds were at boiling point, he said, "This is no time to add up the catalogue of injuries. This is the time to pass the sponge of obligation, merciful oblivion, across the horrid past." And once he said to his friend Walter Graebner, "I look forward to dying. Sleep, endless, wonderful sleep — on a purple velvety cushion. Every so often I will wake up, turn over, and go to sleep again."

Index of Topics

NOTE: The page number here refers to the first page of the article.

Index of Authors

NOTE: The page number here refers to the first page of the article.